Arbind Prasad, Sudipto Datta, J. Paulo Davim (Eds.)

Bioprinting

Advanced Mechanical Engineering

Edited by
J. Paulo Davim

Volume 21

Bioprinting

Artificial Intelligence, Biomaterials, Cells, and Tissue

Edited by
Arbind Prasad, Sudipto Datta and J. Paulo Davim

DE GRUYTER

Editors

Dr Arbind Prasad
Department of Science and Technology
Katihar Engineering College
Govt. of Bihar
Katihar, Hirdayganj
854109 Hajipur
Bihar
India
e-mail: arbind.iitg@gmail.com

Dr Sudipto Datta
Department of Materials Engineering
Indian Institute of Science
C V Raman Road
560012 Bengaluru
Karnataka
India
e-mail: sudiptodatta1990@gmail.com

Prof. Dr J. Paulo Davim
Department of Mechanical Engineering
University of Aveiro
Campus Santiago
3810-193 Aveiro
Portugal
e-mail: pdavim@ua.pt

ISSN 2367-3796
ISBN 978-3-11-171993-1
ISBN 978-3-11-171999-3 (PDF)
ISBN 978-3-11-172057-9 (EPUB)
DOI https://doi.org/10.1515/9783111719993

Library of Congress Control Number: 2026934628

Bibliographic information published by the Deutsche Nationalbibliothek
The Deutsche Nationalbibliothek lists this publication in the Deutsche Nationalbibliografie; detailed bibliographic data are available on the internet at http://dnb.dnb.de.

De Gruyter and Walter de Gruyter GmbH are part of De Gruyter Brill.
www.degruyterbrill.com

Questions about General Product Safety Regulation:
productsafety@degruyterbrill.com

Cover illustration: Sky_blue/iStock/thinkstock
Printing: CPI books GmbH, Leck

FSC www.fsc.org MIX Papier | Fördert gute Waldnutzung FSC® C083411

Preface

The convergence of biology, engineering, and digital intelligence has ushered in a transformative era for regenerative medicine. At the heart of this revolution lies 3D bioprinting, a technology that has evolved from a futuristic concept into a robust scientific discipline capable of fabricating complex, functional living tissues. This edited volume serves as a comprehensive roadmap for this interdisciplinary landscape. It is designed to bridge the gap between fundamental research and clinical application by exploring the four critical pillars (artificial intelligence, biomaterials, cells, and tissue engineering) that define the modern bioprinting workflow.

This book consists of 15 chapters. Chapter 1 deals with background, history, and introduction to bioprinting technology. This chapter also deals with the classification of bioprinting technology. Chapter 2 discusses about process and characterization of the bioink formulation techniques in bioprinting. Chapter 3 explores the application of computer-aided design and manufacturing for bioprinting in organ development. Chapter 4–6 investigate advanced biomaterials for extrusion-based bioprinting in context to scaffold design and cellular compatibility, 3D bioprinting, and also innovative design in 3D bioprinting toward the digital revolution as surface topographies and design have proven enhanced biocompatibility. Chapters 7–10 discuss about biomanufacturing and bioprinting of vasculatures, laser-based bioprinting of skin, and extrusion-based bioprinting. Chapter 11 comprises emerging applications of bioprinting in reformative medicine. Chapter 12 explores bioprinting of structures using viable cells, biomaterials, and living molecules. Chapters 13 and 14 deal with bioprinting, integrating artificial intelligence with bioprinting. Chapter 15 explores the challenges, ethical issues, and perspectives in bioprinting. It will provide in-depth knowledge to readers for easier, faster, efficient, and reliable ways to understand smart design and optimization of tissues construct, presently implemented in research labs and industries. This book has the potential to reach a wide readership, including academics, practitioners, doctors, health professionals, postgraduate students, and researchers working in the bioprinting fields. Authors believe that precise and existing contents of the chapters of the book will open up some of bright minds and will encourage them to take up some of the field for their future research.

Editors
Dr Arbind Prasad
Dr Sudipto Datta
Prof. (Dr) J. Paulo Davim

 | https://doi.org/10.1515/9783111719993-202

Acknowledgments

We express our gratitude to **De Gruyter publishing** and the editorial team for their suggestions and support during completion of this book. We are grateful to all contributors and reviewers for their illuminating views on each book chapter presented in this book.

"This book is dedicated to all engineers, doctors researchers, health professionals and academicians . . . ."

Editors
Dr Arbind Prasad
Dr Sudipto Datta
Prof. (Dr) J. Paulo Davim

 | https://doi.org/10.1515/9783111719993-203

Contents

Editors' Short Biography

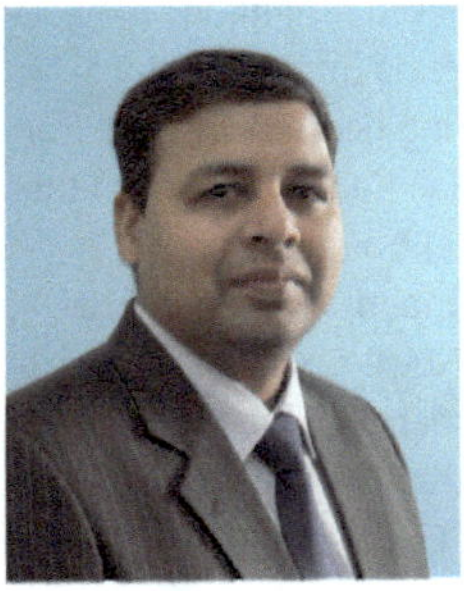

Dr Arbind Prasad has completed his PhD (mechanical engineering) from **the Indian Institute of Technology Guwahati**, Assam, India. He has also earned a **gold medal** in **MTech**. He is currently working as an assistant professor (senior) and head (mechanical engineering) of the Department of Science, Technology and Technical Education, Government of Bihar, at Katihar Engineering College, Katihar, Bihar, India. He has **four granted patents** out of his research work. He has authored 17 international journal papers, and edited numerous books (Wiley, Elsevier, AAP, De Gruyter, and CRC Press (Taylor & Francis) USA), book chapters, and reputed international conference papers to his credit. He has obtained various prestigious awards such as the Sponsored Research Industrial Consultancy (SRIC) award from IIT Kanpur, Best Oral Presentation from the American Chemical Society, and Best Paper awards from IIT Guwahati during Research Conclave. His main areas of research include *resorbable polymers, recycling of biodegradable polymers, waste processing, implant biomaterials, materials processing, and bioenergy generation.* He is also a lifetime member of the Society of Polymer Science India, the Material Research Society of India, the Society of Biomaterials and Artificial Organs of India, the Asian Polymer Association, and the Indian Society of Technical Education.

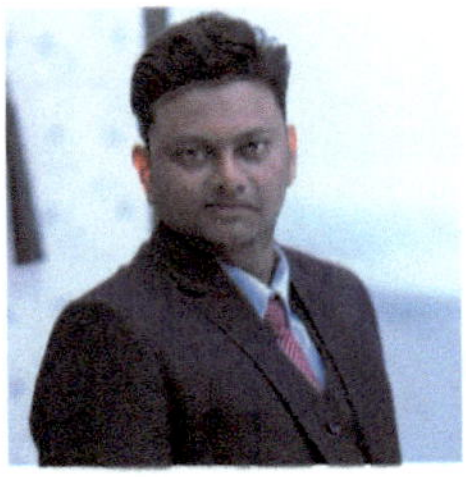

Dr Sudipto Datta is currently working as a research scientist at the All-India Institute of Medical Sciences (AIIMS), New Delhi. His academic journey spans a BTech in electrical and electronics engineering, MTech and PhD in materials engineering and tissue engineering from IIEST Shibpur, and a postdoctoral fellowship at IISc Bangalore. Over the years, he has developed strong expertise in 3D printing, bioprinting, biomaterials, microfluidics, organ on a chip, and biosensors, with a special focus on tissue engineering and regenerative medicine. His research career has allowed him to work across premier institutes such as IIT Roorkee, IISc Bangalore, and AIIMS Delhi, contributing to projects ranging from bioink development and extrusion-based bioprinting to the design of organ-on-chip systems. As a National Postdoctoral Fellow (DST, India), he led a project on the fabrication of a lung-on-a-chip device using bioprinting to study lung fibrosis, which combined his interests in bioprinting, biomaterials, and translational medical research.

 | https://doi.org/10.1515/9783111719993-205

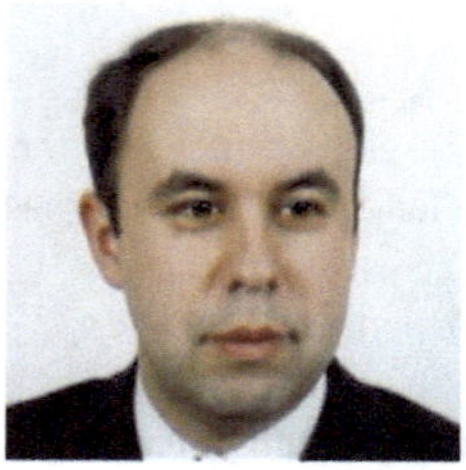

Prof. J. Paulo Davim is a Full Professor at the University of Aveiro, Portugal. He is also distinguished as honorary professor in several universities/colleges/institutes in China, India and Spain. He received his PhD in Mechanical Engineering, MSc in Mechanical Engineering (materials and manufacturing processes) and Mechanical Engineering degree (5 years), from the University of Porto (FEUP), the Aggregate title (Full Habilitation) from the University of Coimbra and the DSc (Higher Doctorate) from London Metropolitan University. He is Fellow (FIET) of IET-London, Fellow (FIMF) of IMF-Birmingham and Eur Ing by Engineers Europe FEANI-Brussels. He is also *Engenheiro Conselheiro* and Specialist Engineer by the Portuguese Order of Engineers with an MBA and Specialist titles in Industrial Management as well as in Metrology. He has more than 35 years of teaching and research experience in Manufacturing, Materials, Mechanical and Industrial Engineering, with special emphasis in Machining, Tribology & Surface Engineering. He has also interest in Design, Management, Sustainability, Industry 5.0, Engineering Education and Higher Education for Sustainability. He has guided large numbers of postdoc, PhD and master's students as well as has coordinated and participated in several financed research projects. He has received several scientific awards and honors. He has worked as evaluator of projects for ERC-European Research Council and other international research agencies as well as examiner of PhD thesis for many universities in different countries. He is the Editor in Chief of several international journals, book Series Editor and Scientific Advisory for many conferences.

List of Contributing Authors

Samir Das
School of Medical Science and Technology
Indian Institute of Technology
Kharagpur 721302
West Bengal
India

Sudipto Datta
Stem Cell Facility/Department of Surgery
All India Institute of Medical Sciences
Ansari Nagar East
Delhi 110029
New Delhi
India

Arbind Prasad
Mechanical Engineering Department
Katihar Engineering College
(Under Department of Science, Technology and Technical Education, Government of Bihar)
Katihar 854109
Bihar
India

P. Sangeetha
Biotechnology Department
University of Madras
Guindy Campus
Chennai 600025
Tamil Nadu
India

K. Logaratshai
Biotechnology Department
University of Madras
Guindy Campus
Chennai 600025
Tamil Nadu
India

Huda Nafees
Department of Saidla
Aligarh Muslim University
Aligarh
Uttar Pradesh
India

S. Nizamudeen
Department of Ilaj bil Tadbeer
Government Unani Medical College
Arumbakkam
Chennai 600106
Tamil Nadu
India

Vicky Subhash Telang
Jawaharlal Nehru Medical College
Datta Meghe Institute of Higher Education and Research, Sawangi (M)
Wardha, 442005
Maharashtra
India

Dr Monika Khatri
Medical Consultant, Primary Health Centre
PDPM Indian Institute of Information Technology, Design and Manufacturing
Jabalpur
India

Mr Mohd. Nadeem
Indian Council of Medical Research
National Institute of Research in Tribal Health
Jabalpur
India

Dr Subhasm Telang
Department of General Medicine,
Government Medical College and Hospital,
Chandrapur
India

Bhupesh Sarode
Jawaharlal Nehru Medical College
Datta Meghe Institute of Higher Education and Research, Sawangi (M)
Wardha 442005
Maharashtra
India

 | https://doi.org/10.1515/9783111719993-206

Prerana Singh
Department of Bioengineering
Indian Institute of Science Bangalore
Bengaluru 560012
Karnataka
India

Ruchi Kaul Pathak
Reconstructive Healthcare Solutions
IMT
Faridabad 121004
Haryana
India

Jonali Das
Raja Peary Mohan College
Hooghly 712258
Uttarpara
West Bengal
India

Ahsan Riaz Khan
Department of Interventional and Vascular Surgery
Shanghai Tenth People's Hospital
Tongji University School of Medicine
Shanghai 200072
China
and
National United Engineering Laboratory for Biomedical Material Modification
Branden Industrial Park
Qihe Economic and Development Zone
Dezhou City
Shandong 251100
China

Pameli Jana
Sri Shankara Cancer Foundation
Bengaluru 560004
Karnataka India

Kanika Nawani
School of Pharmaceutical Sciences
Delhi Pharmaceutical Sciences and Research University
New Delhi
India

Sumit Sharma
School of Pharmaceutical Sciences
Delhi Pharmaceutical Sciences and Research University
New Delhi
India

Navdeep Singh Grewal
University of South Bohemia
Branisovska 1760
37005 Ceske Budejovice
Czech Republic
and
Department of Mechanical Engineering
Guru Kashi University
Talwandi Sabo 151302
Bathinda
Punjab
India

Zhang Hai-Jun
Department of Interventional and Vascular Surgery
Shanghai Tenth People's Hospital
Tongji University School of Medicine
Shanghai 200072
China
and
National United Engineering Laboratory for Biomedical Material Modification
Branden Industrial Park
Qihe Economic and Development Zone
Dezhou City
Shandong 251100
China

Saswata Mitra
Department of Biomedical Engineering
Indian Institute of Technology Ropar
Rupnagar 140001
Punjab
India

Anwesha Mukherjee
Department of Biomedical Engineering
Indian Institute of Technology Ropar
Rupnagar 140001
Punjab
India

Bodhisatwa Das
Department of Biomedical Engineering
Indian Institute of Technology Ropar
Rupnagar 140001
Punjab
India

Menaga S.
Centre for Biomaterials, Cellular and Molecular Theranostics (CBCMT)
Vellore Institute of Technology (VIT)
Vellore 632014
Tamil Nadu
India

Abira R.
Centre for Biomaterials, Cellular and Molecular Theranostics (CBCMT)
Vellore Institute of Technology (VIT)
Vellore 632014
Tamil Nadu
India

Pratima Parulekar
Centre for Biomaterials, Cellular and Molecular Theranostics (CBCMT)
Vellore Institute of Technology (VIT)
Vellore 632014
Tamil Nadu
India

Sushma Kumari
Centre for Biomaterials, Cellular and Molecular Theranostics (CBCMT)
Vellore Institute of Technology (VIT)
Vellore 632014
Tamil Nadu
India

N. Vishnu Devi
Department of Electronics Engineering (VLSI)
Velammal College of Engineering and Technology
Viraganoor
Madurai 625 009
Tamil Nadu
India

M. Vijay
Department of Electrical and Electronics Engineering
Aditya University
Surampalem 533437
Kakinada
Andhra Pradesh
India

Dr Kavita Kumari Thakur
Department of Mechanical Engineering
K. J. Somaiya School of Engineering
(formerly known as K J Somaiya College of Engineering)
Vidyavihar
Mumbai 400 077
Maharashtra
India

Dr Ramesh Lekurwale
Department of Mechanical Engineering
K. J. Somaiya School of Engineering
(formerly known as K J Somaiya College of Engineering)
Vidyavihar
Mumbai 400 077
Maharashtra
India

Tanaya Shyam Salvi
Department of Mechanical Engineering
K. J. Somaiya School of Engineering
(formerly known as K J Somaiya College of Engineering)
Vidyavihar
Mumbai 400 077
Maharashtra
India

Maneesh Dubey
Department of ME
IIT Madras
Chennai
Tamil Nadu
India

Ruchin Kacker
Department of Mechanical Engineering
SISTec
Bhopal
Madhya Pradesh
India

Sanjay Singh
Department of Mechanical Engineering
SISTec
Bhopal
Madhya Pradesh
India

Amit Arora
Department of DEECE
Galgotias University
Greater Noida
Uttar Pradesh
India

Koyel Ghosal
Department of Biomedical Engineering
IIT Ropar
Rupnagar 140001
Punjab
India

Nikita Saini
Department of Biomedical Engineering
IIT Ropar
Rupnagar 140001
Punjab
India

Durba Pal
Department of Biomedical Engineering
IIT Ropar
Rupnagar 140001
Punjab
India

K. Aravinth
Velammal College of Engineering and Technology
Viraganoor
Madurai 625 009
Tamil Nadu
India

B. Krishna Kumar
Velammal College of Engineering and Technology
Viraganoor
Madurai 625 009
Tamil Nadu
India

Bidyanand Mahto
Government Engineering College Vaishali
(Under Department of Science, Technology and Technical Education, Government of Bihar)
Vaishali 844115
Bihar
India

Nisha Shankhwar
Special Centre for Nanoscience
Jawaharlal Nehru University
New Delhi 110067
India

Satyendra Singh
Special Centre for Nanoscience
Jawaharlal Nehru University
New Delhi 110067
India

T. Thenmozhi
Department of Electronics Engineering (VLSI)
Velammal College of Engineering and Technology
Viraganoor
Madurai 625 009
Tamil Nadu
India

S. Vijayasharmila
Department of Electronics Engineering (VLSI)
Velammal College of Engineering and Technology
Viraganoor
Madurai 625 009
Tamil Nadu
India

Samir Das, Sudipto Datta, Arbind Prasad

Chapter 1 Background, History, and Introduction to Bioprinting Technology

Abstract: Bioprinting, an intersection of biology, engineering, and material science, represents a transformative leap in tissue engineering and regenerative medicine. This chapter delves into the origins, historical milestones, and fundamental principles of bioprinting. Starting from traditional 3D printing roots, the evolution toward biologically compatible fabrication systems is explored in detail. The chapter highlights pivotal innovations, early prototypes, and the multidisciplinary convergence that shaped bioprinting into a viable platform for creating living tissues and organ analogues. A foundational understanding of bioprinting modalities, bio-ink development, and application scope is presented, to set the stage for advanced discussions in subsequent chapters. This primer serves researchers, clinicians, and technologists as an essential overview of the landscape of bioprinting technology.

Keywords: Bioprinting, 3D printing, tissue engineering, regenerative medicine, bio-inks, additive manufacturing, organ printing, scaffold fabrication, bioprinter types, biomedical engineering

1.1 Introduction

Bioprinting is a specialized form of additive manufacturing that involves the precise deposition of living cells, biomaterials, and biological molecules in a layer-by-layer manner to fabricate tissue-like structures. The objective is to replicate the form and function of natural tissues or organs [1]. This process uses computer-aided design (CAD) to control the spatial arrangement of components, allowing the creation of complex, three-dimensional biological constructs that support cell viability, proliferation, and differentiation [2]. Unlike traditional printing technologies that deal with inert

*Corresponding authors: **Sudipto Datta,** Stem Cell Facility, All India Institute of Medical Sciences, Ansari Nagar East, New Delhi 110029, Delhi, e-mail: sudiptodatta1990@gmail.com
*Corresponding authors: **Arbind Prasad,** Mechanical Engineering Department, Katihar Engineering College (Under Department of Science, Technology and Technical Education, Government of Bihar), Katihar 854109, Bihar, India, e-mail: arbind.iitg@gmail.com
Samir Das, School of Medical Science and Technology, Indian Institute of Technology, Kharagpur 721302, West Bengal, India

 | https://doi.org/10.1515/9783111719993-001

materials like plastics or metals, bioprinting requires careful handling of fragile and living biological entities. The printing environment must maintain sterility, temperature control, and biochemical compatibility, which adds its potentiality toward biomedical application.

The demand for organ transplants far exceeds the availability of donor organs, leaving many patients without life-saving treatment. Traditional tissue engineering methods face challenges in replicating the microarchitecture and functional integration of native tissues. Bioprinting addresses these challenges by offering patient-specific tissue constructs tailored to individual anatomical and physiological needs. The high-throughput fabrication of tissue models for drug testing reduces reliance on animal models. Controlled cell distribution and vascularization aligns tissue functionality for clinical and research applications. Furthermore, the ability to incorporate multiple cell types and growth factors in a single construct makes bioprinting a highly versatile platform in regenerative medicine, oncology, toxicology, and precision therapeutics [3], as depicted in Figure 1.1.

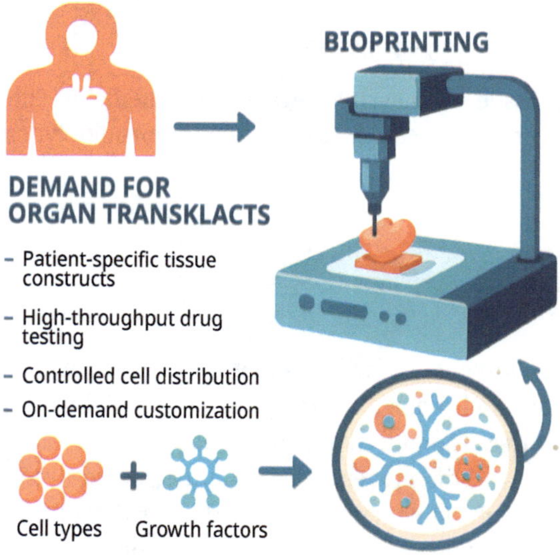

Figure 1.1: Illustration of the urgent need for bioprinting to address organ shortages and enhance personalized, functional tissue fabrication.

While bioprinting shares its foundational principles with conventional 3D printing layer-by-layer fabrication, guided by digital models, the two differ significantly in their materials, objectives, and technological requirements, as mentioned in Table 1.1.

Therefore, bioprinting represents an evolution of 3D printing from mechanical to biological fabrication, where the printed product is not only structural but also functional and dynamic within a living system.

Table 1.1: Comparison between conventional 3D printing and bioprinting in terms of applications and functional goals.

Aspect	Conventional 3D printing	Bioprinting
Materials used	Plastics, metals, and resins	Living cells, hydrogels, and biomolecules [4]
Application	Industrial design, prototyping, and tools	Biomedical: tissues, scaffolds, and organ models [5]
Environmental needs	Ambient	Sterile, temperature- and humidity-controlled [6]
Resolution and complexity	High structural fidelity	Balance between structure and biological function [7]
Goal	Mechanical performance	Biological functionality and integration [8]

1.2 Historical Timeline

The development of bioprinting is deeply rooted in the evolution of traditional 3D printing. Originating in the 1980s, 3D printing, also known as additive manufacturing, initially focused on creating physical prototypes from digital models using polymers and metals. Techniques such as stereolithography (SLA) and fused deposition modeling (FDM) gained popularity in industrial design, manufacturing, and engineering. The transition from printing inert materials to biological ones began in the early 2000s, driven by the increasing need for precision-engineered tissues in medicine [9]. Researchers modified conventional printers to accommodate biological components, such as cells and hydrogels, giving rise to the field now known as bioprinting. The field of bioprinting has evolved rapidly since 2003 when Thomas Boland at Clemson University first modified an inkjet printer to deposit living cells, marking the inception of cell printing [10]. Between 2004 and 2008, extrusion-based bioprinting emerged, allowing for the use of more viscous, cell-laden hydrogels. In 2009, biotech company, Organovo, successfully printed functional liver tissue, showcasing the technology's therapeutic potential. A year later, the first 3D-printed blood vessels were demonstrated using hydrogel scaffolds. The concept of "4D bioprinting" was introduced in 2013, referring to printed constructs capable of undergoing programmed transformations over time. From 2016 onwards, advancements included the integration of machine learning and high-resolution imaging in tissue design, along with the publication of standardized protocols for printing viable, vascularized tissues. Entering the 2020s, bioprinting has seen significant growth in applications such as printable organoids, tumor models, and early-stage clinical trials using printed skin and cartilage [11]. These milestones reflect the growing maturity and interdisciplinary nature of bioprinting research. Bioprinting has flourished through the collaborative contributions of leading researchers and institutions spanning academia, industry, and specialized research centers. Thomas Boland of Clemson University was the first to demonstrate inkjet-based cell printing, laying the foundation for the field. At the Wake Forest Institute for Regenerative Medicine, Anthony Atala pioneered the bioprinting of complex organs such as the bladder and kidney. Jennifer Lewis, at Harvard University's Wyss Institute, significantly advanced the field by developing multi-material bioprinting platforms with integrated vascular networks. Gabor Forgacs, affiliated with the University of Missouri and Organovo, played a key role in commercializing tissue printing technologies, particularly for pharmaceutical testing. In Europe, Dr. Poietis spearheaded innovations in laser-assisted bioprinting, enabling precise, high-resolution cellular patterning. Collectively, these visionaries have shaped the trajectory of bioprinting toward clinical and translational success. Early biofabrication focused on demonstrating that living cells could be printed in 3D without losing function. Key models included skin substitutes, cartilage patches, liver microtissues, and blood vessel constructs (Figure 1.2). These early successes proved the feasibility of bioprinting and aided the foundation for more advanced constructs like vascularized tissues, organoids, and organs on a chip.

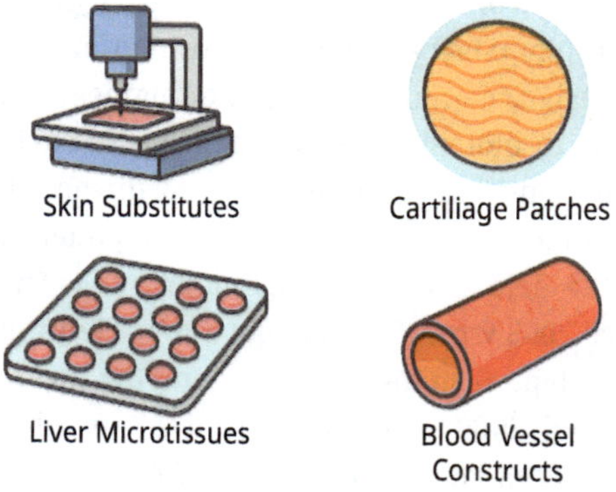

Figure 1.2: Early bioprinting models demonstrating the feasibility of 3D cell deposition, laying the groundwork for complex tissue and organoid development.

1.3 Core Concepts and Terminology

A bioprinter is a specialized device designed to deposit biological materials, including living cells, biomolecules, and biocompatible materials, in a highly controlled, spatially defined manner. It functions similarly to a 3D printer but is engineered to handle delicate biological substances under sterile, temperature-controlled conditions. Bioprinters are equipped with multiple nozzles, precise motion systems, and often real-time imaging modules to ensure accuracy and viability during and after printing. Depending on the printing technique (e.g., inkjet, extrusion, or laser-assisted), bioprinters can fabricate structures layer by layer, creating functional tissue constructs ranging from simple sheets to complex, vascularized organs. In bioprinting, living cells are used as one of the core components of the printing material, i.e., primary cells (directly derived from tissue), stem cells (capable of differentiation into multiple lineages), or cell lines (immortalized for repeated use in research). Cells are often suspended in a hydrogel matrix or bio-ink that mimics the native extracellular matrix (ECM), providing a supportive environment for proliferation and differentiation. The placement of cells in precise geometries allows them to form tissue-like architectures, interact with neighboring cells, and respond to biochemical cues in ways that replicate in vivo conditions. Scaffold-based methods are more common due to their ease of use and tunable properties, but scaffold-free approaches are gaining traction for applications that require minimal interference with native tissue architecture. Table 1.2 describes various aspects for scaffold-based bioprinting techniques.

Table 1.2: Comparative overview of scaffold-based and scaffold-free bioprinting approaches in terms of structure, materials, advantages, and challenges.

Aspect	Scaffold-based bioprinting	Scaffold-free bioprinting
Structure	Uses biomaterials to create a framework or support matrix	Relies on cellular self-assembly and tissue fusion [12]
Materials	Hydrogels, synthetic/natural polymers (e.g., alginate and collagen)	Spheroids, organoids, and cell aggregates [13]
Advantages	Offers mechanical integrity and defined initial shape	Eliminates the use of foreign materials, enabling natural tissue remodeling [14]
Challenges	Issues with material degradation and immune response	Demands high precision in cell placement and viability for structural integrity [15]

Bio-inks are specialized formulations that integrate living cells with biocompatible materials to enable the 3D printing of tissue-like structures. An ideal bio-ink must support printability, biocompatibility, mechanical stability, and promote cell viability and function [16]. Bio-inks are broadly classified into natural-based (e.g., alginate, gelatin, fibrin, and collagen), synthetic-based (e.g., PEG, Pluronic F127, and PCL), and composite types that blend both to enhance performance [17]. Core components include cells as functional tissue units, a hydrogel matrix to mimic the ECM, crosslinkers (such as calcium chloride or UV light) to solidify the printed structure, and bioactive agents like growth factors to guide cell behavior, differentiation, and vascularization [18, 19]. In parallel, computer-aided design (CAD) is fundamental to bioprinting, enabling precise digital modeling of complex biological structures. The CAD workflow involves image acquisition (via MRI, CT, or histology), 3D model reconstruction of target tissues, slicing and toolpath generation to guide nozzle movement, and simulation/optimization to ensure print fidelity, resolution, and biological compatibility, prior to fabrication [20].

1.4 Bioprinting Techniques: An Overview

Bioprinting technologies differ based on the mechanism used to deposit bio-inks, the range of materials supported, resolution, and application specificity. Each method has its own strengths and limitations. The four primary types are inkjet, extrusion-based, laser-assisted, and light-based (e.g., stereolithography), with emerging hybrid systems combining their advantages. Bioprinting technologies have evolved to support various applications through distinct mechanisms and material compatibilities. Inkjet bioprinting utilizes thermal or piezoelectric actuators to deposit bio-ink droplets, offering high resolution and cell viability at low cost, though it is limited to low-viscosity materials and prone to nozzle clogging [21]. Extrusion-based bioprinting, which employs pneumatic or mechanical forces for continuous filament deposition, supports high cell densities and a wide range of bio-inks but typically has lower resolution and may induce shear stress on cells [22]. Laser-assisted bioprinting propels bio-ink droplets using laser-induced pressure, allowing for precise, nozzle-free printing with high cell viability, though it is costly and complex with limited throughput [23], as mentioned in Figure 1.3. SLA/light-based bioprinting, which relies on UV or visible light to cross-link photocurable bio-inks, achieves fine resolution and complex structures rapidly but is restricted to compatible bio-inks and may involve photoinitiator toxicity [24]. Finally, hybrid bioprinting systems, which integrate multiple techniques such as extrusion and inkjet, combine their strengths to fabricate complex, multi-material, or multicellular constructs, although they require sophisticated equipment and are expensive to operate.

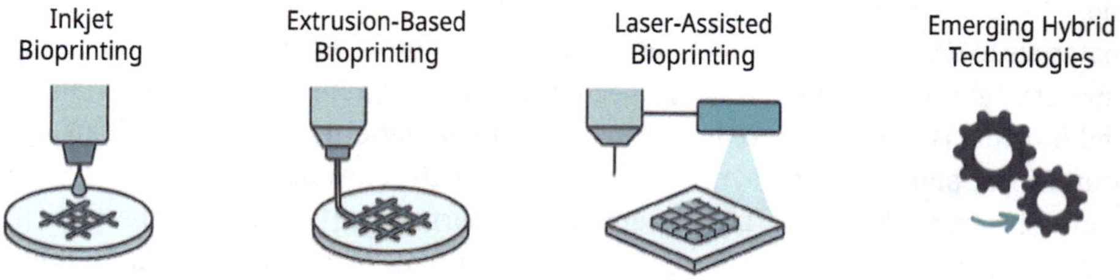

Figure 1.3: Overview of key bioprinting techniques in tissue engineering and regenerative medicine.

1.5 Materials in Bioprinting

The choice of material plays a critical role in bioprinting, directly influencing printability, mechanical strength, biocompatibility, and cellular behavior. Bio-ink formulations used in bioprinting are primarily composed of natural or synthetic biomaterials [25], often with embedded living cells. A well-designed bio-ink must mimic the native ECM while supporting the printing process and maintaining cell viability, using natural or synthetic biomaterials, as mentioned in Table 1.3.

Table 1.3: Aspects of biomaterials toward biomedical applications.

Aspect	Natural biomaterials	Synthetic biomaterials
Source	Derived from biological tissues or ECM like alginate, gelatin, collagen, fibrin, hyaluronic acid	Chemically synthesized polymers like PEG, PLA, PLGA, and PCL [1]
Advantages	High biocompatibility; promotes cell adhesion	Tunable mechanical and degradation properties
Limitations	Low mechanical strength; batch variability	May lack bioactivity; potentially cytotoxic
Applications	Skin, cartilage, liver, and soft tissues	Structural support, bone scaffolds, and hybrid bio-inks

Natural biomaterials are biologically favorable but mechanically weak, whereas synthetic materials offer strength and consistency but may need functionalization to enhance cell interaction. Hybrid bio-inks, combining both types, are increasingly used to balance biological and structural requirements, in which hydrogels are three-dimensional, water-swollen polymer networks that serve as the most common base material for bio-inks. Their high water content and tunable properties make them excellent ECM analogues for supporting embedded cells. Cross-linking stabilizes the printed structure and impacts mechanical properties, degradation rate, and cell behavior. The choice of method must ensure cell compatibility and structural integrity during and after printing. Table 1.4 describes various gelation kinetics for natural and synthetic hydrogel toward live-cell printing.

An ideal bio-ink must exhibit a balance between printability, mechanical performance, and biological function. The success of bioprinting heavily relies on the physicochemical properties of bio-inks, each influencing printability and biological performance. Viscosity is a critical parameter that must be tailored to the bioprinting method, low for droplet-based inkjet systems and higher for extrusion-based techniques [26]. Shear-thinning behavior is desirable as it enables smooth extrusion with minimal damage to cells. Biocompatibility ensures that the bio-ink supports cell viability, proliferation, and differentiation post-printing [27]. The gelation time should align with the printing speed to maintain shape fidelity during and after deposition.

Table 1.4: Classification of common natural and synthetic hydrogels used in bioprinting based on cross-linking methods and mechanisms.

Category	Examples	Cross-linking method	Mechanism/notes
Natural hydrogels	Alginate	Ionic cross-linking (e.g., Ca^{2+})	Rapid gelation via ionic bonding; widely used in cell encapsulation
	Gelatin	Thermal gelation	Gelation occurs upon cooling; reversible and biocompatible
	Collagen	Thermal/pH-dependent gelation	Forms fibrillar networks mimicking native ECM
	Agarose	Thermal gelation	Reversible gelation; good structural support
	Fibrin	Enzymatic cross-linking (thrombin)	Biologically active; mimics natural clotting process
Synthetic hydrogels	PEG-based hydrogels	Photo-cross-linking (UV/visible + PI)	Highly tunable; requires photoinitiator; enables precise spatial control
	Pluronic	Thermal gelation	Gelation at physiological temperatures; useful as sacrificial/support materials

Mechanical strength is especially important for constructs intended to support mechanical loads, while degradability should match the pace of new tissue formation, allowing the scaffold to be gradually replaced by native ECM [28]. Lastly, cell adhesion is vital to promote proper integration and maturation of printed tissues, often enhanced by incorporating natural ECM components.

1.6 Applications

Bioprinting has demonstrated significant success in fabricating tissue models such as skin, cartilage, and bone that replicate the structural and cellular complexity of native human tissues. These engineered constructs serve both as implantable grafts and as platforms for in vitro testing. Bioprinted skin is widely used in wound healing research, burn treatment, and cosmetic testing, while cartilage models support joint regeneration and reconstructive procedures. Bone constructs are applied in craniofacial repair and orthopedic grafting. A key advantage of bioprinting is its ability to produce patient-specific, customizable tissues, reducing reliance on donor sources and improving clinical outcomes. Beyond regenerative medicine, one of the most transformative applications of bioprinting is in creating 3D disease models that better mimic physiological microenvironments than traditional 2D cultures. For instance, bioprinted tumor models replicate cancer heterogeneity and drug resistance, organ-on-chip platforms allow functional studies of liver, kidney, or lung tissues, and patient-specific constructs enable tailored drug testing in personalized medicine. These innovations not only accelerate drug discovery and reduce animal testing but also provide more accurate predictions of therapeutic efficacy and safety. While customization and full fabrication of complex, functional organs remains a long-term goal, significant progress has been made in developing vascularized, multicellular constructs that serve as building blocks for future organ printing. Therefore, the potential future targets include functional mini organs (organoids) for transplantation, bioengineered kidneys, livers, and hearts for use in regenerative medicine, and on-demand organ fabrication to solve global transplant shortages. Though challenges remain, such as immune compatibility, regulatory hurdles, and scalability, the path toward fully functional organ printing is rapidly unfolding through multidisciplinary innovation.

1.7 Ethical and Regulatory Considerations

As bioprinting progresses to clinical implementation, it brings forth critical ethical and regulatory considerations. While the technology offers transformative possibilities, such as enabling personalized therapies and reducing dependence on animal testing, ethical concerns include defining the boundaries of life, differentiating therapeutic use from human enhancement, ensuring equitable access, and addressing issues of ownership and informed consent for bioprinted tissues. Concurrently, global regulatory bodies are working to keep pace, as reflected in efforts to establish standardized testing, approval pathways, and quality protocols specifically tailored for bioprinted constructs. The regulatory basis based on region is mentioned in Table 1.5.

Table 1.5: Overview of regulatory frameworks for bioprinting across key regions and international bodies.

Region	Regulatory authority	Current status
United States	US Food and Drug Administration (FDA)	Regulates bioprinted products under a combination of medical device and biologics guidelines (e.g., 21 CFR Part 1271); no dedicated bioprinting policy yet
Europe	European Medicines Agency (EMA)	Uses Advanced Therapy Medicinal Product (ATMP) classification
India	CDSCO, ICMR, and DBT	Limited formal regulation; guided by ethical biomedical research frameworks
Global	ISO, WHO, and ASTM	Working to define international standards for bioprinted tissue safety and quality

Despite promising advancements in the lab, several challenges continue to hinder the clinical translation of bioprinted tissues. A primary concern is ensuring long-term safety and functionality, including the seamless integration of constructs with host tissues, while avoiding immune rejection or failure. Vascularization remains a critical hurdle, as supplying adequate blood flow in thick or complex tissues is essential for survival and function. Additionally, consistent manufacturing practices for ensuring reproducibility, scalability, and batch uniformity are vital for regulatory approval and clinical reliability. Ethical considerations and the complexity of designing controlled clinical trials for living tissue implants further complicate progress. Moreover, high costs and the need for specialized infrastructure limit access and scalability, particularly in resource-constrained settings, posing significant barriers to widespread adoption.

1.8 Conclusion

Bioprinting has rapidly evolved from its roots in traditional 3D printing to a cutting-edge field at the forefront of regenerative medicine and tissue engineering. Initially adapted from desktop inkjet printers, early bioprinting efforts focused on proving that living cells could survive the printing process. Over the past two decades, this concept has grown into a sophisticated platform capable of fabricating multicellular, anatomically precise, and even vascularized tissue constructs. From early proof-of-concept models like skin and cartilage to advanced organoids and disease models, the field has made remarkable strides, supported by advancements in materials science, cellular biology, and digital manufacturing. The success of bioprinting is deeply rooted in the convergence of multiple disciplines. Engineers design precision printers and computational models; biologists optimize cell behavior and culture conditions; chemists develop novel bio-inks; and clinicians define the translational goals and ethical boundaries. It is this collaborative ecosystem that enables bioprinting to move from laboratory innovation to real-world medical solutions. Collaboration also plays a vital role in overcoming regulatory, ethical, and technical challenges. As new use cases emerge – from personalized tissue grafts to organ-on-chip platforms for drug testing – the synergy between academia, industry, and healthcare systems becomes even more essential. The future of bioprinting holds immense promise, with ongoing advancements aimed at overcoming current limitations and expanding clinical applications. Key areas of focus include the fabrication of fully functional, transplantable organs, with integrated vasculature and sustained physiological function, as well as in situ bioprinting, where tissues are printed directly onto or into the body during surgery. The development of smart bio-inks, capable of responding to biological signals or environmental stimuli, is also gaining momentum. Equally important is the push for regulatory standardization to ensure the safety, reproducibility, and scalability of clinically viable constructs. Despite persistent challenges such as achieving vascular integration, ensuring immune compatibility, and addressing cost-effective large-scale production, bioprinting represents a transformative leap toward personalized and regenerative healthcare solution, moving concepts once deemed science fiction closer to clinical reality.

References

[1] Murphy, S. V., & Atala, A. (2014). 3D bioprinting of tissues and organs. Nature Biotechnology, 32(8), 773–785. https://doi.org/10.1038/nbt.2958.

[2] Groll, J., Boland, T., Blunk, T., Burdick, J. A., Cho, D. W., Dalton, P. D., & Malda, J. (2016). Biofabrication: reappraising the definition of an evolving field. Biofabrication, 8(1), 013001. https://doi.org/10.1088/1758-5090/8/1/013001.

[3] Ozbolat, I. T. (2015). Bioprinting: Past, Present and Future. Biofabrication, 7(2), 023001. https://doi.org/10.1088/1758-5090/7/2/023001.

[4] Murphy, S. V., & Atala, A. (2014). 3D bioprinting of tissues and organs. Nature Biotechnology, 32(8), 773–785. https://doi.org/10.1038/nbt.2958.

[5] Mandrycky, C., Wang, Z., Kim, K., & Kim, D. H. (2016). 3D bioprinting for engineering complex tissues. Biotechnology Advances, 34(4), 422–434.

[6] Groll, J. et al. (2016). A definition of bioinks and their distinction from biomaterial inks. Biofabrication, 11(1), 013001. https://doi.org/10.1088/1758-5090/aaec52.

[7] Ozbolat, I. T. (2016). 3D Bioprinting: Fundamentals, Principles and Applications. Academic Press.

[8] Jakab, K., Norotte, C., Damon, B., Marga, F., Neagu, A., Besch-Williford, C. L., & Forgacs, G. (2008). Tissue engineering by self-assembly of cells printed into topologically defined structures. Tissue Engineering Part A, 14(3), 413–421.

[9] Boland, T., Xu, T., Damon, B., & Cui, X. (2006). Application of inkjet printing to tissue engineering. Biotechnology Journal, 1(9), 910–917. https://doi.org/10.1002/biot.200600081.

[10] Atala, A., Bauer, S. B., Soker, S., Yoo, J. J., & Retik, A. B. (2006). Tissue-engineered autologous bladders for patients needing cystoplasty. The Lancet, 367(9518), 1241–1246. https://doi.org/10.1016/S0140-6736(06)68438-9.

[11] Kolesky, D. B., Truby, R. L., Gladman, A. S., Busbee, T. A., Homan, K. A., & Lewis, J. A. (2014). 3D bioprinting of vascularized, heterogeneous cell-laden tissue constructs. Advanced Materials, 26(19), 3124–3130. https://doi.org/10.1002/adma.201305506.

[12] Moroni, L. et al. (2018). Biofabrication: a guide to technology and terminology. Trends in Biotechnology, 36(4), 384–402. https://doi.org/10.1016/j.tibtech.2017.10.015.

[13] Groll, J. et al. (2016). Bioinks for three-dimensional bioprinting. Nature Reviews Materials, 1(1), 16013. https://doi.org/10.1038/natrevmats.2016.13.

[14] Murphy, S. V., & Atala, A. (2014). 3D bioprinting of tissues and organs. Nature Biotechnology, 32(8), 773–785. https://doi.org/10.1038/nbt.2958.

[15] Ozbolat, I. T. (2015). Scaffold-based or scaffold-free bioprinting: competing or complementing approaches? Journal of Nanotechnology in Engineering and Medicine, 6(2), 021001. https://doi.org/10.1115/1.4030837.

[16] Gungor-Ozkerim, P. S., Inci, I., Zhang, Y. S., Khademhosseini, A., & Dokmeci, M. R. (2018). Bioinks for 3D bioprinting: an overview. Biomaterials Science, 6(5), 915–946. https://doi.org/10.1039/C7BM00765E.

[17] Hospodiuk, M., Dey, M., Sosnoski, D., & Ozbolat, I. T. (2017). The bioink: A comprehensive review on bioprintable materials. Biotechnology Advances, 35(2), 217–239. https://doi.org/10.1016/j.biotechadv.2016.12.006.

[18] Ozbolat, I. T. (2016). Bioprinting scale-up tissue and organ constructs for transplantation. Trends in Biotechnology, 34(9), 695–705. https://doi.org/10.1016/j.tibtech.2016.03.004.

[19] Chimene, D., Lennox, K. K., Kaunas, R. R., & Gaharwar, A. K. (2016). Advanced bioinks for 3D printing: A materials science perspective. Annals of Biomedical Engineering, 44(6), 2090–2102. https://doi.org/10.1007/s10439-016-1638-y.

[20] Zhao, X., Liu, L., Zhang, Y., Liang, Y., Huang, Y., & He, Y. (2020). Three-dimensional printing of Haversian bone–mimicking scaffold for multicellular delivery in bone regeneration. Science Advances, 6(12), eaay6396. https://doi.org/10.1126/sciadv.aay6396.

[21] Derby, B. (2012). Printing and prototyping of tissues and scaffolds. Science, 338(6109), 921–926. https://doi.org/10.1126/science.1226340.

[22] Murphy, S. V., & Atala, A. (2014). 3D bioprinting of tissues and organs. Nature Biotechnology, 32(8), 773–785. https://doi.org/10.1038/nbt.2958.

[23] Guillemot, F. et al. (2010). Laser-assisted bioprinting for tissue engineering. Trends in Biotechnology, 28(9), 492–500. https://doi.org/10.1016/j.tibtech.2010.06.011.

[24] Ma, X. et al. (2018). Rapid 3D bioprinting of cellular structures using light and hydrogel materials. Advanced Materials, 30(1), 1705912. https://doi.org/10.1002/adma.201705912.

[25] Gungor-Ozkerim, P. S., Inci, I., Zhang, Y. S., Khademhosseini, A., & Dokmeci, M. R. (2018). Bioinks for 3D bioprinting: an overview. Biomaterials Science, 6(5), 915–946. https://doi.org/10.1039/C7BM00765E.

[26] Gungor-Ozkerim, P. S., Inci, I., Zhang, Y. S., Khademhosseini, A., & Dokmeci, M. R. (2018). Bioinks for 3D bioprinting: an overview. Biomaterials Science, 6(5), 915–946. https://doi.org/10.1039/C7BM00765E.

[27] Murphy, S. V., & Atala, A. (2014). 3D bioprinting of tissues and organs. Nature Biotechnology, 32(8), 773–785. https://doi.org/10.1038/nbt.2958.

[28] Groll, J. et al. (2016). Biofabrication: reappraising the definition of an evolving field. Biofabrication, 8(1), 013001. https://doi.org/10.1088/1758-5090/8/1/013001.

P. Sangeetha, K. Logaratshai, Huda Nafees, S. Nizamudeen*

Chapter 2
Process and Characterization of Bioink Formulation Techniques in Bioprinting

Abstract: Tissue engineering has experienced significant development in the past few decades through the introduction of 3D (three-dimensional) bioprinting technology, which shows immense potential to transform regenerative medicine. In this engineering field biomaterials, cells, and engineering methods are combined to develop artificial tissue substitutes. The dual objectives of this approach involve the replacement of harmed tissues alongside the development of in vitro models, which serve both to study diseases and to conduct drug screening, thereby enabling researchers to create precise arrangements of live cells and biomaterials in stacked configurations or layer-by-layer scaffold constructs through 3D printing technology. This process involves additive manufacturing technology that shows strong potential to create intricate tissue structures, yet its success depends on multiple variables with the different printing methodologies, and the printed tissue's structure and functionality heavily depends on the selected bioink formulation method making it one of the most important criteria for a successful 3D scaffold fabrication. A bioink functions as a printable biomaterial, which combines living cells and biomolecules in a compatible material that acts as a support for creating tissue-like structures through 3D bioprinting. The material needs to have appropriate rheological properties and cross-linking agents for accurate deposition and biological compatibility to enable cell viability and tissue development before and after printing for stable tissue constructs. Therefore, to produce functional tissue constructs that closely resemble human tissues, the bioink formulation and optimization play a crucial role in 3D printing. Overall, this chapter provides an overview of tissue engineering research that includes both processes and characterization of bioink for bioprinting.

Keywords: Tissue engineering, 3D bioprinting, bioink, scaffolds, rheological tuning

***Corresponding author: S. Nizamudeen**, Post-graduate Department of Ilaj bil Tadbeer (Special Therapy), Government Unani Medical College, Arumbakkam, Chennai 600106, Tamil Nadu, India, e-mail: drnizamgumc@gmail.com
P. Sangeetha, K. Logaratshai, Biotechnology Department, University of Madras, Guindy Campus, Chennai 600025
Huda Nafees, Department of Saidla, Aligarh Muslim University, Aligarh

 | https://doi.org/10.1515/9783111719993-002

2.1 Introduction

Tissue engineering has experienced significant advancements over the past two decades because of the considerable progress due to 3D bioprinting technology [1, 2]. As the global need for tissue and organ replacements has increased, conventional approaches such as donor-based transplants and traditional scaffold-based engineering have faced significant challenges based on immune rejection with the transplanted grafts and donor shortages [1, 3]. Through 3D bioprinting researchers can create complex tissue-mimicking structures by precise layer-by-layer deposition of cells and biomaterials using a bioprinter [4]. This additive manufacturing process has enabled regenerative medicine to transform by making personalized implants for patients, while producing accurate tissue models for research and therapeutic applications [5].

The fundamental component for this technology is the bioink, which is a biological compatibility material that is formulated for tissue or scaffold printing through the bioprinters [1, 2, 5]. The bioink typically functions as a hydrogel-based material, which can be formulated form natural or synthetic compounds and operated through extrusion or deposition to create 3D structures that can support the structure and the growth of living cells [5, 6]. Therefore, successful tissue fabrication requires a bioink that not only supports the cells in the printed scaffolds but also helps in replicating the target tissue's mechanical properties after printing by maintaining the cellular viability and differentiation for tissue maturation [7]. The development of bioink formulations requires scientists to unite knowledge from materials science with cell biology and bioengineering principles. The selection and modification of the base biomaterials for printing requires careful attention to their biocompatibility, mechanical strength, and degradation behavior as well as their ability to support embedded cells based on the tissue that is required for different biomedical application [8].

The bioactivity of ink receives additional components such as growth factors together with nanoparticles and signaling peptides, which enhances the functionality of bioink and provides the printed constructs the stability it needs through cross-linking methods like ionic, enzymatic, thermal, and photoinitiation based on the application requirements and cell sensitivity [7]. Likewise, the printing process also heavily depends on multiple printing parameters such as extrusion pressure, nozzle temperature, print speed and resolution [8–10]. The rheological properties of the bioink also play a crucial role for a successful print. Properties like the shear-thinning behavior together with yield stress and the viscosity of the bioink are essential to ensure both print head flow and printed filament shape preservation [10]. The characterization process includes mechanical tests such as porosity, compressive strength, and Young's modulus, which is combined with biological assays for cell viability, proliferation, and differentiation alongside structural assessments through imaging methods like scanning electron microscopy or confocal microscopy to validate design specifications and helps acquire information about construct functionality during in vitro and in vivo applications [7, 10]. Bioprinting techniques has developed significantly with various material and cellular combinations as summarized in Table 2.1, which presents the types of biomaterials, cell types, source of biomaterials, and crosslinking materials.

In summary, this chapter provides an extensive overview of bioink formulation methods together with essential formulation and printing parameters along with characterization outlines for evaluating the printed constructs offering insight into the evolving landscape of 3D bioprinting.

2.2 Bioink Formulation Techniques

Bioinks exist in many categories based on their material origin and their functional properties and a biomaterial refers to a non-viable material that can be from a natural or synthetic source, or composite substance that is used for the bioink formulations that is used to fabricate biological structures through additive manufacturing that not only provides a structural framework but also supports cell viability and function [7]. The following section explains the bioink formulation process through material classification, additive modifications, rheological property, and base material selection along with the cross-linking mechanisms.

2.2.1 Criteria for Choosing Biomaterials

The selection of appropriate biomaterials for bioink formulation stands as a critical factor because it determines both printing capabilities and the resulting tissue construct [7, 8, 11]. The choice of suitable biomaterials relies on factors such as biocompatibility and does not interfere with the cellular growth while the material must also have the ability to withstand the sterilization process and maintain its mechanical properties [8, 12]. The biomaterial mush also has appropriate porosity or porous architecture for cell migration, gas and nutrient diffusion, and vascularization that matches the target tissue type [8]. When it comes to the mechanical property, the elastic modulus and the Young's modulus of the chosen material must be as close as the biological tissue [7, 11]. Surface chemistry also plays a major role for material selection as it allows for the cell adhesion or modification, with its controlled biodegradability [7]. The rheological behavior of shear-thinning properties along with the viscosity of the formulated material is crucial for maintaining smooth extrusion, shape fidelity, and mechanical integrity after printing to prevent collapse [12]. The optimization of one bioink property typically leads to compromises in other properties, so designers must create specific trade-offs for particular tissue engineering needs.

Table 2.1: Types of biomaterials, cell types, source of biomaterials, and cross-linking materials used for bioprinting.

Material type		Source	Cross-linker	Cross-linking mechanism	References
Natural polymers	Alginate	Brown algae	Ionic cross-linking – $CaCl_2$	Ca^{2+} ions interact with guluronic acid blocks in sodium alginate, forming a 3D network.	[13, 14]
	Gelatin	Porcine	Physical cross-linking – thermal	Gelatin undergoes gelation via cooling on the print bed (25 °C).	[13]
	Collagen (type I most common)	Porcine skin, bovine skin and tendon, rat tail tendon, marine sources	Chemical cross-linking – glutaraldehyde (GTA), EDC/NHS, Genipin, NDGA	Forms covalent bonds between amino/carboxyl groups of collagen chains.	[15]
			Physical cross-linking – UV/thermal	Through UV light or heat.	
			Enzymatic cross-linking – transglutaminase, lysyl oxidase, tyrosinase, laccase	Forms amide bonds or oxidizes and reduce to form covalent cross-links.	
	Hyaluronic acid (HA)	Microbial fermentation –*Streptococcus zooepidemicus* and *Streptococcus* equip	Chemical cross-linking – 1,4-butanediol diglycidyl ether (BDDE).	BDDE contains epoxide groups that react with the hydroxyl (–OH) groups on the HA chains through nucleophilic attack, forming ether bonds and creating a stable cross-linked HA network.	[16]
			Physical cross-linking – methacrylic anhydride (HAMA), UV, LAP	When exposed to UV or visible light in the presence of a photoinitiator, the methacrylate groups undergo free-radical polymerization, forming covalent cross-links.	

	Chitosan	Crustacean shells	Physical cross-linking	It stabilizes through electrostatic interactions and hydrogen bonding, especially when blended with an ionically cross-linked polymer (e.g., alginate).	[17]
	Agarose	Red seaweed	Physical cross-linking	Agarose undergoes physical gelation upon cooling – forms a gel below ~35–40 °C and melts around 85–95 °C.	[17]
	Silk fibroin	Silkworm cocoons	Enzymatic cross-linking – tyrosinase	Tyrosinase oxidizes tyrosine residues in silk fibroin and gelatin to quinones and these reactive quinones then form covalent bonds between protein chains.	[18]
	Decellularized ECM (dECM)	Tissues/organs	Chemical cross-linking – carbodiimide, glutaraldehyde	Formation of covalent bonds between functional groups in the ECM proteins using agents like carbodiimide or glutaraldehyde.	[19]
			Enzymatic cross-linking – Microbial transglutaminase	Microbial transglutaminase form ε-(γ-glutamyl) lysine bonds between ECM proteins	
	Carrageenan	Marine red algae	Ionic cross-linking – K^+, Ca^{2+}	Forms ionotropic gels with K^+ or Ca^{2+} ions.	[20]
Synthetic polymers	Polyethylene glycol (PEG)	Petroleum-derived polymer	Photo-cross-linking – UV/visible light, LAP, Irgacure 2959	UV or visible light activates the photoinitiator, initiating free-radical polymerization of acrylate.	[7, 8]
	Polyvinyl alcohol (PVA)	Polymer derived by hydrolysis of polyvinyl acetate	Chemical cross-linking – glutaraldehyde	Glutaraldehyde forms covalent bonds with hydroxyl groups on PVA, resulting in a stable hydrogel network	[21]
			Physical cross-linking – freeze-thaw	Freeze-thaw cycles can induce crystallite formation and hydrogen bonding, forming physically cross-linked PVA hydrogels.	

(continued)

Table 2.1 (continued)

Material type		Source	Cross-linker	Cross-linking mechanism	References
	Polycaprolactone (PCL)	Aliphatic polyester derived from ε-caprolactone monomer	Physical cross-linking – thermal fusion or cooling-based solidification	The material is melted (usually around 60 °C), extruded, and solidifies as it cools down to room temperature without the need for chemical agents.	[21]
Non-polymer	Ceramics/ bioactive glass	Synthetic ceramic calcium phosphates – hydroxyapatite, β-tricalcium phosphate, amorphous calcium phosphate, and dicalcium phosphate dihydrate	Cross-linked using - UV light + photoinitiators (e.g., for GelMA) Ionic cross-linking with Ca^{2+} (e.g., for alginate) Enzymatic methods (e.g., tyrosinase with hyaluronic acid)	No direct chemical cross-linkers are used on the calcium phosphates themselves but are generally paired with a different polymer material and they are blended into hydrogels.	[22]
	Nanoparticle	Carbon-based, ceramics, polymers, metal oxides, and natural nanofibers	Nanoparticles themselves do not require cross-linkers but in the surrounding hydrogel matrix	Nanoparticles in bioinks are typically stabilized through mechanisms like physical entrapment within hydrogels, covalent bonding (e.g., functionalized CNTs), photo-cross-linking with UV-reactive polymers, ionic interactions (e.g., iron oxide in Ca^{2+}-cross-linked alginate), or self-assembly as seen with peptide nanostructures. These approaches enhance structural integrity, bioactivity, and mechanical reinforcement of printed constructs.	[23]
	Clay-based	Clay mineral –montmorillonite	Ionic cross-linking with polymers (e.g., alginate and gelatin)	Electrostatic interaction, hydrogen bonding; MMT intercalates between polymer chains.	[24]

Bioink	Bioink formulation	Cell type	Target tissue	Rheological Properties	Print parameters	3D print method	References
Alginate	4% sodium alginate in DI water, sometimes blended with 4% gelatin (Alg-Gel), or modified with nanocellulose or dECM; cross-linked with 0.1–0.5 M $CaCl_2$ post-printing	Human mesenchymal stem cells (hMSCs), chondrocytes, myoblasts	Skeletal muscle scaffold engineering	Shear-thinning behavior; viscosity increased with alginate concentration (4–12%); $G''>G'$ indicates viscous nature; peak viscosity at shear rate of 0.1 s^{-1}; Power-law flow behavior modeled as $\eta = m\gamma^{n-1}$	Nozzle: 250 μm; pressure: 10–30 kPa; speed: 15–30 mm/s; layer height: 0.1–0.2 mm; temp.: 25 °C (bed), 37 °C (nozzle); Infill: 25%	Extrusion-based	[13, 17, 25]
Gelatin	3–10% gelatin in aqueous solution; often combined with alginate, collagen, fibrin, or Matrigel; forms hydrogel at 20–30 °C	C2C12 myoblasts, MSCs, A549 epithelial cells; sometimes supplemented with collagen or laminin	Skeletal muscle, skin, lung epithelium, and vascular tissue	Thermosensitive; viscosity adjustable with temperature and concentration; shear-thinning	Temperature-controlled (20–30 °C); nozzle size: 200–400 μm	Extrusion-based	[17, 21]
Collagen	Type I collagen (typically 3–15 mg/mL); sometimes modified (e.g., methacrylated ColMA); or blended with gelatin, alginate, or chitosan; pH adjusted to 7.4; thermally gelled at 20–30 °C	hMSCs, fibroblasts, chondrocytes, keratinocytes; TGF-β for chondrogenesis	Skin, cartilage, bone, cornea, vascular tissue	Shear-thinning; viscosity increases with temp. and concentration; self-assembling fibers form above 20 °C	Temp.: 4–20 °C for prep; 20–30 °C for gelation; nozzle size ~200–400 μm; slow pressure	Mostly extrusion; also inkjet and DLP (if modified)	[15, 17, 20]

(continued)

Table 2.1 (continued)

Bioink	Bioink formulation	Cell type	Target tissue	Rheological Properties	Print parameters	3D print method	References
HA	Native HA or methacrylated HA (HAMA); often combined with alginate or PEGDA; cross-linked via UV and photoinitiators	hMSCs, neural progenitors, fibroblasts; may include bFGF or VEGF for enhanced regeneration	Cartilage, skin, neural, and vascular tissue	Shear-thinning, tunable stiffness, reversible sol–gel behavior; enhanced by methacrylation or ion coordination	25–30 °C for extrusion; UV light (365 nm, 10–60 s) for HAMA; Fe^{3+} or Ca^{2+} used in hybrid blends	Extrusion-based, inkjet, digital light processing (DLP)	[16, 21, 25]
Chitosan	Chitosan derived from crustacean shells (via deacetylation of chitin); usually dissolved in weak acids (acetic acid, pH < 6.2); used alone or blended with gelatin, alginate, or CNTs; sometimes grafted with PEG	Myoblasts, osteoblasts, fibroblasts; can be combined with neural or skin-derived cells	Bone, skin, muscle, nerve tissue	pH-sensitive sol–gel behavior; shear-thinning; low mechanical strength alone	25–30 °C; nozzle ~200–400 µm; acid-dissolved, requires neutralization or post-treatment	Extrusion-based	[17, 21]
Silk	Silk fibroin extracted from *Bombyx mori* cocoons; used alone or blended with gelatin and/or glycerol; can be physically cross-linked or enzymatically via tyrosinase	Chondrocytes, fibroblasts, and stem cells; no growth factor needed in base formulation	Cartilage, soft tissue, ear and facial tissue, and skeletal muscle	Shear-thinning; tunable viscoelasticity depending on SF:gelatin ratio	25–30 °C; nozzle size 200–400 µm; enzymatic or physical curing post-print	Extrusion-based	[17]

dECM	dECM obtained from porcine or human tissues (liver, heart, cartilage, etc.); processed using detergents, enzymes, or freeze-thaw cycles; used alone or blended with polymers like GelMA, alginate, or PEGDA; optionally methacrylated	MSCs, hepatocytes, chondrocytes, cardiac progenitor cells; supports native ECM signaling without added GFs	Cartilage, heart, skin, liver, kidney, esophagus, bone, and colon	Soft, shear-thinning, pH-dependent; mechanically tunable with PEG, gelatin, or SF; porosity and stiffness vary by source	Temp.: ~ 20–37 °C; nozzle: 200–400 μm; UV/photo/enzymatic cross-linking; sometimes dual-nozzle	Extrusion-based, inkjet, DLP, and stereolithography	[19]
Carrageenan	Kappa- carrageenan (κ-CA), 5% w/v, or methacrylated κ-CA (MA-κCA); may be combined with gelatin or collagen; cross-linking via ionic (K^+, Ca^{2+}) or photo (UV) mechanisms	NIH-3T3 fibroblasts, and MSCs	Cartilage, skin, and neural scaffolds	Thermoreversible; shear-thinning; gelation enhanced with cations; improved stiffness via methacrylation	Printed at ~25 °C, cross-linked using K^+/Ca^{2+} or UV light with photoinitiator	Extrusion-based or DLP	[20]
Cellulose	Carboxymethyl cellulose (CMC), hydroxyethyl cellulose, nanocellulose (CNF/CNC), DEAE-cellulose, often blended with alginate, gelatin, or chitosan; sometimes photo- or ionically cross-linked	HeLa, MSCs, hFB4 fibroblasts, ASCs, pancreatic, liver, and cancer cell models; growth factors like EGF or insulin used in some constructs	Skin, bone, liver, pancreas, wound, and tumor models	Shear-thinning; tunable by cellulose content; enhanced shape fidelity, structural integrity	25–37 °C; nozzle diameters typically 200–400 μm; compatible with UV, thermal, ionic, or click-cross-linking	Extrusion-based	[4]

(continued)

Table 2.1 (continued)

Bioink	Bioink formulation	Cell type	Target tissue	Rheological Properties	Print parameters	3D print method	References
GelMA	GelMA is synthesized by reacting gelatin with methacrylic anhydride; used at 3–10% w/v; mixed with photoinitiators like LAP or Irgacure and cross-linked via UV (365 nm) exposure	C2C12 myoblasts, hMSCs, endothelial cells, neural cells; often used with VEGF or laminin	Muscle, cartilage, vascular, neural, skin	Shear-thinning, thermosensitive; tunable stiffness (1–50 kPa); improves with blend concentration	22–25 °C for printability; UV (10–60 s) for cross-linking; LAP concentration ~0.05%	Extrusion, DLP, and inkjet bioprinting	[17, 21]
Hyaluronic acid methacrylate (HAMA)	HAMA synthesized by reacting HA with methacrylic anhydride; often blended with PEGDA, GelMA, or alginate; cross-linked via UV or visible light in presence of photoinitiators (e.g., LAP)	Human mesenchymal stem cells (hMSCs), neural stem cells; sometimes supplemented with bFGF or TGF-β	Cartilage, skin, CNS, bone, vascular tissue	Shear-thinning; low viscosity pre-gel, forms stable hydrogel post-photo-cross-linking; tunable stiffness via degree of methacrylation	UV (365 nm) or visible light; printing temp. ~ 25 °C; nozzle: 200–400 μm	Extrusion, DLP, or inkjet bioprinting	[8, 16, 25]
PEG	PEG-based hydrogels often in the form of PEGDA or PEGMA, cross-linked using UV or visible light with photoinitiators (LAP, Irgacure); PEG frequently blended with GelMA, HAMA, or bioactive ceramics for tissue engineering	MSCs, fibroblasts, endothelial cells; often functionalized with RGD peptides or blended with bioactive cues like VEGF	Cartilage, bone, soft tissue, vascular, and wound healing	Low viscosity pre-cross-linking; tunable stiffness post-cross-linking; good flowability	UV (365 nm), 10–60 s; print temp. ~5 °C; nozzle: 200–400 μm	Extrusion, DLP, stereolithography	[7, 17, 20]

PVA	Water-soluble linear polymer; formulated as 5–15% w/v PVA; optionally blended with alginate; cross-linking by ionic methods, chemical cross-linkers (e.g., glutaraldehyde), or freeze–thaw cycles for physical gelation	Myoblasts, fibroblasts, and other adherent cells; sometimes used with growth-promoting media for wound healing	Skin, muscle, wound healing, and microneedles	Highly crystalline; shear-thinning behavior; elasticity and swelling tunable by degree of hydrolysis and cross-linking	Temp:. ~25 °C; cross-linked by Ca^{2+} (with alginate) or through repeated freeze-thaw cycles	Extrusion-based	[8, 21]
PCL	Thermoplastic polyester from ring-opening polymerization of ε-caprolactone; used as solid filament or molten ink; sometimes combined with GelMA, collagen, or ceramics	MSCs, osteoblasts, fibroblasts; can be loaded with VEGF, NGF for improved bioactivity	Bone, cartilage, muscle, and skin	Non-shear-thinning; melts above 55 °C; solidifies upon cooling; retains shape well	Printing temp. ~60 °C; nozzle 200–400 µm; slow cooling for solidification	Extrusion-based	[8]
PLA (polylactic acid)	PLA is used as a thermoplastic filament or granulate; not a hydrogel-based bioink; typically printed at high temperature; may be blended with bioceramics or used as a support material	Typically used without embedded cells (acellular); sometimes seeded post-print with MSCs or osteoblasts	Bone, orthopedic implants, and dental scaffolds	Non-shear-thinning; thermoplastic flow; hardens rapidly upon cooling	Printing temp.: ~180–220 °C; nozzle size: 0.2–0.4 mm	Melt-extrusion (FDM/FFF)	[21]

(continued)

Table 2.1 (continued)

Bioink	Bioink formulation	Cell type	Target tissue	Rheological Properties	Print parameters	3D print method	References
Ceramics	Hydroxyapatite (HAp), tricalcium phosphate (TCP), or bioactive glass (BG); typically blended with polymers like GelMA, PEG, PCL, or alginate to form printable pastes or composites	Osteoblasts, MSCs; sometimes includes BMP-2 or VEGF to enhance osteogenesis	Bone, dental, and craniofacial	High viscosity; particle-based pastes; non-shear-thinning unless blended with hydrogels	Nozzle ~200–400 µm; room temp. or 60–90 °C for PCL blends	Extrusion-based bioprinting (low temp.), or FDM with ceramic-polymer composites	[22]
Nanoparticles	Nanoparticles (e.g., carbon nanotubes, graphene, nHA, Fe_3O_4) blended with base hydrogels (e.g., GelMA, alginate, and PEGDA); some are functionalized (e.g., CNT–COOH) to allow covalent bonding	hMSCs, neural cells, fibroblasts; may include VEGF or osteogenic factors for directed differentiation	Bone, neural tissue, vascular, and detox platforms	Improved shear-thinning and stiffness; physical or covalent entrapment; conductivity enabled in CNT/GO	Dependent on base matrix (e.g., 25–37 °C); UV light if photo-cross-linking; low-to-mid shear pressure	Extrusion, DLP, inkjet (depends on base hydrogel)	[23]
Clay-based	Clay minerals (e.g., laponite, montmorillonite, Cloisite®, HNTs, PAL) combined with base hydrogels like GelMA, PEGDA, alginate, gelatin, dECM, or methylcellulose (MC); concentrations typically 0.5–5% w/v	MSCs, endothelial cells, cardiac fibroblasts, myoblasts, NIH/3T3 fibroblasts	Bone, cartilage, skeletal muscle, cardiac, and vascular tissue	Adds shear-thinning, increases viscosity, enhances shape fidelity; modifies mechanical behavior of base ink	Room temp. printing; nozzle ~200–400 µm; cross-linked via UV, ionic, or enzymatic methods depending on base hydrogel	Extrusion-based	[24]

2.2.2 Types of Bioinks Based on the Resources

Bioinks can be derived from a wide range of materials in which each class offers distinct advantages and limitations in terms of the biocompatibility, printability, and mechanical tunability. The schematic representation of biomaterials applicable to 3D bioprinting fabrication was depicted in the figure 2.1–2.3.

2.2.2.1 Natural

Natural biomaterials originate from biological systems and can replicate the extracellular matrix (ECM) and aids in cellular attachment and function but their mechanical strength remains limited [11, 12]. Some of the major biomaterials include collagen, gelatin (denatured collagen), fibrin, alginate (from algae), hyaluronic acid (HA), chitosan, and silk fibroin [10, 11]. The main benefit of these materials lies in their bioactivity since they naturally facilitate cell attachment through recognized ligands and cellular environments with adjustable gelation properties. *However*, the mechanical properties of these materials often tend to be weak and degrade quickly [8]. For instance, the pure forms of collagen and gelatin gels lack sufficient mechanical strength to maintain complex structures unless they receive chemical cross-linking or reinforcement while maintaining its biological properties [11].

2.2.2.2 Synthetic

Synthetic biomaterials or man-made polymers often play a crucial role in the formulation of bioinks for 3D bioprinting, offering a range of properties that can be tailored to meet specific tissue engineering needs. The synthetic polymers used in bioprinting applications include polyethylene glycol (PEG), polycaprolactone (PCL), and polylactic-co-glycolic acid (PLGA), and polyurethane and Pluronic materials [7]. The mechanical properties of these materials can be modified through changes in molecular weight and composition, which allows for customization of their degradation rates and chemical properties. The materials generally have strong mechanical properties when creating scaffolds yet need modifications to minimize cytotoxic effects and enhance cell binding capabilities and control degradation rates [1, 21] and face challenges to replicate the ECM for cell attachment and tissue development [26, 27].

2.2.2.3 Composite (Hybrid)

Bioinks made from composite biomaterials combine at least two different materials to produce a single formulation, which benefits from multiple component strengths. The

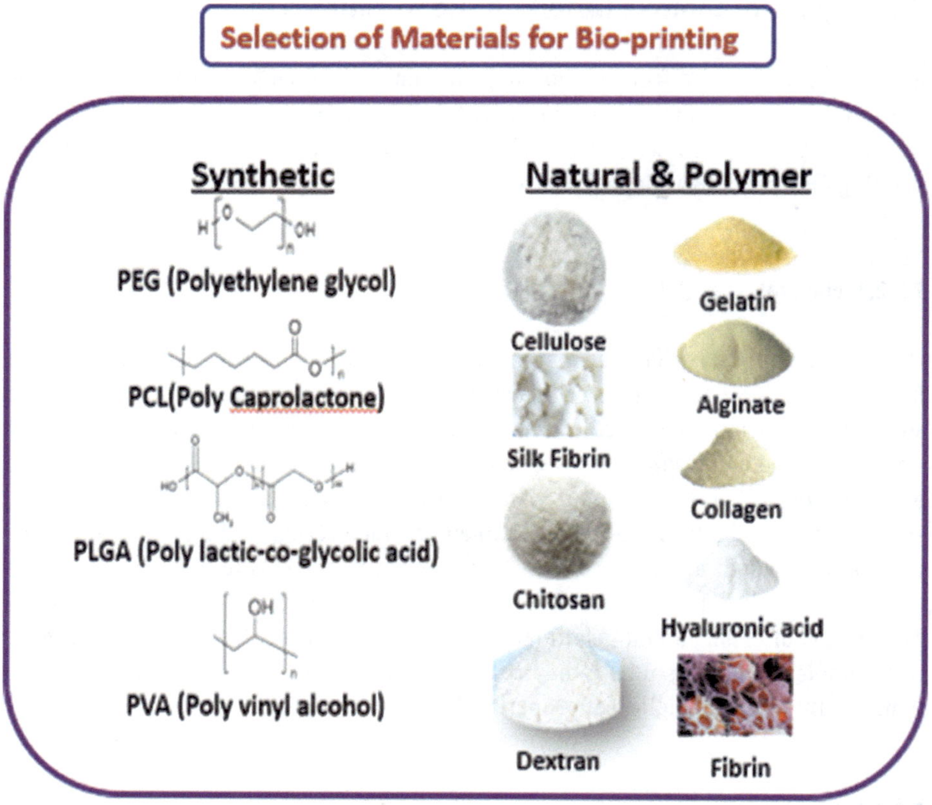

Figure 2.1: Schematic representation of biomaterials used for 3D bioprinting [81, 82].

common example of composite materials is gelatin or collagen combined with PLGA or PCL fibers or reinforcing alginate with nanocellulose [4, 6, 7]. Such composites can attain a point where they balance their bioactive properties with their mechanical strength. The success of composite bioinks depends on achieving chemical or physical compatibility while maintaining printability requirements [8].

2.2.2.4 Decellularized Extracellular Matrix (dECM)

Decellularized extracellular matrix (dECM) is an excellent material for bioink formulation due to its bioactive and tissue-specific properties [1, 28]. This material is derived by decellularization of native tissues through chemical, enzymatic, or physical methods, and it retains the essential biochemical cues and structural proteins such as collagen, laminin, fibronectin, and growth factors needed to direct cellular growth and proliferation [7, 29]. Tissue-specific dECM from different tissue sources like cardiac, hepatic, adipose, or neural demonstrates better outcomes for tissue regeneration than generic hydrogels [29–32].

2.2.2.5 Ceramic Biomaterials

3D bioprinting utilizes ceramic biomaterials extensively for bone and dental tissue engineering because these materials exhibit excellent osteoconductive properties and bio-inert properties and can endure the shear pressure and have load bearing functions similar to the bone [11, 33]. Commonly used ceramics include tricalcium phosphate(TCA), hydroxyapatite (HA), and bioactive glass where these materials are inherently bioactive to bond with surrounding tissue and their integration into bioinks or scaffolds improves mechanical strength and creates an optimal environment with suitable porosity for hard tissue regeneration [11, 12, 33, 34].

2.2.2.6 Smart biomaterials

Smart biomaterials or shape-memory materials have the ability to detect and react when exposed to an external stimulus such as temperature, pH, light, electric or magnetic fields, or biochemical signals and automatically adjust and change its 3D structure based on the exposed time [10, 12, 35]. This technology enables implant deployment through swelling or geometric changes after surgical placement by developing stimuli-responsive bioinks and its responsive and adaptable features enable 4D bioprinting to create tissues that change their shape or stiffness over time while its self-healing properties help fix damage from extrusion and enhance print quality and construct strength.

2.2.3 Classification of Biomaterials Based on Biological Response

The biological response produced by a biomaterial plays an important role for bioink formulations and specific bioprinting applications. So, based on how these materials interact with the cells and tissues around them, they can be broadly classified into three major categories such as bio-inert, bioactive, and bioresorbable. These materials are characterized by their minimal to no interaction with the biological system where they neither provoke an immune response nor promote active cell adhesion or signaling. Instead, they are primarily used as structural or supportive frameworks in bioink formulations by using of both natural and synthetic polymers, which can be tailored to meet the specific requirements of different bioprinting applications [7, 11]. Materials such as unmodified PEG, PVA, and Pluronic F127 do not inherently interact with cells or the biological setting as they lack cell-recognition sites and thus do not promote adhesion, proliferation, or differentiation unless chemically modified (e.g., by adding RGD peptides) [7]. Their advantage lies in their predictable behavior, structural tunability, and stability, but they are inherently non-bioactive unless functionalized. Bioactive biomaterials, in contrast, engage in dynamic and purposeful physicochemical interactions. It does not interact with the cells or tissues and often mimicking the native extracellular matrix (ECM) to improve cellular adhesion, proliferation, and differentiation [12]. These materials have the ability to degrade gradually within a certain period of time or when it is present in a biological environment, and it gives the necessary support for the cells attachment and growth allowing them to be replaced by regenerating tissues while the materials themselves degrade over time leaving behind the tissue construct [11, 36]. Moreover the material degradation can be chemically tuned to match the timeframe for tissue growth rates, which is very advantageous in many biomedical applications such as bone scaffolds and skin regeneration [7, 8, 11].

2.2.4 Additives and Functionalization

Apart from the biomaterials for formulations some additional components are essential to help control the materials gelation, viscoelasticity, its structural integrity, while improving cell growth and tissue formation.

2.2.4.1 Cross-Linkers and Initiators

After printing a bioink into the shape of a tissue or organ, from its gel-like state it turns into a solid form that maintains its shape after printing a tissue or organ. This has been carried out through a process called cross-linking, which creates a network of bonds inside the material. The bonds within the structure determine its strength while influencing cell growth patterns and cellular behavior within the printed construct. These cross-linking methods are categorized into three major classes, namely physical, chemical, and photo-cross-linking, and many bioinks today use a combination of these methods known as dual cross-linking to achieve optimal results.

Physical cross-linking methods do not involve strong chemical bonds but instead depends on weak reversible bonds between polymer chains, which include hydrogen bonding, electrostatic forces, and hydrophobic interactions. Common example such as alginate, can turn into a gel when interacting with calcium ion while gelatin and agarose solidifies through cooling called thermal cross-linking mechanism. However, one main drawback with this mechanism is that the mechanical strength of these gels remains weak while their dissolution rate increases when exposed to biological environments. Therefore, this technique is commonly paired with one or more cross-linking process for stable printed structures [39].

Chemical cross-linking mechanism forms covalent bonds, which result in more durable gels and provides good mechanical strength for the scaffolds by using chemical reagents and enzymes, which acts as a catalyst that facilitates the covalent bonds to form within the polymer or material leading to the cross-linking mechanism offering efficient control over the cross-linking density and mechanical properties of the resulting hydrogels. For instance, gelatin for its biocompatibility melts at body temperature thus making it unstable for long-term cell culture with poor mechanical stability, so the gelatin is chemically modifying with methacrylic anhydride, introducing methacryloyl ($-CH_2=C(CH_3)-CO^-$) groups onto the gelatin backbone. Another category of chemical cross-linking called photo-cross-linking uses either UV or visible light to initiate the bond formation in the material by inducing free radicals from the photoinitiators such as Irgacure 2959 (UV), LAP and Eosin Y (visible light) that are added to the biomaterial for the covalent bond formation, but excessive UV exposure must be carefully controlled to avoid cellular damage when compared to visible light cross-linking [40].

While chemical cross-linking offers higher stiffness and long-term stability, care must be taken with the type and amount of chemicals used, as some may harm cells or interfere with nutrients moving through the gel. For enzymatic cross-linking mechanism, common examples such as horseradish peroxidase (HRP) or transglutaminase catalyze the formation of covalent bonds within the polymer. Enzymatic methods are safe for cells, relatively fast, and often occur at body temperature and neutral pH. Photo-cross-linking is one of the most precise and popular methods in bioprinting. It uses light (UV or visible) and photoinitiators, which are light-sensitive chemicals that generate free radicals or reactive species when exposed. These reactive species start a chain reaction that links up polymer molecules into a solid gel. The main advantage is control – you can cure the bioink exactly where and when you want, which is great for creating complex structures or layer-by-layer printing. Common photo-cross-linkable materials include GelMA (gelatin modified with methacrylate groups), PEGDA (a synthetic polymer), and HAMA (methacrylated hyaluronic acid). Typical photoinitiators include LAP (which works with 405 nm blue light), Irgacure 2959 (activated by UV), and eosin Y (green light, with co-initiators). Photo-cross-linking is fast and can produce strong, stable hydrogels, but the light exposure and chemicals used must be carefully managed to avoid cell damage. For example, too much UV light or too many free radicals can harm living cells. This is why many systems now use visible light and low-toxicity photoinitiators. Also, the amount of photoinitiator is kept low – just enough to get the job done without compromising cell health.

In addition, one or more cross-linking mechanisms are combined to balance out the different drawbacks that come with a singular cross-linking approach. This method is called dual or multimode cross-linking mechanism that can combine different combinations of these cross-linking mechanisms and frame different strategies to balance printability, tunability, and biomechanical stability. A common example is alginate-GelMA bioinks where the alginate is ionically cross-linked with calcium exposure while the GelMA part of the scaffold is then exposed to UV light for photo-cross-linking. Therefore, the process of cross-linking serves as a critical step in bioprinting because it transforms soft bioinks into stable structures, which provide cell support and structural integrity. The most effective results emerge from using multiple strategies together to achieve both printability and functional requirements for successful tissue engineering.

2.2.4.2 Growth Factors

Growth factors (GFs) play a critical role in regulating cellular behavior and tissue development within the bioprinted constructs and they promote specific cellular responses such as proliferation, differentiation, migration, and tissue maturation. A wide variety of GFs including, TGF-β, bFGF, EGF, PDGF, and BMPs have been utilized to support angiogenesis, chondrogenesis, osteogenesis, and epithelial repair depending on the target tissue [7, 12, 21, 28, 37].

2.2.5 Cell-Laden Versus Acellular Bioinks

Bioinks can be prepared with cells suspended in the matrix prior to printing (cell-laden), or without cells (acellular), with cells introduced later by seeding or infiltration. The cells are embedded in the bioink, so there is a simultaneous deposition of cells and matrix, thereby resulting in cell placement within the printed structure [31]. This approach allows cells to interact and start maturing *in situ* during the printing process, which requires the bioink to be cytocompatible along with the appropriate printing conditions such as shear stresses, cross-linking chemicals, pressure, and nozzle diameter based on the type of cells used and the biomaterial to maintain cell viability and avoid cell damage. These bioinks are printed as scaffold structures without cells, and cells are seeded post-printing or the construct are directly implanted to allow cell infiltration from the body. A cellular printing is common when creating complex scaffold architectures, which are later exposed so cell culture for cell migration and differentiations through the porous structure of the constructs, but a major drawback is ensuring efficient cell migration into the dense scaffold and achieving uniform cell distribution afterward to prevent irregular tissue formation [67].

2.2.6 Rheological Tuning of Bioinks

The rheological property of a bioink describes how a material deforms and flows when stress is applied and how well they retain their structure after deposition during and after printing. Parameters such as viscosity, shear-thinning behavior, yield stress, thixotropic, and viscoelastic moduli such as storage modulus G′ and loss modulus G″, and all of these properties must be optimized to ensure that the bioink can be extruded smoothly and maintain its structural integrity. So, if a bioink shows shear thinning it becomes easy during printing by aligning macromolecules and reducing viscosity, while thixotropy is another parameter that is a time-dependent property, which allows the ink to remain fluid under stress and recover its structure post-printing. However, excessive shear stress or prolonged residence time in the nozzle can reduce cell viability, making shear conditions and cell survival critical parameters in bioink formulation. High viscosity can aid in the printed filament to hold its shape, but too much viscosity can make extrusion difficult or can clog the nozzles [38]. If a bioink behaves too much like a Newtonian fluid with constant viscosity, it may either fail to maintain shape by being too fluid or become too difficult to extrude with high viscosity.

The yield stress is another important parameter, which is defined as the minimum applied stress required to initiate flow in the material. A slight yield stress in a bioink is advantageous because it allows the material to remain stationary and maintain shape under its own weight but flow easily once the yield point is exceeded by applied extrusion pressure. Viscoelastic is defined by properties such as storage modulus (G'), which is the elastic behavior that defines the energy stored in the material, while the loss modulus (G'') is the viscous behavior that shows the energy dissipated or lost. So, a higher G' than G'' at rest indicates that the material behaves more like a soft solid, suitable for retaining printed structures. During extrusion, the viscous behavior (G'') is the desired property to ensure stable flow, whereas after printing, elastic recovery (G') becomes important for the structural integrity [41].

2.3 Processing and Printing Parameters

In this section, we discuss the various bioprinting methods and the key parameters that influence printing outcomes. Different bioprinting methods have different requirements for bioink formulation and the preparations needed before printing and the factors that determine print quality.

2.3.1 Bioprinting Methods

There are various bioprinting techniques such as extrusion-based, inkjet, laser-assisted, stereolithography, and digital light processing. Each of these techniques consists of a unique bioink formulation that is suitable for the chosen biological application and printing technique that have been chosen.

Most commonly used technique is extrusion-based bioprinting, which elutes the bioink continuously by giving air or mechanical pressure, which requires the bioinks to have proper viscosity and shear-thinning properties to enable smooth flow through the nozzle, which helps to maintain the shape after deposition. These bioinks must also express rapid recovery and adequately adapt stress to confirm the material sta-

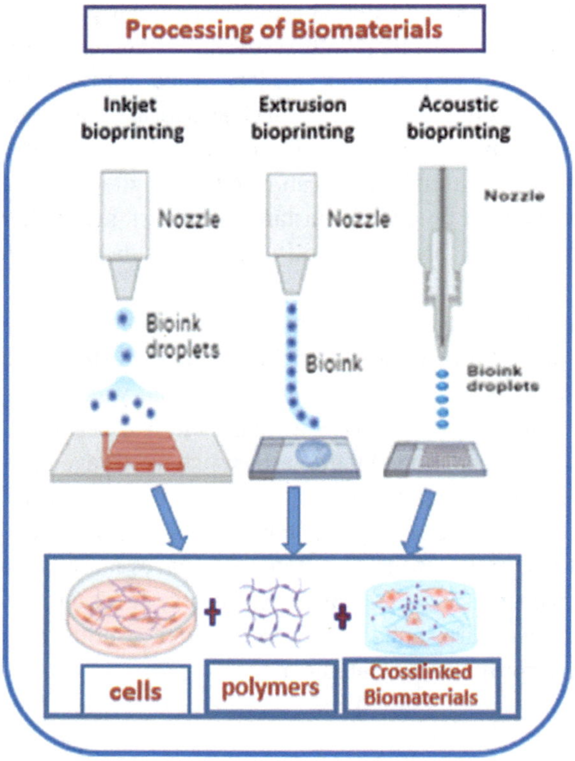

Figure 2.2: Preparation of biomaterials prior to cross-linking using different bioprinters [82, 83].

bility; excess shear stress must be avoided to protect implanted cells. The inkjet bioprinting necessitate the use of low viscous materials for the formulation of the bioink. This bioprinting employs droplet-based deposition via thermal, piezoelectric, or electrostatic actuators [42]. Laser-assisted bioprinting employs high-energy to expel droplets, which enables accurate implication of cell-rich bioinks without direct nozzle contact. Anyhow due to the high energy exposure, it may facilitate formulations that are photothermally sensitive and stable during laser exposure, while also taking cellular compatibility into consideration. Conversely, digital light processing and stereolithography depend on photo-cross-linkable polymers as Iragure photoinitiators or lithium phenyl-2,4,6-trimethylbenzoylphosphinate (LAP) or methacrylated gelatin (GelMA) or polyethylene glycol-diacrylate (PEGDA) [43, 51]. To facilitate effective cross-linking, these bioinks need to have low absorbance and light-scattering capacity. The degree of functionalization, light intensity, and exposure duration affects the mechanical properties of the bioink. Femtosecond lasers are used in two-photon polymerization, which produces ultra-high-resolution printing by nonlinear absorption. In contrast, three-material printing in core middle shell format creates complicated structures, while coaxial and triaxial bioprinting techniques use a concentric nozzle to deposit several materials simultaneously (e.g., core-shell configurations) [41, 42].

Finally, electro hydrodynamic bioprinting methods acquire electric fields to control jetting of bioinks at sub-micron resolution. Hence, all the methods have their own distinct advantages like extrusion, which offers versatility and scalability, inkjet extinguishing in speed and resolution, laser-assisted method assures non-contact precision, and stereolithography provides unmatched spatial control all the while demanding carefully tuned rheological, chemical, biological parameters in the bioink formulation to finalize printing fidelity, stability and high cell viability [40].

2.3.2 Preprinting Considerations

The following paragraph enumerates various bioprinting methods extrusion, inkjet, laser-assisted and stereolithography, which require different bioink formulations altogether with essential parameters, which provides unique advantages over the resolution speed and cell management capabilities.

2.3.2.1 Sterilization and Aseptic Setup

Using sterile materials in bioprinting is very crucial since the methodology involves living cells and appropriate sterilization of all the materials such as bioinks nozzles, print bed, etc., is essential for each and every successful print. The sterilization of bioink components includes filtration (0.22 µm sterile filters), autoclaving, UV irradiation, ethanol treatment, or gamma irradiation. Filter sterilization is the commonly used sterilization method for bioinks, solutions, and solvents by passing them through a 0.22-µm membrane filter. Composition for bioink formation and heat-sensitive polymer solutions like gelatin, alginate, or polyethylene glycol (diacrylate) (PEGDA) are filter-sterilized before cells are added. Solid materials, tools, laminar hood minimal volume of bioinks are even sterilized under UV light before the cell encapsulation procedure to remove microbiological contaminants but also excessive exposure can break down the structure of polymer and makes the photoinitiators unstable [47]. Steam-based sterilization also known as autoclaving at high pressure and temperature (usually 121 °C for 15–20 min), are used to sterilize the heat-stable components such as empty syringe barrels and stainless steel nozzles and sometimes to dry polymers without any cellular content. This heat-based method of sterilization is not appropriate for hydrogels or bioactive components that break down under exposure to high temperatures. Other materials such as tools, print beds, nozzles, support frames, and containers must be frequently sterilized with 70% ethanol [48].

After printing, the printed structures must be handled sterilely by transferring them to culture media; the printing procedure is carried inside a biosafety cabinet or in an enclosed sterile printer chamber. Filtering or utilizing commercially available pre-sterilized materials are recommended while handling inks that contain proteins or growth factors because of exposure to heat and other heat-based sterilization techniques can cause denaturation.

2.3.2.2 Temperature Control

Due to the use of live cells and temperature-sensitive materials, the manufacturing of bioink and bioprinting require proper temperature control. Because gelatin, collagen, and agarose-based bioink display temperature-dependent gelation, they require particular temperature conditions to get transit from liquid to a gel state or vice versa [52]. The gelatin-based inks remains at liquid state even at high temperatures until the temperatures fall below 30 °C reach gelation state. For example, in order to completely dissolve the gelatin, these materials must be handled between the temperatures of 37–60 °C to prevent premature gel formation. Therefore, to prevent nozzle obstructions and guarantee uniform extrusion, the bioink solutions are placed under temperature-controlled system. Extreme temperature variations during this stage could induce cell death; hence the printing procedure is carried at room temperature or under slightly varying temperature. Temperature control is an essential physical factor in bioprinting workflows, because it affects the cross-linking rate of bioinks that use thermal or enzymatic activation at 37 °C. Additionally, photopolymerization can result in local heating, and improper temperature control causes cartridge gelation and nozzle blockages, as well as decreased resolution and loss of viable cells. Therefore, few printing systems have a temperature-controlled stage in the bioprinter or a printhead heater [53].

2.3.2.3 Nozzle Selection and Compatibility

The selection of nozzles in bioprinting influences both printing resolution and the rate of cell survival. The nozzles differ among the inner diameter measurements such as 150 µm, 250 µm, etc. The needle gauges with small nozzle produce precise lines; even then it generates high shear stress that potentially clogs the nozzle due to viscous inks causing cell aggregation. The important concern while working with cell-laden bioinks is the nozzle diameter that should also prevent excessive shear stress, which will develop the intended print. Few bioprinters contain specialized nozzles like coaxial needles to create hollow tubes where the core receives a particular form of bioink and the shell receives another form of bioink like cross-linker. The nozzle material must be sterile and the bioink should not react with it [54].

2.3.3 Printability and Fidelity

It is important to evaluate and finalize the print materials regardless of the printer settings that are optimal for well-formulated bioink. The ability of a bioink to build structures exactly as intended without problems like spreading, sagging, or clogging is known as printability.

Important aspects include:

2.3.3.1 Shape Fidelity

An effective bioink for printing must prevent extreme dispersion or structural collapse after deposition; optimizing viscosity and yield stress, along with supportive measures such as freeform reversible embedding of suspended hydrogels (FRESH) using a slurry gel support medium, it improves shape fidelity; cross-linking at the exact time is the most important factor because alginate filaments will retain their shape but gelation occurs quickly in calcium-enriched solutions.

Excessive fluidity in a bioink can lead to two possible issues: either adjacent strands will merge (reducing resolution) or the layers will flatten. Measuring strand width, pore dimensions, and angular retention in experimental configurations that have printed, the dimensions of a 3D scaffold (including strand thickness and spacing) exhibit high fidelity when they match the computer-aided design (CAD) model [55].

2.3.3.2 Resolution and Precision

The resolution is determined by the printer capacity to produce consistent features, while accuracy determines the emplacement of the special features in the printer. Different printing methods have unique intrinsic resolution capacities. However extrusion techniques require a minimum strand of 200 μm; inkjet and laser-assisted printing can deposit droplets as small as 50–100 μm. Effective resolution is determined by the rheological characteristics of the bioink since tiny droplets or filaments will develop into bigger sizes. The synchronization of a precisely adjusted nozzle with a fast-reacting bioink necessitates attaining high resolution printing. Because any inconsistencies in stage movements or extrusion rates may result in feature blurring, precision is determined by the printers' mechanical precision as well as consistent flow of bioink. Calibration pattern testing and the production of self-supporting test geometry, including lattice structures, are used to emancipate the actual resolution of the printing system. The capacity of a bioink to print parallel filaments that remain distinct at a given distance indicates its lateral resolution [54].

2.3.3.3 Layer-by-Layer Stacking (Vertical Fidelity)

The systematic building of biomaterials required for the bioprinting manufacturing process necessitates adequate adhesion between each new layer and sufficient support from previous layers. The bioinks' ability to withstand weight instantaneously after the application determines the effective stacking. The underlying layers will deform when further layers are added if the bioink persists fragile or extends the gelation period. Due to this phenomenon, and when the height increases, the construct develops outward "bulging" or structural collapse. To rectify this issue three alternatives are identified such as printing at lower speeds or employing smaller *z*-increments for partial solidification, embedding the structure in supportive media, using sacrificial scaffold materials that can be taken off after printing, or putting additional cross-linking techniques into practice by installing rapid UV flashes between layers [56]. To create complex geometries without deviations, the printer requires precise calibration to guarantee that each layer correctly aligns with the previous layer. Because overhanging parts require either sacrificial support inks or precise ink stiffness optimization, printing them assumes importance. In research on printability, the highest possible self-supporting structure and the maximum number of layers that can be printed without failing for specific bioinks are determined. The process of turning bioink into a three-dimensional structure is dependent on printability, which facilitates using standardized geometric shape-like grids and tubes to test novel bioink formulations for certain accuracy levels [57].

2.4 Characterization Techniques

Characterization is necessary after making a bioink and printing a construct to ascertain whether the bioink and tissue construct meet the standards of the biomaterial. In order to perform the characterization process, the bioink and its associated hydrogel mandatorily have their physical and chemical characteristics are measure. Additionally the scaffolds' mechanical features such as tensile strength and elasticity testing and structural integrity evaluation with a focus on microarchitecture and fidelity must be done. This section explains basic characterization techniques that are applicable to several fields [62].

2.4.1 Physicochemical Characterization

Methods to examine the fundamental physical and chemical properties of the bioink material and the resulting hydrogel network:

2.4.1.1 Rheological Measurements

Rheometer tests the viscosity and viscoelastic behavior, which are used to measure the rheological characteristics of bioink prior to printing. In order to verify shear-thinning behavior, shear rheometry with shear rate sweeps aids in determining viscosity changes brought on by shear rate variations. When displaying gel-like characteristics, the pre-cross-linked ink and completely cross-linked hydrogel can be examined using oscillatory rheology, which calculates the storage modulus (G') and loss modulus (G''). Because the ink keeps its shape ($G \gg G''$ implies solid-like behavior), a well-printable gel usually displays $G' > G''$, which denotes solid-like behavior at rest. Through thixotrophic behavior assessment (recovery testing after high shear) and yield stress measurement (Stress ramp) the behavior of bioink during extrusion can be better understood [49].

2.4.1.2 Swelling Ratio and Water Content

Hydrogel-based bioinks hold the capacity to absorb aqueous solutions and it undergoes the process of volumetric expansion. The swelling ratio (Q) is determined by submerging the gel in a buffered solution after a bioink has cross-linked into its gel state and measuring the increase in weight.

A traditional methodology includes: initial weight of the freshly prepared gel (wet weight), subsequently drying the sample (dry weight) and calculating Q = (wet weight/dry weight). This particular computation provides insights into the water content and the porosity within the polymeric network [58]. Elevated swelling ratios ($\gg$1) denote the high level hydration and porous network, which is regularly observed in the natural polymers; conversely, smaller ratios suggest a more condensed network topology. The swelling phenomenon plays a pivotal role in influencing nutrient diffusion and cellular migration with the structured construct. The swelling regulation is important, for example, a bioink aimed for cartilage applications may be engineered to prevent excessive swelling to conserve the dimensional integrity during the culture. This evaluation is also a measure of density of the cross-link material, which forms a network with more cross-links showing less swelling [59].

2.4.1.3 Degradation and Stability Testing

In tissue engineering applications, it is necessary to precisely evaluate the rate of scaffold degradation from bioink for a certain period.

Hydrogel samples prepared for printing kept for incubation in physiological buffers or biological enzyme solutions (collagenase for collagen or lysozyme for alginate) and then measuring mass loss and changes in mechanical properties over the research period are necessary steps in evaluating degradation. After four weeks of PBS incubation at 37 °C, the mass of an alginate/gelation hydrogel created by cross-linking would eventually decrease to a certain amount [60]. When the cellular entities are present, the enzymatic activity of these entities, such as matrix metalloproteinases, causes the bioink to degrade naturally. In order to prevent both delayed degradation that prevents tissue remodeling and premature structural breakdown prior to tissue creation, the degradation process should be carefully managed. Hence the spectroscopic characterization to analyze the chemical parameters are acquired such as bond cleavage and gel permeation chromatography to examine if polymer molecular weight can support physical measurements of loss in the mass [61].

2.4.1.4 Porosity and Microstructure

The distribution of nutrients and the rates of cellular growth are determined by the architectural design of the pores in scaffolds cross-linked bioink. To check the porosity both the overall void percentage and the distribution of pore sizes must be measured. Techniques followed by the researchers aid in detecting the porous framework by combining freeze-dried hydrogel specimens with scanning electron microscopy (SEM). SEM photography produces the foam-like appearance of desiccated hydrogel clear. Micro-computed tomography (μCT) can be used to scan dry or polymerized scaffolds in three dimensions and determine the pore sizes for the whole structure of the material. The structure with large pore dimensions, mercury intrusion porosimetry, and the related techniques offer a way to calculate the volume of the pores. Porosity is often expressed using percentage calculation. However the mesh size of the hydrogel differs from scaffold macropores, which measure hundreds of microns between printed filaments, the macroporosity of bioinks can be computed from the spacing of the print strand when they form a grid pattern. Both the scales are extremely important. Moreover the macropores facilitate tissue integration, cell migration, and molecular transport, and the availability of cells attached is determined with the nano- to microscale mesh size [50].

2.4.1.5 Cross-Linking Density and Chemical Analysis

Mechanical stiffness of the bioink produced for the hydrogel and structural integrity of the gel directly depends on the mechanism of cross-linking within the material. The Flory-Rehner model represents the technique for determining the density of the cross-link [63].

FTIR spectroscopy depicts the specific chemical functionalities through spectral peak changes when the methacrylate C=C bond disappears during polymerization. NMR spectroscopy aids the researchers in quantifying functional groups that modify during cross-linking reactions [64]. The level of double bond conversion during photo-cross-linking serves as an indicator to measure bioinks' cross-link density. In mechanical evaluations (Section 4.3), the Young's modulus measurement serves as a stand-in indicator to demonstrate that higher values correspond to increased cross-link density for specific base polymers. The analytical techniques support the confirmation of proper network architecture from printing and curing processes because reproducibility still depends on achieving uniform cross-link density [64, 65].

2.4.2 Biological Characterization

It is crucial to assess the bioink and the printed constructs biological performance once cells are utilized. Longer-term cell functions, cell viability following printing, and any particular tissue evaluation assays are mentioned.

2.4.2.1 Cell Viability and Cytocompatibility

Cell viability is the percentage of living cells that remain after the bioprinting process. It is typically assessed using live/dead staining methods (e.g., ethidium homodimer for nonviable cells and Calcein-AM for viable cells) in conjunction with fluorescence microscopy or confocal imaging to measure the proportion of living to dead cells as soon as possible after printing (within 24 h) [66]. A specific bioink and printer combination must often have an acceptable viability threshold that exceeds 80% for the non-disruption of the cells. It is possible to improve cell viability by improvising the printing-related parameters (such as needle gauge, pressure, and exposure to cross-linking agents). Cytocompatibility is more than just viability of the cells. It strictly means that the substance and the by-products breakdown do not cause cytotoxicity to the cells. Cellular metabolic activity in the following printing process can be evaluated by assays such as MTT, XTT, or AlamarBlue as a measure of cellular health. A bioink designed for implantation, in vitro cytocompatibility evaluations in accordance with ISO standards, for instance, extract cytotoxicity tests may be conducted to confirm that zero leachable molecules from the hydrogel adversely affect the cells. Hiked levels of viability and cytocompatibility exhibit that the bioink composes a favorable microenvironment for cells immediately following the printing [68].

2.4.2.2 Cell Proliferation and Growth

Cells' capacity to divide leads to an increase in the number of printed constructs over the course of prolonged culture periods, which can last anywhere from days to many weeks. Quantitative information about cell proliferation is obtained by serial viability/metabolic assays or DNA content assays utilizing PicoGreen to detect the number of cells. Ki-67 labeling is used to identify dividing cells and imaging techniques are employed to count cells at various intervals to give the information about cellular proliferation [69]. Bioink that promotes active cell growth will exhibit increased metabolic activity or proliferation. When proliferation levels stay constant, the bioink matrix either exhibits too many cells being restricted into quiescence or many signaling cues. Maintaining a certain cell type (such as primary cells, which must remain nondividing) may be the primary emphasis of the research rather than proliferation; however cell division studies enumerate the values of the tissue engineering applications [70].

2.4.2.3 Differentiation and Functionality

The characterization of cell differentiation into certain level of lineages and functional capabilities remains essential for bioprinting constructs, which aim to proliferate specific tissue types. In order to produce bone tissue from stem cells then researchers must quantify osteogenic differentiation by measuring calcium deposition and alkaline phosphatase (ALP) activity using Alizarin Red staining and proceed with the osteocalcin gene expression analysis [71]. General techniques for measuring gene expression include RT-PCR and qPCR, while particular enzymatic assays offer additional information, and protein markers are used in immunohistochemistry and immunofluorescence techniques. Safranin O staining can be used to quantify the amount of glycosaminoglycan matrix synthesized in a bioprinted cartilage component [72].

Biomarker expression analysis and contraction measurement are used to evaluate the functions of tissues in the muscle. According to this procedure, the bioink environment must help cells develop their specific characteristic of target tissue. Performing control trials by different bioprinted constructions with ordinary hydrogels' 2D cultures are essential. In order to investigate the tissue formation and examine the functional capabilities of bioprinted constructions in vivo, further the researchers implant them into animal models.

2.4.2.4 In Vitro and In Vivo Biocompatibility

The construct can be considered for clinical use and before that it must pass substantial biocompatibility studies in complicated systems. Studying the biomaterial's ability to trigger immunological responses requires in vitro tests that involve co-cultivation of immune cells and assessments of inflammatory cytokine production. Researchers can examine the evolution of the immune response, including fibrosis and inflammation, and host tissue integration by implanting materials in small animal models using subcutaneous techniques and other approaches [73]. Before histological analysis indicates the existence of inflammation or successful tissue integration, a bioink disk made by extrusion can be implanted in rodents for a few weeks. Whether the bioink exhibits the potency for cellular activities and ensures compatibility with humans is determined by the characterization processes in future [73, 74].

2.4.3 Mechanical Characterization

Mechanical integrity is necessary for printed tissue structures, particularly scaffolds used in load-bearing applications. Criteria including stiffness, strength, and elasticity measured by mechanical testing are essential for preparation of the construct and promoting tissue function.

Important mechanical tests include:

2.4.3.1 Compressive and Tensile Testing

Young's modulus, also known as elastic modulus, is calculated by subjecting the printed hydrogel to uniaxial stress, either compressive or tensile, and then measuring the outcome of the strain. Due to their fragility, soft hydrogels are mostly used for compression testing for tensile evaluations [64]. The amount of stress, measured in pascal, which corresponds to a given strain, can be determined using a rheometer in compression mode or using a dynamic mechanical analyzer. The modulus is indicated by the slope of the linear portion of this link. For instance, a bioink intended to replicate the mechanical characteristics of brain tissue would have a modulus between 0.5 and 1 kPa, while a bioink intended to replicate cartilage might have moduli in the range of 10 kPa. Additionally, it is possible to fix factors like maximal strain – the amount of compression that a material can withstand before breaking or permanently undergo compression and deformation [75]. At the time of testing, tensile properties including ultimate tensile strength and elongation at break are evaluated employing dog-bone shaped specimens or other standardized geometries, although many hydrogels does not possess sufficient strength to undergo such testing. Aligning the mechanical modulus of the scaffold with that of the target tissue is often a primary design objective, particularly given the responsiveness of cells to variations in substrate stiffness. These measurements are most important for validating that the printed scaffold can withstand handling any physiological forces that may be encountered in vivo.

2.4.3.2 Viscoelastic (Dynamic) Testing

The time-dependent deformation characteristics of many hydrogels reveal their viscoelastic behavior. To determine the storage and loss the moduli that differentiate elastic from viscous behavior, the fully cross-linked constructions are subjected to oscillatory rheological investigation. The ability of the material to dissipate stress, which defines its performance under continuous loading, is determined by stress relaxation testing, which implies a fixed load to the material and observes stress decay after compression [76]. Dynamic mechanical analysis (DMA) is used in the testing process to simulate repeating stresses, such as heartbeats on cardiac patches, by applying cyclic loads to the sample. By measuring the stress-strain phase difference, the material response provides important insights on its damping behavior [77]. The specific viscoelastic behaviors that cartilage and other biological tissues exhibit are the main focus of research. Because fatigue testing entails exposing scaffolds to various compressive stresses in order to evaluate their structural integrity over a number of cycles, it is a crucial evaluation technique for implantable grafts. The assessments helps determining if the printed construct can effectively pass on the cellular mechanical signals and withstand mechanical stress until the next tissue integration.

2.4.3.3 Elasticity and Recoverability

A key component of mechanical characterization is the capacity of the bioprinted material to regain its original shape during deformation, as this characteristic is crucial for tissues that undergo mechanical strain (e.g., skin during stretching or lungs during inflation). To examine for elastic recovery through springing back or plastic deformation retention, the specimen is unloaded after the compressive tests [78]. High-elasticity materials, like elastin or polyethylene glycol have a tendency to regain their shape, whereas brittle materials, like high-concentration alginate, will either break or remain distorted. The elastic limit measurement in muscle and vascular tissue engineering applications determines the enduring capacity of a stretching material before losing its original shape. The local stiffness of soft hydrogels can be analyzed using atomic force microscopy, which is important for evaluating the cellular tendency to perceive matrix stiffness. Bioink scaffolds that are rigid will hinder cell movement and also have poor tissue integration, while bioink scaffolds that are very weak will probably tear during transplantation. Mechanical characterization of the printed construct is necessary to ensure that it matches native tissue properties or at least basic parameters and culture requirements [79].

2.4.4 Structural and Morphological Characterization

To examine the microscale structure, various imaging and analysis techniques are employed:

2.4.4.1 Microscopy (2D and 3D Imaging)

In order to observe filament continuity and layer alignment, optical microscopy is used to rapidly evaluate printed structures. Researchers can examine cell distribution patterns in bioink by using the sophisticated imaging technique of confocal laser scanning microscopy (CLSM), which can observe marked components under three dimensions with fluorescence such as DAPI-tagged cell nuclei and phalloidin-labeled F-actin. The spatial distribution of cells throughout a large construct becomes visible through the confocal stacks proving that the cells are evenly distributed throughout the entire structure instead of being present only on the surface. The structural features of the matrix surrounding cells become perceptible when the bioink contains autofluorescent or labeled matrix components. SEM provides excellent surface and cross-sectional imaging capabilities at high resolution and magnification, which makes it suitable for studying pore structures of the scaffolds after freeze drying or critical-point drying. The images captured through SEM are generally used in scientific publications to represent the measurements of dimensions of the pores in scaffolds and fiber diameters. Environmental SEM or cryo-SEM techniques are used to study cell-containing constructs while keeping them hydrated because they help retain the structure of the cell [45, 46]. Particularly fluorescence microscopy serves mainly two purposes in research by helping scientists evaluate cellular viability through live/dead staining and by examining cell morphology through the comparisons of spreading of the cells and the round shape in three-dimensional constructs.

2.4.4.2 Tomography and Whole-Structure Imaging

Micro-CT (micro-computed tomography) is one of the imaging modalities required to evaluate large-scale 3D structure. Micro-CT provides scanning capabilities for the centimeter-scale scaffolds with resolutions ranging from 10 to 50 μm, allowing the observation of massive holes or channels, printed lattice architecture. Researchers can use the imaging technique to quantify structural characteristics, such as the interlayer pore dimensions and filament diameter distribution throughout the construct, to identify any structural integrity issues like the layer misalignment. Bioink material that exhibits low X-ray contrast requires either sample drying or the use of a contrast for imaging. MRI is a rarely used technique for scaffolds imaging since it can track water diffusion and is used to analyze the hydrated structures. Optical coherence tomography (OCT), a nondestructive imaging technology, allows real-time monitoring of several millimeters within transparent hydrogel scaffolds by viewing the material (OCT has been used to monitor layer-by-layer growth during printing for some systems) [45]. Through nondestructive techniques, these imaging technologies demonstrate the entire geometry and internal details of the construct, extending the extreme uses of microscopy.

2.4.4.3 3D Reconstruction and Image Analysis

The information recorded from confocal *z*-stacks and micro-CT slices can be used to generate a three-dimensional tissue model. The volumetric data is produced using sophisticated software programs that allow quantitative study parameters, including comparison of the printed morphology to the original digital model and enumeration to quantify porosity and channel continuity. Complete measurement capacity is provided by image analysis to ascertain strand thickness, cell orientation, and distribution patterns.

Analysis through microscopic images makes it possible to identify any line coalescence and determine the true distance between two parallel printed lines, which may differ from their theoretical 500-µm separation. The examination of pore connectivity, the designing complex anatomical structures, the ability to scan objects and compare them to CAD drawings is crucial for identifying aberrations linked to material behavior [44]. Hence researchers can forecast transport patterns using three-dimensional reconstructions of tissue constructs.

The evaluation of the structure through the analytical characterization becomes essential to approve the true form–function alignment with material properties and finally the biological performance of the material.

2.5 Summary and Future Directions

The chapter enumerates the direction methods and identification procedures for bioink formulations, which are very essential for the 3D bioprinting applications. Bioinks function as the essential printing material in bioprinting due to their compatibility with the cellular components-made hydrogels, which can be natural or synthetic or composite materials and sometimes include cross-linkers and bioactive additives.

Bioinks can be produced with or without cell inclusions, but their development demands changes to printability through shear-thinning behavior and appropriate gelation kinetics. This book chapter considered four main bioprinting methods, namely, extrusion, inkjet, laser-assisted, and stereolithography. Each of these methods has its own advantages in terms of speed, resolution, and managing cells, but they also require very unique and varying printing conditions. Other parameters and conditions such as maintaining sterility, regulating temperature, and choosing the right nozzle/printer settings are mandate for both printing success and cell survival. Shape integrity and layer-stacking are crucial printability parameters that must be evaluated for the bioink optimization and printing process to work well together. The abovementioned analyses and multiple characterization techniques are required for evaluating bioinks and bioprinted constructs. The material properties are selected after checking the suitability and uniformity through physicochemical evaluations which include rheology, swelling, and degradation tests. The bioink environment is proven to be safe for cells through different biological evaluations that demonstrate its ability to support tissue development. The three-dimensional architecture and microstructure of printed constructs receive verification through structural examinations, which include microscopy and imaging techniques. The conjunction of characterization instruments provides a complete understanding of bioink operational effectiveness. The practical application of these principles is approved after numerous research studies, which include a bioprinted cardiac patch and commercially implanted auricle while highlighting commercially available bioinks that support best practices for broader bioprinting adoption. The major advancement of bioprinting toward the clinical implementation requires addressing classification challenges while meeting strict quality and safety regulations.

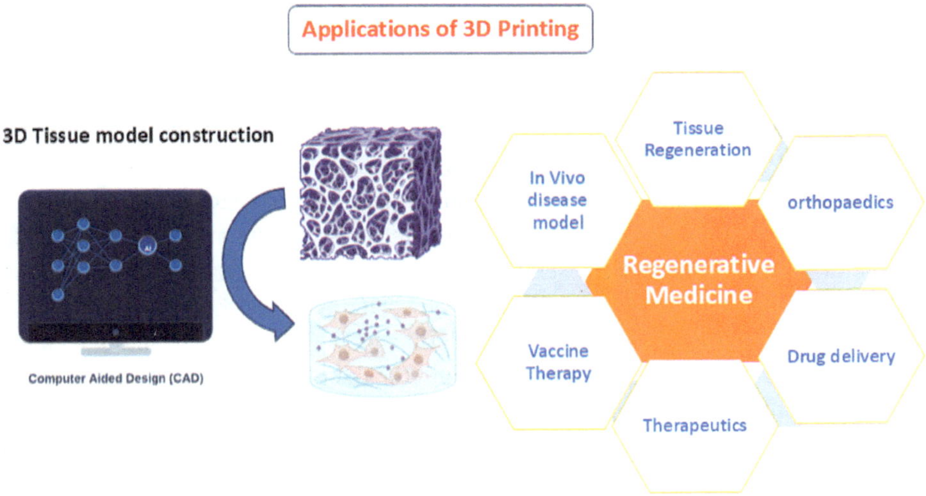

Figure 2.3: Diverse applications of 3D bioprinting in medical field [84, 85].

In summary, achieving successful bioprinting requires a thoughtful integration of multiple scientific disciplines working in harmony: Material science plays a foundational role in developing bioinks that possess the right flow behavior and the ability to cross-link effectively, ensuring structural integrity throughout the printing process. Particularly, cell biology ensures that the bioink maintains cellular viability and the necessary cellular functions; engineering the biomaterials carefully than the material fine-tunes the printing process to ensure accuracy and viability; analytical science rigorously assesses that the printed structures meet the required standards. Each of these elements must be thoroughly understood and optimized by the bioprinting industry to achieve the laboratory-based experimental creations of effective tissue substitutes for the human in the medical field.

2.6 Future Directions

The field of bioprinting and bioinks is rapidly evolving. Looking forward, several trends and research frontiers are emerging that promise to enhance the capabilities and applications of bioprinted tissues:

- The development of "smart" bioinks will focus on developing materials, which can identify different stimuli or actively participate in tissue maturation processes. Bioinks in the future will change their mechanical properties through cellular remodeling activities while simultaneously controlling the release of growth factor through enzyme-dependent mechanisms. The current research fidelity focuses on developing 4D printing technology that enables printed constructs to change their shape or functional properties after fabrication, which also includes temporal factors as a fourth dimension. A system of bioink that swells or contracts through external triggers would enable tissue construct morphogenetic processes, that is, change in the after printing. Researchers are currently investigating hydrogels, which are self-healing because these materials have the potential to improve tissue structural integrity after implantation.
- Higher Complexity Tissues and Organs: The current state of bioprinting technology makes it possible to create tiny organ precursors as well as basic tissue architectures like cartilage and skin layers. The bioengineering of complete organ systems or intricate tissue constructs including fully differentiated hepatic and renal structures, remains a central objective in regenerative medicine and tissue engineering. In order to facilitate the integrity of vascular structures and huge cell populations in printed constructs, there must be a continuous progress in the bioink development. In the construction of unique bioinks that use sacrificial material to create channels through disintegration or coaxial printing for simultaneous blood vessel formation, research is aiming to develop methodologies for developing networks. Modern printer architectures with multiple printheads are

emerging to develop the creation of heterogeneous tissues through multicellular and multi-material printing for example, producing livers and kidneys with nephrons and vascular elements. The organ level development and its functionality require either integration of neural structure or composite architecture development, which includes bone marrow. The field of organoid development and stem cell differentiation will integrate bioprinting methods by using miniature organoids as bioink components, which will eventually develop into mature organs.

- The development of standardized bioink libraries that perform similarly to accepted cell culture medium standards is anticipated in the near future. After the production of well-characterized materials, the development would expedite regulatory approval procedures and proceed with the compatibility studies and testing across several laboratories.
- Initiatives for the development of online databases to catalog bioink formulations with their inherent qualities would be beneficial to researchers since they will enable them to choose appropriate inks for particular applications without any demand to start from the initial stage. The standardized testing methods that were previously covered in the regulatory forum will develop into either an established rheological protocol for bioinks or an ASTM standard for a "printability test." These developments will improve the biomaterial field and encourage the developers for the acquisition of information.
- Bioinks are a key component of the paradigm change in bioprinting is now under progression. The creation and description of bioinks has made it possible to print biological tissues with improved functionality and fidelity. Even though there are still issues (vascularization, innervation, long-term functionality, and regulatory approval), the progress made so far is extremely essential.
- Bioprinting will transmit the phase of clinical research to life saving applications with the ongoing innovations in materials science, tissue engineering, biological integration coupled with rigorous characterization, and technical validation. Each progressive enhancement in bioink technology represents a significant stride toward that transformational goal.

References

[1] Al-Hatamleh, M. A. I., Alshaer, W., Hatmal, M. M., Lambuk, L., Ahmed, N., Mustafa, M. Z., Low, S. C., Jaafar, J., Ferji, K., Six, J., Uskoković, V., & Mohamud, R. (2022). Applications of alginate-based nanomaterials in enhancing the therapeutic effects of bee products. Frontiers in Molecular Biosciences, 9. https://doi.org/10.3389/fmolb.2022.865833.

[2] Ali, M. E. A., Aboelfadl, M. M. S., Selim, A. M., Khalil, H. F., & Elkady, G. M. (2018). Chitosan nanoparticles extracted from shrimp shells, application for removal of Fe(II) and Mn(II) from aqueous phases. Separation Science and Technology, 53(18), 2870–2881. https://doi.org/10.1080/01496395.2018.1489845.

[3] Banach-Kopeć, A., Mania, S., Tylingo, R., Wawrzynowicz, A., Pawłowska, M., Czerwiec, K., Deptuła, M., & Pikuła, M. (2024). Thermosensitive composite based on agarose and chitosan saturated with carbon dioxide. Preliminary study of requirements for production of new CSAG bioink. Carbohydrate Polymers, 336, 122120. https://doi.org/10.1016/j.carbpol.2024.122120.

[4] Benwood, C., Chrenek, J., Kirsch, R. L., Masri, N. Z., Richards, H., Teetzen, K., & Willerth, S. M. (2021). Natural biomaterials and their use as bioinks for printing tissues. Bioengineering, 8(2), 27. https://doi.org/10.3390/bioengineering8020027.

[5] Bercea, M. (2023). Rheology as a tool for fine-tuning the properties of printable bioinspired gels. Molecules, 28(6), 2766. https://doi.org/10.3390/molecules28062766.

[6] Blanco, J. C. G., Macías-García, A., Rodríguez-Rego, J. M., Mendoza-Cerezo, L., Sánchez-Margallo, F. M., Marcos-Romero, A. C., & Pagador-Carrasco, J. B. (2024). Optimising bioprinting nozzles through computational modelling and design of experiments. Biomimetics, 9(8), 460. https://doi.org/10.3390/biomimetics9080460.

[7] Bonda, U., Jaeschke, A., Lighterness, A., Baldwin, J., Werner, C., De-Juan-Pardo, E. M., & Bray, L. J. (2020). 3D quantification of vascular-like structures in z stack confocal images. STAR Protocols, 1(3), 100180. https://doi.org/10.1016/j.xpro.2020.100180.

[8] Brusentsev, Y., Yang, P., King, A. W. T., Cheng, F., Ruiz, M. F. C., Eriksson, J. E., Kilpeläinen, I., Willför, S., Xu, C., Wågberg, L., & Wang, X. (2023). Photocross-linkable and shape-memory biomaterial hydrogel based on methacrylated cellulose nanofibres. Biomacromolecules, 24(8), 3835–3845. https://doi.org/10.1021/acs.biomac.3c00476.

[9] Budharaju, H., Sundaramurthi, D., & Sethuraman, S. (2025). Insights on the role of cryoprotectants in enhancing the properties of bioinks required for cryobioprinting of biological constructs. Journal of Materials Science Materials in Medicine, 36(1). https://doi.org/10.1007/s10856-024-06855-2.

[10] Carvalho, V., Gonçalves, I., Lage, T., Rodrigues, R. O., Minas, G., Teixeira, S. F. C. F., Moita, A. S., Hori, T., Kaji, H., & Lima, R. A. (2021). 3D printing techniques and their applications to organ-on-a-chip platforms: A systematic review. Sensors, 21(9), 3304. https://doi.org/10.3390/s21093304.

[11] Cengiz, I. F., Oliveira, J. M., & Reis, R. L. (2018). Micro-CT – A digital 3D microstructural voyage into scaffolds: A systematic review of the reported methods and results. Biomaterials Research, 22(1). https://doi.org/10.1186/s40824-018-0136-8.

[12] Chakraborty, J., Roy, C., Kalogeropoulou, M., Mota, C., Ghosh, S., & Moroni, L. (2024a). Protocol for developing shape-morphing 4D bioprinted magnetic constructs to promote articular cartilage regeneration using silk fibroin-gelatin bioink. STAR Protocols, 5(4), 103332. https://doi.org/10.1016/j.xpro.2024.103332.

[13] Chakraborty, J., Roy, C., Kalogeropoulou, M., Mota, C., Ghosh, S., & Moroni, L. (2024b). Protocol for developing shape-morphing 4D bioprinted magnetic constructs to promote articular cartilage regeneration using silk fibroin-gelatin bioink. STAR Protocols, 5(4), 103332. https://doi.org/10.1016/j.xpro.2024.103332.

[14] Chandra, C. S. J., Sasi, S., & Sharmila, T. K. B. (2023). Material applications of gelatin. In: Thomas, S., Ajitha, AR, Jose Chirayil, C., & Thomas, B. (eds). Material Applications of Gelatin. Handbook of Biopolymers Springer, Singapore. (pp. 749–782). https://doi.org/10.1007/978-981-19-0710-4_28.

[15] Chen, H., Xue, H., Zeng, H., Dai, M., Tang, C., & Liu, L. (2023). 3D printed scaffolds based on hyaluronic acid bioinks for tissue engineering: A review. Biomaterials Research, 27(1). https://doi.org/10.1186/s40824-023-00460-0.

[16] Cheng, Q., Liu, C., Zhao, J., Li, W., Guo, F., Qin, J., & Wang, Y. (2023). Unlocking the potential of hyaluronic acid: Exploring its physicochemical properties, modification, and role in food applications. Trends in Food Science & Technology, 142, 104218. https://doi.org/10.1016/j.tifs.2023.104218.

[17] Di Marzio, N., Eglin, D., Serra, T., & Moroni, L. (2020). Bio-fabrication: Convergence of 3D bioprinting and nano-biomaterials in tissue engineering and regenerative medicine. Frontiers in Bioengineering and Biotechnology, 8. https://doi.org/10.3389/fbioe.2020.00326.

[18] Fang, W., Yang, M., Wang, L., Li, W., Liu, M., Jin, Y., Wang, Y., Yang, R., Wang, Y., Zhang, K., & Fu, Q. (2023). Hydrogels for 3D bioprinting in tissue engineering and regenerative medicine: Current progress and challenges. International Journal of Bioprinting, 9(5), 759. https://doi.org/10.18063/ijb.759.

[19] Field, E. H., Ratcliffe, J., Johnson, C. J., Binger, K. J., & Reynolds, N. P. (2024). Self-healing, 3D printed bioinks from self-assembled peptide and alginate hybrid hydrogels. Biomaterials Advances, 169, 214145. https://doi.org/10.1016/j.bioadv.2024.214145.

[20] Freitas-Rodríguez, S., Folgueras, A. R., & López-Otín, C. (2017). The role of matrix metalloproteinases in aging: Tissue remodeling and beyond. Biochimica Et Biophysica Acta (BBA) – Molecular Cell Research, 1864(11), 2015–2025. https://doi.org/10.1016/j.bbamcr.2017.05.007.

[21] Gadre, M., Kasturi, M., Agarwal, P., & Vasanthan, K. S. (2024). Decellularization and their significance for tissue regeneration in the era of 3D bioprinting. ACS Omega. https://doi.org/10.1021/acsomega.3c08930.

[22] Galante, R., Pinto, T. J. A., Colaço, R., & Serro, A. P. (2017). Sterilization of hydrogels for biomedical applications: A review. Journal of Biomedical Materials Research Part B Applied Biomaterials, 106(6), 2472–2492. https://doi.org/10.1002/jbm.b.34048.

[23] Galocha-León, C., Antich, C., Voltes-Martínez, A., Marchal, J. A., Mallandrich, M., Halbaut, L., Souto, E. B., Gálvez-Martín, P., & Clares-Naveros, B. (2024). Human mesenchymal stromal cells-laden crosslinked hyaluronic acid-alginate bioink for 3D bioprinting applications in tissue engineering. Drug Delivery and Translational Research. https://doi.org/10.1007/s13346-024-01596-9.

[24] García-Villén, F., Ruiz-Alonso, S., Lafuente-Merchan, M., Gallego, I., Sainz-Ramos, M., Saenz-Del-Burgo, L., & Pedraz, J. L. (2021). Clay minerals as bioINK ingredients for 3D printing and 3D bioprinting: Application in tissue engineering and regenerative medicine. Pharmaceutics, 13(11), 1806. https://doi.org/10.3390/pharmaceutics13111806.

[25] Godau, B., Stefanek, E., Gharaie, S. S., Amereh, M., Pagan, E., Marvdashti, Z., Libert-Scott, E., Ahadian, S., & Akbari, M. (2022). Non-destructive mechanical assessment for optimization of 3D bioprinted soft tissue scaffolds. iScience, 25(5), 104251. https://doi.org/10.1016/j.isci.2022.104251.

[26] Gorgieva, S., & Kokol, V. (2012a). Preparation, characterization, and in vitro enzymatic degradation of chitosan-gelatine hydrogel scaffolds as potential biomaterials. Journal of Biomedical Materials Research Part A, 100A(7), 1655–1667. https://doi.org/10.1002/jbm.a.34106.

[27] Gorgieva, S., & Kokol, V. (2012b). Preparation, characterization, and in vitro enzymatic degradation of chitosan-gelatine hydrogel scaffolds as potential biomaterials. Journal of Biomedical Materials Research Part A, 100A(7), 1655–1667. https://doi.org/10.1002/jbm.a.34106.

[28] Gungor-Ozkerim, P. S., Inci, I., Zhang, Y. S., Khademhosseini, A., & Dokmeci, M. R. (2018). Bioinks for 3D bioprinting: An overview. Biomaterials Science, 6(5), 915–946. https://doi.org/10.1039/c7bm00765e.

[29] Hanna, H., Mir, L. M., & Andre, F. M. (2018). In vitro osteoblastic differentiation of mesenchymal stem cells generates cell layers with distinct properties. Stem Cell Research & Therapy, 9(1), https://doi.org/10.1186/s13287-018-0942-x.

[30] Jovic, T. H., Nicholson, T., Arora, H., Nelson, K., Doak, S. H., & Whitaker, I. S. (2023). A comparative analysis of pulp-derived nanocelluloses for 3D bioprinting facial cartilages. Carbohydrate Polymers, 321, 121261. https://doi.org/10.1016/j.carbpol.2023.121261.

[31] Jusoh, W. N. L. W., Sajab, M. S., Abdul, P. M., & Kaco, H. (2022). Recent advances in 3D bioprinting: A review of cellulose-based biomaterials ink. Polymers, 14(11), 2260. https://doi.org/10.3390/polym14112260.

[32] Kafy, A., Kim, H. C., Zhai, L., Kim, J. W., Van Hai, L., Kang, T. J., & Kim, J. (2017). Cellulose long fibers fabricated from cellulose nanofibers and its strong and tough characteristics. Scientific Reports, 7(1). https://doi.org/10.1038/s41598-017-17713-3.

[33] Kakarla, A. B., Kong, I., Nguyen, T. H., Kong, C., & Irving, H. (2022). Boron nitride nanotubes reinforced gelatin hydrogel-based ink for bioprinting and tissue engineering applications. Biomaterials Advances, 141, 213103. https://doi.org/10.1016/j.bioadv.2022.213103.

[34] Kesti, M., Müller, M., Becher, J., Schnabelrauch, M., D'Este, M., Eglin, D., & Zenobi-Wong, M. (2014). A versatile bioink for three-dimensional printing of cellular scaffolds based on thermally and photo-triggered tandem gelation. Acta Biomaterialia, 11, 162–172. https://doi.org/10.1016/j.actbio.2014.09.033.

[35] Kim, J. (2023). Characterization of biocompatibility of functional bioINKs for 3D bioprinting. Bioengineering, 10(4), 457. https://doi.org/10.3390/bioengineering10040457.

[36] Klimek, K., Terpilowska, S., Michalak, A., Bernacki, R., Nurzynska, A., Cucchiarini, M., Tarczynska, M., Gaweda, K., Głuszek, S., & Ginalska, G. (2025). Modern approach to testing the biocompatibility of osteochondral scaffolds in accordance with the 3Rs principle—preclinical in vitro, ex vivo, and in vivo studies using the biphasic curdlan-based biomaterial. ACS Biomaterials Science & Engineering. https://doi.org/10.1021/acsbiomaterials.4c01107.

[37] Krakos, A., Cieślak, A., Hartel, E., Łabowska, M. B., Kulbacka, J., & Detyna, J. (2023). 3D bio-printed hydrogel inks promoting lung cancer cell growth in a lab-on-chip culturing platform. Microchimica Acta, 190(9). https://doi.org/10.1007/s00604-023-05931-8.

[38] Layrolle, P., Payoux, P., & Chavanas, S. (2022). Message in a scaffold: Natural biomaterials for three-dimensional (3D) bioprinting of human brain organoids. Biomolecules, 13(1), 25. https://doi.org/10.3390/biom13010025.

[39] Li, Z., Li, T., Yang, H., Ding, M., Chen, L., Yu, S., Meng, X., Jin, J., Sun, S., Zhang, J., & Tian, H. (2024). Design and fabrication of viscoelastic hydrogels as extracellular matrix mimicry for cell engineering. Chem & Bio Engineering, 1(11), 916–933. https://doi.org/10.1021/cbe.4c00129.

[40] Loi, G., Stucchi, G., Scocozza, F., Cansolino, L., Cadamuro, F., Delgrosso, E., Riva, F., Ferrari, C., Russo, L., & Conti, M. (2023). Characterization of a bioink combining extracellular matrix-like hydrogel with osteosarcoma cells: Preliminary results. Gels, 9(2), 129. https://doi.org/10.3390/gels9020129.

[41] Lorson, T., Ruopp, M., Nadernezhad, A., Eiber, J., Vogel, U., Jungst, T., & Lühmann, T. (2020). Sterilization methods and their influence on physicochemical properties and bioprinting of alginate as a bioINK component. ACS Omega, 5(12), 6481–6486. https://doi.org/10.1021/acsomega.9b04096.

[42] Lu, H., Froidevaux, C., Biermann, I., Kaňková, H., Büchner, M., Schubert, D. W., Salehi, S., & Boccaccini, A. R. (2025). Printable ADA-GEL-based composite inks containing Zn-doped bioactive inorganic fillers for skeletal muscle biofabrication. Biomaterials Advances, 172, 214233. https://doi.org/10.1016/j.bioadv.2025.214233.

[43] Maan, Z., Masri, N. Z., & Willerth, S. M. (2022). Smart bioINKs for the printing of human tissue models. Biomolecules, 12(1), 141. https://doi.org/10.3390/biom12010141.

[44] Malafaia, A. P., Sobreiro-Almeida, R., Rodrigues, J. M. M., & Mano, J. F. (2024). Thiol-ene click chemistry: Enabling 3D printing of natural-based inks for biomedical applications. Biomaterials Advances, 167, 214105. https://doi.org/10.1016/j.bioadv.2024.214105.

[45] Malashin, I., Masich, I., Tynchenko, V., Gantimurov, A., Nelyub, V., Borodulin, A., Martysyuk, D., & Galinovsky, A. (2024). Machine learning in 3D and 4D printing of polymer composites: A review. Polymers, 16(22), 3125. https://doi.org/10.3390/polym16223125.

[46] Mazzoldi, E. L., Gaudenzi, G., Ginestra, P. S., Ceretti, E., & Giliani, S. C. (2024). Evaluating cells metabolic activity of bioinks for bioprinting: The role of cell-laden hydrogels and 3D printing on cell survival. Frontiers in Bioengineering and Biotechnology, 12. https://doi.org/10.3389/fbioe.2024.1450838.

[47] Montanari, M., Korkeamäki, J. T., Campodoni, E., Mohamed-Ahmed, S., Mustafa, K., Sandri, M., & Rashad, A. (2025). Effects of magnesium-doped hydroxyapatite nanoparticles on bioINK formulation for bone tissue engineering. ACS Applied Bio Materials. https://doi.org/10.1021/acsabm.4c01418.

[48] Morgan, F. L. C., Fernández-Pérez, J., Moroni, L., & Baker, M. B. (2021). Tuning hydrogels by mixing dynamic cross-linkers: Enabling cell-instructive hydrogels and advanced bioINKs. Advanced Healthcare Materials, 11(1). https://doi.org/10.1002/adhm.202101576.

[49] Mouser, V. H. M., Melchels, F. P. W., Visser, J., Dhert, W. J. A., Gawlitta, D., & Malda, J. (2016). Yield stress determines bioprintability of hydrogels based on gelatin-methacryloyl and gellan gum for cartilage bioprinting. Biofabrication, 8(3), 035003. https://doi.org/10.1088/1758-5090/8/3/035003.

[50] Mukasheva, F., Adilova, L., Dyussenbinov, A., Yernaimanova, B., Abilev, M., & Akilbekova, D. (2024). Optimizing scaffold pore size for tissue engineering: Insights across various tissue types. Frontiers in Bioengineering and Biotechnology, 12. https://doi.org/10.3389/fbioe.2024.1444986.

[51] Ouiyangkul, P., Hirun, N., Suknuntha, K., & Tantishaiyakul, V. (2023). Development and characterization of 3D bioprintable and mechanically reinforced hydrogel based on gellan gum/methylcellulose/cellulose nanocrystals. Polymers for Advanced Technologies, 35(1). https://doi.org/10.1002/pat.6206.

[52] Park, H. E., Gasek, N., Hwang, J., Weiss, D. J., & Lee, P. C. (2020). Effect of temperature on gelation and cross-linking of gelatin methacryloyl for biomedical applications. Physics of Fluids, 32(3). https://doi.org/10.1063/1.5144896.

[53] Paxton, N., Smolan, W., Böck, T., Melchels, F., Groll, J., & Jungst, T. (2017). Proposal to assess printability of bioinks for extrusion-based bioprinting and evaluation of rheological properties governing bioprintability. Biofabrication, 9(4), 044107. https://doi.org/10.1088/1758-5090/aa8dd8.

[54] Puistola, P., Kethiri, A., Nurminen, A., Turkki, J., Hopia, K., Miettinen, S., Mörö, A., & Skottman, H. (2024). Cornea-specific human adipose STEM cell-derived extracellular matrix for corneal stroma tissue engineering. ACS Applied Materials & Interfaces, 16(13), 15761–15772. https://doi.org/10.1021/acsami.3c17803.

[55] Rajabimashhadi, Z., Gallo, N., Salvatore, L., & Lionetto, F. (2023). Collagen derived from fish industry waste: Progresses and challenges. Polymers, 15(3), 544. https://doi.org/10.3390/polym15030544.

[56] Ratheesh, G., Vaquette, C., & Xiao, Y. (2020). Patient-specific bone particles bioprinting for bone tissue engineering. Advanced Healthcare Materials, 9(23). https://doi.org/10.1002/adhm.202001323.

[57] Risangud, N., Lertwimol, T., Sitthisang, S., Wongvitvichot, W., Uppanan, P. & Tanodekaew, S. (2024). The preparation of 3D-printed self-healing hydrogels composed of carboxymethyl chitosan and oxidized dextran via stereolithography for biomedical applications. International Journal of Biological Macromolecules, 292, 139251. https://doi.org/10.1016/j.ijbiomac.2024.139251.

[58] Sabetkish, S., Currie, P., & Meagher, L. (2024). Recent trends in 3D bioprinting technology for skeletal muscle regeneration. Acta Biomaterialia, 181, 46–66. https://doi.org/10.1016/j.actbio.2024.04.038.

[59] Salih, T., Caputo, M., & Ghorbel, M. T. (2024). Recent advances in hydrogel-based 3D bioprinting and its potential application in the treatment of congenital heart disease. Biomolecules, 14(7), 861. https://doi.org/10.3390/biom14070861.

[60] Salthouse, D., Novakovic, K., Hilkens, C. M., & Ferreira, A. M. (2022). Interplay between biomaterials and the immune system: Challenges and opportunities in regenerative medicine. Acta Biomaterialia, 155, 1–18. https://doi.org/10.1016/j.actbio.2022.11.003.

[61] Schweinitzer, S., Kadousaraei, M. J., Aydin, M. S., Mustafa, K., & Rashad, A. (2024). Measuring cell proliferation in bioprinting research. Biomedical Materials, 19(3), 031001. https://doi.org/10.1088/1748-605x/ad3700.

[62] Shi, W., Zhang, Z., & Wang, X. (2024). The prospect of hepatic decellularized extracellular matrix as a bioINK for liver 3D bioprinting. Biomolecules, 14(8), 1019. https://doi.org/10.3390/biom14081019.

[63] Siwach, A., Baliyan, V., Sharma, A., Ahlawat, S., Chaudhary, S., & Chakraborty, E. (2025). Current standing and future potential of 3D bioprinting and biomaterials. Biomaterials Connect. https://doi.org/10.69709/biomatc.2025.198090.
[64] Sonaye, S. Y., Ertugral, E. G., Kothapalli, C. R., & Sikder, P. (2022). Extrusion 3D (bio)printing of alginate-gelatin-based composite scaffolds for skeletal muscle tissue engineering. Materials, 15(22). 7945. https://doi.org/10.3390/ma15227945.
[65] Song, Y. E., Eckman, N., Sen, S., Jons, C. K., Saouaf, O. M., & Appel, E. A. (2025). Highly extensible physically crosslinked hydrogels for high-speed 3D bioprinting. Advanced Healthcare Materials. https://doi.org/10.1002/adhm.202404988.
[66] Stepanovska, J., Supova, M., Hanzalek, K., Broz, A., & Matejka, R. (2021). Collagen bioINKs for bioprinting: A systematic review of hydrogel properties, bioprinting parameters, protocols, and bioprinted structure characteristics. Biomedicines, 9(9), 1137. https://doi.org/10.3390/biomedicines9091137.
[67] Stone, R. N., Reeck, J. C., & Oxford, J. T. (2023). Advances in cartilage tissue engineering using bioinks with decellularized cartilage and three-dimensional printing. International Journal of Molecular Sciences, 24(6), 5526. https://doi.org/10.3390/ijms24065526.
[68] Thomas, O., Priester, R. D. Jr, Hinze, K. J., & Latham, D. D. (1994). Effect of cross-link density on the morphology, thermal and mechanical properties of flexible molded polyurea/urethane foams and films. Journal of Polymer Science Part B Polymer Physics, 32(13), 2155–2169. https://doi.org/10.1002/polb.1994.090321304.
[69] Tolmacheva, N., Bhattacharyya, A., & Noh, I. (2024). Calcium phosphate biomaterials for 3D bioprinting in bone tissue engineering. Biomimetics, 9(2), 95. https://doi.org/10.3390/biomimetics9020095.
[70] Tripathi, S., Mandal, S. S., Bauri, S., & Maiti, P. (2022). 3D bioprinting and its innovative approach for biomedical applications. MedComm, 4(1). https://doi.org/10.1002/mco2.194.
[71] Tsui, J. H., Leonard, A., Camp, N. D., Long, J. T., Nawas, Z. Y., Chavanachat, R., Smith, A. S., Choi, J. S., Dong, Z., Ahn, E. H., Wolf-Yadlin, A., Murry, C. E., Sniadecki, N. J., & Kim, D. (2021). Tunable electroconductive decellularized extracellular matrix hydrogels for engineering human cardiac microphysiological systems. Biomaterials, 272, 120764. https://doi.org/10.1016/j.biomaterials.2021.120764.
[72] Volpi, M., Paradiso, A., Costantini, M., & Święszkowski, W. (2022). Hydrogel-based fiber biofabrication techniques for skeletal muscle tissue engineering. ACS Biomaterials Science & Engineering, 8(2). 379–405. https://doi.org/10.1021/acsbiomaterials.1c01145.
[73] Wang, X., Zhang, D., Singh, Y. P., Yeo, M., Deng, G., Lai, J., Chen, F., Ozbolat, I. T., & Yu, Y. (2024). Progress in organ bioprinting for regenerative medicine – article. Engineering. https://doi.org/10.1016/j.eng.2024.04.023.
[74] Wang, Z., Sun, Y., & Li, C. (2024). Advances in 3D printing technology for preparing bone tissue engineering scaffolds from biodegradable materials. Frontiers in Bioengineering and Biotechnology, 12. https://doi.org/10.3389/fbioe.2024.1483547.
[75] Wu, C. A., Zhu, Y., Venkatesh, A., Stark, C. J., Lee, S. H., & Woo, Y. J. (2023). Optimization of freeform reversible embedding of suspended hydrogel microspheres for substantially improved three-dimensional bioprinting capabilities. Tissue Engineering Part C Methods, 29(3), 85–94. https://doi.org/10.1089/ten.tec.2022.0214.
[76] Xu, H., Casillas, J., Krishnamoorthy, S., & Xu, C. (2020). Effects of Irgacure 2959 and lithium phenyl-2,4,6-trimethylbenzoylphosphinate on cell viability, physical properties, and microstructure in 3D bioprinting of vascular-like constructs. Biomedical Materials, 15(5), 055021. https://doi.org/10.1088/1748-605x/ab954e.

[77] Yue, K., Santiago, G. T., Alvarez, M. M., Tamayol, A., Annabi, N., & Khademhosseini, A. (2015). Synthesis, properties, and biomedical applications of gelatin methacryloyl (GelMA) hydrogels. Biomaterials, 73. 254–271. https://doi.org/10.1016/j.biomaterials.2015.08.045.

[78] Zhang, T., Yan, K. C., Ouyang, L. & Sun, W. (2013). Mechanical characterization of bioprinted in vitro soft tissue models. Biofabrication, 5(4), 045010. https://doi.org/10.1088/1758-5082/5/4/045010.

[79] Zhang, Y. S., & Khademhosseini, A. (2017). Advances in engineering hydrogels. Science, 356(6337). https://doi.org/10.1126/science.aaf3627.

[80] Zhang, Y., Wang, Z., Sun, Q., Li, Q., Li, S., & Li, X. (2023). Dynamic hydrogels with viscoelasticity and tunable stiffness for the regulation of cell behavior and fate. Materials, 16(14), 5161. https://doi.org/10.3390/ma16145161.

[81] Zhang, Y., Zhou, D., Chen, J., Zhang, X., Li, X., Zhao, W., & Xu, T. (2019). Biomaterials based on marine resources for 3D bioprinting applications. Marine Drugs, 17(10). 555. https://doi.org/10.3390/md17100555.

[82] Zhao, W., Hu, C., & Xu, T. (2023). In vivo bioprinting: Broadening the therapeutic horizon for tissue injuries. Bioactive Materials, 25. 201–222. https://doi.org/10.1016/j.bioactmat.2023.01.018.

[83] Zheng, K., Ma, Y., Chiu, C., Xue, M., Zhang, C., & Du, D. (2024). Enhanced articular cartilage regeneration using costal chondrocyte-derived scaffold-free tissue engineered constructs with ascorbic acid treatment. Journal of Orthopaedic Translation, 45. 140–154. https://doi.org/10.1016/j.jot.2024.02.005.

[84] Zhou, X., Yu, X., You, T., Zhao, B., Dong, L., Huang, C., Zhou, X., Xing, M., Qian, W., & Luo, G. (2024). 3D printing-based hydrogel dressings for wound healing. Advanced Science, 11(47). https://doi.org/10.1002/advs.202404580.

[85] Zingale, E., Weaver, E., Bertelli, P. M., Lengyel, I., Pignatello, R., & Lamprou, D. A. (2024). Development of dual drug loaded-hydrogel scaffold combining microfluidics and coaxial 3D-printing for intravitreal implantation. International Journal of Pharmaceutics, 124700. https://doi.org/10.1016/j.ijpharm.2024.124700

Vicky Subhash Telang, Monika Khatri, Mohd. Nadeem,
Subhasm Telang, Bhupesh Sarode

Chapter 3
Computer-Aided Design and Manufacturing for Bioprinting in Organ Development

Abstract: The integration of computer-aided design (CAD) and computer-aided manufacturing (CAM) technologies has catalyzed significant advancements in the field of 3D bioprinting, particularly in the fabrication of complex, patient-specific tissues and organs. This chapter presents a comprehensive overview of the role of CAD/CAM systems in biofabrication, emphasizing their capabilities in translating anatomical and cellular data into precision-driven bioprinted constructs. It explores how CAD tools support geometric modeling, scaffold architecture optimization, and toolpath generation, while CAM platforms facilitate controlled material deposition and real-time process monitoring. The synergy between these systems enables the production of biomimetic structures that closely replicate the mechanical, architectural, and functional characteristics of native tissues. The chapter outlines key technical aspects of CAD modeling for bioprinting, including segmentation of medical imaging data, lattice generation, and multi-material design approaches. It also delves into CAM functionalities, such as slicer algorithms adapted for bioinks, actuator synchronization, and support for hybrid biofabrication strategies. Furthermore, the emerging integration of AI-driven algorithms for design optimization and the application of digital twins are discussed as pivotal innovations enhancing model predictability and functional outcomes. Despite these advancements, several challenges persist. Technical limitations include insufficient printing resolution, restricted bio-ink compatibility, and difficulties in incorporating cellular and molecular data into CAD frameworks. The chapter critically examines these hurdles and proposes adaptive, feedback-controlled CAM systems as future solutions. It further emphasizes the importance of multidisciplinary

Vicky Subhash Telang, Jawaharlal Nehru Medical College, Datta Meghe Institute of Higher Education and Research, Sawangi (M), Wardha, 442005, Maharashtra, India, e-mail: vickytelang@iiitdmj.ac.in, 9823706292, Orcid Id:0000-0001-7967-2464
Monika Khatri, Medical Consultant, Primary Health Centre, PDPM Indian Institute of Information Technology, Design and Manufacturing, Jabalpur, India, e-mail: drmonika.k@iiitdmj.ac, 9039369215, Orcid Id: 0009-0001-0254-9860
Mohd. Nadeem, Indian Council of Medical Research – National Institute of Research in Tribal Health, Jabalpur, India e-mail: mohdnadeem351@gmail.com, 9823656050, Orcid Id: 0009-0008-7588-5903
Subhasm Telang, Department of General Medicine, Government Medical College and Hospital, Chandrapur e-mail: subhamtelang96@gmail.com, 9765300876, Orcid Id: 0009-0001-8478-314X
Bhupesh Sarode, Jawaharlal Nehru Medical College, Datta Meghe Institute of Higher Education and Research, Sawangi (M), Wardha, 442005, Maharashtra, India e-mail: bhupeshdsarode@gmail.com, 9096040327, Orcid Id: 0000-0002-5131-8292

 | https://doi.org/10.1515/9783111719993-003

collaboration, underscoring how effective integration between engineers, biologists, clinicians, and data scientists is essential for achieving clinically viable bioprinted constructs. Co-design strategies and translational research ecosystems are highlighted as effective mechanisms to align cross-disciplinary objectives. In conclusion, this chapter positions CAD/CAM systems not merely as supportive tools but as central enablers of next-generation 3D bioprinting. Their evolution, when coupled with technological innovation and interdisciplinary synergy, holds the potential to overcome existing limitations and reshape the future of personalized, regenerative medicine.

Keywords: CAD, CAM, biofabrication, computational fluid dynamics, bioprinting

3.1 Introduction

The increasing global medical problem of organ failure and the chronic shortage of donor organs have accelerated the exploration of next-generation solutions in regenerative medicine, among which bioprinting has emerged as one of the most promising solutions [1]. Bioprinting, a subset of additive manufacturing, enables the precise layer-by-layer deposition of bio-inks, complex formulations comprising living cells, biomaterials, and signaling molecules, to fabricate functional tissue analogs and organ-like constructs [2]. With the potential to engineer fully vascularized, patient-specific, and immuno-compatible tissues, bioprinting is poised to revolutionize organ transplantation, drug testing, and disease modeling [3]. At the heart of this transformative technology lies the seamless integration of computer-aided design (CAD) and computer-aided manufacturing (CAM) systems, which serve as the digital-to-physical bridge in the fabrication of biological structures with anatomical and physiological relevance. CAD/CAM, originally conceived to enhance accuracy and automation in mechanical engineering, has undergone a significant evolution to meet the demands of biofabrication [4]. CAD enables researchers and clinicians to convert medical imaging data into intricate 3D models, design internal architectures such as vasculature networks, and perform predictive simulations that evaluate structural integrity and biological performance. CAM, in turn, translates these virtual designs into executable instructions for bioprinters, optimizing parameters like extrusion speed, deposition path, bio-ink switching, and environmental conditions [5, 6]. This digital pipeline not only facilitates reproducibility and scalability, but also supports real-time quality control and adaptive printing, crucial for translating lab-scale bioprinting into clinical-grade applications [2]. Furthermore, the emergence of AI-enhanced CAD tools, cloud-based simulation platforms, and machine learning-guided CAM algorithms has significantly improved the precision, efficiency, and personalization of organ fabrication workflows.

Bioprinting is inherently multidisciplinary, drawing upon the collective expertise of mechanical and biomedical engineers, computational modelers, materials scientists, biologists, and clinicians. The convergence of these domains is essential for addressing the multifaceted challenges associated with replicating the structural, mechanical, and functional complexity of human tissues [7]. For instance, while engineers develop the hardware and software frameworks for high-resolution printing, materials scientists engineer develop novel bio-inks with tunable rheology and bioactivity, and cell biologists investigate the optimal conditions for cell survival, differentiation, and integration within the printed constructs [8]. Moreover, clinicians provide critical input in defining the anatomical and physiological benchmarks that bioprinted tissues must meet to be considered viable for implantation or diagnostic use. As such, the success of organ bioprinting hinges not only on biological innovation but also on the optimization of digital design and manufacturing technologies that govern the translation of biological blueprints into functional constructs. Despite substantial progress, a key limitation in current literature and research practice is the disproportionate focus on biological aspects such as stem cell behavior, growth factors, and scaffold biodegradation, often at the expense of technical methodologies that underpin the design and manufacturing process. While these biological parameters are certainly critical, a significant understanding of CAD/CAM workflows is equally vital for ensuring accuracy, functionality, and reproducibility in bioprinted constructs. The integration of design automation, topology optimization, multi-scale modeling, and feedback-controlled manufacturing has already begun to transform the bioprinting landscape, but widespread adoption is contingent upon greater awareness and cross-disciplinary collaboration.

This chapter addresses the knowledge gap by offering a comprehensive overview of CAD/CAM strategies in the context of bioprinting for organ development [7]. The chapter is structured to reflect the digital workflow that inspires a successful bioprinting process from anatomical data acquisition to construct realization. The discussion begins with an exploration of the historical evolution and current capabilities of CAD/CAM technologies, emphasizing how these tools have been adapted from traditional engineering applications to suit the demands of biological manufacturing. The next section focuses on imaging and data capture techniques, including the use of high-resolution medical imaging modalities such as MRI, CT, and 3D ultrasound, as well as recent advancements in AI-enhanced image segmentation and automated model reconstruction [9]. Following this, we delve into design and simulation methodologies, including finite element analysis (FEA), computational fluid dynamics (CFD), and biophysical modeling, which are used to optimize structural and functional properties of organ constructs prior to printing.

Subsequent sections address the preparation of printable files, highlighting the role of slicing algorithms, material-specific print path generation, and multi-material interface design. Here, we discuss the transition from virtual design to machine-readable code, with emphasis on bio-CAM software development, print parameter optimization, and real-time adaptive control using embedded sensors and AI feedback systems. The final portion of the chapter presents an analysis of current challenges, such as the lack of standardized bio-CAD file formats, resolution limitations, and the need for regulatory-compliant digital workflows. We also explore emerging trends such as generative design algorithms, digital twin models for bioprinting, cloud-integrated collaborative platforms, and the potential role of quantum computing in future design and simulation tasks. Throughout the chapter, special attention is placed on equipping readers, particularly those from the life sciences, with the technical literacy required to engage with CAD/CAM platforms and collaborate effectively in multidisciplinary teams. By demystifying the computational and engineering aspects of bioprinting, this chapter aims to foster synergistic collaborations across scientific domains, ultimately accelerating the translation of bioprinted organs from research prototypes to clinical therapies. The goal is not only to inform but also to inspire the development of new tools, workflows, and standards that will define the future of regenerative medicine [10].

It serves as a gateway into the digital foundations of bioprinting, illustrating how CAD/CAM technologies are not mere auxiliary tools but central components in the design, validation, and realization of functional organ constructs. By tracing the path from medical imaging to printer execution, we highlight both the technical sophistication and the interdisciplinary cooperation necessary for successful organ biomanufacturing. As the field matures, the importance of such digital workflows will only increase, making CAD/CAM literacy an essential skill set for the next generation of tissue engineers and regenerative medicine specialists.

3.2 Historical Context of CAD/CAM in Bioprinting

The evolution of **CAD/CAM** technologies has been a cornerstone in the transformation of design and fabrication practices across a broad range of disciplines. Initially rooted in the engineering sector, these digital tools have evolved from basic graphical interfaces and numerical controllers into sophisticated, integrated platforms that now support the digital fabrication of highly complex structures – including living tissues and organs. Understanding this historical trajectory is essential to appreciate how the same foundational technologies that revolutionized aerospace and automotive industries have, over the past two decades, been adapted and refined for bioprinting in regenerative medicine.

3.2.1 Evolution of CAD/CAM Technologies

The genesis of CAD/CAM technology can be traced back to the late 1950s and early 1960s with two landmark innovations. In 1957, **Dr Patrick J. Hanratty** developed **PRONTO (Program for Numerical Tooling Operations)** [11], the first commercial system for numerical control programming. PRONTO marked a pivotal moment in automated manufacturing, laying the groundwork for computer-controlled machining and later, full-fledged CAM systems [12]. In parallel, the field of graphical computing witnessed a breakthrough in 1963 with **Dr Ivan Sutherland's** development of **Sketchpad**, a revolutionary graphical interface created as part of his PhD research at the Massachusetts Institute of Technology (MIT) [13]. Sketchpad enabled direct interaction between a human and a computer via a graphical user interface – a feat that fundamentally changed how design tasks were approached. Sutherland's work is widely regarded as the inception of modern CAD, introducing principles of interactive design, constraint management, and graphical manipulation that still underpin contemporary CAD software.

Initially, the adoption of CAD/CAM was limited to high-investment industries such as **aerospace, defense, and automotive engineering**, due to the prohibitive cost of early computing hardware [14]. Aerospace manufacturers like Boeing and automotive giants such as General Motors were among the first to embrace CAD for designing aircraft fuselages and automotive bodies, where geometric precision and mechanical performance were mission-critical. The CAM counterpart followed suit, enabling automated tool path generation and numerical control for machining parts directly from digital blueprints. As computational power increased through the 1970s and 1980s, driven by the advent of **microprocessors** and **personal computing**, CAD/CAM systems became more accessible and customizable. Software packages such as **AutoCAD**, **CATIA**, and **SolidWorks** emerged, allowing broader implementation in industrial design, product development, and architecture.

By the late twentieth century, the utility of CAD/CAM began extending into **biomedical engineering**, driven by a confluence of technological readiness and growing demand for patient-specific solutions. The integration of **medical imaging** with digital modeling opened new frontiers in personalized healthcare. CAD/CAM was first utilized in the biomedical context for designing dental prosthetics and orthopedic implants, where anatomical fidelity and customization were crucial [15]. For example, in dental applications, intraoral scanners and CAD-based digital impressions began replacing conventional mold techniques, improving fit, aesthetics, and fabrication speed. Similarly, in orthopedics, pre-surgical planning tools allowed surgeons to visualize and simulate joint replacements using patient-specific anatomical data derived from **CT and MRI scans**.

3.2.2 Emergence of 3D Bioprinting

The paradigm shift, however, came with the rise of **additive manufacturing (AM)** or **3D printing**, which complemented CAD/CAM by enabling the fabrication of complex geometries that were previously unachievable with subtractive techniques. Unlike traditional manufacturing that relied on material removal, AM allowed layer-by-layer deposition, based directly on CAD models, eliminating many intermediate steps and opening the door for biological applications. Early biomedical 3D printing efforts focused on producing anatomical models for education and surgical planning [16]. However, as printing materials evolved to include biocompatible polymers, hydrogels, and even living cells, the concept of bioprinting emerged as a logical extension of existing CAD/CAM workflows into the domain of regenerative medicine [17].

In bioprinting, CAD/CAM systems serve as the central nervous system of the entire digital biofabrication workflow. The CAD process now includes sophisticated tasks such as segmentation of medical images, mesh reconstruction of anatomical features, and computational design of vascular networks and tissue microarchitecture [18]. These digital blueprints are not mere static shapes; they must account for biomechanical constraints, diffusion gradients, and cell viability zones, making the design process inherently more complex than conventional engineering applications. Innovations such as parametric modeling, FEA, as shown in Figure 3.1, and topology optimization, originally developed for mechanical design, are now being repurposed to ensure that engineered tissues can sustain physiological loads and biological functions [19].

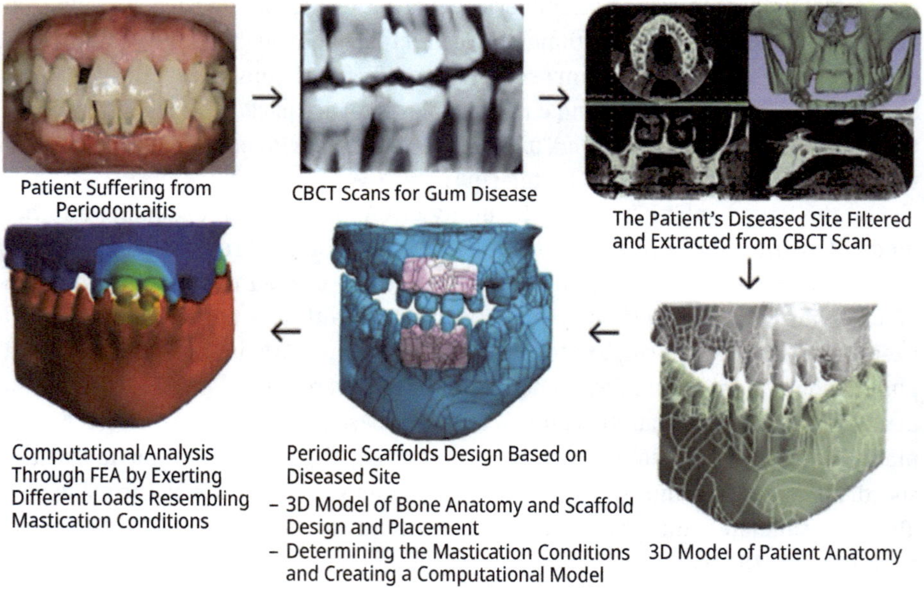

Figure 3.1: Workflow for patient-specific periodontal scaffold design and evaluation. A patient diagnosed with periodontitis undergoes cone-beam computed tomography (CBCT) scanning to capture diseased sites. The pathological regions are segmented and extracted from the CBCT dataset to generate a 3D anatomical model of the affected jaw. Scaffold designs are created based on the patient's bone anatomy and disease site, followed by finite element analysis (FEA) to simulate mastication-induced loads and assess mechanical feasibility of the scaffold placement [18].

On the manufacturing side, bio-CAM systems have emerged as a distinct subdomain that translates digital tissue models into precise printer instructions compatible with extrusion-based, inkjet, or laser-assisted bioprinters. CAM modules for bioprinting must handle variable material compositions (i.e., different bioinks), delicate dispensing mechanisms, and spatiotemporal control of cell deposition. Unlike conventional CAM, where tool paths are optimized for machining efficiency, bio-CAM must prioritize cell viability, cross-linking conditions, and layer fidelity [20]. Recent developments have also integrated closed-loop feedback systems, utilizing computer vision and machine learning algorithms, to correct for nozzle deflection, temperature deviations, or bio-ink inconsistencies in real-time, vastly improving printing reliability and reproducibility [21].

Furthermore, recently, the CAD/CAM platforms in bioprinting are increasingly embracing cloud computing and collaborative design environments, enabling researchers across the globe to co-develop and iterate on organ designs [22]. Digital twin frameworks, where a virtual replica of the bioprinted organ is maintained and updated in real-time, are being tested for predictive modeling of tissue growth and functional maturation. Similarly, generative design tools, powered by AI, are now capable of producing hundreds of structural variants based on user-defined biological constraints, accelerating the design discovery process.

Parallel to technological growth, regulatory considerations are beginning to shape CAD/CAM systems in biomedical domains. Agencies such as the US FDA and EMA are developing frameworks that require digital traceability, model validation, and risk assessment protocols for devices and constructs manufactured using CAD/CAM pipelines [23]. This has led to a push for standardized file formats (e.g., DICOM-to-STL pipelines), interoperability among design tools, and compliance-driven simulation features within CAD platforms. These developments not only facilitate regulatory approval but also support ethical data management and reproducibility, which are vital for the clinical translation of bioprinted constructs.

The shift from traditional engineering to biological applications has also prompted the education and training of a new generation of bio-CAD/CAM specialists. This integration is essential, as the future of bioprinting lies in the hands of professionals who can navigate both the digital and biological domains. In response, open-source platforms like 3D Slicer, FreeCAD, and BioCAM are lowering entry barriers and allowing early-career researchers to engage with state-of-the-art CAD/CAM tools without the burden of high software costs. The evolution of CAD/CAM from its inception in mid-twentieth-century industrial applications to its present-day role in bioprinting for organ development represents a profound technological arc. From Hanratty's numerical control routines and Sutherland's graphical innovations to today's AI-driven, cloud-integrated biofabrication pipelines, CAD/CAM has demonstrated its adaptability, resilience, and transformative potential [24, 25]. As bioprinting continues to mature, the historical foundation and continued refinement of CAD/CAM technologies will remain instrumental in overcoming the remaining challenges in tissue complexity, scalability, and clinical translation [26]. The next phase of innovation will likely see deeper integration of real-time biosensing, AI-driven adaptive design, and regulatory-compliant digital workflows, ensuring that CAD/CAM systems not only support but actively drive the future of regenerative medicine.

3.3 Medical Imaging for Bioprinting

3.3.1 Imaging Modalities

In the domain of biomedical engineering and regenerative medicine, the accurate visualization and reconstruction of internal anatomical structures are difficult to achieve effectively for patient-specific bioprinted constructs [27]. Imaging modalities serve as the foundational step in the computer-aided tissue design (CATD) and bioprinting pipeline, providing the raw spatial and morphological data necessary to generate precise three-dimensional (3D) models of organs, tissues, and vasculature. The selection of appropriate imaging technology is thus critically important, influencing not only the fidelity of the reconstructed models but also the overall clinical applicability of the biofabricated construct. Among the various imaging techniques, computed tomography (CT), magnetic resonance imaging (MRI), and ultrasound stand out as principal modalities used for bioprinting applications due to their complementary capabilities in capturing soft and hard tissue features, vascular topologies, and dynamic physiological states. These imaging techniques convert biological complexity into digital geometry, enabling subsequent segmentation, mesh reconstruction, and 3D modeling essential for additive manufacturing in tissue engineering.

3.3.1.1 Computed Tomography (CT)

CT is one of the most widely utilized imaging techniques in clinical and research settings due to its high spatial resolution and rapid acquisition time. CT imaging, as shown in Figure 3.2, is based on the differential attenuation of X-rays as they pass through various tissue densities in the body [28]. The resulting two-dimensional (2D) projections are computationally reconstructed into a volumetric dataset comprising thousands of voxels, each representing a discrete volume of tissue, with associated attenuation coefficients. This imaging modality excels in capturing skeletal structures, dental anatomy, and calcified tissues, making it particularly useful in applications such as craniofacial reconstruction, bone scaffold fabrication, and dental implant planning [29, 30]. In the context of bioprinting, CT data is frequently converted into stereolithography (STL) or other CAD-compatible formats, enabling the design of anatomically accurate scaffolds and implants.

Recent advances in micro-CT (μCT) and dual-energy CT (DECT) have expanded the capability of traditional CT systems. Micro-CT offers voxel resolutions in the micrometer range, providing more details in the internal microarchitecture of bone and engineered scaffolds, which is important for evaluating porosity, interconnectivity, and mechanical strength [31, 32]. Dual-energy CT, on the other hand, enables material differentiation based on atomic number, enhancing soft-tissue contrast and allowing for more nuanced segmentation of heterogeneous biological materials. Moreover, low-dose CT protocols and iterative reconstruction algorithms are now being implemented to reduce radiation exposure, making CT more feasible for longitudinal studies in bioprinting research involving live subjects or repeated imaging sessions.

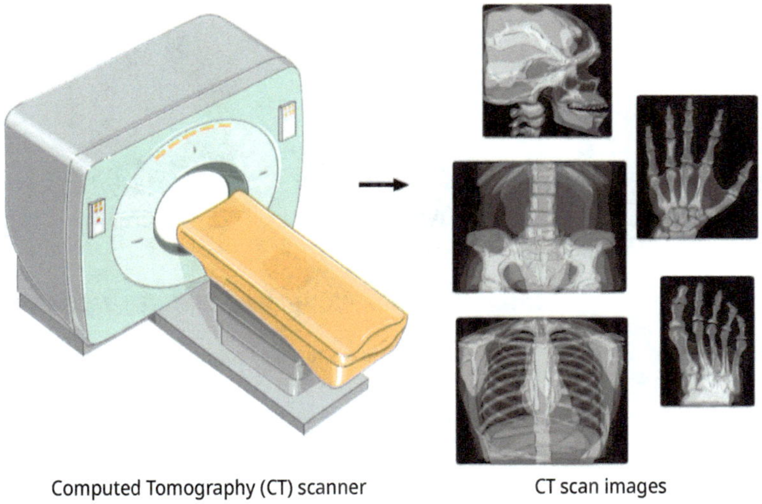

Figure 3.2: Medical imaging workflow using computed tomography (CT). Illustration of a CT scanner with representative radiographic outputs, including cranial, thoracic, abdominal, and appendicular skeletal images, highlighting the role of CT in generating high-resolution anatomical data for diagnostic, surgical planning, and computational modeling applications. Image provided by Servier Medical Art.

3.3.1.2 Magnetic Resonance Imaging (MRI)

MRI is a noninvasive imaging modality that offers superior soft-tissue contrast without the use of ionizing radiation, making it particularly advantageous for applications involving the brain, muscles, cartilage, and internal organs [33]. MRI, shown in Figure 3.3, operates based on the principles of nuclear magnetic resonance (NMR), wherein hydrogen nuclei in the body align with an applied magnetic field and subsequently emit radiofrequency signals, upon excitation. These signals are spatially encoded to generate high-resolution cross-sectional images.

For bioprinting applications, MRI provides critical data on tissue morphology, hydration states, and functional dynamics, all of which are essential for designing biomimetic constructs [34, 35]. For example, the layered architecture of the myocardium, the complex structure of cartilage, and the fiber orientation in muscles can be accurately visualized and reconstructed. In addition to standard T1- and T2-weighted imaging, advanced MRI techniques such as diffusion tensor imaging (DTI) and magnetic resonance elastography (MRE) are being increasingly utilized [36]. DTI enables the visualization of anisotropic diffusion in fibrous tissues such as nerves and muscles, providing insight into microstructural orientation that can be translated into fiber-guided bioprinting [37]. MRE, meanwhile, assesses tissue stiffness, which can inform the biomechanical design of printed constructs to mimic native viscoelastic properties.

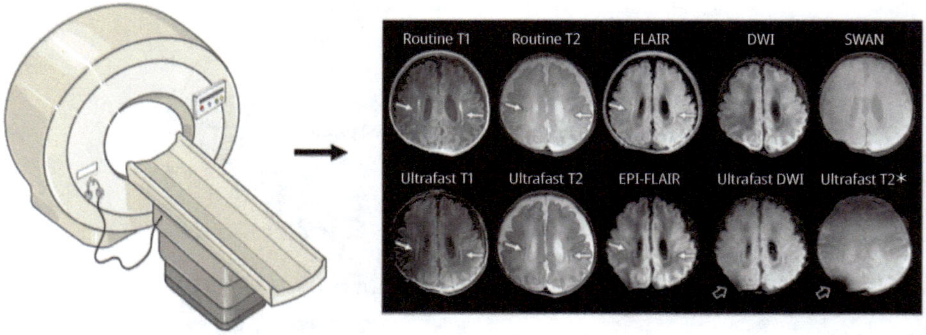

Magnetic resonance imaging machine **Magnetic resonance imaging of the brain**

Figure 3.3: Magnetic resonance imaging (MRI) modalities for brain assessment. Schematic representation of an MRI scanner (Image provided by Servier Medical Art), alongside routine and ultrafast MRI sequences, including T1, T2, FLAIR, diffusionweighted imaging (DWI), and susceptibility-weighted angiography (SWAN). These modalities provide complementary diagnostic information, enhancing visualization of structural and pathological features within the brain [122].

Functional MRI (fMRI) extends these capabilities by measuring hemodynamic responses associated with neural activity [38]. Though predominantly used in neuroscience, fMRI holds potential in dynamic modeling of vascularized tissues, capturing spatiotemporal blood flow patterns which can be integrated into vascular scaffold design. Innovations in real-time MRI and ultra-high-field MRI (≥7 T) are pushing the boundaries of spatial and temporal resolution, offering near-histological detail that can be invaluable in bioprinting applications requiring high precision, such as retinal, hepatic, and renal tissue constructs [39].

3.3.1.3 Ultrasound Imaging

Ultrasound imaging, or medical ultrasonography, employs high-frequency acoustic waves to visualize soft tissue interfaces in real-time as shown in figure 3.4. It is used for its portability, cost-effectiveness, and safety profile, as it does not involve ionizing

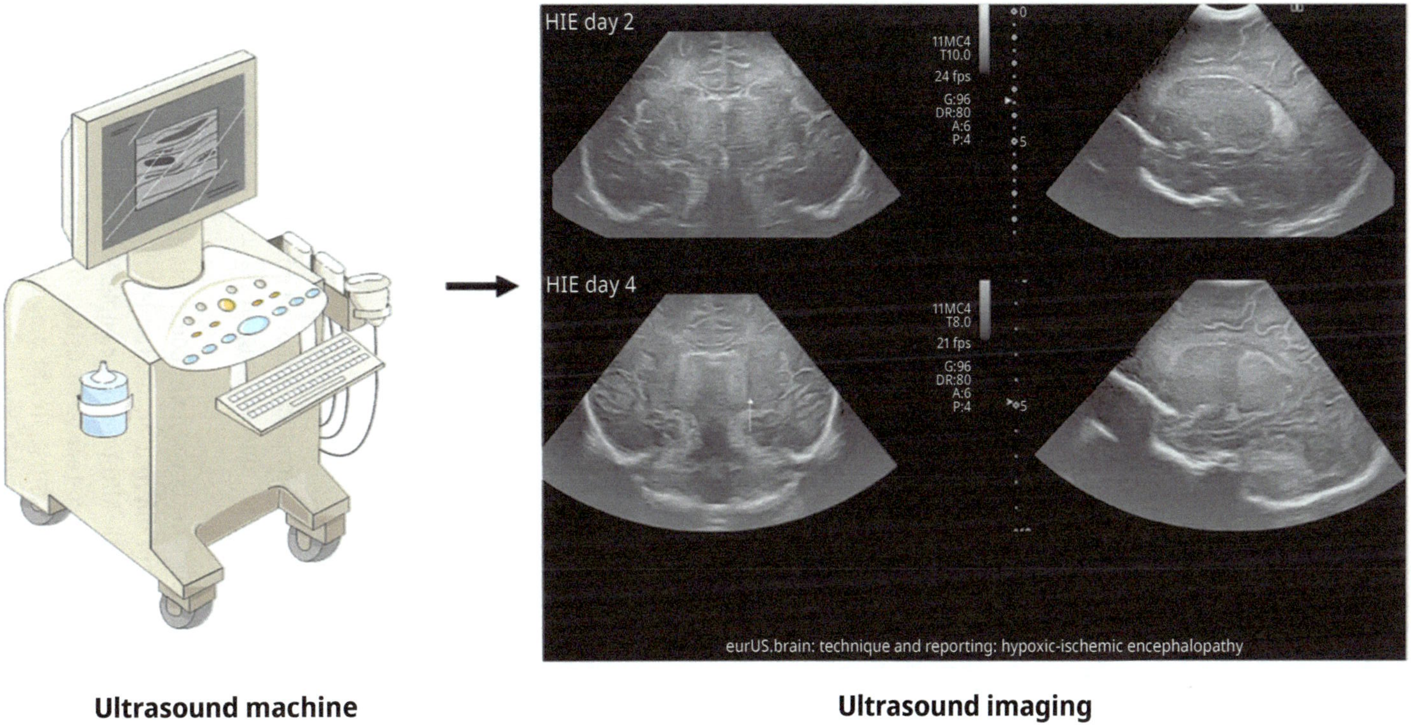

Figure 3.4: Schematic representation of an ultrasound ((Image provided by Servier Medical Art)) brain imaging, sonography equipment to clinical interpretation of cerebral ultrasound scans [123].

radiation [40]. Unlike CT or MRI, which are often constrained to large, immobile systems, ultrasound devices range from cart-based systems to handheld probes, making them ideal for point-of-care applications. Ultrasound is extensively used in cardiac, obstetric, and vascular imaging, as well as in real-time guidance of needle biopsies and surgical interventions.

In bioprinting, the dynamic nature of ultrasound imaging can be particularly useful for intraoperative tissue acquisition, assessment of mechanical deformation, and monitoring of printed constructs in vivo [41]. For example, 3D and 4D ultrasound techniques enable the visualization of moving structures, such as beating hearts or peristaltic intestines, which can be captured and modeled in near real time [42]. Furthermore, elastography, an advanced ultrasound modality, allows mapping of tissue stiffness and is being investigated for the design of mechanosensitive scaffolds [43]. Recent integration of AI-enhanced image analysis in ultrasound has enabled automated feature extraction and segmentation, facilitating the rapid creation of 3D models suitable for biofabrication.

Emerging developments in photoacoustic imaging, a hybrid technique combining optical contrast with ultrasound detection, have shown promise in visualizing oxygenation, vascular density, and biomolecular composition, offering a new dimension of functional imaging for bioengineered tissues. In addition, ultrasound-sensitive hydrogels and acoustically tunable bio-inks are being explored for feedback-controlled bioprinting, underscoring the growing interdependence between imaging and biofabrication technologies.

3.3.1.4 Comparative Utility and Workflow Integration

Each imaging modality presents distinct advantages and limitations, and their selection depends on the target tissue, resolution requirements, and clinical context [44]. CT is unparalleled in imaging mineralized tissues and generating high-fidelity anatomical models quickly, but its reliance on ionizing radiation makes it less suitable for serial imaging or pediatric cases. MRI, while offering superior soft-tissue resolution and safety, is time-consuming and cost-intensive, often requiring specialized infrastructure and long scan durations [45]. Ultrasound, though limited by operator dependence and lower resolution, offers real-time imaging and is uniquely suited for dynamic or bedside applications.

In contemporary bioprinting workflows, multimodal imaging is increasingly employed to leverage the strengths of different modalities [46]. For instance, CT can be used to model bone structures, while MRI provides complementary data for adjacent soft tissues. These datasets are then co-registered using image fusion algorithms to generate hybrid models that guide multi-material bioprinting. Furthermore, deep learning algorithms are being deployed to automate segmentation and enhance image quality, improving the efficiency and accuracy of digital model generation from imaging data [47].

3.3.1.5 Recent Trends and Innovations

A prominent trend in this space is the movement towards noninvasive, high-throughput imaging platforms tailored for tissue engineering applications. The contrast agents, such as nanoparticle-based MRI tracers, optical dyes, and targeted microbubbles, are enhancing the specificity and sensitivity of imaging modalities [48]. These agents enable selective visualization of cell populations, extracellular matrices, and metabolic activity within engineered tissues, allowing more informed design and monitoring of bioprinted constructs.

Another frontier is the integration of AI-driven image reconstruction techniques that allow super-resolution imaging from lower-quality inputs, thereby reducing scan time, radiation exposure, and costs. For example, generative adversarial networks (GANs) have been used to reconstruct high-resolution 3D models from sparse CT or MRI slices [49]. Similarly, reinforcement learning algorithms are being investigated for optimizing probe positioning and acquisition parameters in real-time ultrasound imaging, making the process more reproducible and operator-independent.

The convergence of imaging with wearable biosensors and organ-on-chip platforms is also redefining the scope of what imaging can capture in terms of tissue physiology, micro environmental changes, and cell signaling dynamics [50, 51]. These data streams can be fed back into the design loop for adaptive bioprinting, where construct geometry or bio-ink composition is dynamically modified in response to real-time feedback. The standardization of imaging-to-print workflows remains a major focus. Initiatives aimed at developing open-source platforms and interoperable file formats (e.g., DICOM-to-STL pipelines, Bio-CAD frameworks) are addressing the long-standing gap between medical imaging and biofabrication [52]. These efforts are expected to streamline the transition from patient scan to personalized implant or tissue graft, ultimately enhancing the reproducibility, scalability, and clinical translation of bioprinted products [53].

CT, MRI, and ultrasound each offers unique strengths in terms of resolution, tissue contrast, and operational logistics. The choice of modality is dictated by the specific anatomical and physiological characteristics of the target tissue, as well as the clinical setting in which imaging occurs. Continued advancements in image acquisition, data integration, and AI-driven analysis are rapidly closing the loop between diagnosis and therapeutic fabrication. As the field progresses, the fusion of imaging science with regenerative medicine will play a pivotal role in translating bioprinting from a laboratory technique into a mainstream clinical solution.

3.3.2 Image Processing and Denoising

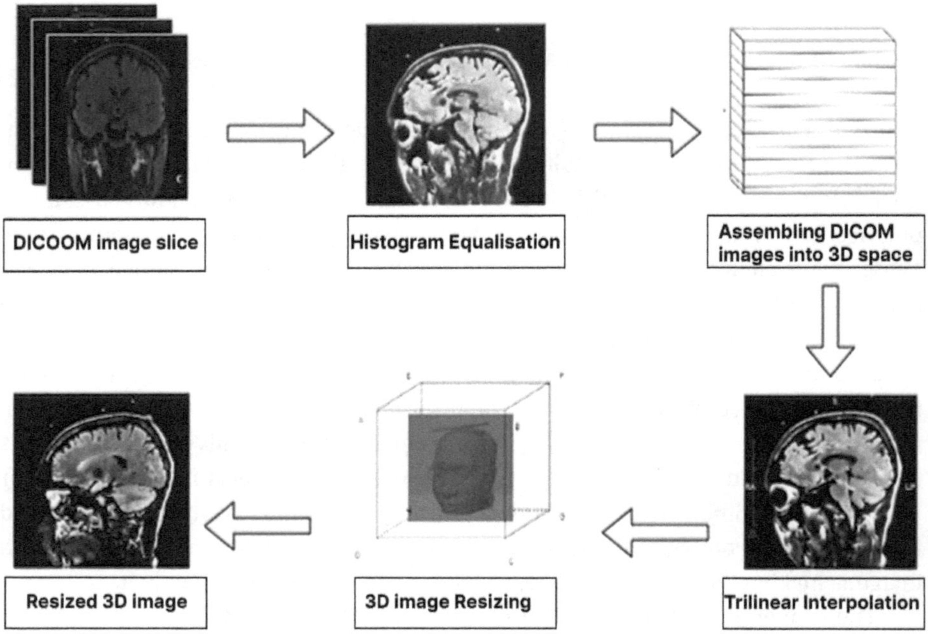

Figure 3.5: DICOM-to-3D medical image processing pipeline: A workflow diagram illustrating the conversion of DICOM image slices through histogram equalization, 3D space assembly, trilinear interpolation, and 3D image resizing to generate resized 3D medical images [124].

In the workflow of patient-specific 3D bioprinting, the quality of medical imaging data is paramount, serving as the basis for geometric modeling, scaffold generation, and spatial planning of bio-inks and cell-laden materials [54]. However, raw medical images acquired from modalities such as CT, MRI, and ultrasound are often corrupted by various types of noise originating from both hardware limitations and physiological sources. Such noise, ranging from thermal fluctuations and photon scatter to motion artifacts and undersampling, can obscure anatomical detail, distort boundary definitions, and ultimately compromise the fidelity of the 3D reconstructed model [55]. Therefore, image denoising is a critical preprocessing step that enhances signal quality and preserves essential structural features required for segmentation and bioprinting [56].

In CT imaging, quantum noise and electronic noise arise due to the stochastic nature of X-ray photon detection and limitations in detector sensitivity [57]. Lower radiation doses, though preferred for patient safety, affects it by reducing signal-to-noise ratios (SNR), necessitating sophisticated denoising techniques to compensate [58]. This challenge is particularly critical within the DICOM-to-3D medical image processing pipeline shown in figure 3.5, where sequential steps such as histogram equalization, 3D space assembly, trilinear interpolation, and image resizing amplify the impact of noise on the final reconstructed 3D model. In MRI, thermal noise, gradient-induced artifacts, and susceptibility variations distort fine features, particularly at high field strengths or in regions with air–tissue interfaces [59, 60]. Ultrasound images, meanwhile, are heavily affected by speckle noise, an interference pattern resulting from the coherent nature of the acoustic wave reflections, which masks small-scale anatomical structures [61]. Regardless of modality, if left uncorrected, such noise can introduce significant redundant data during image segmentation, leading to morphological inaccuracies and geometric distortions in the final 3D model used for printing. A wide array of denoising techniques has been developed, each tailored to the specific characteristics of different noise types and imaging modalities. Traditional approaches such as Gaussian smoothing and median filtering offer computational simplicity but often compromise structural details and blur anatomical boundaries. To address these limitations, more advanced edge-preserving algorithms have been introduced [62]. Anisotropic diffusion filtering, also known as Perona–Malik diffusion, applies directional smoothing, guided by image gradients, allowing for noise suppression, while preserving edges and local contrasts [63]. This method has been successfully adapted for CT and MRI images to retain bone–soft tissue interfaces and organ boundaries, essential for CAD modeling [64].

Anisotropic diffusion solves a partial differential equation (PDE) [65]:

$$\frac{\partial I(x,y,t)}{\partial t} = \nabla \cdot (c(x,y,t) \cdot \nabla I(x,y,t))$$

- $I(x, y, t)$: image intensity at time
- ∇I: gradient of image (direction of intensity change)
- ∇: divergence operator
- $c(x, y, t)$: conductance function, which controls diffusion rate

A commonly used conductance function:

$$c(x,y,t) = e^{-\left(\frac{|\nabla I|}{K}\right)^2}$$

where K is the edge-stopping threshold when small gradients (noise) are smoothed, while large gradients (edges) are preserved. For instance, if we have an MRI brain image with noise around gray-white matter boundaries, using anisotropic diffusion, we can set $K = 15$, and iterate for 10 time steps [66]. The result is denoised images, where the gyri-sulci edges are preserved, critical for generating accurate cortical surface models in neurosurgical bioprinting.

Similarly, bilateral filtering, another nonlinear method, combines spatial and intensity information to achieve selective smoothing. It has proven particularly effective in preserving fine textures and gradients, especially in MRI scans used for neurological or musculoskeletal modeling [67]. Adaptive filters, such as the Wiener filter and Kalman filter, estimate noise characteristics dynamically and tailor their response based on local image statistics, offering improved results in heterogeneous tissues [68]. Non-local means (NLM) filtering, a more recent advancement, enhances denoising by leveraging pixel similarity over the entire image domain rather than local neighborhoods, making it highly effective in reducing random noise, while preserving repetitive anatomical patterns. NLM is especially useful in low-dose CT and volumetric MRI, where voxel-wise consistency is vital for 3D reconstruction. The innovations in machine learning and deep learning into the forefront of medical image denoising. Convolutional neural networks (CNNs) trained on paired noisy-clean datasets have demonstrated superior performance in eliminating complex noise patterns, without sacrificing structural integrity [69]. Architectures such as DnCN-N, U-Net-, and ResNet-based denoisers have been adapted to medical imaging tasks, outperforming classical methods in terms of peak signal-to-noise ratio (PSNR) and structural similarity index (SSIM) [70]. These models are capable of learning context-aware features, enabling them to distinguish between noise and genuine anatomical variability. Some studies have even proposed unsupervised or self-supervised learning frameworks (e.g., Noise2Void and Noise2Self) that eliminate the need for clean ground-truth data, a major advantage, given the scarcity of high-quality annotated medical images [71].

Moreover, GANs have been explored for noise reduction, particularly in low-dose CT imaging [72]. These networks generate high-fidelity denoised outputs by pitting a generator against a discriminator, resulting in reconstructions that are not only statistically accurate but also perceptually realistic. CycleGANs and Pix2Pix models have also been applied to ultrasound and PET scans, producing images with enhanced clarity, suitable for anatomical modeling [73]. Beyond static denoising, emerging approaches are targeting temporal coherence in dynamic imaging (e.g., 4D ultrasound or fMRI), ensuring noise reduction across time points, without compromising motion information, critical for dynamic bioprinting applications [74]. The impact of effective denoising on the bioprinting pipeline is substantial. High-quality, denoised images facilitate more accurate segmentation, which in turn leads to better mesh generation and smoother surface rendering in the CAD model. Structural details such as vascular bifurcations, trabecular bone microarchitecture, and cartilage–ligament interfaces, which are crucial for functional fidelity, can be preserved only when the underlying imaging data is of high clarity [75]. Denoising also contributes to the precision of printing toolpaths, ensuring that the spatial arrangement of multiple bio-inks and embedded cells mimics native anatomical complexity. Moreover, noise-free models reduce computational load during mesh optimization and FEA, accelerating the design iteration cycle and reducing manufacturing errors. Additionally, denoising plays a critical role in automated image analysis and AI-assisted segmentation [76]. Many contemporary pipelines use deep neural networks to identify organ boundaries, classify tissues, or label pathological features. The performance of these models is highly sensitive to image quality; noisy data can lead to misclassifications or failure in feature recognition. By incorporating denoising as a preprocessing step, the robustness and generalizability of AI models can be significantly improved, enhancing the reliability of automated model generation for bioprinting. Another emerging trend is the development of modality-specific denoising strategies, wherein algorithms are fine-tuned based on the physics and statistical noise characteristics of a particular imaging modality. For instance, deep residual learning has been optimized for low-dose CT, while transform-domain sparsity models have been applied to MRI and diffusion-weighted imaging [77]. These specialized algorithms not only improve image quality but also reduce the dependency on manual intervention during downstream processing stages. Moreover, multiscale and multi-resolution frameworks, which operate at various levels of image granularity, have demonstrated improved adaptability across different organ systems and anatomical scales – from small neural tracts to large abdominal structures.

The integration of real-time denoising is also gaining traction, particularly in intraoperative imaging or bedside scanning scenarios where rapid acquisition and interpretation are necessary. Lightweight neural networks and edge computing platforms are being developed to perform denoising on the fly, enabling near-instant feedback for image-guided interventions and immediate CAD modeling for urgent tissue engineering needs. Image denoising is an indispensable component of the medical imaging workflow, particularly in the context of bioprinting where structural fidelity and anatomical precision are nonnegotiable. As imaging technologies evolve toward higher resolution, faster acquisition, and broader accessibility, the parallel advancement of denoising techniques – spanning classical filters, statistical models, and deep learning frameworks – will continue to play a pivotal role in ensuring that raw imaging data can be reliably transformed into accurate, high-quality 3D models. The pursuit of denoising algorithms that balance computational efficiency with anatomical preservation remains a vibrant area of research, with direct implications for the quality, safety, and clinical applicability of bioprinted constructs.

3.3.3 Segmentation and 3D Reconstruction

In the context of patient-specific 3D bioprinting, image segmentation and 3D reconstruction are critical steps that bridge raw imaging data and printable anatomical models [78, 79]. Segmentation refers to the computational process of partitioning medical images into meaningful regions that correspond to anatomical structures such as organs, bones, or pathological lesions. This step is essential for isolating the tissues of interest from surrounding structures, enabling accurate modeling and downstream processing for scaffold fabrication and bioprinting as shown in figure 3.6. Given the inherent variability of human anatomy, pathology, and imaging modalities, segmentation must be robust, precise, and adaptive. In practice, segmentation begins with the acquisition of tomographic data in the form of 2D image slices from CT, MRI, PET, or ultrasound modalities. These images often require preprocessing steps such as denoising, contrast enhancement, and normalization to improve signal-to-noise ratio and enhance boundary detection. Traditional segmentation methods – such as thresholding, region-growing, and edge detection have been widely used in clinical applications due to their simplicity and computational efficiency. However, these techniques are often limited by their sensitivity to noise, contrast variation, and anatomical ambiguity, particularly in heterogeneous tissues.

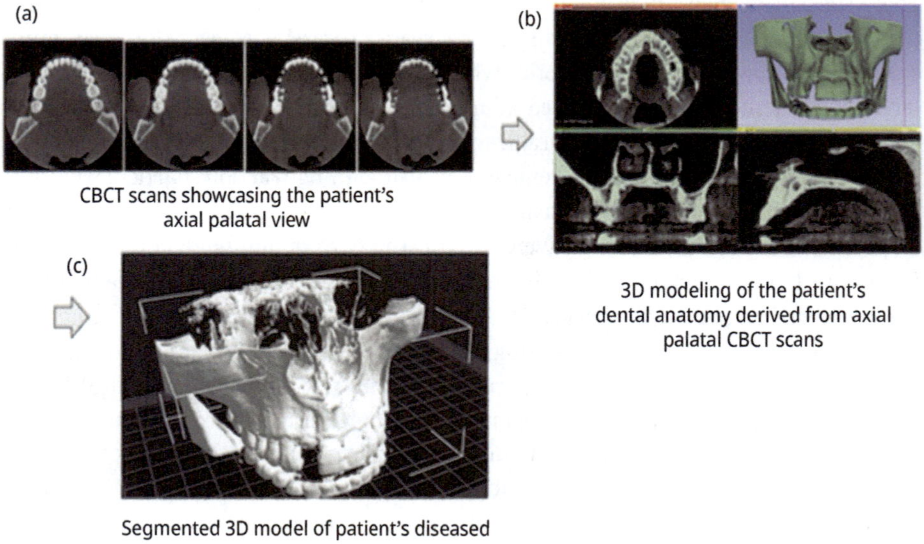

Figure 3.6: (a) CBCT scans showcasing the patient's axial palatal view, (b) 3D modeling of the patient's dental anatomy, derived from axial palatal CBCT scans, (c) Segmented 3D model of patient's diseased site [18].

To overcome these limitations, more advanced techniques have emerged. Level-set methods and active contour models provide semiautomated segmentation by evolving a contour over time to fit the target boundary based on image gradients and curvature constraints. These approaches are effective in delineating complex anatomical structures with irregular boundaries, such as vasculature and soft tissue interfaces. Similarly, graph-based methods, which model image pixels or voxels as graph nodes, with edge weights based on intensity similarity and spatial proximity, offer globally optimal solutions for tissue partitioning using algorithms like Graph Cut or Random Walker. However, the field has undergone a significant transformation with the advent of machine learning and deep learning, which now represent the state-of-the-art in medical image segmentation [80]. CNNs, especially architectures like U-Net, 3D U-Net, and V-Net, have shown remarkable success in segmenting complex anatomical structures across different modalities [81–84]. These networks are trained on annotated datasets to learn hierarchical feature representations, enabling them to segment organs with high accuracy, even in the presence of imaging noise, artifacts, or anatomical variations. Furthermore, multitask learning approaches, which simultaneously learn segmentation and auxiliary tasks (e.g., organ classification or boundary detection), have been shown to improve robustness and generalizability.

Recent innovations have also focused on multi-organ and whole-body segmentation, shifting the paradigm from organ-specific models to comprehensive systems that can process full-body scans. For example, fully automated pipelines now exist that can segment over 100 anatomical structures from CT or MRI volumes using deep ensemble networks or hybrid approaches, combining CNNs with transformers [79]. Such systems are being actively integrated into bioprinting workflows to enable multi-tissue scaffold design for complex applications, including musculoskeletal regeneration and organ-on-chip models. A key challenge in segmentation lies in dealing with ambiguous boundaries or overlapping tissue intensities, especially in regions with pathological alterations such as tumors or necrosis. In these scenarios, attention mechanisms have been employed in segmentation networks to selectively focus on relevant regions and suppress irrelevant background signals. Additionally, self-supervised learning frameworks, such as SimCLR or BYOL, have demonstrated promise in reducing dependency on large annotated datasets by leveraging unlabeled medical images for pretraining.

Following successful segmentation, 3D reconstruction entails the conversion of segmented 2D image slices into a volumetric 3D model. This process typically involves voxel stacking, surface meshing, and volume rendering [85]. While voxel-based reconstructions offer high fidelity, they are memory-intensive and may include staircase artifacts. Surface-based approaches, such as marching cubes and Poisson surface reconstruction, are widely used to generate polygonal meshes suitable for CAD modeling and bioprinting. The resulting mesh may undergo smoothing, decimation, and topological correction to ensure watertightness and printability. Recent advances in differentiable rendering and neural implicit representations (e.g., neural radiance fields or NeRFs) have introduced new paradigms for 3D reconstruction [86]. These methods learn continuous volumetric fields from 2D projections, offering smooth and photorealistic 3D outputs. They are particularly useful in reconstructing anatomically accurate models from sparse or incomplete data, which is common in pediatric or emergency imaging scenarios.

Another emerging approach involves federated learning, wherein segmentation and reconstruction models are trained collaboratively across multiple institutions without data sharing, preserving patient privacy while increasing dataset diversity [87]. This has significantly improved the generalizability of 3D models across different demographics and scanner types. Despite these advancements, accuracy and reproducibility remain critical concerns, especially when the reconstructed models serve as templates for bioprinted tissues. Sub-millimeter errors in segmentation can translate into functional deficits in the printed scaffold. Hence, validation against ground-truth annotations, cross-modality comparisons, and in silico simulations are essential quality control measures. Moreover, integration with semiautomatic proofreading interfaces allows expert intervention when needed, striking a balance between automation and precision. Segmentation and 3D reconstruction form the backbone of bioprinting-ready anatomical modeling. With continued integration of AI, domain adaptation, and multimodal fusion, these technologies are poised to deliver high-precision, patient-specific models that meet the stringent demands of regenerative medicine and surgical planning

3.4 Design and Modeling in CAD

3.4.1 CAD Tools for Bioprinting

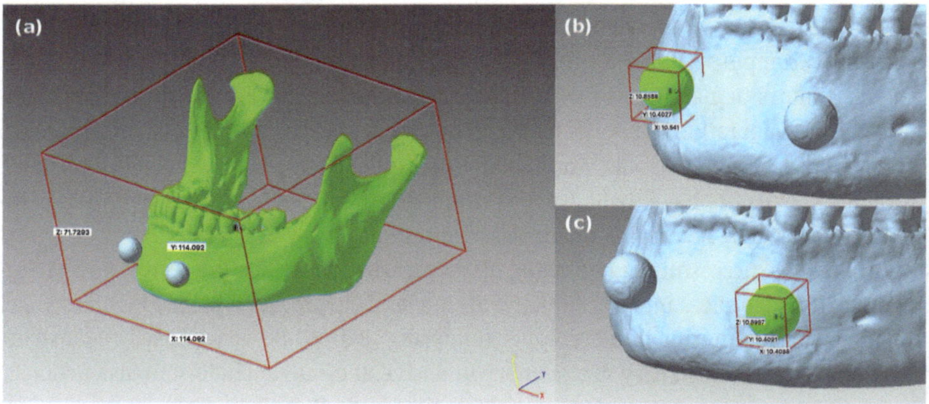

Figure 3.7: Progressive 3D reconstruction of dental structures: (a) geometric wireframe with coordinate system, (b-c) surface-rendered models, demonstrating integration of anatomical features with spatial positioning [125].

The development and application of CAD tools in the field of bioprinting have revolutionized how complex tissue and organ structures are conceptualized, designed, and realized. Traditional CAD platforms, originally developed for mechanical engineering, have evolved through the incorporation of biodesign modules, enabling the accurate modeling of heterogeneous biological architectures [88]. Modern CAD systems for bioprinting support anatomical precision, geometrical complexity, and multi-material configurations, essential for the fabrication of tissue scaffolds and functional organs. One of the core capabilities of CAD software in bioprinting lies in parametric design [89]. This approach allows for the modulation of model parameters, such as pore size, strut thickness, and curvature, thereby facilitating the customization of scaffolds tailored to individual patient anatomies. Tools such as SolidWorks, with biomedical plugins, Autodesk Fusion 360, with Bio-CAD extensions, and specialized platforms like BioCAD and 3D Slicer have gained traction in biomedical research. These platforms not only permit the design of biomimetic structures but also integrate anatomical data derived from DICOM files to enhance biological relevance as shown in figure 3.7.

Bio-CAD software, specifically developed for tissue engineering applications, allows the generation of models with compartmentalized structures representing different tissue types (e.g., vascularized versus non-vascularized regions). These platforms can integrate anatomical landmarks and biomechanical constraints to produce functional organ replicas. Innovations like voxel-based modeling, implemented in software such as Mimics and Simpleware, provide improved resolution and control over micro architectural features. This is particularly crucial for gradient-based tissue constructs where variations in mechanical or biochemical properties are critical for tissue regeneration. Further enhancements include machine learning-driven design tools that utilize large datasets of anatomical and pathological models to predict optimal scaffold geometries. AI-assisted CAD tools are capable of suggesting design modifications based on predicted deformation patterns, growth behavior, or vascular requirements. Additionally, cloud-based collaborative platforms allow for multidisciplinary inputs, ensuring that biological, mechanical, and clinical perspectives are embedded into the final model.

Simulation capabilities embedded within modern CAD platforms further enrich the design process. Integrated modules for stress analysis, porosity estimation, and diffusion modeling help predict the behavior of the scaffold during in vivo conditions [89]. These pre-manufacturing validations reduce trial-and-error effort during physical printing and ensure alignment with clinical performance expectations. Recent trends have also pushed toward generative design, a computational approach where algorithms autonomously generate design alternatives that meet defined criteria. This is particularly valuable for creating scaffolds with optimized mechanical integrity and nutrient diffusion, often resulting in highly nonintuitive, yet biologically favorable architectures.

The convergence of CAD design with bioinformatics and tissue informatics holds promise for further innovations. For example, gene expression patterns and histological data can now be integrated into the CAD models to predict cell behavior post-printing. Such multidimensional design integration transforms the scaffold from a structural replica to a biologically functional entity. In summary, CAD tools tailored for bioprinting have matured significantly, transitioning from mere shape generators to biologically intelligent platforms. These tools now facilitate the comprehensive modeling of patient-specific, functionally graded, and multi-material constructs, marking a critical milestone in personalized regenerative medicine.

3.4.2 Biomechanical Simulations

Biomechanical simulations have become an indispensable component of the bioprinting workflow, enabling the prediction, analysis, and optimization of the mechanical and physiological behavior of bioprinted constructs [19]. These simulations, primarily grounded in FEA and CFD, serve as virtual testbeds for evaluating structural integrity,

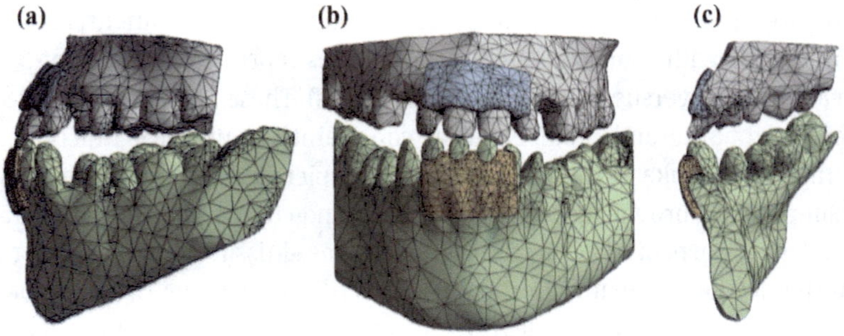

Figure 3.8: Finite element discretization of mandibular geometry: (a) lateral view, (b) anterior view with implant region (highlighted), (c) sagittal section showing internal mesh topology [18].

cellular microenvironments, and long-term functionality before the actual fabrication of tissue or organ models.

FEA divides complex geometries into finite elements, allowing for the solution of mechanical problems under defined boundary conditions [90]. In bioprinting, FEA is widely used to simulate the mechanical behavior of scaffolds under physiological loads. This includes assessing stress distribution, deformation, and failure zones within bone, cartilage, and vascular graft models. A representative example of such discretization is illustrated in figure 3.8, where mandibular geometry is partitioned into finite elements, highlighting implant regions and internal mesh topology for accurate biomechanical analysis. FEA assists in optimizing scaffold porosity and architecture, ensuring that constructs maintain mechanical support, while facilitating tissue ingrowth and nutrient diffusion. CFD, on the other hand, models the behavior of fluids within and around the printed constructs. This is especially critical for vascularized tissues, where CFD is used to predict shear stress, flow velocity, and pressure gradients within bioprinted vascular networks. The coupling of FEA and CFD provides a holistic view of the scaffold performance, especially in dynamic environments such as the cardiovascular system or bioreactor conditions. Advanced simulations are now moving beyond static analysis. Dynamic simulations, which consider time-dependent loading, cell proliferation, and matrix deposition, offer insights into how constructs evolve over time. Multiphysics modeling frameworks that combine fluid flow, mass transport, and mechanical deformation have been developed to simulate the complex interplay between biological and physical phenomena during tissue maturation.

In cardiac tissue engineering, for instance, electromechanical FEA simulations allow researchers to model the synchronous contraction of engineered myocardium and predict its interaction with surrounding tissues [91]. Similarly, in orthopedic applications, simulations are employed to analyze osteointegration and stress shielding, guiding the design of load-bearing scaffolds that promote bone regeneration, while minimizing the risk of implant loosening [92]. Emerging approaches such as agent-based modeling and machine learning-enhanced simulations offer new avenues for predictive modeling. Agent-based models simulate the behavior of individual cells or molecules within the scaffold, providing detailed insights into cellular interactions and migration [93]. Machine learning algorithms trained on large experimental datasets can predict scaffold degradation rates, tissue growth kinetics, and even suggest optimal scaffold designs based on desired outcomes.

The application of digital twins, virtual replicas of physical constructs that continuously update based on real-time data, is gaining momentum in bioprinting. Digital twins enable continuous monitoring and adjustment of printing parameters, environmental conditions, and biological responses, thereby bridging the gap between simulation and actual fabrication. Furthermore, simulation-based validation of constructs before implantation is crucial for regulatory approval and clinical translation. Simulated fatigue testing, perfusion efficiency, and mechanical compliance assessments ensure that the constructs meet safety and performance standards. Another innovative trend involves the integration of patient-specific data into simulation pipelines. Personalized biomechanical models based on MRI or CT data allow for individualized design and validation of implants or tissue constructs, ensuring better clinical outcomes. This is particularly relevant in reconstructive surgery, where anatomical variations can significantly influence the performance of grafts or scaffolds. Biomechanical simulations offer a powerful, noninvasive strategy to optimize scaffold design, ensure biocompatibility, and predict in vivo performance. The continued evolution of simulation techniques, fueled by advances in computational power and data-driven modeling, is set to further enhance the reliability and effectiveness of bioprinted tissues and organs.

3.5 Manufacturing with CAM

3.5.1 Slicing and Toolpath Generation

The transition from digital CAD models to physical bioprinted constructs is mediated through the process of slicing and toolpath generation, which forms the core of computer-aided manufacturing (CAM) in bioprinting [94]. This process involves converting a 3D model into printer-executable commands, commonly known as G-code. The slicing algorithm dissects the volumetric CAD model into a series of planar layers, each representing a horizontal cross section of the intended structure. These 2D slices are translated into sequential movement and extrusion instructions for the bioprinter. Slicing is not merely a geometric exercise but a material-aware and machine-specific process. Given the complex rheological and biological behavior of bio-inks, slicing algorithms must incorporate information such as viscosity, gelation temperature, cross-linking behavior, and printability windows [95]. Moreover, the parameters such as layer height, infill density, and print speed are optimized to maintain structural fidelity, while minimizing cellular stress and deformation during extrusion. The innovations in slicing tools include adaptive slicing techniques, where the layer thickness varies depending on the curvature and resolution requirements of the geometry [96]. This not only enhances the surface smoothness and reduces stair-stepping artifacts but also accelerates the printing process by allowing thicker layers in less critical regions. Machine learning-driven slicers are also being explored, where historical print data is used to predict and optimize parameters for new constructs.

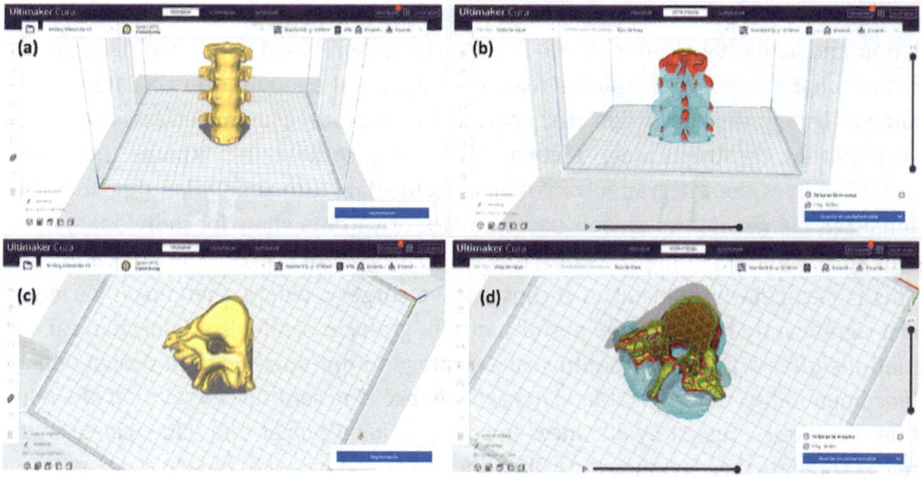

Figure 3.9: Steps in digital preparation of vertebral and cranial anatomical models for 3D printing, showing segmentation, support visualization, and slicing in Ultimaker Cura.

Toolpath generation must also account for nonstandard features common in biofabrication, such as hollow vascular networks, overhangs requiring sacrificial supports, and multi-material transitions. Advanced slicers allow the assignment of specific printheads to individual regions, facilitating heterogeneous tissue constructs with spatially controlled material deposition as shown in figure 3.9. Support structures are designed with biocompatible or removable materials to prevent interference with post-print maturation.

Furthermore, slicing software is evolving to simulate the deposition process in silico. These simulations predict the thermal and mechanical stresses during printing, allowing adjustments before actual fabrication. In bioprinting, where errors can result in cell death or loss of function, such predictive slicing ensures high fidelity and reproducibility. Integration with feedback loops, where real-time data from sensors is used to modify slicing parameters on the fly, is becoming a hallmark of intelligent bioprinting systems.

3.5.2 3D Printing Technologies

3D printing technologies have diversified to accommodate a wide array of bioinks and tissue types, each with its specific CAM requirements [96]. The five primary categories of 3D printing, Wire arc additive manufacturing process, Paste extrusion process, Friction stir additive manufacturing process, Powder bed fusion process, and Binder jetting technique, differ in their deposition mechanisms, resolution capabilities, and compatibility with cells and biomaterials as shown in the figure 3.10 [97].

Extrusion-based bioprinters dominate the field due to their ability to deposit viscous, cell-dense bio-inks. CAM systems for these printers must control syringe pressure, screw rotation speed, or pneumatic force to ensure consistent flow. Recent advancements include coaxial and triaxial extrusion systems for producing core-shell structures, enabling the fabrication of vascularized tissues [98]. These complex geometries require CAM systems capable of synchronizing multiple extruders and generating simultaneous toolpaths with interleaving materials. Inkjet bioprinting, known for its high speed and droplet precision, requires CAM algorithms that manage thermal or piezoelectric actuation for droplet ejection. Toolpaths in this context focus on raster scanning, droplet frequency modulation, and substrate cooling. These printers are ideal for printing low-viscosity bio-inks and cellular suspensions, often used in skin and neural tissue engineering. Laser-assisted bioprinting (LAB) offers high-resolution deposition through laser-induced forward transfer mechanisms. CAM requirements for LAB include precise laser pulse coordination, beam focusing, and energy modulation. The absence of nozzles reduces clogging risks, making it suitable for printing fragile or rare cell types. However, LAB systems demand intricate calibration of timing and spatial resolution, managed through high-fidelity CAM protocols.

Other emerging technologies such as acoustic [99], electrohydrodynamic [100], and volumetric bioprinting introduce novel CAM challenges [101]. Acoustic droplet ejection requires control of sound wave parameters, while electrohydrodynamic printing manipulates electric fields for ultrafine deposition. Volumetric bioprinting, where the entire construct is polymerized in a single step using light patterns, requires a paradigm shift from traditional layer-by-layer toolpath planning to volumetric data modulation and light-field patterning. Printer-specific considerations in CAM include resolution constraints, nozzle diameters, heating/cooling elements, stage stability, and biocompatibility of components. Multi-material capabilities introduce synchronization complexities, necessitating time-staggered extrusion or active material switching. CAM systems must therefore incorporate printer-specific firmware configurations, actuation feedback, and fail-safe protocols to ensure precision and safety.

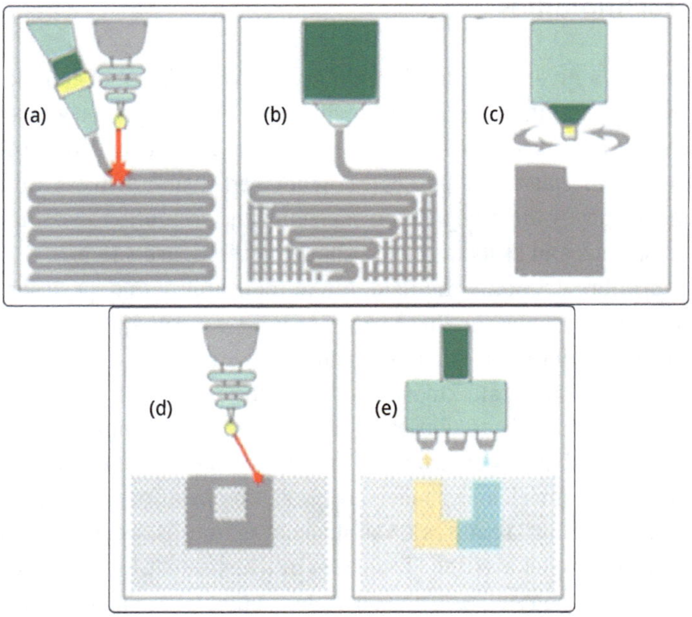

Figure 3.10: Types of additive manufacturing process used to fabricate bio-implants. (a) Wire arc additive manufacturing process. (b) Paste extrusion process. (c) Friction stir additive manufacturing process. (d) Powder bed fusion process. (e) Binder jetting technique [97].

3.5.3 Data Management and Optimization

The digitization of biological systems through medical imaging and CAD modeling produces massive datasets, posing significant challenges for data management in CAM workflows. These datasets often originate from high-resolution modalities like MRI, CT, or confocal microscopy and may exceed several gigabytes per patient. Efficient handling of this data is critical for maintaining print fidelity and ensuring clinical scalability.

One of the primary challenges lies in maintaining data integrity during compression and transfer. Lossless compression techniques, such as those based on JPEG2000 or HDF5, are preferred to prevent degradation of spatial resolution, especially in regions of high anatomical complexity [102]. CAM systems must interface seamlessly with data standards such as DICOM, ensuring that volumetric imaging data is accurately translated into printable geometries [103]. To manage this complexity, advanced preprocessing pipelines involving segmentation, surface reconstruction, and mesh optimization are employed. Mesh decimation, smoothing, and error correction algorithms help reduce data size without compromising critical features. The use of surface versus volumetric representations (e.g., STL vs. AMF or 3MF formats) is guided by the complexity of the construct and the need for metadata such as material type, color, or print order [104]. Real-time processing has become feasible with the integration of GPUs and parallel computing frameworks into CAM software [105]. These enable rapid segmentation, real-time rendering, and dynamic toolpath updates based on intraoperative imaging or sensor feedback. Cloud-based data management platforms offer collaborative design capabilities and facilitate the integration of patient data from electronic health records for personalized bioprinting.

Optimization algorithms, including evolutionary strategies and reinforcement learning, are increasingly used to determine optimal print parameters. These algorithms iterate through large parameter spaces – such as nozzle temperature, print speed, and infill density – to identify configurations that maximize cell viability and structural fidelity. Predictive modeling using digital twins further enhances optimization by simulating outcomes based on current data. Another critical aspect is the security and regulatory compliance of biomedical data. CAM systems must ensure encryption, controlled access, and audit trails for sensitive patient data. As bioprinting moves closer to clinical applications, adherence to standards such as HIPAA and GDPR becomes imperative [106]. The effective CAM integration in bioprinting involves more than just translating CAD models into G-code. It requires a deep understanding of bio-ink behavior, printer mechanics, data science, and real-time optimization. The confluence of slicing algorithms, printer-specific control, and intelligent data handling ensures that bioprinted constructs are not only structurally accurate but also biologically functional and clinically viable.

3.6 Challenges and Future Directions

3.6.1 Technical Challenges

Despite significant advances in bioprinting technologies and CAD/CAM integration, technical challenges continue to hinder the realization of fully functional, patient-specific tissues and organs [107]. One major limitation lies in the current capabilities of CAD/CAM systems, particularly in terms of resolution, processing speed, and the range of compatible materials. Most slicing algorithms and toolpath generators, originally developed for thermoplastics and metals, lack the sensitivity and precision required for soft, heterogeneous bio-inks [108]. Achieving microscale fidelity while maintaining cell viability remains a major bottleneck. Resolutions below 50 μm are often necessary to replicate fine vascular and neural architectures, yet such precision compromises printing speed and structural stability.

CAM systems often struggle to accommodate the unique rheological and cross-linking behaviors of bio-inks, particularly those with temperature- or pH-sensitive components. Current hardware and software configurations limit the effective co-printing of multiple materials with distinct physical and chemical properties. Moreover, the lack of standardized characterization data for emerging bio-inks impedes the development of predictive printability models and dynamic parameter tuning [109]. A particularly complex challenge is the integration of cellular-level and molecular data into the CAD modeling process [110]. While medical imaging modalities such as MRI and CT provide macroscale anatomical templates, they do not capture cellular distributions, matrix composition, or tissue-specific gradients. High-content imaging and spatial omics are emerging as tools to inform model heterogeneity, but translating these datasets into actionable printing instructions is still in early development. The transition from anatomical data to functional, biomimetic models requires advanced algorithms that incorporate cell–matrix interactions, mechanotransduction feedback, and micro environmental cues.

In addition, bioprinting technologies still face limitations in hardware capabilities. Extruder clogging, inconsistent droplet formation, limited multi-material switching speeds, and inadequate temperature or humidity control all negatively impact print fidelity [111]. These problems are exacerbated in constructs with internal voids, overhangs, or vascular channels [112]. Although support materials and coaxial nozzles offer partial solutions, reliable and automated handling of complex features remains a work in progress [113]. To address these challenges, future CAM systems must evolve toward adaptive, feedback-controlled platforms that incorporate real-time sensing, AI-driven decision-making, and closed-loop control architectures. Integration with digital twins and predictive simulation environments can enable iterative optimization of both structural and biological parameters, paving the way toward more robust and clinically relevant bioprinting.

3.6.2 Multidisciplinary Collaboration

The progress of bioprinting from laboratory research to clinical application necessitates seamless collaboration across multiple disciplines, including engineering, biology, materials science, medicine, and data science [114]. Each stakeholder brings a unique set of knowledge and objectives, yet aligning these into a unified workflow remains a formidable task. A persistent issue lies in the communication barriers between disciplines. Engineers and CAD designers may prioritize manufacturability and mechanical performance, while biologists focus on cellular viability, differentiation, and biomolecular signaling. Clinicians, on the other hand, are primarily concerned with functional outcomes and regulatory compliance. Misalignments in priorities and terminology can result in suboptimal designs, delays, and costly iterations.

Bridging these gaps requires standardized protocols, shared vocabularies, and collaborative design environments. Tools such as multidisciplinary design optimization (MDO) frameworks, digital health platforms, and common data standards (e.g., DICOM, FHIR) help foster better integration [115]. Additionally, cross-training programs and translational research centers have emerged to promote interdisciplinary literacy and collaborative problem-solving. Another essential strategy is the implementation of co-design methodologies, where end-users (e.g., surgeons or patients) actively participate in the design and development process. This user-centric approach not only ensures clinical relevance but also accelerates regulatory acceptance and patient outcomes. Feedback from clinicians during the early design phases can guide CAD modeling decisions, material selection, and post-processing requirements.

Ethical considerations also underscore the need for multidisciplinary discourse. Questions surrounding the use of human cells, long-term implant effects, patient consent, and data privacy require input from ethicists, legal experts, and healthcare policymakers. Thus, the roadmap to successful bioprinting demands not only technical and biological integration but also societal and regulatory alignment. Digital platforms for collaborative modeling and cloud-based CAM software can facilitate real-time interaction among geographically dispersed teams. These platforms enable the sharing of high-fidelity models, simultaneous editing, and integration with electronic health records (EHRs), thereby fostering a truly connected bioprinting ecosystem. Ultimately, the success of this field hinges on dismantling disciplinary silos and fostering a cooperative, iterative innovation process.

3.6.3 Future Innovations

The future of CAD/CAM in bioprinting is poised for a paradigm shift, driven by emerging technologies such as artificial intelligence (AI), machine learning (ML), and 4D bioprinting [116]. AI is increasingly being employed to optimize slicing parameters, predict print outcomes, and identify material combinations that maximize structural fidelity and biological function. Reinforcement learning algorithms are capable of adapting to new bio-ink behaviors by iteratively refining toolpaths in response to real-time sensor data.

4D bioprinting represents a transformative innovation, wherein printed constructs can change their shape, properties, or function over time in response to external stimuli [117]. These dynamic constructs often leverage smart materials, such as shape-memory polymers or hydrogel composites, which respond to thermal, pH, or biochemical triggers. CAD/CAM systems are being adapted to model and simulate these time-dependent behaviors, requiring integration of finite element modeling (FEM) and stimulus-response mapping into the design workflow. Another frontier is volumetric bioprinting, which challenges the traditional layer-by-layer paradigm by enabling simultaneous cross-linking of entire 3D structures using light patterns [118]. This approach drastically reduces printing time while improving cell viability, by minimizing shear stresses. CAM systems must evolve to incorporate tomographic reconstruction algorithms and voxel-wise control mechanisms to manage such processes. Quantum computing, though still nascent, is being explored for solving complex optimization problems in multi-material deposition, cellular arrangement, and vascular network integration. Similarly, advances in spatial transcriptomics and single-cell sequencing are expected to influence the customization of bio-inks and construct geometries at unprecedented resolution.

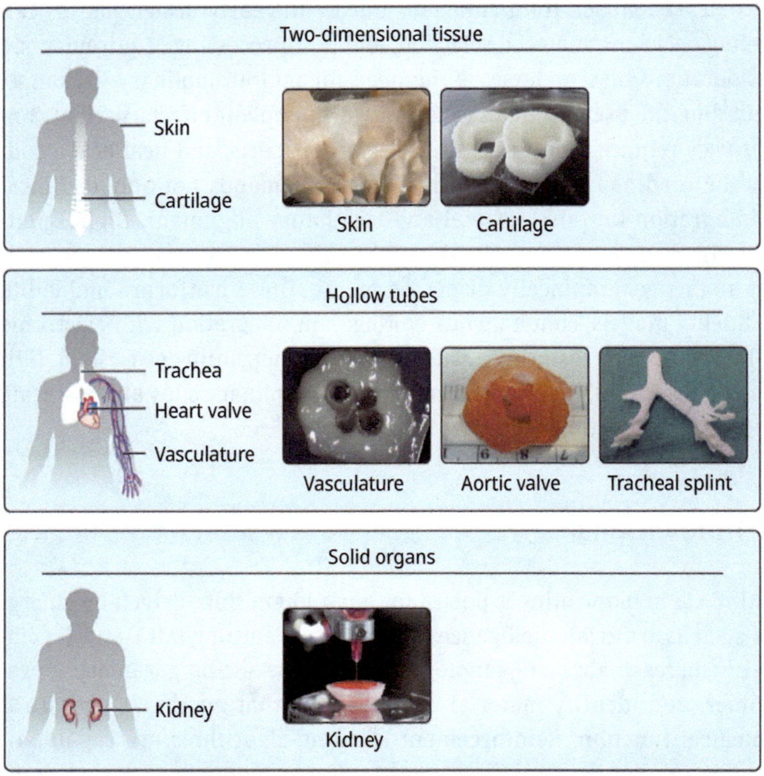

Figure 3.11: Bioprinted tissue constructs, including skin and cartilage substitutes, (inkjet bioprinting) [126], vascular grafts (microextrusion of fused cellular rods) [127], aortic valves (dual-cell microextrusion bioprinting), and airway splints (laser bioprinting) [128]. An early-stage kidney prototype was also fabricated using microextrusion bioprinting [129]. These examples highlight the integration of multiple bioprinting approaches to achieve functional [130], anatomically relevant tissues [131].

The vision of printing fully functional organs such as kidneys, hearts, or lungs (shown in figure 3.11) demands not only structural mimicry but also integrated vascularization, innervation, and immune compatibility [119]. It is anticipated that in future, bioprinted organoids and mini-tissues will enter routine preclinical testing and drug screening workflows [120]. Fully functional, transplant-ready organs may become a clinical reality within two to three decades, contingent on advancements in biomanufacturing, immunoengineering, and regulatory frameworks. In parallel, bioprinting is being integrated with organ-on-chip systems, enabling the creation of dynamic microenvironments that replicate physiological responses. These hybrid platforms can be used for precision medicine, toxicology testing, and personalized therapy development. As computational power, biofabrication methods, and biological understanding converge, the future of CAD/CAM-guided bioprinting appears not only promising but transformative [121]. While significant technical, collaborative, and conceptual challenges remain, the trajectory of innovation in CAD/CAM bioprinting is aligned with the grand vision of regenerative and precision medicine. Strategic investment in interdisciplinary research, data integration, and adaptive manufacturing platforms will be pivotal in realizing the full potential of bioprinting for next-generation healthcare solutions.

3.7 Conclusion

The integration of CAD and CAM systems has emerged as a cornerstone in the advancement of bioprinting technologies, enabling a transformative shift from static scaffold fabrication to the generation of dynamic, functional biological constructs. CAD/CAM frameworks facilitate precise spatial control over cellular and material placement, allowing researchers to mimic native tissue architecture with unprecedented fidelity. This synergy not only accelerates the prototyping of patient-specific implants and tissues but also enhances reproducibility and scalability, critical prerequisites for clinical translation. The role of CAD/CAM in bioprinting extends beyond geometric modeling; it encompasses a comprehensive pipeline including imaging integration, structural optimization, print-path planning, and process simulation. By bridging anatomical imaging data with print-ready design files, these digital tools create a seamless workflow that is both personalized and biologically informed. With the advent of high-resolution imaging modalities, advanced slicing algorithms, and multimaterial printing strategies, CAD/CAM platforms have evolved to accommodate the complexity inherent in living systems. Importantly, this evolution has laid the groundwork for printing vasculature, tissue gradients, and even organ-specific microarchitectures capabilities that are indispensable for viable organ fabrication.

Technological innovation has been central to these advancements. Machine learning algorithms are now being deployed to automate toolpath optimization, predict print fidelity, and adapt printing parameters in real time based on sensor feedback. Likewise, 4D bioprinting and volumetric fabrication techniques demand a reimagining of CAM frameworks to incorporate temporal dynamics and tomographic control, respectively. These forward-leaning innovations underscore the necessity of continuous evolution in CAD/CAM platforms to keep pace with the multifaceted challenges of biofabrication. However, the translation of bioprinting from bench to bedside is not a purely technological endeavor. It necessitates robust interdisciplinary collaboration among biologists, engineers, clinicians, materials scientists, and regulatory experts. The convergence of these domains fosters innovation that is not only technically sound but also clinically relevant and ethically grounded. Design protocols that integrate biological requirements with engineering constraints, informed by clinician input and patient data, are essential for producing implants and organs that meet real-world needs.

Looking ahead, the promise of CAD/CAM-enabled bioprinting is immense. It holds the potential to redefine therapeutic paradigms by enabling the fabrication of autologous, immunocompatible tissues and organs on demand. In the near term, bioprinted constructs will likely see widespread use in drug screening, disease modeling, and preclinical testing. Over the longer horizon, breakthroughs in vascularization, innervation, and organ-level integration may culminate in the routine clinical use of bioprinted organs – alleviating organ shortages and transforming transplantation medicine. The CAD/CAM systems have transitioned from being mere design tools to becoming integral enablers of regenerative medicine. Their continued refinement, informed by cross-disciplinary insights and empowered by intelligent automation, will be crucial in realizing the full potential of bioprinting. As the field progresses, it is clear that CAD/CAM-guided bioprinting stands at the frontier of biomedical innovation – poised to reshape the landscape of personalized and precision healthcare.

References

[1] G. Huang, Y. Zhao, D. Chen, L. Wei, Z. Hu, J. Li, X. Zhou, B. Yang, Z. Chen, Applications, advancements, and challenges of 3D bioprinting in organ transplantation, Biomater Sci 12 (2024) 1425–1448. https://doi.org/10.1039/D3BM01934A.

[2] H. Chen, B. Zhang, J. Huang, B. Zhang, J. Huang, Recent advances and applications of artificial intelligence in 3D bioprinting, (2024). https://doi.org/10.1063/5.0190208.

[3] G. Huang, Y. Zhao, D. Chen, L. Wei, Z. Hu, J. Li, X. Zhou, B. Yang, Z. Chen, Applications, advancements, and challenges of 3D bioprinting in organ transplantation, Biomater Sci 12 (2024) 1425–1448. https://doi.org/10.1039/D3BM01934A.

[4] P.P. Ikubanni, A.A. Adeleke, O.O. Agboola, C.T. Christopher, B.S. Ademola, J. Okonkwo, O.S. Adesina, P.O. Omoniyi, E.T. Akinlabi, Present and Future Impacts of Computer-Aided Design/Computer-Aided Manufacturing (CAD/CAM), Journal Europeen Des Systemes Automatises 55 (2022) 349–357. https://doi.org/10.18280/JESA.550307.

[5] S.G. Dennis, M.J. Yost, Deposition of Cell-Laden Hydrogels in a Complex Geometry Using a 3D BioPrinter, (1927). https://doi.org/10.1007/s00253-013-4853-6.

[6] P.S. Ginestra, R. Rovetta, A. Fiorentino, E. Ceretti, Bioprinting process optimization: Evaluation of parameters influence on the extrusion of inorganic polymers, Procedia CIRP 89 (2020) 104–109. https://doi.org/10.1016/J.PROCIR.2020.05.125.

[7] A. Rossi, T. Pescara, A.M. Gambelli, F. Gaggia, A. Asthana, Q. Perrier, G. Basta, M. Moretti, N. Senin, F. Rossi, G. Orlando, R. Calafiore, Biomaterials for extrusion-based bioprinting and biomedical applications, Front Bioeng Biotechnol 12 (2024) 1393641. https://doi.org/10.3389/FBIOE.2024.1393641/XML/NLM.

[8] M. Rocca, A. Fragasso, W. Liu, M.A. Heinrich, Y.S. Zhang, Embedded Multimaterial Extrusion Bioprinting, SLAS Technol 23 (2018) 154–163. https://doi.org/10.1177/2472630317742071.

[9] V. Filippou, C. Tsoumpas, Recent advances on the development of phantoms using 3D printing for imaging with CT, MRI, PET, SPECT, and ultrasound, Med Phys 45 (2018) e740–e760. https://doi.org/10.1002/MP.13058,.
[10] R.S. Veeravalli, B. Vejandla, S. Savani, A. Nelluri, N.C. Peddi, Three-Dimensional Bioprinting in Medicine: A Comprehensive Overview of Current Progress and Challenges Faced, Cureus 15 (2023) e41624. https://doi.org/10.7759/CUREUS.41624.
[11] B. Flachsbart, D. Shuey, G.P.-E. of C. Science, undefined 2003, Computer-aided design/computer-aided manufacturing (CAD/CAM), Dl.Acm.Org (n.d..). https://doi.org/10.5555/1074100.1074238.
[12] SandersNorman, An industry perspective on the beginnings of CAD, ACM SIGCSE Bulletin 40 (2008) 128–134. https://doi.org/10.1145/1383602.1383652.
[13] I.E. Sutherland, Sketch pad a man-machine graphical communication system, Proc Des Autom Conf (1964). https://doi.org/10.1145/800265.810742.
[14] N. Sanders, A possible first use of CAM/CAD, IFIP Adv Inf Commun Technol 387 (2012) 43–56. https://doi.org/10.1007/978-3-642-33899-1_3.
[15] I. Susic, M. Travar, M. Susic, The application of CAD / CAM technology in Dentistry, IOP Conf Ser Mater Sci Eng 200 (2017) 012020. https://doi.org/10.1088/1757-899X/200/1/012020.
[16] S. Derakhshanfar, R. Mbeleck, K. Xu, X. Zhang, W. Zhong, M. Xing, 3D bioprinting for biomedical devices and tissue engineering: A review of recent trends and advances, Bioact Mater 3 (2018) 144–156. https://doi.org/10.1016/J.BIOACTMAT.2017.11.008.
[17] I. Donderwinkel, J.C.M. Van Hest, N.R. Cameron, Bio-inks for 3D bioprinting: Recent advances and future prospects, Polym Chem 8 (2017) 4451–4471. https://doi.org/10.1039/C7PY00826K.
[18] R. Pemmada, V.S. Telang, P. Tandon, V. Thomas, Patient-specific mechanical analysis of PCL periodontal membrane: Modeling and simulation, J Mech Behav Biomed Mater 151 (2024) 106397. https://doi.org/10.1016/J.JMBBM.2024.106397.
[19] A. Ahmadi Soufivand, S.J. Lee, T. Jüngst, S. Budday, Challenges and perspectives in using finite element modeling to advance 3D bioprinting, Progress in Biomedical Engineering 7 (2025) 032004. https://doi.org/10.1088/2516-1091/ADDB19.
[20] A. Malekpour, X Chen undefined 2022, Printability and cell viability in extrusion-based bioprinting from experimental, computational, and machine learning views, Journal of Functional Biomaterials, 2022•mdpi.Com (n.d.). https://www.mdpi.com/2079-4983/13/2/40 (accessed September 20, 2025).
[21] S. Freeman, S. Calabro, R. Williams, S. Jin, K. Ye, Bioink formulation and machine learning-empowered bioprinting optimization, Frontiers in Bioengineering and Biotechnology frontiersin. Org 10 (2022). https://doi.org/10.3389/FBIOE.2022.913579/FULL.
[22] R. Rezende, V. Kasyanov, V. Mironov, JVL Da Silva undefined 2015, Organ printing as an information technology, Procedia Engineering, 2015•Elsevier (n.d.). https://www.sciencedirect.com/science/article/pii/S1877705815012643 (accessed September 20, 2025).
[23] P. Kyratsis, K. Kakoulis, A. Markopoulos, Advances in cad/cam/cae technologies, 2020. https://books.google.com/books?hl=en&lr=&id=TSbnDwAAQBAJ&oi=fnd&pg=PP7&dq=Advances+in+CAD/CAM/CAE+Technologies&ots=dsYzBwXoVi&sig=njhjQ9S4gQJlQbK0SOkiz6M4Xtg (accessed September 20, 2025).
[24] P. Ikubanni, A. Adeleke, . . . O.A.-J.E., undefined 2022, Present and future impacts of computer-aided design/computer-aided manufacturing (CAD/CAM), Academia.Edu (n.d.). https://www.academia.edu/download/99758731/55.03_07.pdf (accessed September 20, 2025).
[25] A.u.- Leonardo, undefined 2013, Early Visions of Interactivity: The in (put) s and Out (put) s of Real-Time Computing, Direct.Mit.EduA UttersonLeonardo, 2013•direct.Mit.Edu (n.d.). https://direct.mit.edu/leon/article-abstract/46/1/67/45560 (accessed September 20, 2025).
[26] D.G.-E.W. on R. Techniques, Undefined 1999, Disruptive Technologies in Computer Graphics: Past, Present, and Future, SpringerDP GreenbergEurographics Workshop on Rendering Techniques, 1999•Springer (1999) 1–3. https://doi.org/10.1007/978-3-7091-6809-7_1.

[27] M. Wegner, D. Krause, 3D printed phantoms for medical imaging: Recent developments and challenges, Journal of Mechanical Science and Technology 38 (2024) 4537–4543. https://doi.org/10.1007/S12206-024-2407-8/METRICS.

[28] S. Hatamikia, I. Gulyas, W. Birkfellner, G. Kronreif, A. Unger, G. Oberoi, A. Lorenz, E. Unger, J. Kettenbach, M. Figl, J. Patsch, A. Strassl, D. Georg, A. Renner, Realistic 3D printed CT imaging tumor phantoms for validation of image processing algorithms, Physica Medica 105 (2023) 102512. https://doi.org/10.1016/J.EJMP.2022.102512.

[29] S.T. Gokdeniz, A. Buyuksungur, M.E. Kolsuz, Production of heterogenous bone radiopacity phantom using 3D printing, Phys Eng Sci Med 48 (2024). https://doi.org/10.1007/S13246-024-01500-2,.

[30] K. Baer, Quantitative spectral photon-counting computed Tomography imaging of bone and cartilage degradation in osteoarthritis and repair strategies, (2022). https://ourarchive.otago.ac.nz/esploro/outputs/doctoral/Quantitative-spectral-photon-counting-computed-Tomography-imaging/9926479060901891 (accessed September 20, 2025).

[31] S. Handschuh, U. Reichart, S. Kummer, S. Gabner, B. Ruthensteiner, A. Sombke, T. Schwaha, C.J. Beisser, P. Lemell, D. Haberthür, R. Hlushchuk, R. Glueckert, B.D. Metscher, M. Glösmann, Microscopic dual-energy computed tomography (microDECT) imaging of animal tissues: The colour of X-rays, Methods in Microscopy (2025). https://doi.org/10.1515/MIM-2025-0006.

[32] I. Buchanan, M. Esposito, A. Astolfo, T. Partridge, G. Lioliou, M. Endrizzi, D. Bate, C.H. Hagen, A. Olivo, Fast dual-energy micro-CT with reliable detection of iodine in thin vessels, Biomed Phys Eng Express 11 (2025) 045011. https://doi.org/10.1088/2057-1976/ADDD26.

[33] Y. Wang, 3D-printing inherently MRI-visible accessories in aiding MRI-guided biopsies, 3D Print Med 10 (2024). https://doi.org/10.1186/S41205-024-00227-W,.

[34] H. Haag, P.D. Dalton, V. Bloemen, The Synergy of Biomimetic Design Strategies for Tissue Constructs, Adv Funct Mater 32 (2022) 2201414. https://doi.org/10.1002/ADFM.202201414.

[35] F. Pupilli, A. Ruffini, M. Dapporto, M. Tavoni, A. Tampieri, S. Sprio, Design Strategies and Biomimetic Approaches for Calcium Phosphate Scaffolds in Bone Tissue Regeneration, Biomimetics 2022, Vol. 7, Page 112 7 (2022) 112. https://doi.org/10.3390/BIOMIMETICS7030112.

[36] S.D. Serai, Basics of magnetic resonance imaging and quantitative parameters T1, T2, T2*, T1rho and diffusion-weighted imaging, Pediatr Radiol 52 (2022) 217–227. https://doi.org/10.1007/S00247-021-05042-7/FIGURES/11.

[37] F. Bruno, F. Arrigoni, S. Mariani, A. Splendiani, E. Di Cesare, C. Masciocchi, A. Barile, Advanced magnetic resonance imaging (MRI) of soft tissue tumors: Techniques and applications, Radiologia Medica 124 (2019) 243–252. https://doi.org/10.1007/S11547-019-01035-7/FIGURES/4.

[38] F. Kruggel, D von C.-H. brain mapping, undefined 1999, Temporal properties of the hemodynamic response in functional MRI, Wiley Online LibraryF Kruggel, DY von CramonHuman Brain Mapping, 1999•Wiley Online Library (n.d.). https://doi.org/10.1002/(SICI)1097-0193(1999)8:4.

[39] M.L. Seghier, 7 T and beyond: Toward a synergy between fMRI-based presurgical mapping at ultrahigh magnetic fields, AI, and robotic neurosurgery, Eur Radiol Exp 8 (2024) 1–12. https://doi.org/10.1186/S41747-024-00472-Y/FIGURES/3.

[40] L. Lee, J.M. DeCara, Point-of-Care Ultrasound, Curr Cardiol Rep 22 (2020) 1–10. https://doi.org/10.1007/S11886-020-01394-Y/TABLES/1.

[41] A.M. Hasson, R.D. Patel, C.A. Sissoko, L. Brattain, G.R. Dion, 3D-printed neck phantoms with detailed anatomy for ultrasound-guided procedure and device testing, Laryngoscope Investig Otolaryngol 9 (2024). https://doi.org/10.1002/LIO2.1309,.

[42] J. Seo, Y Sun Kim, Ultrasound imaging and beyond: Recent advances in medical ultrasound, Biomed Eng Lett 7 (2017) 57–58. https://doi.org/10.1007/S13534-017-0030-7/METRICS.

[43] C.J. Harvey, J.M. Pilcher, R.J. Eckersley, M.J.K. Blomley, D.O. Cosgrove, Advances in ultrasound, Clin Radiol 57 (2002) 157–177. https://doi.org/10.1053/crad.2001.0918.

[44] A. Butt, H. Bach, Nanomedicine and clinical diagnostics part I: Applications in conventional imaging (MRI, X-ray/CT, and ultrasound), Nanomedicine 20 (2025) 167–182. https://doi.org/10.1080/17435889.2024.2439776.
[45] F. Alshomrani, Recent Advances in Magnetic Resonance Imaging for the Diagnosis of Liver Cancer: A Comprehensive Review, Diagnostics 2025, Vol. 15, Page 2016 15 (2025) 2016. https://doi.org/10.3390/DIAGNOSTICS15162016.
[46] B. VanBerlo, J. Hoey, A. Wong, A survey of the impact of self-supervised pretraining for diagnostic tasks in medical X-ray, CT, MRI, and ultrasound, BMC Medical Imaging 2024 24:1 24 (2024) 1–24. https://doi.org/10.1186/S12880-024-01253-0.
[47] T.B. Nguyen-Tat, T.Q. Hung, P.T. Nam, V.M. Ngo, Evaluating pre-processing and deep learning methods in medical imaging: Combined effectiveness across multiple modalities, Alexandria Engineering Journal 119 (2025) 558–586. https://doi.org/10.1016/J.AEJ.2025.01.090.
[48] H. Hyun, C.c.-t.e. and R. Medicine, Undefined 2019, Updates in Molecular Imaging Techniques, SpringerH Hyun, CS Cho Tissue Engineering and Regenerative Medicine, 2019•Springer 16 (2019) 431–432. https://doi.org/10.1007/S13770-019-00222-X.
[49] G. Zhu, B. Jiang, L. Tong, Y. Xie, G. Zaharchuk, M. Wintermark, Applications of deep learning to neuro-imaging techniques, Front Neurol 10 (2019) 459874. https://doi.org/10.3389/FNEUR.2019.00869/BIBTEX.
[50] K. Fetah, P. Tebon, M.J. Goudie, J. Eichenbaum, L. Ren, N. Barros, R. Nasiri, S. Ahadian, N. Ashammakhi, M.R. Dokmeci, A. Khademhosseini, The emergence of 3D bioprinting in organ-on-chip systems, Progress in Biomedical Engineering 1 (2019) 012001. https://doi.org/10.1088/2516-1091/AB23DF.
[51] F. Yu, D. Choudhury, Microfluidic bioprinting for organ-on-a-chip models, Drug Discov Today 24 (2019) 1248–1257. https://doi.org/10.1016/J.DRUDIS.2019.03.025.
[52] M. Allenby, M.W.-J. of C. Fibrosis, undefined 2019, Biofabrication of personalised anatomical models and tools for the clinic, Cysticfibrosisjournal.Com (n.d.). https://www.cysticfibrosisjournal.com/article/S1569-1993(19)30023-2/fulltext (accessed September 22, 2025).
[53] D.W.-J. of 3D P. in Medicine, undefined 2017, Translation of 3D bioprinting into medical practice: Learning from related fields to focus our efforts, Taylor & FrancisDJ Williams Journal of 3D Printing in Medicine, 2017•Taylor & Francis 1 (2017) 3–4. https://doi.org/10.2217/3DP.15.1.
[54] A. MacAdam, E. Chaudry, C.D. McTiernan, D. Cortes, E.J. Suuronen, E.I. Alarcon, Development of in situ bioprinting: A mini review, Frontiers in Bioengineering and Biotechnology, 2022•frontiersin.Org 10 (2022). https://doi.org/10.3389/FBIOE.2022.940896/FULL.
[55] S. Rahmani Dabbagh, M. Rezapour Sarabi, M.T. Birtek, N. Mustafaoglu, Y.S. Zhang, S. Tasoglu, 3D bioprinted organ-on-chips, Aggregate 4 (2023) e197. https://doi.org/10.1002/AGT2.197.
[56] I. Ludwig, A. Ernst, . . . P.G.-T. on, undefined 2019, Clinical workflow in medical additive manufacturing, Journals.Infinite-Science.DeI Ludwig, A Ernst, P Gromzig, J Wolff Transactions on Additive Manufacturing Meets Medicine, 2019•journals.Infinite-Science.De 1 (2019) 1–02. https://doi.org/10.18416/AMMM.2019.1909S01T02.
[57] D.W.-J. of 3D P. in Medicine, undefined 2017, Translation of 3D bioprinting into medical practice: Learning from related fields to focus our efforts, Taylor & FrancisDJ WilliamsJournal of 3D Printing in Medicine, 2017•Taylor & Francis 1 (2017) 3–4. https://doi.org/10.2217/3DP.15.1.
[58] S. Narayan, S.M.-I.J. of, undefined 2023, An approach for radiation dose reduction in computerized tomography, Academia.EduSB Narayan, SH Mahabaleshwara International Journal of Electrical and Computer Engineering, 2023 academia.Edu (n.d.). https://www.academia.edu/download/94382583/112_27348_EMr_23Sep22_2feb22_N.pdf (accessed September 22, 2025).
[59] M.J. Mackinnon, S. Song, T.-H.H. Chao, L.-M. Hsu, S.T. Albert, Y. Ma, T. Shnitko, T.-W.W. Wang, R.J. Nonneman, C.D. Freeman, S.S. Ozarkar, U.E. Emir, M.D. Shen, B.D. Philpot, A.W. Hantman, S.-H.

Lee, W.-T. Chang, Y.-Y.I. Shih, SORDINO for Silent, Sensitive, Specific, and Artifact-Resisting fMRI in awake behaving mice, BioRxiv (2025) 2025.03.10.642406. https://doi.org/10.1101/2025.03.10.642406.
[60] Y.-H. Tung, Highly-accelerated diffusion magnetic resonance imaging at ultrahigh field, (2024). https://doi.org/10.25673/118929.
[61] D. Vilimek, J. Kubicek, M. Golian, R. Jaros, R. Kahankova, P. Hanzlikova, D. Barvik, A. Krestanova, M. Penhaker, M. Cerny, O. Prokop, M. Buzga, Comparative analysis of wavelet transform filtering systems for noise reduction in ultrasound images, PLoS One 17 (2022) e0270745. https://doi.org/10.1371/JOURNAL.PONE.0270745.
[62] S. Sharma, S. Rani, A. Dogra, M.W. Bhatt, Edge-aware multisensor brain image fusion via guided filtering in Laplacian domain, Discover Artificial Intelligence 5 (2025) 1–34. https://doi.org/10.1007/S44163-025-00446-Y/FIGURES/16.
[63] B. Maiseli, Nonlinear anisotropic diffusion methods for image denoising problems: Challenges and future research opportunities, Array 17 (2023) 100265. https://doi.org/10.1016/J.ARRAY.2022.100265.
[64] A.A. Yahya, J. Tan, B. Su, K. Liu, A.N. Hadi, Image edge detection method based on anisotropic diffusion and total variation models, The Journal of Engineering 2019 (2019) 455–460. https://doi.org/10.1049/JOE.2018.5345.
[65] J. Weickert, B.g.t. Stuttgart, Anisotropic Diffusion in Image Processing, (n.d.).
[66] H. S. Kim and Y. J. Cho, "Anisotropic diffusion for preserving boundary-edge," 2010 12th International Conference on Advanced Communication Technology (ICACT), Gangwon-Do, South Korea, 2010, pp. 375–378.
[67] N. Joshi and S. Jain, "An Improved Anisotropic Diffusion Filtering Approach for noise reduction in MRI," 2021 9th International Conference on Reliability, Infocom Technologies and Optimization (Trends and Future Directions) (ICRITO), Noida, India, 2021, pp. 1022–1027, doi: 10.1109/ICRITO51393.2021.9596244.
[68] Kubicek, J., Strycek, M., Cerny, M., Penhaker, M., Prokop, O., & Vilimek, D. (2021). Quantitative and comparative analysis of effectiveness and robustness for enhanced and optimized non-local mean filter combining pixel and patch information on MR images of musculoskeletal system. Sensors, 21(12), 4161. https://doi.org/10.3390/s21124161.
[69] Z. Li, Image Denoising based on Deep Learning, Highlights in Science, Engineering and Technology 39 (2023) 1245–1251. https://doi.org/10.54097/HSET.V39I.6749.
[70] H. Kang, C. Park, H. Yang, Evaluation of Denoising Performance of ResNet Deep Learning Model for Ultrasound Images Corresponding to Two Frequency Parameters, Bioengineering 11 (2024) 723. https://doi.org/10.3390/BIOENGINEERING11070723.
[71] W.C. Wang, E. Ahn, D. Feng, J. Kim, A review of predictive and contrastive self-supervised learning for medical images, Machine Intelligence Research, 2023 Springer 20 (2023) 483–513. https://doi.org/10.1007/S11633-022-1406-4.
[72] W. Du, H. Chen, H. Yang, Y. Zhang, Disentangled generative adversarial network for low-dose CT, EURASIP J Adv Signal Process 2021 (2021) 1–16. https://doi.org/10.1186/S13634-021-00749-Z/TABLES/4.
[73] J. Sun, Y. Du, C.Y. Li, T.H. Wu, B.H. Yang, G.S.P. Mok, Pix2Pix generative adversarial network for low dose myocardial perfusion SPECT denoising, Quant Imaging Med Surg 12 (2022) 3539–3555. https://doi.org/10.21037/QIMS-21-1042/COIF).
[74] Q. Huang, Y. Xian, D. Yang, H. Qu, J. Yi, P. Wu, D.N. Metaxas, Dynamic MRI reconstruction with end-to-end motion-guided network, Med Image Anal 68 (2021). https://doi.org/10.1016/j.media.2020.101901.
[75] K. Ranat, H. Phan, S. Ellythy, M. Kenter, A. Akkouch, Advancements in Musculoskeletal Tissue Engineering: The Role of Melt Electrowriting in 3D-Printed Scaffold Fabrication, Journal of Functional Biomaterials 2025, Vol. 16, Page 163 16 (2025) 163. https://doi.org/10.3390/JFB16050163.

[76] X. Li, Y. Jiang, J.J. Rodriguez-Andina, H. Luo, S. Yin, O. Kaynak, When medical images meet generative adversarial network: Recent development and research opportunities, Discover Artificial Intelligence 1 (2021) 1–20. https://doi.org/10.1007/S44163-021-00006-0/TABLES/4.

[77] S. Bin Park, Advances in deep learning for computed tomography denoising, World J Clin Cases 9 (2021) 7614. https://doi.org/10.12998/WJCC.V9.I26.7614.

[78] P. Ravi, Advanced Image Segmentation and Modeling – A Review of the 2021–2022 Thematic Series, 3D Print Med 9 (2023) 1–5. https://doi.org/10.1186/S41205-022-00163-7/FIGURES/6.

[79] Y. Yu, C. Wang, Q. Fu, R. Kou, F. Huang, B. Yang, T. Yang, M. Gao, Techniques and Challenges of Image Segmentation: A Review, Electronics 2023, Vol. 12, Page 1199 12 (2023) 1199. https://doi.org/10.3390/ELECTRONICS12051199.

[80] I. Domingues, G. Pereira, P. Martins, H. Duarte, J. Santos, P.H. Abreu, Using deep learning techniques in medical imaging: A systematic review of applications on CT and PET, Artif Intell Rev 53 (2020) 4093–4160. https://doi.org/10.1007/S10462-019-09788-3/TABLES/7.

[81] F. Neha, D. Bhati, D.K. Shukla, S.M. Dalvi, N. Mantzou, S. Shubbar, U-Net in Medical Image Segmentation: A Review of Its Applications Across Modalities, (2024). https://arxiv.org/pdf/2412.02242 (accessed September 23, 2025).

[82] N.S. Punn, S. Agarwal, Modality specific U-Net variants for biomedical image segmentation: A survey, Artif Intell Rev 55 (2022) 5845–5889. https://doi.org/10.1007/S10462-022-10152-1/FIGURES/8.

[83] W. Jiangtao, N.I.R. Ruhaiyem, F. Panpan, A Comprehensive Review of U-Net and Its Variants: Advances and Applications in Medical Image Segmentation, IET Image Process 19 (2025) e70019. https://doi.org/10.1049/IPR2.70019.

[84] Y. Zhang, Q. Yang, T. Li, F. Zhang, Y. Ren, Y. Li, C. Xu, V-UNet: Medical Image Segmentation Based on Variational Attention Mechanism, CAAI Trans Intell Technol (2025). https://doi.org/10.1049/CIT2.70053.

[85] U. Khan, A.U. Yasin, M. Abid, I.S. Awan, S.A. Khan, A Methodological Review of 3D Reconstruction Techniques in Tomographic Imaging, J Med Syst 42 (2018) 1–12. https://doi.org/10.1007/S10916-018-1042-2/FIGURES/12.

[86] A. Tewari, J. Thies, B. Mildenhall, P. Srinivasan, E. Tretschk, W. Yifan, C. Lassner, V. Sitzmann, R. Martin-Brualla, S. Lombardi, T. Simon, C. Theobalt, M. Nießner, J.T. Barron, G. Wetzstein, M. Zollhöfer, V. Golyanik, Advances in Neural Rendering, Computer Graphics Forum 41 (2022) 703–735. https://doi.org/10.1111/CGF.14507.

[87] W. Zhang, W. Jin, S. Rho, F. Jiang, C. fu Yang, A Federated Learning Framework for Brain Tumor Segmentation Without Sharing Patient Data, Int J Imaging Syst Technol 34 (2024) e23147. https://doi.org/10.1002/IMA.23147.

[88] F. Górski, Computer Aided Design of 3D Printable Anatomically Shaped Medical Devices: Methodologies and Applications, Computer Aided Design of 3D Printable Anatomically Shaped Medical Devices: Methodologies and Applications (2025) 1–356. https://doi.org/10.1201/9781003386544/COMPUTER-AIDED-DESIGN-3D-PRINTABLE-ANATOMICALLY-SHAPED-MEDICAL-DEVICES-FILIP-GORSKI/RIGHTS-AND-PERMISSIONS.

[89] A.H. Foroughi, C. Valeri, M.J. Razavi, A review of computational optimization of bone scaffold architecture: Methods, challenges, and perspectives, Progress in Biomedical Engineering 7 (2024) 012003. https://doi.org/10.1088/2516-1091/AD879A.

[90] R. Pemmada, V.S. Telang, P. Tandon, V. Thomas, Patient-specific mechanical analysis of PCL periodontal membrane: Modeling and simulation, J Mech Behav Biomed Mater 151 (2024) 106397. https://doi.org/10.1016/J.JMBBM.2024.106397.

[91] A. Jean, G.C. Engelmayr, Finite element analysis of an accordion-like honeycomb scaffold for cardiac tissue engineering, J Biomech 43 (2010) 3035–3043. https://doi.org/10.1016/J.JBIOMECH.2010.06.032.

[92] M. Abbasi, M.S. Barakat, K. Vahidkhah, A.N. Azadani, Characterization of three-dimensional anisotropic heart valve tissue mechanical properties using inverse finite element analysis, J Mech Behav Biomed Mater 62 (2016) 33–44. https://doi.org/10.1016/J.JMBBM.2016.04.031.

[93] A. Salih, F. Hamandi, T. Goswami, Advancements in Finite Element Modeling for Cardiac Device Leads and 3D Heart Models, Bioengineering 2024, Vol. 11, Page 564 11 (2024) 564. https://doi.org/10.3390/BIOENGINEERING11060564.

[94] M.S. Chaudhry, A. Czekanski, Surface slicing and toolpath planning for in-situ bioprinting of skin implants, Biofabrication 16 (2024) 025030. https://doi.org/10.1088/1758-5090/AD30C4.

[95] S.J. Lee, W. Jeong, A. Atala, 3D Bioprinting for Engineered Tissue Constructs and Patient-Specific Models: Current Progress and Prospects in Clinical Applications, Advanced Materials 36 (2024) 2408032. https://doi.org/10.1002/ADMA.202408032.

[96] C.D. Fay, Computer-Aided Design and Manufacturing (CAD/CAM) for Bioprinting, Methods in Molecular Biology 2140 (2020) 27–41. https://doi.org/10.1007/978-1-0716-0520-2_3.

[97] V.S. Telang, R. Pemmada, V. Thomas, S. Ramakrishna, P. Tandon, H.S. Nanda, Harnessing additive manufacturing for magnesium-based metallic bioimplants: Recent advances and future perspectives, Curr Opin Biomed Eng 17 (2021) 100264. https://doi.org/10.1016/J.COBME.2021.100264.

[98] K. Pawar, V. Telang, H.Y. Shahare, P. Tandon, Numerical Analysis of Progressive Cavity Pump Extruder for 3D Printing of High Viscosity Ceramic Paste, Comput Aided Des Appl 21 (2024) 171–178. https://doi.org/10.14733/CADAPS.2024.171-178.

[99] S. Jentsch, R. Nasehi, C. Kuckelkorn, B. Gundert, S. Aveic, H. Fischer, S. Jentsch, R. Nasehi, C. Kuckelkorn, B. Gundert, S. Aveic, H. Fischer, Multiscale 3D bioprinting by nozzle-free acoustic droplet ejection, Wiley Online Library 5 (2021). https://doi.org/10.1002/SMTD.202000971.

[100] Y. Zhang, B. Wang, J. Hu, T. Yin, T Yue, N Liu . . . undefined 2020, 3D composite bioprinting for fabrication of artificial biological tissues, International Journal of Bioprinting, 2020•pmc.Ncbi.Nlm. Nih.Gov (n.d.). https://pmc.ncbi.nlm.nih.gov/articles/PMC7875057/ (accessed September 23, 2025).

[101] B. Zhang, Y. Luo, L. Ma, L. Gao, Y. Li, Q. Xue, H. Yang, Z. Cui, 3D Bioprinting: An Emerging Technology Full of Opportunities and Challenges, Springer 1 (2018) 2–13. https://doi.org/10.1007/S42242-018-0004-3.

[102] V.B.-I.J. of A.R. in, undefined 2017, The Role and Challenges of Compression in Medical Image Communication., Academia.EduVK BairagiInternational Journal of Advanced Research in Computer Science, 2017•academia.Edu (n.d.). https://www.academia.edu/download/88343112/3647-8148-1-PB.pdf (accessed September 23, 2025).

[103] A.A. Giannopoulos, T. Pietila, Post-processing of DICOM Images, 3D Printing in Medicine: A Practical Guide for Medical Professionals (2017) 23–34. https://doi.org/10.1007/978-3-319-61924-8_3.

[104] T.M. Bücking, E.R. Hill, J.L. Robertson, E. Maneas, A.A. Plumb, D.I. Nikitichev, From medical imaging data to 3D printed anatomical models, PloS One, journals.Plos.Org 12 (2017). https://doi.org/10.1371/JOURNAL.PONE.0178540.

[105] Real-time adaptive control of additive manufacturing processes using machine learning, (2017).

[106] A. Hasselgren, P.K. Wan, M. Horn, K. Kralevska, D. Gligoroski, A. Faxvaag, GDPR Compliance for Blockchain Applications in Healthcare, (2020) 23–35. https://doi.org/10.5121/csit.2020.101303.

[107] S.J. Lee, W. Jeong, A. Atala, 3D Bioprinting for Engineered Tissue Constructs and Patient-Specific Models: Current Progress and Prospects in Clinical Applications, Advanced Materials 36 (2024) 2408032. https://doi.org/10.1002/ADMA.202408032.

[108] A.M. Jorgensen, J.J. Yoo, A. Atala, Solid Organ Bioprinting: Strategies to Achieve Organ Function, Chem Rev 120 (2020) 11093–11127. https://doi.org/10.1021/ACS.CHEMREV.0C00145.

[109] A. Schwab, R. Levato, M. D'Este, S. Piluso, D. Eglin, J. Malda, Printability and Shape Fidelity of Bioinks in 3D Bioprinting, Chem Rev 120 (2020) 11028–11055. https://doi.org/10.1021/ACS.CHEMREV.0C00084.

[110] C. Mota, S. Camarero-Espinosa, M.B. Baker, P. Wieringa, L. Moroni, Bioprinting: From Tissue and Organ Development to in Vitro Models, Chem Rev 120 (2020) 10547–10607. https://doi.org/10.1021/ACS.CHEMREV.9B00789.
[111] E. Davoodi, E. Sarikhani, H. Montazerian, S. Ahadian, M. Costantini, W. Swieszkowski, S.M. Willerth, K. Walus, M. Mofidfar, E. Toyserkani, A. Khademhosseini, N. Ashammakhi, Extrusion and microfluidic-based bioprinting to fabricate biomimetic tissues and organs Advanced Materials Technologies, 2020•Wiley Online Library 5 (2020). https://doi.org/10.1002/ADMT.201901044.
[112] E. Davoodi, E. Sarikhani, H. Montazerian, S. Ahadian, M. Costantini, W. Swieszkowski, S.M. Willerth, K. Walus, M. Mofidfar, E. Toyserkani, A. Khademhosseini, N. Ashammakhi, Extrusion and Microfluidic-Based Bioprinting to Fabricate Biomimetic Tissues and Organs, Adv Mater Technol 5 (2020) 1901044. https://doi.org/10.1002/ADMT.201901044.
[113] J. Yang, P.b.-t. on Additive, undefined 2020, Novel co-axial extrusion printing head for tissue engineering, Journals.Infinite-Science.DeJ Yang, P Bartolo Transactions on Additive Manufacturing Meets Medicine, 2020 journals.Infinite-Science.De 2 (2020). https://doi.org/10.18416/AMMM.2020.2009023.
[114] C. Mota, S. Camarero-Espinosa, M.B. Baker, P. Wieringa, L. Moroni, Bioprinting: From Tissue and Organ Development to in Vitro Models, Chemical Reviews, 2020•ACS Publications 120 (2020) 10547–10607. https://doi.org/10.1021/ACS.CHEMREV.9B00789.
[115] L. Mendoza-Cerezo, . . . M.j.-i., undefined 2023, Evolution of bioprinting and current applications, Pmc.Ncbi.Nlm.Nih.GovL Mendoza-Cerezo, MRR Jesús, A Macías-García, AC Marcos-Romero, A Díaz-Parralejo International Journal of Bioprinting, 2023•pmc.Ncbi.Nlm.Nih.Gov (n.d.). https://pmc.ncbi.nlm.nih.gov/articles/PMC10261138/ (accessed September 23, 2025).
[116] P. Ikubanni, A. Adeleke, . . . O.A.-J.E., undefined 2022, Present and future impacts of computer-aided design/computer-aided manufacturing (CAD/CAM), Academia.Edu (n.d.). https://www.academia.edu/download/99758731/55.03_07.pdf (accessed September 23, 2025).
[117] N. Ashammakhi, S. Ahadian, F. Zengjie, K. Suthiwanich, F. Lorestani, G. Orive, S. Ostrovidov, A. Khademhosseini, Advances and future perspectives in 4D bioprinting, Biotechnology Journal, 2018 Wiley Online Library 13 (2018). https://doi.org/10.1002/BIOT.201800148.
[118] S. Mohammadi, G. Cidonio, Unravelling hierarchical patterning of biomaterial inks with 3D microfluidic-assisted spinning: A paradigm shift in bioprinting technologies, Frontiers in Biomaterials Science 2 (2023) 1279061. https://doi.org/10.3389/FBIOM.2023.1279061.
[119] S. Aminabee, Printing Organs with 3D Technology, Integrating Metaheuristics in Computer Vision for Real-World Optimization Problems (2024) 55–70. https://doi.org/10.1002/9781394230952.CH3.
[120] G. Zhang, T. Zhang, F.F. Yin, A roadmap for the implementation of 3D-printed organs in healthcare, Device 0 (2025). https://doi.org/10.1016/J.DEVICE.2025.100847.
[121] M.W. Ullah, M. Ul-Islam, A. Shehzad, S. Manan, S.U. Islam, A. Fatima, A.K. Al-Saidi, M.E.H. El Nokab, J.Q. Sanchez, K.O. Sebakhy, From Bioinks to Functional Tissues and Organs: Advances, Challenges, and the Promise of 3D Bioprinting, Macromol Mater Eng (2025) e00251. https://doi.org/10.1002/MAME.202500251.
[122] J.Y. Ha, H.J. Baek, K.H. Ryu, B.H. Choi, J. Il Moon, S.E. Park, T.B. Kim, J.Y. Ha, H.J. Baek, K.H. Ryu, B.H. Choi, J. Il Moon, S.E. Park, T.B. Kim, One-Minute Ultrafast Brain MRI With Full Basic Sequences: Can It Be a Promising Way Forward for Pediatric Neuroimaging?, https://Www.Ajronline.Org/ 215 (2020) 198–205. https://doi.org/10.2214/AJR.19.22378.
[123] J. Dudink, S. Jeanne Steggerda, S. Horsch, T. Agut, A. Alarcon, R. Arena, M. Bartocci, M. Bravo, F. Cabañas, N. Carreras, O. Claris, J. Dudink, M. Fumagalli, P. Govaert, S. Horsch, A. Parodi, A. Pellicer, L. Ramenghi, C.C. Roehr, S. Steggerda, E. Valverde, State-of-the-art neonatal cerebral ultrasound: Technique and reporting., Pediatr Res 87 (2020) 3–12. https://doi.org/10.1038/S41390-020-0776-Y.

[124] A. Fajar, R. Sarno, C. Fatichah, A. Fahmi, Reconstructing and resizing 3D images from DICOM files, Journal of King Saud University – Computer and Information Sciences 34 (2022) 3517–3526. https://doi.org/10.1016/J.JKSUCI.2020.12.004.
[125] T. Kamio, M. Suzuki, R. Asaumi, T. Kawai, DICOM segmentation and STL creation for 3D printing: A process and software package comparison for osseous anatomy, 3D Print Med 6 (2020) 1–12. https://doi.org/10.1186/S41205-020-00069-2/FIGURES/10.
[126] X. Cui, K. Breitenkamp, M.G. Finn, M. Lotz, D.D. D'Lima, Direct human cartilage repair using three-dimensional bioprinting technology, Tissue Engineering Part A, 2012 liebertpub.Com 18 (2012) 1304–1312. https://doi.org/10.1089/TEN.TEA.2011.0543.
[127] F. Marga, K. Jakab, C. Khatiwala, . . . B.S.-, undefined 2012, Toward engineering functional organ modules by additive manufacturing, Biofabrication. Iopscience.Iop.OrgF Marga, K Jakab, C Khatiwala, B Shepherd, S Dorfman, B Hubbard, S Colbert, G Forgacs, 2012•iopscience.Iop.Org (n.d.). https://doi.org/10.1088/1758-5082/4/2/022001/META.
[128] B. Duan, L.A. Hockaday, K.H. Kang, J.T. Butcher, 3D bioprinting of heterogeneous aortic valve conduits with alginate/gelatin hydrogels, Wiley Online LibraryB Duan, LA Hockaday, KH Kang, JT Butcher Journal of Biomedical Materials Research Part A, 2013 Wiley Online Library 101 A (2013) 1255–1264. https://doi.org/10.1002/JBM.A.34420.
[129] D. Zopf, S. Hollister, . . . M.N.-N.E.J., undefined 2013, Bioresorbable airway splint created with a three-dimensional printer, Mass Medical SocDA Zopf, SJ Hollister, ME Nelson, RG Ohye, GE GreenNew England Journal of Medicine, 2013 Mass Medical Soc (n.d.). https://doi.org/10.1056/NEJMC1206319.
[130] F. Marga, K. Jakab, C. Khatiwala, . . . B.S.-, undefined 2012, Toward engineering functional organ modules by additive manufacturing, Biofabrication. Iopscience.Iop.OrgF Marga, K Jakab, C Khatiwala, B Shepherd, S Dorfman, B Hubbard, S Colbert, G Forgacs, 2012•iopscience.Iop.Org (n.d.). https://doi.org/10.1088/1758-5082/4/2/022001/META.
[131] B. Duan, L.A. Hockaday, K.H. Kang, J.T. Butcher, 3D bioprinting of heterogeneous aortic valve conduits with alginate/gelatin hydrogels, Journal of Biomedical Materials Research Part A, 2013 Wiley Online Library 101 A (2013) 1255–1264. https://doi.org/10.1002/JBM.A.34420.

Samir Das, Prerana Singh, Ruchi Kaul Pathak, Jonali Das, Pameli Jana, Bidyanand Mahto, Sudipto Datta*

Chapter 4
Advanced Biomaterials for Extrusion-Based Bioprinting: Scaffold Design and Cellular Compatibility

Abstract: Bioprinting has wide applicability in generating three-dimensional living tissue constructs, replicating both the structure of real tissue and its biological function. Extrusion-based bioprinting constructs structures with defined mechanical properties, as the technique affords the creation of laminations and layering of bioinks. Patient-specific tissue constructs, implants, and disease and drug test models can be manufactured. Bioprinting can use a heterogeneous mix of bioinks with different polymer characteristics, cells, and additives that need to be extruded with control, in either pneumatic, screw, or piston extruders, for the construction of complex, robust tissue constructs. To achieve successful bioprinting, print resolution, print speed, cell viability, and the composition of bioinks need to be determined. During the bioprinting process, the bioinks also need to be compatible with the bioprinting methods and with tissue engineering, and then closely controlled during cross-linked post extrusion for bioprinting to achieve functional tissue constructs. Bioprinting has to improve cell viability/end-cell apoptosis, custom no bioink cross-linking methods, and bioprinting resolution and speed. New methods to control bioprinting, including coaxial or multi-material approaches, 4D bioprinting, and the use of AI have the potential to significantly improve the ability to bioprint in clinically relevant sizes and have a functional construct ready for implantation. Out of all the possible platforms in bioprinting, extrusion appears to be the most relevant in generating the bioprinting constructs needed for regenerative medicine, where the speed and throughput are more important than the resolution.

***Corresponding author: Sudipto Datta,** Reconstructive Healthcare Solutions IMT, Faridabad 121004, Haryana; Department of Surgery, All India Institute of Medical Sciences, New Delhi 110029, India, e-mail: sudiptodatta1990@gmail.com
Samir Das, School of Medical Science and Technology, Indian Institute of Technology Kharagpur, Kharagpur 721302, West Bengal, India
Prerana Singh, Department of Bioengineering, Indian Institute of Science Bangalore, Bengaluru 560012, India
Ruchi Kaul Pathak, Reconstructive Healthcare Solutions IMT, Faridabad 121004, Haryana; Department of Surgery, All India Institute of Medical Sciences, New Delhi 110029, India
Jonali Das, Raja Peary Mohan College, Hooghly, Uttarpara 712258, West Bengal
Pameli Jana, Sri Shankara Cancer Foundation, Bengaluru 560004, Karnataka
Bidyanand Mahto, Government Engineering College, Vaishali (Under Department of Science, Technology and Technical Education, Government of Bihar), Vaishali 844115, Bihar, India

 | https://doi.org/10.1515/9783111719993-004

Keywords: Extrusion-based bioprinting, bioinks, tissue engineering, cross-linking, regenerative medicine

4.1 Introduction

Extrusion-based bioprinting is one of the most widely used additive manufacturing approaches for fabricating three-dimensional biological constructs that closely represent the tissue architecture and function of living tissues. It enables the accurate deposition of cell-laden biomaterials, known as bioinks, through a controlled extrusion nozzle [1]. By following a digital design, the printer builds multilayered structures that provide a supportive microenvironment for cellular organization, differentiation, and tissue maturation [2]. This technology has gained strong momentum in biomedical engineering because it offers material versatility, allows high cell loading, and can create patient-specific constructs that align with personalized medical needs [3]. It also combines engineering principles with biological requirements. The process typically uses pneumatic pressure, mechanical pistons, or screw-driven systems to push bioinks through a fine nozzle [4]. The extruded filaments are deposited in a predefined pattern and gradually form a stable three-dimensional geometry. During or after printing, cross-linking is applied to solidify the printed layers and maintain mechanical integrity [5, 6]. This workflow is well-suited for hydrogels, thermoplastic polymers, and composite bioinks that mimic the physical and biochemical properties of native extracellular matrix [6].

The relevance of extrusion-based bioprinting in tissue engineering is linked to its compatibility with a broad range of materials and cell types [7]. Natural polymers such as alginate, gelatin, collagen, and hyaluronic acid provide favorable biological cues but often lack mechanical strength [8]. Synthetic polymers, including polyethylene glycol [9] and polycaprolactone [10], offer tunable properties and slower degradation. Blended or reinforced bioinks combine these advantages and support load-bearing tissues such as bone and cartilage. The selection of suitable bioinks is closely tied to printability, rheological behavior, biocompatibility, and post-printing cell viability. Another reason for increasing interest in this technique is its ability to fabricate constructs of clinically relevant size [11–13].

Other methods, including inkjet bioprinting or laser-assisted printing, offer high resolution but struggle with high viscosity materials and high cell densities [14]. Extrusion systems do not face these limitations, which enables the development of thick, heterogeneous structures with controlled microarchitectures, internal channels, and porosity. These features are essential for the diffusion of nutrients and oxygen, especially in large constructs intended for regenerative medicine [15, 16].

Extrusion-based bioprinting has transformed preclinical research and personalized treatment strategies [17]. In regenerative medicine, it is employed to fabricate bone grafts, cartilage implants, vascular grafts, skin substitutes, and soft tissues for reconstructive surgery [18]. In pharmacological testing, patient-derived tissues allow more accurate drug response evaluation and disease modeling by reducing the reliance on animal studies. The long-term vision is to produce fully functional, vascularized organs suitable for transplantation, although this goal still faces significant technical and biological challenges. Continued progress depends on improvements in bioink development, printing resolution, automation, and cell viability control [19]. Integration with imaging, artificial intelligence, and microfluidic technologies is expected to enhance fabrication precision and accelerate clinical translation. Overall, extrusion-based bioprinting stands as a foundational tool in modern biofabrication and continues to shape the future of tissue engineering and personalized healthcare [20].

4.2 Principles of Extrusion Bioprinting

Extrusion-based bioprinting operates on the principle of controlled material flow, in which bioinks are extruded through a nozzle by the application of mechanical force. This printing modality closely integrates engineering design with biological requirements, making it suitable for constructing tissues with defined geometry and biological function. The technique is driven by computer-aided design (CAD) [21], enabling the precise reproduction of complex structures derived from patient imaging data, such as CT or MRI scans [22]. Through defined toolpaths, extrusion bioprinters deposit continuous filaments to build three-dimensional constructs that can support cell adhesion, proliferation, and tissue organization.

4.2.1 Basic Working Mechanism

The process begins with a digital 3D model, which is sliced into individual layers using specialized software. The printer interprets this data to guide nozzle movement along the X, Y, and Z axes [23]. Mechanical pressure pushes the bioink through the nozzle as a continuous filament, rather than as discrete droplets, allowing the formation of stable strands. Shear-thinning properties of many bioinks help them flow easily through the nozzle and regain viscosity, upon deposition. The printed filaments accumulate layer by layer, forming a construct with internal porosity that supports nutrient transport and cellular communication [24].

4.2.2 Components of Extrusion Systems

A typical extrusion bioprinter includes a material reservoir that maintains the bioink under controlled pressure and temperature, an extrusion mechanism such as pneumatic, piston-driven, or screw-driven systems to regulate flow, and a nozzle assembly that sets filament diameter and affects the shear stress experienced by cells, as depicted in Figure 4.1. It also features temperature control units to support thermosensitive materials, a motor-controlled

Stage, or printhead for accurate positioning, guided by CAD instructions, and a cross-linking system that stabilizes the printed structure through chemical, thermal, or photoinitiated methods. Together, these components must work in synchrony to ensure print fidelity, structural stability, and high cell viability [25].

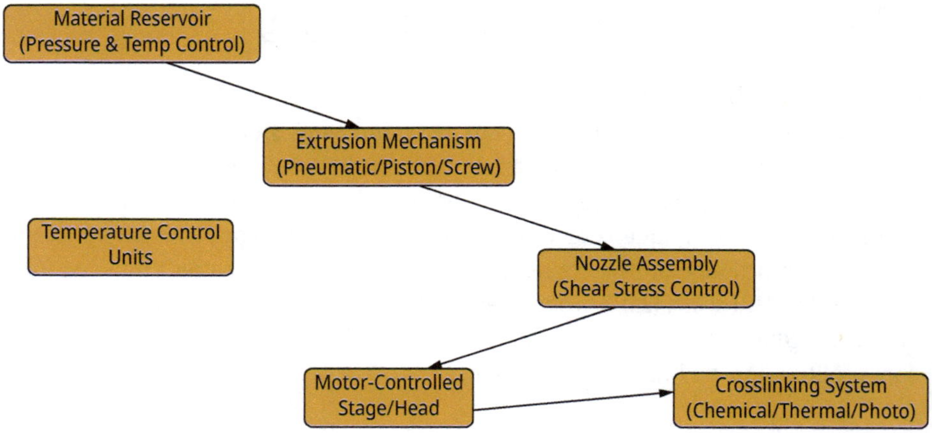

Figure 4.1: Key components and functional layout of a typical extrusion bioprinter.

4.2.3 Layer-by-Layer Fabrication

The core principle of extrusion bioprinting is additive manufacturing. Each printed layer serves as the foundation for subsequent deposition, forming a volumetric construct. The thickness of individual layers depends on the nozzle diameter, flow rate, and bioink rheology. Insufficient viscosity may result in filament spreading and loss of shape accuracy, while excessive viscosity may cause nozzle clogging or high shear stress that damages cells. Therefore, optimizing printing parameters is necessary to achieve structural integrity without compromising cellular health [26].

4.2.4 Cross-Linking Methods

Post-extrusion stabilization is essential because freshly deposited bioinks are typically weak and may deform under their own weight. Cross-linking improves mechanical strength and preserves geometry [27]. Methods vary, depending on the chemical nature of the bioink, as depicted in Table 4.1.

Table 4.1: Comparison of cross-linking methods with respect to bioink composition.

Cross-linking method	Example bioinks	Mechanism	Advantages	Limitations
Ionic	Alginate	Divalent cation binding (e.g., Ca^{2+})	Rapid gelation	Weak mechanics, reversible
Photo-cross-linking	GelMA, PEGDA	Light-activated polymerization using photoinitiators	Strong mechanical tuning, spatial control	UV may affect cell viability
Thermal gelation	Gelatin and Pluronic	Phase transition with temperature change	Simple and reversible	Poor strength at body temperature
Enzymatic	Fibrin and collagen	Enzyme-initiated polymerization	High biocompatibility	Slower reaction kinetics

4.3 Types of Extrusion Mechanisms

Extrusion-based bioprinting systems differ by the process of applying mechanical force over the bioink flow through the nozzle. The choice of extrusion mechanism affects printing resolution, shear stress on embedded cells, compatibility with high-viscosity bioinks, and level of control over deposition rate. The three most common extrusion mechanisms include pneumatic, piston-driven, and screw-driven systems. Selection is based on the specific bioink rheology and the functional requirements of the printed construct [28].

4.3.1 Pneumatic Extrusion

Pneumatic extrusion systems use regulated compressed air to pressurize the cartridge containing the bioink. This pressure forces the material through the nozzle as a continuous filament. Pressure settings are carefully optimized to maintain a stable flow without excessive shear forces. Pneumatic systems are widely used due to their structural simplicity, low cost, and compatibility with sterile, closed cartridges. One of the main advantages is the ability to rapidly adjust flow by modifying pressure in real time, which improves printing continuity during complex movements. Pneumatic extrusion is ideal for low- to moderate-viscosity hydrogels such as alginate or collagen. However, a major limitation is the delayed response time between pressure input and filament output, which can reduce accuracy near corners or at printing start/stop points. Additionally, handling highly viscous or particle-laden bioinks is less efficient because greater pressure increases shear stress on cells [29].

4.3.2 Mechanical (Piston-Driven) Extrusion

Piston- or plunger-based extrusion applies direct mechanical force to the bioink using a motor-controlled rod. This mechanism offers improved responsiveness and more precise control of flow rate compared to pneumatic systems. It is well-suited for bioinks that require consistent extrusion pressure, including cell-laden hydrogels with higher viscosity. Mechanical systems provide a nearly instantaneous correlation between actuator displacement and material flow, resulting in better print fidelity during geometric transitions. They are especially beneficial when printing structures with rapid directional changes or variable filament thickness. A drawback is that piston-based systems experience increasing back pressure with more viscous formulations, which can increase mechanical load and cell shear exposure if not calibrated well [30].

4.3.3 Screw-Driven Extrusion

Screw-driven systems incorporate a rotating screw to continuously push the bioink toward the nozzle. This mechanism supports precise volumetric flow control and uniform mixing throughout the printing process. It is the preferred approach for highly viscous bioinks, composite systems containing ceramics or fibers, and formulations with high cell density. The screw design reduces pulsation and ensures homogeneous extrusion, even for heterogeneous materials, making it promising for bone, cartilage, and multi-material constructs. Despite its advantages, prolonged screw rotation may induce localized shear, which could potentially affect cell viability. Furthermore, material retention inside the screw chamber can increase waste and complicate sterilization procedures. Various types of extrusion-based printers are mentioned in Figure 4.2 [4, 31].

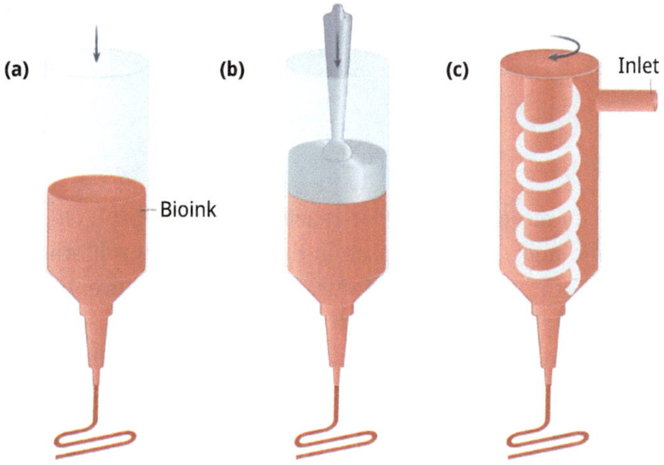

Figure 4.2: Different types of extrusion printers: (a) Pneumatic; (b) piston-driven; and (c) screw-driven (figure courtesy: Zhang, Y.S., Haghiashtiani, G., Hübscher, T. et al. 3D extrusion bioprinting. Nat Rev Methods Primers 1, 75 (2021). https://doi.org/10.1038/s43586-021-00073-8).

4.4 Bioink Requirements

Bioinks serve as the foundational materials in extrusion-based bioprinting, functioning both as a temporary support matrix and as a biological microenvironment for embedded cells. For a bioink to be suitable, it must satisfy multiple criteria that ensure smooth extrusion performance, structural integrity after printing, and favorable cell responses. The interplay between material chemistry, rheology, and biological compatibility determines how well the printed construct performs during fabrication and subsequent tissue maturation [7, 32].

4.4.1 Rheological Characteristics

Rheology plays a critical role in extrusion printing because it governs how a material flows under force and how it behaves, once deposited. Ideal bioinks exhibit shear-thinning behavior, meaning viscosity decreases under shear stress during extrusion and quickly recovers when the stress is removed. This enables smooth flow through the nozzle while still maintaining shape, once printed. If viscosity is too low, printed filaments may spread, deform, or collapse. Conversely, overly viscous bioinks can increase extrusion pressure, impose excessive shear forces on cells, and cause nozzle clogging. Yield stress is another essential parameter. A material must resist deformation caused by its own weight, after deposition, but still allow extrusion at the applied pressure. Proper control of viscoelastic properties is crucial for creating layered structures with high shape fidelity, especially in constructs requiring fine geometries or large vertical height [33].

4.4.2 Biocompatibility

A bioink must not induce toxicity or adverse cellular reactions. To support biological function, the formulation should allow cells to maintain their viability, proliferation, and phenotype throughout the printing process and during long-term culture. Hydrogels derived from natural biomaterials such as collagen, gelatin, hyaluronic acid, and fibrin offer inherent bioactivity and cell recognition motifs that facilitate matrix remodeling, adhesion, and differentiation. Sterility, nutrient diffusion, and oxygen permeability are also biological considerations. A biocompatible bioink must create a supportive environment immediately after printing, reducing stress on cells transitioning from a liquid to gel state. In some cases, biochemical cues such as growth factors or peptides are incorporated to enhance specific cell behavior and promote functional tissue regeneration [32].

4.4.3 Printability

Printability refers to the ability of a bioink to be extruded smoothly and form precise, continuous filaments. It depends on nozzle diameter, extrusion pressure, printing speed, and ink formulation. Good printability ensures that material deposition follows the intended CAD design and produces reproducible architectures with defined pore structure and mechanical properties. A printable bioink must balance ease of extrusion with the ability to maintain a stable geometry. Structural fidelity after printing is critical for applications like load-bearing tissues, vascular networks, or scaffolds with controlled porosity for perfusion. Printability testing methods include filament collapse assays, strand fusion tests, and assessment of construct fidelity compared to digital designs [34].

4.4.4 Cross-Linking Properties

Cross-linking transitions the printed bioink from a soft, flowable material into a stable, cell-supportive scaffold. The mechanism of cross-linking depends on the polymers' chemical structure, as shown in Table 4.2. Effective cross-linking must occur rapidly enough to preserve construct geometry, while protecting cell viability. Mechanical strength, degradation rate, and nutrient diffusion are all influenced by cross-linking density. Tunable cross-linking allows designers to match specific tissue requirements, such as stiffness for cartilage or elasticity for soft tissues [35].

Table 4.2: Summary of common cross-linking strategies used in bioprinting and their influence on construct stability and cell compatibility.

Cross-linking methods	Description
Ionic bonding	Ionic cross-linking relies on electrostatic interactions between charged polymers and multivalent ions. A common example is alginate, which forms a gel when exposed to calcium ions. This process is fast and gentle on cells, making it useful for maintaining printed shape, but the mechanical stability can be limited unless reinforced or secondary cross-linking is applied [36].
Photopolymerization	Photopolymerization uses light-sensitive initiators that activate polymer bonding when exposed to UV or visible light. Materials like GelMA benefit from spatial and temporal control of cross-linking, allowing precise stabilization after deposition. Care must be taken to control light exposure and free-radical formation to avoid cell damage while achieving suitable stiffness [37].
Thermal gelation	Thermal gelation allows temperature-responsive polymers such as gelatin to transition from a liquid state to a solid hydrogel when cooled after printing. This method is cell-friendly and does not require chemical additives, though the thermal sensitivity can result in limited long-term stability unless combined with another cross-linking mechanism [38].
Enzymatic cross-linking	Enzymatic systems use biological catalysts, such as transglutaminase or thrombin, to form stable networks in natural polymers like fibrin or collagen. This approach supports cell viability and mimics natural tissue environments, though reaction speed and stiffness may vary, depending on enzyme concentration and environmental conditions [39].

4.5 Materials for Extrusion Bioprinting

A versatile selection of biomaterials is essential for extrusion-based bioprinting, as different tissues require distinct mechanical, biochemical, and structural characteristics. Bioinks are broadly classified into natural polymers, synthetic polymers, composites, and support or sacrificial materials [40]. The choice of material influences cell behavior, printability, and the long-term performance of the printed construct in vivo or in vitro. Various types of natural and synthetic polymers for extrusion-based printing are detailed below:

4.5.1 Composite Bioinks

Composite materials combine bioactive natural polymers with strong synthetic components to improve printability, cell survival, and mechanical performance, such as alginate-GelMA systems that allow both ionic and photo-cross-linking for better stabil-

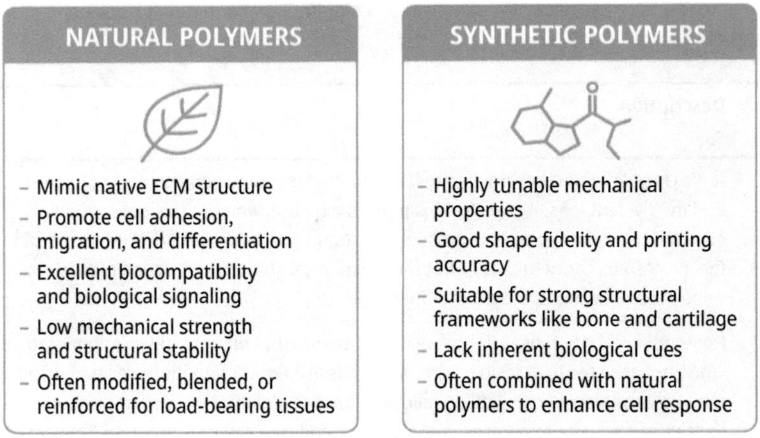

Figure 4.3: Description of natural and synthetic polymers.

ity, PEG-fibrin composites that promote vascularized tissues, or ceramic-reinforced hydrogels that support bone formation, while added cells, growth factors, nanoparticles, or ECM-derived cues help mimic native tissue complexity [41]. The figure 4.3 shows the characteristics properties of natural polymers and synthetic polymers.

4.5.2 Support and Sacrificial Bioinks

Support and sacrificial bioinks act as temporary structural aids that allow extrusion bioprinting to fabricate complex geometries that would otherwise deform under gravity or remain unstable during early gelation. These materials are printed around or within the primary bioink to provide shape retention, and then removed after the construct gains mechanical integrity, leaving behind detailed internal architectures such as hollow channels or interconnected vascular networks. Pluronic F127 is one of the most widely used options, taking advantage of its thermoresponsive behavior to form a solid structure during printing and later liquefying for easy removal without harming embedded cells [42]. Other methods, including gelatin slurry baths that stabilize soft hydrogels during deposition and carbohydrate glass fibers that dissolve to form perfusable conduits, further extend design possibilities [43]. By enabling the formation of branched vascular pathways and fragile or overhanging features, support bioinks significantly enhance the structural and biological functionality of printed tissues [44].

4.6 Process Parameters Affecting Print Quality

Process parameters affecting print quality and control filament consistency, resolution, and cell health. Proper optimization ensures accurate geometry, structural stability, and minimal shear-induced cell damage, leading to high-fidelity bioprinted constructs suitable for tissue engineering applications, as described in Table 4.3 [45].

Table 4.3: Key process parameters influencing print quality in extrusion-based bioprinting.

Parameter	Influence on printing	Effects on cells and construct	Typical optimization strategies
Nozzle diameter	Determines filament thickness and resolution [46]	Smaller nozzles increase shear stress and may damage cells	Select nozzle size based on cell type and required resolution; use shear-thinning bioinks
Extrusion rate	Controls material extrusion rate and strand uniformity [47]	Excess pressure causes high shear, cell damage, and filament swelling	Adjust pressure to match viscosity; maintain stable flow without pulsation
Print speed	Influences filament deposition and layer adhesion [48]	Imbalance can cause filament thinning or irregularity	Balance with flow rate to avoid gaps or overdeposition
Temperature (bioink and nozzle)	Modulates viscosity and gelation for thermosensitive materials [46]	Incorrect temperature may delay cross-linking or increase cell stress	Maintain physiological range for cell viability; control gelation timing
Layer height	Affects pore size and structural accuracy [49]	Too high leads to weak layer bonding; too low causes strand fusion	Match layer height with nozzle size and filament diameter
Cross-linking conditions	Stabilizes printed structure during and after printing [50]	Over-cross-linking reduces nutrient diffusion and cell spreading	Optimize cross-linking intensity, duration, and initiator concentration
Infill pattern and density	Determines mechanical strength and nutrient transport pathways [51]	High density may reduce porosity and limit oxygen diffusion	Use design strategies appropriate for tissue type (e.g., vascularized vs. load-bearing)
Environmental conditions (humidity and sterility)	Affects drying behavior, contamination, and material performance [52]	Protects cells from desiccation and contamination during printing	Controlled biosafety environments and proper hydration

4.7 Cell Viability Considerations

Maintaining high cell viability during and after extrusion-based bioprinting is essential for successful tissue development. Cells embedded within bioinks are exposed to complex mechanical and environmental stresses that can influence their survival, behavior, and long-term functionality. One of the primary factors affecting cell health is shear stress generated during material extrusion. As bioink moves through the nozzle, cells experience deformation and compression forces [53]. High viscosity, narrow nozzle diameters, or excessive extrusion pressure can lead to membrane damage, apoptosis, or altered cell phenotype. Therefore, shear-thinning bioinks are commonly used to reduce viscosity under flow and recover structural stability after deposition [54]. Modifying nozzle geometry and controlling flow rate are also critical strategies to minimize mechanical stress.

4.7.1 Post-printing Efficacy

Post-printing viability depends heavily on mass transport properties. Immediately after fabrication, cells rely on passive diffusion of oxygen and nutrients from the surrounding media. In thick or densely packed constructs, insufficient perfusion may lead to hypoxia and cell death in the construct core. To address this, printing designs often incorporate controlled porosity, perfusable channels, or early vascularization strategies to enhance oxygen exchange and waste removal. Maintaining physiological temperature and sterile conditions further supports early cell survival [55].

4.7.2 Optimization Strategy

Various optimization strategies exist to ensure favorable biological outcomes [56]. Protective additives such as shear-reducing agents or extracellular matrix [57] components can form a cushioning environment around cells. Dynamic cross-linking methods [58], gentler actuation forces [59], and real-time process monitoring can reduce stress during fabrication. Additionally, post-printing culture protocols, including bioreactor conditioning [60], perfusion flow, and growth factor supplementation, promote cell recovery and maturation [61]. Ultimately, balancing printability with cell-friendly conditions is essential for successful tissue engineering applications.

4.8 Applications of Extrusion-Based Bioprinting

Extrusion bioprinting has emerged as a critical technology in translational research and regenerative medicine, thanks to its compatibility with diverse biomaterials and ability to print clinically relevant tissue sizes [62, 63]. A major application is tissue and organ engineering. Load-bearing tissues such as bone [64] and cartilage [65] benefit from mechanically reinforced composite bioinks, while soft tissues like skin [66, 67] and muscle [68, 69] are printed using hydrogels that mimic native extracellular structure. Layer-by-layer deposition enables the fabrication of anatomically personalized implants, offering promising solutions in reconstructive surgery and trauma repair. In disease modeling, bioprinted constructs containing patient-derived cells enable realistic simulations of pathological environments [70]. Cancer models with tumor–stroma interactions [71, 72] and neural tissue mimics [73] for neurological disorders help researchers understand disease progression more accurately than traditional 2D cultures. These platforms provide ethical and biologically relevant alternatives to animal testing. Extrusion bioprinting also plays a growing role in drug testing and pharmaceutical research [74, 75]. Bioprinted tissues with physiological architecture allow controlled studies of drug penetration, toxicity, and therapeutic response. Personalized testing platforms can inform treatment decisions for individual patients, moving medicine toward precision therapy [76].

Another rapidly evolving field is customized implant development. Using patient imaging data, constructs can be fabricated with tailored shape, porosity, and mechanical characteristics that match the defect site [77]. This is particularly valuable in maxillofacial reconstruction [78], orthopedic implants [79], and soft-tissue restoration [80]. Biodegradable materials allow implants to gradually integrate and be replaced by newly formed tissue. Overall, extrusion-based bioprinting is transforming experimental and clinical strategies by enabling the fabrication of biologically instructive, structurally accurate, and patient-specific tissues. As bioreactors, vascularization techniques, and regulatory standards continue to evolve, the translation of printed implants into routine clinical practice becomes increasingly realistic [81].

4.9 Advantages

Extrusion-based bioprinting offers several advantages that make it one of the most widely adopted approaches for biofabrication. One of its most significant strengths is the ability to print high cell-density bioinks, allowing closer representation of native tissue cellularity. The technique is compatible with a broad spectrum of biomaterials, including hydrogels, polymer melts, and composite formulations [82]. This versatility enables engineering of both soft tissues, like skin and liver, and more mechanically demanding tissues such as cartilage and bone. Another benefit is the relatively simple and cost-effective instrumentation, which makes extrusion bioprinters accessible in research and clinical settings. In addition, extrusion printing supports large-scale constructs with macroporous architectures that facilitate nutrient diffusion, vascular ingrowth, and structural integration, when implanted [83]. The ability to co-print multiple materials and cell types within a single construct enables the creation of heterogeneous, biomimetic tissue environments [84–86]. Collectively, these strengths position extrusion bioprinting as a foundational platform in advanced tissue fabrication.

4.10 Limitations and Challenges

Despite its extensive utility, extrusion-based bioprinting faces several limitations. Compared to laser-assisted and inkjet bioprinting, the spatial resolution is lower, making it more difficult to achieve fine microarchitectures such as capillary-scale features. The reliance on high-viscosity bioinks to maintain shape-fidelity increases shear stress during extrusion, potentially reducing cell viability and altering cell behavior. The major challenge is the fabrication of fully functional, long-term viable tissues. Large printed constructs require vascular and neural networks to support nutrient distribution and functional integration with host systems. Current strategies, such as sacrificial channels and growth factor incorporation, show progress but remain insufficient for organ-scale complexity. Moreover, balancing mechanical strength and biological compatibility is still difficult when designing bioinks for load-bearing applications. Standardization, long-term stability, and regulatory approval for clinical use also remain unresolved barriers. Addressing these challenges is necessary for widespread therapeutic translation [87, 88].

4.11 Recent Advances

Rapid advancements are increasing the performance and complexity of extrusion-based bioprinting. Coaxial extrusion enables fabrication of hollow or tubular structures for vascular grafts and perfusable channels, while microfluidic-assisted systems allow multi-material control [89] and gradient formation with greater precision. Smart materials used in 4D bioprinting introduce dynamic shape changes in response to environmental stimuli, supporting more physiologically relevant tissue behavior. Additionally, artificial intelligence and machine learning are being integrated to optimize printing parameters, enhance reproducibility, and predict tissue development [90]. Together, these innovations strengthen both biological functionality and manufacturing reliability in bioprinted constructs.

4.12 Future Perspectives

Future evolution of extrusion-based bioprinting is expected to focus on increased automation, biofunctionality, and clinical integration. Real-time imaging and sensor feedback could provide closed-loop control for improved accuracy and reduced failure rates. Next-generation bioinks may include ECM-derived formulations [91], immunomodulatory factors [92], and vascular-promoting components tailored for specific target tissues. Major research efforts are directed toward developing fully vascularized, innervated, and metabolically active tissues capable of long-term function in vivo [93]. Patient-specific implants, supported by computational modeling and point-of-care manufacturing, could transform reconstructive medicine [94]. As regulatory frameworks evolve and bioprinter costs continue to decline, translation from research laboratories to hospitals becomes increasingly feasible [95].

Ultimately, the goal is to fabricate implantable organs, such as liver or kidney constructs, to address donor shortages and improve patient survival outcomes [96].

4.13 Conclusion

Extrusion-based bioprinting has established itself as a key enabling technology in regenerative medicine and biomedical engineering. Its ability to print high cell-density bioinks, support diverse materials, and fabricate clinically relevant structures makes it indispensable for tissue and organ fabrication. Although challenges remain in increasing resolution, reducing shear-induced damage, and supporting long-term tissue functionality, ongoing advances in material science, automation, and biofabrication strategies are rapidly closing these gaps [97].

Continued innovation is likely to accelerate clinical translation and redefine therapeutic possibilities, making extrusion-based bioprinting a cornerstone of personalized medicine and future healthcare technologies.

References

[1] Ozbolat, I. T. & Hospodiuk, M. (2016). Current advances and future perspectives in extrusion-based bioprinting. Biomaterials.
[2] Zhang, Y. S. et al. (2021). 3D extrusion bioprinting. Nature Reviews Methods Primers.
[3] Qiu, K. et al. (2018). 3D printed organ models with physical properties of tissue and integrated sensors. Advanced Materials Technologies.
[4] Ravanbakhsh, H. et al. (2021). Emerging technologies in multi-material bioprinting. Advanced Materials.
[5] Theus, A. S. et al. (2020). Bioprintability: Physiomechanical and biological requirements of materials for 3D bioprinting processes. Polymers.

[6] Chopin-Doroteo, et al. (2020). Tailoring of the rheological properties of bioinks to improve bioprinting and bioassembly for tissue replacement. Biochimica Et Biophysica Acta – General Subjects.
[7] Groll, J. et al. (2018). A definition of bioinks and their distinction from biomaterial inks. Biofabrication.
[8] Skardal, A. et al. (2015). A hydrogel bioink toolkit for mimicking native tissue biochemical and mechanical properties in bioprinted tissue constructs. Acta Biomater.
[9] Mazzeo, M. S. et al. (2018). Characterization of the Kinetics and Mechanism of Degradation of Human Mesenchymal Stem Cell-Laden Poly(ethylene glycol) Hydrogels. ACS Appl. Bio Mater.
[10] Kundu, et al. (2015). An additive manufacturing-based PCL–alginate–chondrocyte bioprinted scaffold for cartilage tissue engineering. Journal of Tissue Engineering and Regenerative Medicine.
[11] Somasekhar, L. et al. (2021). Three-dimensional printing of cell-laden microporous constructs using blended bioinks. Journal of Biomedical Materials Research Part A.
[12] Loukelis, K. et al. (2025). Extrusion-Based 3D Bioprinted Gellan Gum/Poly (vinyl alcohol)/Nano-Hydroxyapatite Composite Bioinks Promote Bone Regeneration. Advanced Healthcare Materials.
[13] Yuan, Z. et al. (2025). Multimaterial and Multidimensional Bioprinting in Regenerative Medicine: Advances, Limitations, and Future Directions. Advanced Healthcare Materials.
[14] Singh, M. et al. (2010). Inkjet Printing – Process and Its Applications. Advanced Materials.
[15] Placone, J. K. et al. (2017). Recent Advances in Extrusion-Based 3D Printing for Biomedical Applications. Advanced Healthcare Materials.
[16] Kantaros, A. (2022). 3D Printing in Regenerative Medicine: Technologies and Resources Utilized. International Journal of Molecular Sciences.
[17] Moroni, L. et al. (2018). Biofabrication strategies for 3D in vitro models and regenerative medicine. Nature Reviews Materials.
[18] Kalidindi, S. (2024). The role of three-dimensional (3D) printing in plastic and reconstructive surgery: Innovations and applications. European Journal of Plastic Surgery.
[19] Azad, M. A. et al. (2020). Polymers for Extrusion-Based 3D Printing of Pharmaceuticals: A Holistic Materials–Process Perspective. Pharmaceutics.
[20] Seoane-Viaño, I. et al. (2021). Semi-solid extrusion 3D printing in drug delivery and biomedicine: Personalised solutions for healthcare challenges. Journal of Controlled Release.
[21] Kosik-Kozioł, A. et al. (2019). 3D bioprinted hydrogel model incorporating β-tricalcium phosphate for calcified cartilage tissue engineering. Biofabrication.
[22] Haghiashtiani, G. et al. (2020). 3D printed patient-specific aortic root models with internal sensors for minimally invasive applications. Science Advances.
[23] Brown, N. C. et al. (2025). Multimaterial extrusion 3D printing printheads. Nature Reviews Materials.
[24] Amorim, P. A. et al. (2021). Insights on shear rheology of inks for extrusion-based 3D bioprinting. Bioprinting.
[25] Fu, Z. et al. (2021). Printability in extrusion bioprinting. Biofabrication.
[26] Ramesh, S. et al. (2021). Extrusion bioprinting: Recent progress, challenges, and future opportunities. Bioprinting.
[27] Nejad, A. G. et al. (2020). Crosslinking Strategies for 3D Bioprinting of Polymeric Hydrogels. Small.
[28] Jiang, T. et al. (2019). Extrusion bioprinting of soft materials: An emerging technique for biological model fabrication. Applied Physics Reviews.
[29] O'Connell, C. et al. (2020). Characterizing Bioinks for Extrusion Bioprinting: Printability and Rheology. In: Crook, J. M. (ed). 3D Bioprinting. Methods in Molecular Biology, Vol. 2140. Humana, New York, NY.
[30] Waalkes, L. et al. (2020). Feasibility study on piston-based feedstock fabrication with Ti-6Al-4V metal injection molding feedstock. Additive Manufacturing.

[31] Malda, J. et al. (2013). 25th anniversary article: Engineering hydrogels for biofabrication. Advanced Materials.
[32] Gungor-Ozkerim, et al. (2018). Bioinks for 3D bioprinting: An overview. Biomaterials Science.
[33] Lemarié, L., Anandan, et al. (2021). Rheology, simulation, and data analysis toward bioprinting cell viability awareness. Bioprinting.
[34] Hospodiuk, M., Dey, et al. (2017). The bioink: A comprehensive review on bioprintable materials. Biotechnology Advances.
[35] Ghavaminejad, A. et al. (2020). A. Crosslinking strategies for 3D bioprinting of polymeric hydrogels. Small.
[36] Chimene, D. et al. (2018). Nanoengineered ionic–covalent entanglement (nice) bioinks for 3D bioprinting. ACS Applied Materials and Interfaces.
[37] Ying, G. et al. (2018). Three-dimensional bioprinting of gelatin methacryloyl (GelMA). Biodesign and Manufacturing.
[38] Kesti, M. et al. (2015). A versatile bioink for three-dimensional printing of cellular scaffolds based on thermally and photo-triggered tandem gelation. Acta Biomater.
[39] Fisch, P. et al. (2021). Bioprinting of cartilaginous auricular constructs utilizing an enzymatically crosslinkable bioink. Advanced Functional Materials.
[40] Betancourt, N. et al. (2022). Review of extrusion-based multi-material bioprinting processes. Bioprinting.
[41] Michel, R. et al. (2020). Hydrogel-Colloid Composite Bioinks for Targeted Tissue-Printing. Biomacromolecules.
[42] Liu, S. et al. (2022). Application Status of Sacrificial Biomaterials in 3D Bioprinting. Polymers.
[43] Mirdamadi, E. et al. (2019). Agarose Slurry as a Support Medium for Bioprinting and Culturing Freestanding Cell-Laden Hydrogel Constructs. 3D Printing and Additive Manufacturing.
[44] McCormack, A. et al. (2020). 3D Printing in Suspension Baths: Keeping the Promises of Bioprinting Afloat. Trends in Biotechnology.
[45] Wu, Y. et al. (2024). Dissecting the Interplay Mechanism among Process Parameters toward the Biofabrication of High-Quality Shapes in Embedded Bioprinting. Advanced Functional Materials.
[46] Lee, A. et al. (2019). 3D bioprinting of collagen to rebuild components of the human heart. Science.
[47] Li, Q. et al. (2022). Regulable Supporting Baths for Embedded Printing of Soft Biomaterials with Variable Stiffness. ACS Applied Materials and Interfaces.
[48] Prendergast, M. E. et al. (2022). Computational Modeling and Experimental Characterization of Extrusion Printing into Suspension Baths. Advanced Healthcare Materials.
[49] Jeon, O. et al. (2019). Individual cell-only bioink and photocurable supporting medium for 3D printing and generation of engineered tissues with complex geometries. Materials Horizons.
[50] Ning, L. et al. (2020). Embedded 3D Bioprinting of Gelatin Methacryloyl-Based Constructs with Highly Tunable Structural Fidelity. ACS Applied Materials and Interfaces.
[51] Becker, M. et al. (2022). Aqueous Two-Phase Enabled Low Viscosity 3D (LoV3D) Bioprinting of Living Matter. Advanced Science.
[52] Ouyang, L. et al. (2020). Expanding and optimizing 3D bioprinting capabilities using complementary network bioinks. Science Advances.
[53] Loebel, C. et al. (2017). Shear-thinning and self-healing hydrogels as injectable therapeutics and for 3D-printing. Nature Protocols.
[54] Müller, S. J. et al. (2020). Flow and hydrodynamic shear stress inside a printing needle during biofabrication. PLoS ONE.
[55] Petta, D. et al. (2018). Three-dimensional printing of a tyramine hyaluronan derivative with double gelation mechanism for independent tuning of shear thinning and postprinting curing. ACS Biomaterials Science & Engineering.

[56] Kyle, S., Jessop, et al. (2017). 'Printability' of candidate biomaterials for extrusion-based 3D printing: State-of-the-art. Advanced Healthcare Materials.

[57] Kim, B. S. et al. (2020). Decellularized extracellular matrix-based bioinks for engineering tissue-and organ-specific microenvironments. Chemical Reviews.

[58] Morgan, F. L. C. et al. (2020). Dynamic bioinks to advance bioprinting. Advanced Healthcare Materials. 9, 1901798.

[59] Zhou, C. et al. (2021). Ferromagnetic soft catheter robots for minimally invasive bioprinting. Nature Communications.

[60] Parrish, J. et al. (2019). New frontiers for biofabrication and bioreactor design in microphysiological system development. Trends in Biotechnology.

[61] Freeman, F. E. et al. (2020). 3D bioprinting spatiotemporally defined patterns of growth factors to tightly control tissue regeneration. Science Advances.

[62] Moroni, L. et al. (2018). Biofabrication strategies for 3D in vitro models and regenerative medicine. Nature Reviews Materials.

[63] Levato, R. et al. (2020). From shape to function: The next step in bioprinting. Advanced Materials.

[64] Daly, A. C. et al. (2018). 3D printed microchannel networks to direct vascularisation during endochondral bone repair. Biomaterials.

[65] Kang, H.-W. et al. (2016). A 3D bioprinting system to produce human-scale tissue constructs with structural integrity. Nature Biotechnology.

[66] Cheng, R. Y. et al. (2020). Handheld instrument for wound-conformal delivery of skin precursor sheets improves healing in full-thickness burns. Biofabrication.

[67] Ying, G. et al. (2020). An open-source handheld extruder loaded with pore-forming bioink for in situ wound dressing. Materials Today Bio.

[68] Samandari, M. et al. (2021). Controlling cellular organization in bioprinting through designed 3D microcompartmentalization. Applied Physics Reviews.

[69] Russell, C. S. et al. (2020). In situ printing of adhesive hydrogel scaffolds for the treatment of skeletal muscle injuries. ACS Applied Bio Materials.

[70] Maharjan, S. et al. (2019). Three-dimensional bioprinting for tissue and disease modeling. Materials Matters.

[71] Neufeld, L. et al. (2022). 3D bioprinted cancer models: From basic biology to drug development. Nature Reviews Cancer.

[72] Datta, P. et al. (2020). 3D bioprinting for reconstituting the cancer microenvironment. Npj Precision Oncology.

[73] Cadena, M. et al. (2020). 3D Bioprinting of Neural Tissues. Advanced Healthcare Materials.

[74] Budharaju, H. et al. (2025). Bioprinting for drug screening: A path toward reducing animal testing or redefining preclinical research?. Bioactive Materials.

[75] Mota, C. et al. (2020). Bioprinting: From Tissue and Organ Development to in Vitro Models. Chemical Reviews.

[76] Mladenovska, T. et al. (2023). The Regulatory Challenge of 3D Bioprinting. Regenerative Medicine.

[77] Alam, M. I. et al. (2025). 3D-Printed Medical Implants: Recent Trends and Challenges. Biomedical Materials & Devices.

[78] Matheus, H. R. et al. (2024). The state of 3D printing of bioengineered customized maxillofacial bone scaffolds: A narrative review. Frontiers of Oral and Maxillofacial Medicine.

[79] Prządka, M. et al. (2025). Advances in 3D Printing Applications for Personalized Orthopedic Surgery: From Anatomical Modeling to Patient-Specific Implants. Journal of Clinical Medicine.

[80] Nagarajan, N. et al. (2018). Enabling personalized implant and controllable biosystem development through 3D printing. Biotechnology Advances.

[81] Kennedy, S. M. et al. (2025). 4D Bioprinting for Personalized Medicine, Innovations in Implant Fabrication and Regenerative Therapies. Polymer-Plastics Technology and Materials.

[82] Kačarević, Ž. P. et al. (2018). An Introduction to 3D Bioprinting: Possibilities, Challenges and Future Aspects. Materials.
[83] Ng, W. L. et al. (2025). Advanced bioprinting strategies for fabrication of biomimetic tissues and organs. International Journal of Extreme Manufacturing.
[84] Donoughue, M. et al. (2025). Material and surface roughness effects on adhesion of thermoplastic-elastomeric interfaces for dissimilar material 3D printing. Npj Advanced Manufacturing.
[85] Uzel, S. G. M. et al. (2022). Multimaterial Multinozzle Adaptive 3D Printing of Soft Materials. Advanced Materials Technologies.
[86] Zhu, C. et al. (2024). Toward Multiscale, Multimaterial 3D Printing. Advanced Materials.
[87] Zandrini, T. et al. (2023). Breaking the resolution limits of 3D bioprinting: Future opportunities and present challenges. Trends in Biotechnology.
[88] Vu, M. et al. (2022). Progress and challenges on extrusion-based three-dimensional (3D) printing of biomaterials. Bioprinting.
[89] Brown, N. C. et al. (2025). Multimaterial extrusion 3D printing printheads. Nature Reviews Materials.
[90] Robazzi, J. V. S. et al. (2025). The Synergy of Artificial Intelligence and 3D Bioprinting: Unlocking New Frontiers in Precision and Tissue Fabrication. Advanced Functional Materials.
[91] Jergitsch, M. et al. (2025). 3D extrusion bioprinting: Rational bioink design and advanced fabrication techniques. Trends in Biotechnology.
[92] Ma, Z. et al. (2022). 3D bioprinting of proangiogenic constructs with induced immunomodulatory microenvironments through a dual cross-linking procedure using laponite incorporated bioink. Composites Part B: Engineering.
[93] Zhu, J. et al. (2021). Advances in tissue engineering of vasculature through three-dimensional bioprinting. Developmental Dynamics.
[94] Zhang, C. et al. (2024). Machine learning-based prediction and optimisation framework for as-extruded cell viability in extrusion-based 3D bioprinting. TFO.
[95] Gu, Y. et al. (2021). Biobridge: An Outlook on Translational Bioinks for 3D Bioprinting. Advanced Science.
[96] Qiao, T. et al. (2025). Bioink design for organ-scale projection-based 3D bioprinting. Nat. Protoc.
[97] Lindner, N. et al. (2022). Scalable Biofabrication: A Perspective on the Current State and Future Potentials of Process Automation in 3D-Bioprinting Applications. Frontiers in Bioengineering and Biotechnology.

Mohammad Aftab Alam Ansari*, Kanika Nawani, Sumit Sharma*

Chapter 5
3D Bioprinting of Scaffolds and Implants for Orthopedics

Abstract: The repair of critically sized bone defects continues to be a clinical challenge, frequently necessitating advanced bone substitutes or grafts. Despite the progress made in biomaterials, conventional biomaterials cannot provide the required strength and porosity for supporting bone regeneration, along with withstanding static and cyclic mechanical loads. With advances in biofabrication, topologically designed porous structures and biomaterials, novel scaffolds and implants have been developed that aim to mimic the physical and chemical nature of bone, with appropriate mechanical strength. The integration of polymer blends, polymer-ceramic composites, and polymer-degradable metal alloys has enabled researchers to create high-strength, porous biomaterials that promote vascularization and bone formation. 3D printing these composite biomaterials requires printable bioink and sometimes involves pre- and post-processing methods. 3D printing not only ensures a precise fit of the graft into the defect site but also enhances cell attachment and bone regeneration. This chapter highlights recent progress in porous structures inspired by natural bone structure, developments in 3D printed composite scaffolds, and strategies for creating bioink solutions to achieve functional and biomechanically competent bone substitutes.

Keywords: Additive manufacturing, composite biomaterials, topologically optimized scaffolds, bioprinting, implants, scaffolds

5.1 Introduction

The regenerating capacity of bone tissue is remarkable, but it is often limited when it comes to critical-size defects (CSDs). Treating large bone defects remains a significant clinical challenge in orthopedics. Critical-sized bone defects are defined as those that will not heal on their own throughout a patient's lifetime, caused by trauma, tumor

***Corresponding author: Mohammad Aftab AlamAnsari**, Biomaterials and Biomanufacturing Laboratory, Mechanical Engineering Lab, PDPM Indian Institute of Information Technology Design and Manufacturing, Jabalpur 482005, Madhya Pradesh, India, e-mail: ansari.aftab.in@gmail.com
***Corresponding author: Sumit Sharma,** School of Pharmaceutical Sciences, Delhi Pharmaceutical Sciences and Research University, New Delhi, India, e-mail: sumit.ssharma17@gmail.com
Kanika Nawani, School of Pharmaceutical Sciences, Delhi Pharmaceutical Sciences and Research University, New Delhi, India

 | https://doi.org/10.1515/9783111719993-005

removal, or metabolic disorders [1]. The size of a critical defect varies depending on the patient, injury type, and location. Bone defects larger than 2 cm are considered CSDs because they do not achieve at least 30% mineralization within 52 weeks of healing. Generally, a CSD is defined as a bone injury exceeding 2 cm that fails to regenerate naturally into a stable, mineralized bony structure, resulting in a nonunion defect. The need for persistent bone repair options is increasing worldwide due to musculoskeletal conditions, sports injuries, accidents, and aging populations. Currently, several conventional methods are used to treat CSDs. The main autogenous, allogeneic, and xenogeneic grafts are used clinically. Autogenous grafts are considered the gold standard because they are obtained from the patient's own body and have excellent regenerative properties without provoking an immune response. However, they require an additional surgical procedure to harvest bone from a secondary site, such as the iliac crest, which may cause donor site pain, infection, and other complications [2]. Alternatively, cadaveric allogeneic grafts can accelerate recovery, but if not properly sterilized, they pose risks of rejection or disease transmission. Xenografts, derived from animals such as cows, offer both osteoconductivity and structural stability compared to human bone, making them suitable scaffolds for bone regeneration. Despite these benefits, xenografts have disadvantages. Residual proteins in the graft may trigger immunological responses, raising concerns about cross-species disease transmission. Additionally, their resorption in the body can be delayed or incomplete due to high-temperature processing, which hampers long-term integration. Artificial medical implants such as bone plates and scaffolds are increasingly popular due to their effectiveness, although their success depends mainly on how well they integrate with the host tissue and the precision of manufacturing. In load-bearing applications, bone plates are often preferred over allografts because they provide quick, efficient mechanical fixation essential for early weight-bearing and stabilization in severe injuries. However, these metallic implants often do not biodegrade nor are they bioactive, which can lead to poor tissue integration and the need for secondary procedures for CSDs [3].

To overcome the limitations of current grafting methods, tissue-engineered grafts, which are still in the experimental stage, offer a promising substitute that incorporates stem cells, biomaterials, and 3D bioprinting. Bone tissue engineering (BTE) is the process of grafting functional cells onto biocompatible scaffolds that have been grown in vitro before implantation in order to accelerate bone regeneration. As new bone grows, these scaffolds gradually break down to support waste clearance, gas exchange, and nutrient supply [4]. The best scaffold materials should have excellent porosity and bioactivity, be nontoxic, biocompatible, and biodegradable, mimicking the natural bone properties. These scaffolds are designed to replicate the bone porosity and mechanics by incorporating nature-inspired designs, including Voronoi structures, honeycomb geometries, and trabecular lattices into the scaffold design. The resulting scaffolds withhold both the mechanical stability and biological integration after being computationally modeled. For the fabrication of such a complex structure, nonconventional additive manufacturing (AM) techniques are employed to create high-resolution scaffolds. Bioprinting is a special type of AM technique, which enables layer-by-layer deposition of bioinks (a blend of biomaterials, cells, and bioactive compounds) into prefabricated structures that mimic the complex structure of tissue. For BTE, this method allows for the careful positioning of different materials to produce multi-material, heterogeneous scaffolds that closely resemble the trabecular and cortical layers of native bone. While bioprinting offers fabrication of any complex geometries and scaffolds, bioink plays a crucial role in deciding the fate of the resulting 3D printed scaffolds. The bioink is primarily responsible for promoting cell survival and development, maintaining a biocompatible environment, ensuring ease of printability, and maintaining the 3D shape. Alginate, collagen, gelatin, and other hydrogels are frequently mixed with structural elements such as magnesium alloys, PCL, or hydroxyapatite to improve the shape fidelity of the ink. In order to promote healing, bioinks may additionally be loaded with drugs such as growth factors (e.g., BMP-2), antibiotics, or anti-inflammatories [5].

Despite advancements in bioprinting, optimal vascularization, anisotropic mechanical characteristics, and hierarchical organization of bone are challenging to imitate in artificial scaffolds. Ongoing challenges include complexities in post-processing, difficulties in scaling for clinical applications, inadequate control over material degradation rates, and reduced cell viability during the bioprinting process. Integration of composite biomaterials and 3D bioprinting has the potential to be a groundbreaking technique for CSD repair. Personalized bone regeneration is reaching new heights via biomimetic scaffold design and sophisticated fabrication. More recently, scaffold design and print settings are being optimized with the application of artificial intelligence (AI) and machine learning. AI can provide real-time feedback for 3D bioprinting by predicting mechanical and biological performance based on patient-specific imaging data [6].

In an extremely developing discipline, this chapter addresses material selection, design approach, fabrication techniques, and the role of pharmaceutics and therapeutics for improved bone regeneration, culminating in their potential clinical application.

5.1.1 Current Challenges in 3D Bioprinting of Bone Scaffolds

Existing clinical scaffolds are challenged with great difficulty in regenerating the intricate structure and functionality of bone tissue. There are three general ways in which these challenges manifest themselves: (a) It becomes difficult to select scaffold materials capable of meeting both biological and mechanical performance at the same time. Ceramics and polymers possess high biocompatibility but low capacity for support, while metal materials possess good load-carrying capacity but low tissue compatibility. Recent reviews highlight that no single class of material is sufficient; hybrid composites and surface-modified biomaterials are being explored to address this gap [7]. (b) Several drawbacks plague printing techniques, such as poor resolution, sluggish manufacturing speed, complicated shape creation, limited material options, and a lack of soft tissue simulation. Jakus et al. proved that hyperelastic bone scaffolds 3D-printed could mimic trabecular-like structures, but resolution and fidelity to the microarchitecture remained too low for mimicking native bone [8]. Likewise, Temple et al. pointed out that extrusion-based printing, although a versatile technique is disadvantaged by a compromise between nozzle diameter (resolution) and speed of printing [9]. (c) The integration of regenerative cells within bone scaffolds during bioprinting and their maturation to tissue repair levels, while ensuring recipient acceptance, relies on local cell contacts and self-organization, which is a significant challenge. There are still challenges in printing speed, resolution, material degradation properties, biocompatibility, cell supply, and co-culturing, which necessitate increased attention and solutions. Kang et al. demonstrated the ability to bioprint human-sized, stem cell-filled constructs, while Levato et al. identified that long-term survival, spatial organization, and self-organization of cells within scaffolds are still difficult to achieve [10].

5.1.2 Mechanical Strength Versus Biodegradability Trade-Off

The design of 3D-printed bone scaffolds for tissue engineering requires meticulous investigation of the trade-off between mechanical strength and biodegradability. The degrading behavior of biodegradable 3D-printed scaffolds in a physiologically realistic environment is important for bone tissue engineering. The scaffolds' ability to calcify in vitro is linked to their bonding in vivo. When the surface of the scaffold is exposed to a physiological environment during implantation, it must facilitate the creation of an apatite layer. Layers of apatite that form on the scaffold's surface aid in the mineralization of bone. The degradation, dissolution, and desorption of the scaffold surfaces are what primarily determine the kinetics of the antibiotic release profile from 3D scaffolds [11]. Scaffold degradation is initiated by a series of chemical reactions at the exposed surface in the physiological environment, followed by the formation of a long-term layer upon implantation. Such bioactivity plays a pivotal role in anchoring the bond to natural bone. Biodegradable polymers such as polycaprolactone (PCL), polylactic acid or polylactide (PLA), and poly(lactic-co-glycolic acid) (PLGA) degrade in a physiologically simulated environment via the hydrolytic biodegradation pathway/path. However, their overall degradation rates are slow compared to the pace of bone healing. Zhou et al. indicated that PLA scaffolds had high initial strength but degraded slowly, with remaining fragments causing impairment in bone ingrowth. Likewise, Wei et al. [12] found that PLGA scaffolds degraded non-uniformly, providing poor mechanical support.

To overcome this mismatch, approaches such as blending, copolymerization, surface modification, and incorporation of inorganic phases have been employed to modulate degradation while maintaining strength and biocompatibility. For example, Wu et al. reported that PCL-β-TCP scaffolds degraded faster than neat PCL, while Brown et al. showed that magnesium-incorporated PLA improved strength, degradation, and osteogenic activity [13].

5.1.3 Interfacial Bonding in Composite Bioinks

Even though 3D bioprinting has made significant strides, there are still certain obstacles to be addressed. Weak interlayer adhesion is one of the most critical problems that occur often while designing a composite ink containing both organic and inorganic phases, affecting the printability, shape fidelity, and mechanical qualities [14]. Dehydration, swelling, or contraction can also make it challenging to maintain shape after printing soft hydrogel mixed with stiff polymer or ceramics [15]. For high-strength composite materials, factors such as mismatch of chemical groups, insufficient cross-linking at the phase boundary, and the heterogeneity in the surface area lead to an overall decrease in the toughness of scaffolds and thus limit their ability to combine high mechanical strength with biological functionalities. For example, the hydrophobic/hydrophilic mismatch among the polymers and ceramics (such as hydroxyapatite) causes brittle behavior and early failure of composite scaffolds. These difficulties emphasize the necessity of strengthening the interfacial bonding in composite bioinks to preserve biological functioning and structural integrity, which are crucial for printing intricate, functional tissues. Methods such as chemical surface modification (such as plasma treatment, wet chemical activation, or grafting bioactive motifs), layer-by-layer assembly approach, and co-extrusion of hybrid inks are being explored to minimize this problem and enhance the overall performance of the composite scaffold. In-situ dual cross-linking methods (thermal/chemical or ionic/photo or any combination) have been reported to stabilize the interfaces, resulting in improved mechanical strength and benefits long-term cell response.

5.1.4 Limitations of Clinical Translation of 3D Bioprinting

Bioprinting faces significant challenges in striking the right balance between mechanical functionality and scaffold degradability. Degradation that is too quick can compromise tissue support, while degradation that is too sluggish can cause inflammation. Elasticity, fatigue resistance, compressive strength, and tensile strength must all be carefully considered for mechanical performance to be satisfactory. Despite being perfect for 3D bioprinting and cell encapsulation because of their porous structure, hydrogels typically lack mechanical strength [16]. Future strategies include hybrid bioinks with inorganic fillers or thermoplastic frameworks. Yang et al. [17] proposed hollow fiber hydrogel scaffolds with high elasticity, rapid shape recovery, and excellent fatigue resistance.

The VP (vat photopolymerization), BJ (binder jetting), and ME (material extrusion) techniques used in bioprinting raise issues with cell viability. Although VP presents a danger of cell damage from free radicals, it enables the production of high-resolution tissues employing photoactivatable resins [18]. Although BJ's DOD (drop-on-demand) technique maximizes noncontact deposition, it necessitates regulated droplet velocity, print time, and cell concentration to guarantee survivability. Damage from ME is caused by shear stress and is impacted by ink viscosity, nozzle size, and pressure [19]. Internal biomimicry is limited by STL's (stereolithography) geometric-only format, which also frequently contains mesh defects. Although AMF (additive manufacturing file format) utilizes internal structure, color, and texture information to address these issues, its adoption is limited. Standardizing formulas and printing settings through a community-driven bioink database could improve scaffold fidelity, speed up bioprinting advancements, and improve reproducibility [20].

Complicated regulatory processes involving organizations like the US Food and Drug Administration (FDA), the National Institutes for Food and Drug Control (NIFDC) in China, and the European Medicines Agency (EMEA) limit the application of 3D bioprinting technologies in clinical settings. The process encompasses concept development, laboratory viability, regulatory testing, approval, GMP-compliant manufacturing, and post-market surveillance. Data demonstrating safety, effectiveness, and biocompatibility are essential for regulatory approval. Timelines for bio-printed scaffolds can be lengthy; FDA clearances for medicines typically take 11 years, biologics 9 years, and devices 6 years. Robust preclinical studies and clearly defined usage guidelines, including details on target patient demographics, intended indications, and clinical settings, are vital to expedite translation. Early attention to these factors may facilitate regulatory clearance, allowing for easier market access and improved patient care [21].

5.2 Biological and Mechanical Requirements: Bone Tissue Regeneration

The regeneration process of tissue is very complex, and it is practically impossible to completely mimic the natural tissue. However, understanding their biological requirement, engineers and doctors can mimic their physiological environment. Bone is not an exception to this. Successful bone regeneration requires scaffolds that balance biological cues along with mechanical competence. The scaffold should mimic the target tissue, provide initial support without causing stress-shielding, and maintain the structural integrity during the early healing phase, while also degrading at the rate of new bone deposition. The bone has a multilayer hierarchical structure with gradient porosity, as depicted in Figure 5.1. For reference, the elastic modulus of cortical bone ranges between 10 and 30 GPa and its compressive strength in the range of 50–150 MPa, whereas the inner part of the bone, i.e., the trabecular bone, exhibits a modulus of 0.1–2 GPa and a compressive strength of 2–20 MPa. The scaffold should include multiscale porosity with macropores ranging between ~200 µm and 600 µm to allow the blood vessels and bone ingrowth, and microporosity of the order <50 µm, to allow protein adsorption through its highly interconnected pores. The surface of the scaffolds should be functionalized using chemistry to enable communication between the scaffold surface and the cells. Biochemically, the release of Ca^{2+}, Si^{4+}, or Sr^{2+} ions, and controlled delivery of osteogenic and angiogenic factors (e.g., BMP-2 and VEGF) significantly enhances the differentiation and neovascularization of mesenchymal stem cells [22, 23]. Moreover, the role of mechanobiology is also critically important to consider. For example, a scaffold subjected to a shear stress of 0.1–0.5 MPa on its inner walls due to the fluid flow through it and a cyclic strain of 1–10% has been reported to promote osteogenesis and matrix organization in the scaffold [24].

Another important consideration is the role of immune modulation, i.e., how the body's immune system responds after the scaffold has been implanted. The body's immune cells naturally trigger inflammation to clear the debris and defend against the infection, and therefore play a decisive role in the success of a scaffold. The scaffold should be designed in such a way that the initial pro-inflammatory M1 response must shift into a pro-M2 phase to initiate tissue repair, promote angiogenesis, and bone deposition [25]. Therefore, it is practically very challenging to incorporate all these essential cues into a single artificial graft. The traditional manufacturing techniques lack multi-material and multidirectional manufacturing, hindering the incorporation of multiple chemical and biological factors into a single scaffold. Thanks to the advanced manufacturing techniques, which open the door for an innovative design approach to develop a scaffold with multi-tailored properties.

5.3 Advanced Manufacturing Techniques: 3D Bioprinting for BTE

In order to develop efficient bone regeneration methods, bone tissue engineering (BTE) relies heavily on simulating the intricacy of natural structures and functions. Designing 3D bio-printed bone constructions mainly relies on biomimetic ideas, which draw inspiration from natural creatures. These designs serve as novel models for BTE because they include complex porous architectures, hierarchical arrangements, and gradient distributions that resemble those observed in nature. 3D bio printing enables patient-specific designs with intricate geometries that closely resemble natural bone (Figure 5.2). In contrast to conventional techniques, it offers tailored therapeutic solu-

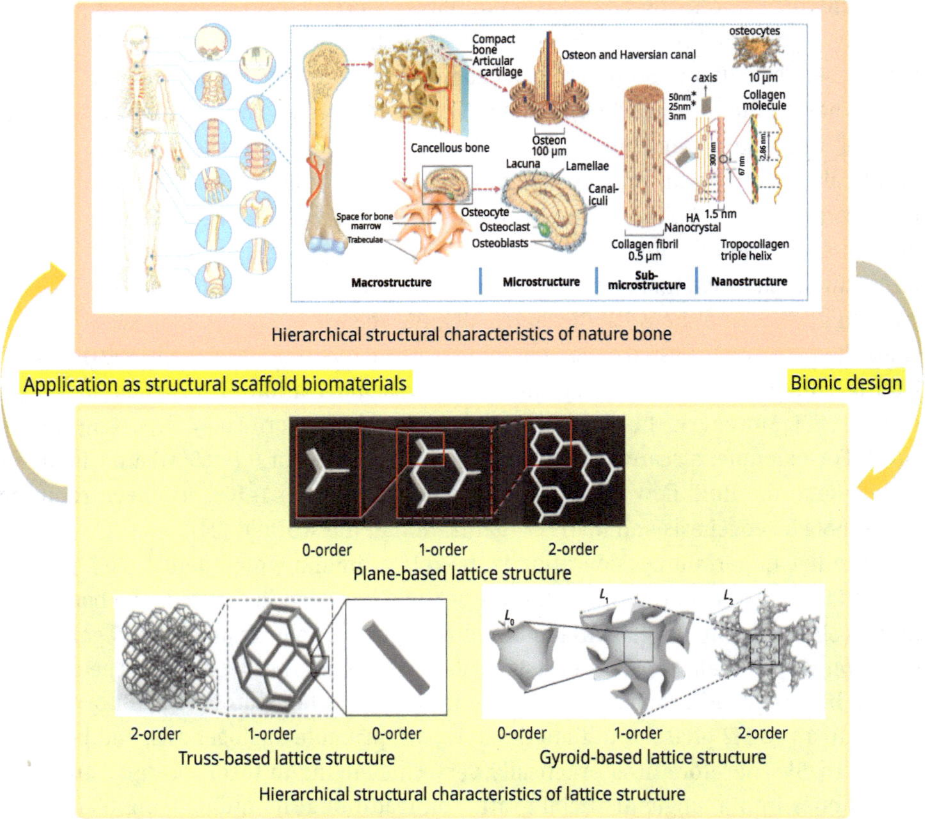

Figure 5.1: Graphical representation of human bone with a hierarchical structure and a lattice structure inspired by the natural structure of bone. Scaffolds containing plane-based, truss-based, and gyroid-based lattice structures can be designed for use in BTE applications. Adapted with permission from ref. [92]. Copyright 2024 Elsevier Ltd.

tions for bone injuries, particularly for CSDs that exceed the body's innate regenerative capacity. By combining physiologically compatible materials with precise construction, it enhances regeneration and overcomes the drawbacks of standard grafts [26, 27]. Moreover, in silico simulations can be utilized to examine mechanical behavior, while surface morphological deviations can be digitally assessed. The two prevalent 3D bioprinting techniques for orthopedic applications are hybrid bioprinting and multi-material co-extrusion. 3D bioprinting based on multi-material co-extrusion provides a one-step method for creating physiologically active, structurally strong, and biomimetic structures for orthopedic applications. The constraints of weak hydrogel-only systems and labor-intensive sequential printing are overcome by enabling the simultaneous deposition of thermoplastic and hydrogel bioinks. Due to the strong interfacial bonding that is encouraged by this method, integrated scaffolds with improved structural integrity and functionality are produced. Hence, multi-material bioprinting offers a potent instrument for producing therapeutically useful bone grafts that are both biologically compatible and mechanically strong [28]. Hybrid bioprinting has become a viable method for reproducing the structural and biological complexity of bone by co-printing soft, cell-rich hydrogels with mechanically durable bioinks [29]. This method fabricates mechanically robust, vascularized bone grafts with clinically relevant geometry. The reinforcing bioink forms a porous scaffold supporting large tissue bioprinting, enhancing biocompatibility, and enabling constructs to endure mechanical loads in vivo while supporting living cells and vascular integration [30].

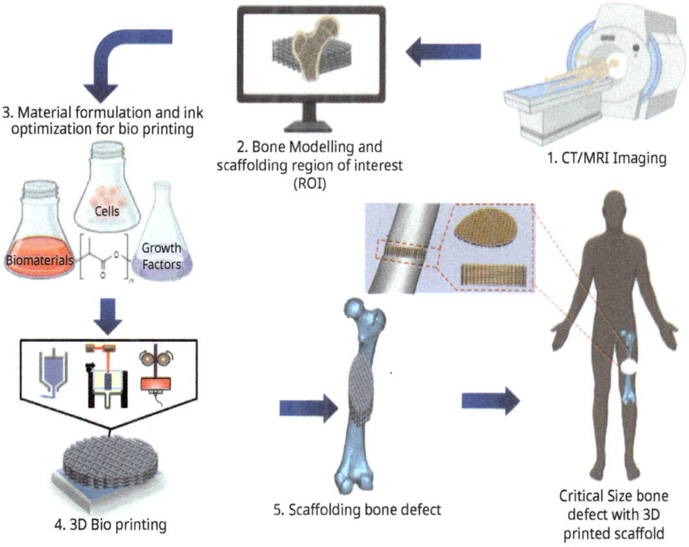

Figure 5.2: Steps involved in 3D bioprinting for critical bone defect repair.

5.3.1.1 Fused Deposition Modeling (FDM)

Fused deposition modeling (FDM) is an extrusion-based 3D printing process where thermoplastic filaments are melted and deposited layer by layer following a prescribed trajectory. Some of the critical parameters, like layer thickness, infill density, internal structure, and nozzle/bed temperature, significantly affect the print fidelity, resolution, and biomechanical performance of scaffolds, splints, and patient-specific orthopedic implants [31]. Recent research confirms the possibility of using FDM in bone tissue engineering: Li et al. printed fibronectin-modified PLA scaffolds that stimulated osteoblast adhesion, proliferation, and osteogenic differentiation in vitro;, SEM analysis indicated that S1, S2, and S4 scaffolds had uniform pores (~250 μm diameter with ~300 μm spacing), with S1 having a relatively smoother surface than S2 and S4

(Figure 5.3) Consistent with previous work, incorporating nHA gave the S2 scaffold a rougher surface, whereas incorporation of nHA and composite hydrogels increased the surface area without sacrificing the porosity of dECM hydrogels. These nHA/PLA/dECM/β-CD-CHX composite scaffolds not only offered better substrates for cell adhesion but also facilitated osteoblast proliferation and bone regeneration without loss of antibacterial activity and mechanical strength [32]. Mi et al. [33] created PEEK/HA scaffolds presenting improved osteogenesis and good biocompatibility . Among the thermoplastics, the best is perhaps PEEK (polyether-ether-ketone), which has an elastic modulus close to that of cortical bone and, therefore, causes less stress shielding, and in addition, is radiolucent and does not cause imaging artefacts. Its low cytotoxicity, slow release of toxic ions, and corrosion resistance make it an ideal candidate for surgical implants [34, 35]. FDM with PEEK and other polymer composites is therefore a very versatile platform for developing patient-specific orthopedic scaffolds and implants with both mechanical ability and biological function [36].

Limitations: The low cost and accessibility of FDM make it popular, but it also has some disadvantages. FDM prints' surface finish frequently exhibits obvious layer lines, which may detract from the appearance and may require sanding for a smooth finish. Compared to resin printing, it falls short when it comes to small or intricately complex components. Due to uneven cooling, warping is another problem, particularly with larger prints or certain materials. If high precision is needed, printing

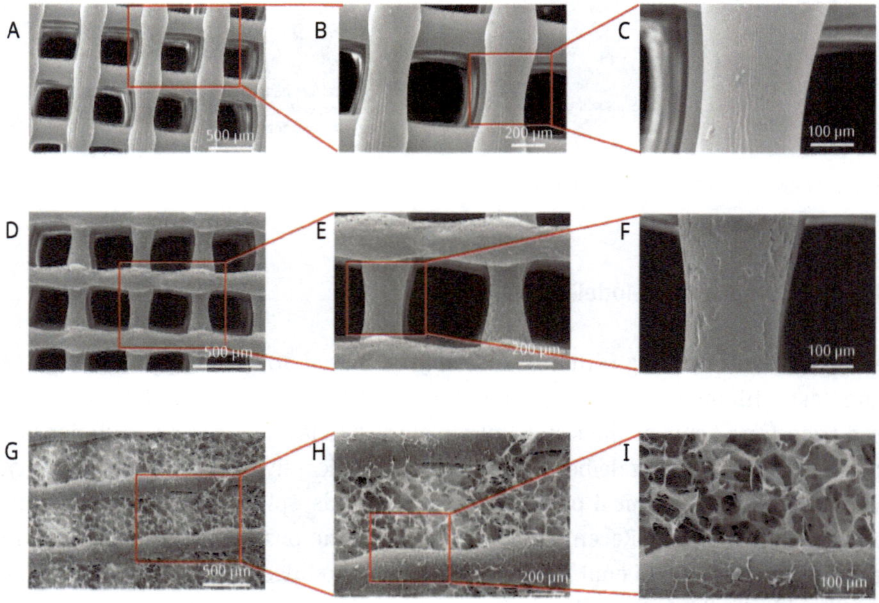

Figure 5.3: SEM analysis images: S1 (A–C). S2 (D–F). S4 (G–I). (A, D, and G) 100×, (B, E, and H) 200×, and (C, F, and I) 500×.

could be slow. Support structures can be challenging to remove and may cause harm to the printed product. Despite its support for a wide range of materials, FDM still falls short of other methods in terms of fine detail and durability [37].

5.3.1.2 Digital Light Processing (DLP)

Digital light processing (DLP) is an advanced photopolymerization-based 3D printing technique that cures complete layers at once by projecting a pattern of digital light onto the resin surface. This allows intricate shapes with precise features to be fabricated quickly [38]. DLP has emerged as an essential instrument for creating biocompatible and useful tissues and organs when combined with bioprinters. However, the limited material characteristics of the biomaterials used in this technique represent a major restriction [39]. Utilizing an assortment of material classes, such as hydrogels, nanocomposites, polymer-based materials, and bioceramics, DLP technology has recently seen increased need in biomaterials. The advantages of this technology include a wide range of biocompatible material alternatives, high resolution, and quick manufacturing. However, there are drawbacks to DLP. For example, unequal light intensity can cause deformation, shrinkage, or interlayer delamination in big structures during light-based curing [40]. Overheating and projector edge fall-off are additional factors that contribute to these mechanical constraints [41].

Limitation: 3D printing with DLP has significant drawbacks despite providing detailed, high-resolution prints. Because printed models are frequently brittle, they are inappropriate for components that must endure mechanical force or stress. The total cost is increased by the comparatively high cost of the liquid resins used in DLP. Each item must undergo post-processing after printing, which might take a while and involves UV light exposure and alcohol cleaning. These resins also need careful handling and adequate ventilation because they can produce strong scents and irritate skin. Because most desktop DLP printers have a small build area, the print size is often small. Additionally, DLP-made components are susceptible to weather and UV rays, which could eventually cause deterioration [42].

5.3.1.3 Direct Ink Writing (DIW) for Bioinks

Direct ink writing (DIW) is an extrusion-based AM process that employs viscoelastic inks to fabricate intricate 3D structures at meso- and microscales. Using a computer-controlled stage, material is extruded layer by layer through a nozzle, solidifying into the desired shapes. DIW is categorized into two classes: continuous extrusion and droplet. The steps include ink deposition, slicing for path planning, and CAD-based modeling. Resolution (typically 100–1,200 µm in x–y and 100–400 µm in z) is affected by essential parameters such as nozzle size and speed. DIW utilizes ink rheology, rather than heat, to ensure printability at room temperature. Evaporation, gelation, and curing are some methods of solidification [43].

Limitation: Lower resolution than other AM techniques, nozzle clogging with fine inks, slow printing speed, restricted material compatibility, structural instability during printing, and the requirement for exact ink rheology control are some of the drawbacks of DIW [44].

5.3.1.4 Stereolithography

The process of layered curing a photopolymer resin in a stereolithography apparatus (SLA), an ultraviolet (UV) light-based 3D printing technique, enables the creation of accurate, high-resolution structures [45]. A mixture of ceramic particles and photopolymer resin, and a subsequent debinding and sintering process, can also be employed to fabricate bioceramic components using SLA [46]. Based on in vitro SLA biocompatibility tests, such scaffolds provide a microenvironment for osteogenic differentiation and proliferation of many cell types, including human embryonic stem cells [47], human periosteal-derived stem cells, and human mesenchymal stem cells. SLA-fabricated scaffolds have exhibited high effectiveness in inducing angiogenesis, the formation of new bone, and osseointegration of the scaffold into calvarial defects in rabbits and mice in vivo. Lee et al. [93] indicated that the incorporation of microspheres containing BMP-2 into the scaffold caused successful bone formation in mouse calvarial lesions with a blend of poly(propylene fumarate) and diethyl fumarate (DEF) as the raw materials for the SLA scaffold. Wei and coworkers [49] demonstrated that, when BMSC-seeded scaffolds made from calcium phosphate/monoalcohol ethoxylate phosphate slurry were implanted in dorsal muscles, they resulted in effective angiogenesis and ectopic bone formation using a dog mode. SLA-generated scaffolds are highly effective in inducing angiogenesis, new bone formation, and osseointegration of the scaffold within calvarial defects in rabbits and mice in vivo [50]. Lee et al. demonstrated that the incorporation of microspheres with BMP-2 into the scaffold resulted in successful bone regeneration in mouse calvarial defects with the use of a combination of poly(propylene fumarate) and diethyl fumarate (DEF) as precursor materials for the SLA scaffold (Figure 5.3). Wei et al. demonstrated that when BMSC-seeded scaffolds made from calcium phosphate/monoalcohol ethoxylate phosphate slurry were implanted into dorsal muscles, they resulted in excellent angiogenesis and ectopic bone formation with a canine model.

Limitation: SLA printers haven't reached mainstream use mainly due to their high cost compared to FDM printers. While FDM models typically range from \$300 to \$500, SLA printers often start at \$1,000. Additionally, resin used in SLA printing is significantly pricier than FDM filaments like PLA. A liter of resin, costing around \$50, is more expensive than a spool of PLA and yields fewer prints. Moreover, SLA prints are usually brittle and degrade outdoors, limiting their practical use to prototypes or display items [51].

5.3.2 Biomaterials and Bioinks for Orthopedic Applications

5.3.2.1 Biomaterials for Cartilage Repair and Regeneration

Recent developments in 3D printing have allowed the creation of scaffolds that closely resemble the native cartilage environment, offering mechanical support and facilitating chondrogenesis. For example, Ghobadi et al. [52] created multiphasic alginate-gelatin scaffolds with 1% graphene oxide and platelet-rich plasma (PRP), with the 2% PRP formulation exhibiting improved glycosaminoglycan production and chondrogenic marker expression. Similarly, Liu and coworkers [53] synthesized collagen type I/II-hyaluronic acid (CI/II-HyA) scaffolds combined with a 3D-printed poly(glycerol sebacate) (PGS) framework, reaching a compressive modulus of 167 kPa and superior fatigue resistance, while supporting excellent cartilage-like matrix deposition in vitro (Figure 5.4). These reports show how the combination of sophisticated biomaterials with 3D printing approaches can generate scaffolds that successfully direct cartilage regeneration without compromising structural integrity.

5.3.2.2 Composite Biomaterials for Bone Restoration

Biomaterials are the backbone of BTE, and therefore biomaterial-based scaffolds have emerged as an indispensable tool for improving osteogenesis, restoring biomechanical functions, while delivering the bioactive molecules. In order to perform such a multifunctional task, composite biomaterials with a focus on synthetic polymer-based biocomposites have gained significant interest over the past few decades, whereas those using natural polymers as matrices or scaffolds for osteogenic substitutes are relatively limited. The natural polymers, e.g., chitosan, alginate, and collagen, have inherent biocompatibility and biological signaling, while the synthetic polymers, such as but not limited to polylactic acid (PLA), poly(ethylene glycol) (PEG), and PCL, offer mechanical strength and controllable degradation rate. Therefore, through combining these various classes, a researcher seeks to replicate the chemical, structural, and biological signals of the extracellular matrix (ECM), leading to bioactive scaffolds that induce cell adhesion, proliferation, and differentiation.

For example, a deacetylated version of chitin, chitosan, is both biodegradable and biocompatible and falls under the natural bioink category. It is often used alongside ceramics to balance the brittleness of ceramics and the weakness of polymers. A 3D nanocomposite of chitosan, gelatin, and nano-silica demonstrated enhanced cell adhesion and mineralization. Similarly, chitosan/gelatin/CEL2 and α-chitin/nHA scaffolds

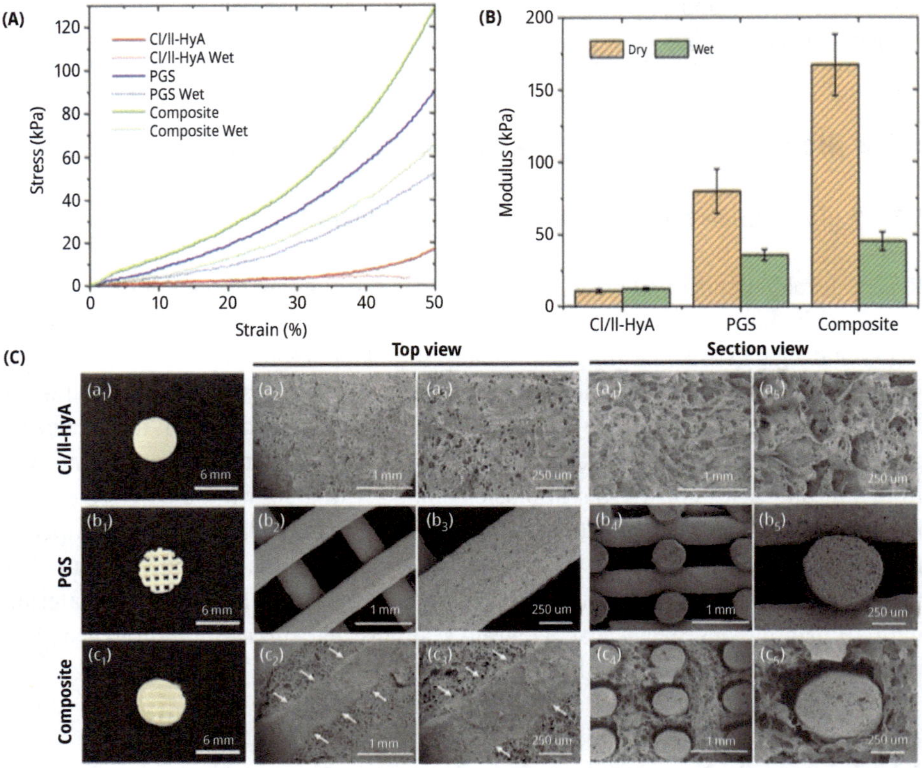

Figure 5.4: (A) Compressive strength of the scaffold measured at a speed of 0.1 mm/s; (B) the corresponding compressive modulus of CI/II-HyA, PGS, and composite scaffolds under dry and wet conditions; (C) The SEM image CI/II-HyA scaffold, followed by PGS and composite scaffolds, taken from top and side views. Adapted with permission from ref. [53]. Copyright 2024 Elsevier Ltd.

improve osteogenic properties. Chitosan-alginate-fucoidan scaffolds enhanced proliferation and ALP secretion. The proliferation of osteoblasts was boosted by chitosan coatings on Ti-6al-4 v [54].

Collagen, the most prevalent animal protein, constitutes the ECM. OCP/collagen sponges displayed good resorbability and osteogenesis. In mice, collagen-apatite composite (Col-Ap) scaffolds mineralized with simulated bodily fluid supported fresh bone growth. Collagen, alginate, and silica scaffolds facilitated pre-osteoblast activity. Collagen is denaturated to produce gelatin, a naturally occurring protein with minimal toxicity. The proliferation of human MSCs hMSCs on a porous gelatin-covered HA scaffold increased by 163%. After being submerged in SBF, a gelatin-bioactive glass scaffold displayed bone formation.

PEG is a synthetic polymer bioink produced through the polymerization of ethylene oxide. It can be fashioned into various topologies, including linear or multi-armed architectures and different chain lengths. Due to its mechanical qualities, which are generally strong but can be customized, it is a preferred synthetic material for bioprinting and for maintaining the shape of deposited constructions. Additionally, PEG is non-immunogenic and non-cytotoxic (at higher molecular weights). It must be combined with other biologically active hydrogels, as it is a bio inert substance that is difficult for cells to adhere to. The degrading properties of PEG-based structures are enhanced by blends of PEG and natural biomaterials. For osteoblasts, a PEG-PPG-PEG/pregelatinized starch composite was found to be innocuous. Rats' bone growth was enhanced by PVA/gelatin fiber mats containing BCP nanoparticles. In mice, a 3D combination of gelatin, hyaluronan, and alginate demonstrated osseointegration and decreased inflammation [55].

PCL is a biodegradable, biocompatible polyester with excellent mechanical properties and a slow degradation rate, making it an ideal support material for load-bearing tissue constructs such as cartilage. Its thermoplastic nature allows for easy processing and precise control during extrusion-based bioprinting. When combined with soft hydrogels like HAMA, PCL provides the necessary structural integrity to the printed constructs while fostering an environment conducive to cell proliferation and differentiation. The hydrogel was co-printed with PCL and HAMA to raise the constructs' stiffness to a degree equivalent to that of native cartilage.

In another study, articular cartilage tissue constructs were formed by using thio-functionalized HA cross-linked with allyl-functionalized poly(glycidol)s (P(AGE-co-G)) as a bioink. Poly(glycidol)s (PG) are structurally analogous to PEGs but have additional side groups that can be further functionalized. An extrusion-based bioprinter was used for bioprinting. PG-based bioinks incorporating HA showed enhanced cell viability and differentiation than PG-alone bioinks. Polyvinylpyrrolidone (PVP) has been studied as a bioink additive in a separate study [56]. Concentrations of 2–2.5% (w/v) enhanced printability, lessened cell sedimentation, and resulted in a more uniform distribution of cells. In addition, these PVP-based bioinks exhibited enhanced long-term cell viability (up to 96 h after printing) with no print-induced injury, indicating their potential as a constituent of future bioinks.

Ceramics are nonmetallic and inorganic biomaterials, such as hydroxyapatite and β-tricalcium phosphate (β-TCP), extensively used in bone regeneration due to their biocompatibility, osteoconductivity, and chemical resemblance to bone mineral. According to a study by Wen et al., in rabbit models with segmental defects, 3D-printed scaffolds with a 3:7 hydroxyapatite/β-TCP ratio effectively stimulated bone regeneration, exhibiting improved bone union and osteointegration [57]. In a similar vein, Sun et al. found that gelatin-coated porous β-TCP scaffolds made them appropriate for load-bearing applications by dramatically increasing osteoblast proliferation and compressive strength. In accordance with Zhang et al., hydroxyapatite/β-TCP bioceramics demonstrated greater osteoinductive potential in environments with shattered bones, indicating the relevance of biological and mechanical cues in promoting regeneration. These results emphasize the significance of local circumstances, coating, and composition in maximizing the effectiveness of ceramic scaffolds for bone healing.

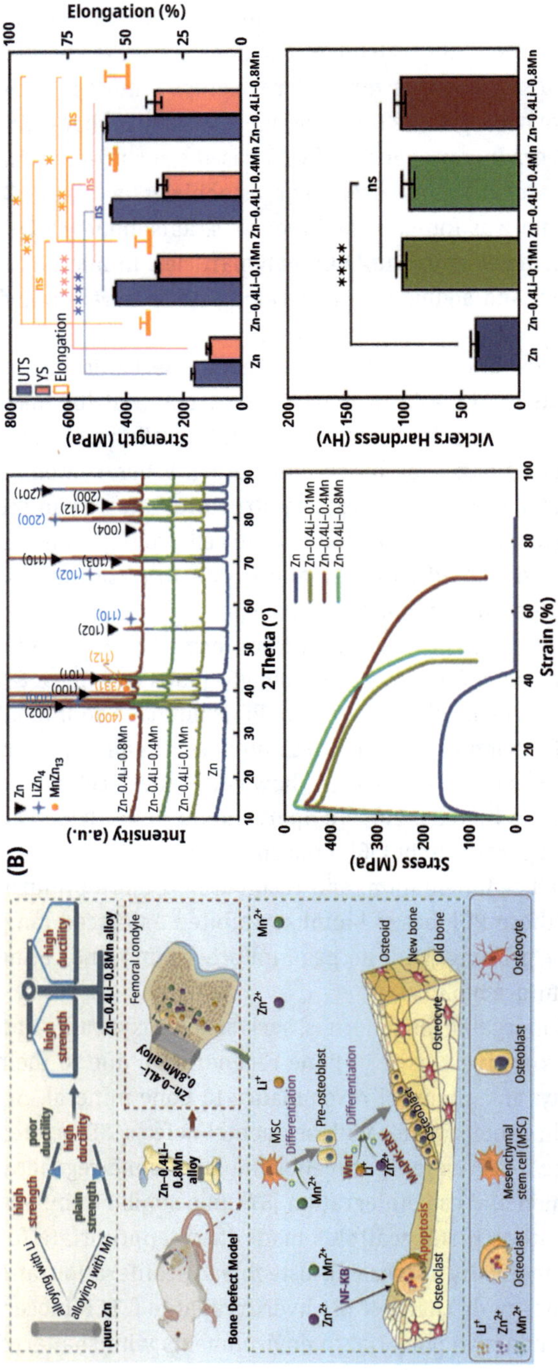

Figure 5.5: (A) Schematic of Zn-0.4 Li-0.8 Mn alloy, promoting the osseointegration effect; (B) The characterization results of the developed materials, such as X-ray diffraction pattern, Mechanical strength, stress-strain curve, and Vickers hardness, respectively. Adapted with permission from ref. [58]. Copyright 2025 Published by Elsevier Inc. on behalf of Acta Materialia Inc.

Biodegradable metals, particularly alloys of magnesium (Mg) and zinc (Zn), are becoming increasingly prevalent for orthopedic applications simply due to their slow degradation in vivo and mechanical compatibility with bone. Magnesium alloys are strong and encourage osteogenesis, but they have problems since they corrode quickly and produce hydrogen gas. Alloying with elements such as zinc and calcium enhances biocompatibility and corrosion resistance. Mg-0.5Ca-1.5Zn alloys, for instance, encouraged osseointegration and indicated excellent degradation rates. Zn-based alloys, including Zn-Li-Mn, also demonstrated the best mechanical strength and degradation behavior for bone regeneration. In vivo measurements of Zn-0.05 Mg alloys have revealed reduced inflammatory responses and improved bone regeneration. Magnesium and zinc alloys work together to create biodegradable scaffold materials that balance bioactivity and mechanical integrity for effective bone healing [58].

5.3.2.3 Bioinks with Pro-angiogenic Additives

The fabrication of bone scaffold has reached to mature stage where multiple biological and chemical cues have been incorporated to achieve optimal tissue growth. However, the lack of proper vascularization persists, and it remains a major challenge for the BTE communities. The lack of a functional vascular network leads to a compromised cellular survival within the engineered constructs, beyond a diffusion limit of (~~200 μm), causing nutrient and oxygen deficiency. The function of pro-angiogenic additives thus becomes extremely important in the design of any bioink, in order to induce vascular growth and maintain the long-term survival of the engineered bone scaffold. To that end, the growth factors like vascular endothelial growth factor (VEGF) and basic fibroblast growth factor (bFGF) have been shown to directly cause angiogenesis, thus substantially increasing the proliferation, migration, and vessel formation. However, their long-term efficacy has been hindered by their short half-life and rapid diffusion from the hydrogel, necessitating the use of controlled release carriers such as microspheres. These growth factors are released gradually to encourage endothelialization. Co-printing with pericytes, mesenchymal stem cells, or endothelial cells promotes remodeling and angiogenesis. Endothelial adhesion and network development are naturally supported by natural polymers such as collagen, decellularized ECM (dECM), and gelatin. Furthermore, the printing method and ideal rheological characteristics need to coincide. To ensure lifetime and functionality, scaffold degradation for biohybrid vascular grafts should correspond with tissue development. Co-printing with pericytes, MSCs, or endothelial cells enhances remodeling and angiogenesis within engineered bone scaffolds. For example, one study illustrated that co-culturing MSCs and endothelial cells yielded human-derived microvessels throughout the construct, with increased vascularization and bone formation [59, 60]. Endothelial network formation and adhesion are inherently promoted by natural polymers like gelatin, collagen, and dECM. Studies have demonstrated that scaffolds with the inclusion of dECM of immature porcine aorta showed better cell infiltration and increased angiogenesis, indicating the significance of ECM structure in scaffold composition.

Furthermore, the printing process and rheological optimum properties should be coordinated to offer structural support and functionality to the scaffold. Studies emphasized that the scaffolds' degradation rate must be coordinated with tissue growth to offer mechanical properties and promote tissue regeneration [61].

To guarantee functionality and lifetime, scaffold degradation of biohybrid vascular grafts must match tissue growth. A recently published study emphasized that the profile of degradation of scaffolds is an important factor in the remodeling and integration of tissues, supporting that synchronized degradation is necessary to provide long-term functionality.

5.4 Design and Optimization of Bioinks

The formulation of bioinks for 3D bioprinting requires careful tuning of physicochemical and rheological properties to ensure both cell viability and printed construct integrity. Critical rheological properties that control printability and accuracy of CAD models are thixotropic recovery, storage modulus (G'), zero-shear viscosity, shear-thinning behavior, and gelation kinetics; these significantly impact extrusion behavior and retention of shape post-printing. Biocompatibility and dispensing modality compatibility (inkjet, extrusion, or light-based modalities) are just as important when choosing or designing bioinks, especially for intricate tissues that need accurate cell positioning, high viability, vascularization, and innervation. Recent research has applied statistical multi-objective optimization (MOO) to balance low extrusion pressures (<30 kPa) for cell protection with high shape fidelity (<5% deformation of CAD geometries). Resampled DoE models generated synthetic datasets that trained artificial neural networks (ANNs) using rheological features alone, achieving high printability prediction accuracy (MAE ≈ 6.3%). Collectively, these findings highlight that integrating rheology, MOO, and machine learning offers a practical strategy to design bioinks that preserve cell viability, improve fidelity, and reduce trial-and-error in bioprinting [62].

5.5 Role of Pharmaceuticals in BTE

Scaffold-based delivery of osteoinductive drugs and small molecules has shown significant potential in BTE. For example, adding rhBMP-2 to calcium silicate/calcium phosphate cement scaffolds markedly increased osteogenic differentiation in vitro and improved the repair of critical-sized bone lesions in vivo. Similarly, rhBMP-2 delivered via perlecan-functionalized PCL electrospun scaffolds maintained growth factor releases and promoted osteogenesis in bone marrow stromal cells. Furthermore, simvastatin and other small compounds have been successfully incorporated into scaffolds made from chitosan or calcium sulfate, demonstrating bone regeneration in rabbit defect models like that of rhBMP-2. It has also been demonstrated that dual drug scaffolds containing simvastatin and dexamethasone within PCL-collagen nanofibers can enhance osteoblastic development and regulate inflammation [63, 64].

By employing functionalized bioinks to incorporate pharmaceuticals into 3D-bioprinted scaffolds, localized, sustained drug release is made possible. The scaffold's usefulness in cancer treatment, wound healing, and bone regeneration is increased by hydrogels such as gelatin methacryloyl (GelMA) or HAMA, which have a high drug-loading capacity and act as both drug reservoirs and cell carriers [65].

The application of scaffolds as delivery platforms for bioactive small molecules and osteoinductive compounds has gained considerable attention in BTE. For instance, the inclusion of recombinant human bone morphogenetic protein-2 (rhBMP-2) into calcium silicate/calcium phosphate cement (CSPC) scaffolds induced more osteogenic differentiation in vitro and superior repair of critical-sized bone defects in vivo. In a similar way, rhBMP-2 released from perlecan-functionalized PCL electrospun scaffolds induced sustained growth factor release and osteogenesis in bone marrow stromal cells. In addition, simvastatin and other small molecules were effectively loaded within scaffolds prepared from chitosan or calcium sulfate and reported bone regeneration in rabbit defect models. It has also been shown that dual-drug scaffolds with simvastatin and dexamethasone incorporated into PCL-collagen nanofibers can promote osteoblastic growth and modulate inflammation. New technologies have provided new biomaterials and 3D-printed scaffolds for drug delivery in BTE. In a study, a novel modified glue gun was developed that 3D prints synthetic bone grafts in situ on living tissue during surgery, employing a biodegradable polymer (PCL) blended with hydroxyapatite. The technique yields a bone scaffold that stimulates natural bone growth and is more acceptable than conventional bone cement [66, 67].

Another innovation is the use of mesoporous bioactive glass/PCL (MBG/PCL) scaffolds that allow for controlled drug release due to the porous structure of the scaffolds. Such scaffolds have been shown to support bone regeneration by enhanced osteoblast activity and inhibition of osteoclast-mediated bone resorption.

Furthermore, scaffolds made of silk proteins that can be 3D printed have been studied for bone tissue engineering. These scaffolds support a favorable environment for osteoblast proliferation and mineralization by offering mechanical strength and biocompatibility [68].

Through the use of functionalized bioinks to load therapeutic agents (such as drugs, growth factors, and biomolecules) in 3D-bioprinted scaffolds, localized and controlled release is enabled. Hydrogels like GelMA or HAMA with high drug-loading capacity can be used as drug reservoirs and carriers of cells, thus enhancing the scaffold's application in cancer therapy, wound healing, and bone tissue engineering [69].

5.6 Commercially Available Bioinks

Commercial bioinks are essential to the advancement of 3D bioprinting as they provide ready-to-use, standardized formulations designed for structural integrity, printability, and cell survival. By mimicking the ECM, these bioinks encourage tissue growth, cell adhesion, and proliferation. Examples of widely used commercial formulations include hyaluronic acid HA, which promotes cell migration and proliferation, alginate, valued for its biocompatibility and ionic cross-linking ability, and GelMA, which allows for photo-cross-linking to ensure structural stability. Collagen-based bioinks, such as those produced by CollPlant and CELLINK, replicate the natural tissue microenvironment, while fibrin supports tissue regeneration and cell adhesion. Rich in growth hormones, Matrigel is frequently employed in cancer and stem cell research. Clinical research, medication development, and tissue modeling all rely on these commercial inks, as they provide consistency, reproducibility, and properties specific to particular applications [70].

5.7 Nature-Inspired Geometries and Design Strategies to target CSBDs

5.7.1 Biomimetic Structures: Trabecular and Cortical Bone

Biomimetic scaffolds enhance integration, vascularization, and regeneration by mimicking the porous, hierarchical structures of bone. This has been proven to enhance scaffold performance and outcomes in clinical trials. The natural composition of bones can serve as a stimulus for creating innovative bone scaffold structures in the science of BTE and regenerative medicine, but the inherent structure of the bone itself also deserves adequate investigation and use in bone constructs. In bone, trabeculae are intricate, beam-like structures that are particularly prevalent in cancellous bone [77]. The effectiveness of bone defect restoration can be greatly increased by creating biomimetic structures that mimic the texture and shape of genuine bone [78]. The recent development in AM and computational modeling has made complex, multilayer porous scaffolds resembling the two different regions of a bone possible. For instance, Zhao et al. [79] created a porous scaffold based on triply periodic minimal surface geometries, with enhanced mechanical strength and near-natural bone mechanics. Many studies have reported combining polymers, ceramics, and bioactive glasses to modulate the stiffness of the cortical bone while still maintaining the porosity and the permeability of the trabecular bone Bose et al., 2012 [94]. Corresponding to the mechanical characteristics of real cancellous bone, 3D-printed constructs with irregular and linked porous structures have been created by simulating the internal network of trabeculae [80, 81]. The complex layered structure of cortical bone represents what

S. no	Commercial bioinks	Trade name	Composition	Key properties	Advantages	Limitations	Applications	References
1.	Bone-mimetic GelMA Bioink	GelXA® BONE	Gelatin methacrylate. Xanthan gum. Alginate. Tricalcium phosphate. Hydroxyapatite.	Light-curable, mimics bone extracellular matrix and promotes cell proliferation and mineralization.	stimulates osteoblast differentiation and makes high-resolution printing feasible.	UV light is required for crosslinking; insufficient for deep tissue scaffolds alone	Long bone scaffolds, osteoinductive matrices, and bone defect repair	[70]
2.	Recombinant Human Collagen Bioink	ColliK® 3D	Recombinant human type I collagen (rhCollagen)	The human-origin protein is biocompatible and provides excellent matrix signaling and cell adhesion.	Non-immunogenic, ideal for clinical use, chemically defined	Requires blending with other biomaterials for mechanical strength	Osteochondral structures, soft-hard tissue contact, and cartilage regeneration	[70]
3.	Gelatin Methacrylate Bioink	GelMA BioGel™	Gelatin methacrylate (GelMA)	Light-activated, adjustable stiffness which promotes cell growth and adhesion	High print fidelity and compatibility with MSCs and osteoblasts	Requires photoinitiators and post-curing	Cartilage engineering, subchondral bone repair	[71].
4.	Silk Protein Bioink	SilkGel™	Regenerated silk fibroin	Exhibits mechanical strength, slow degradation, and protein bioactivity	Excellent stability, adaptable degradation, and compatibility with cells	Limited spontaneous gelation; printability requires adjustment	Bone-ligament interface, joint repair, orthopedic mesh	[72]
5.	Bone ECM Based Bioink	dECM-Bone™	Bone-derived decellularized extracellular matrix	maintains osteogenic cell fate and native bone proteins and growth signals.	improves mineral deposition and bone-specific cell activity.	Soft mechanical profile, donor variability	Bone regeneration, orthopedic scaffold functionalization	[73].

(continued)

(continued)

S. no	Commercial bioinks	Trade name	Composition	Key properties	Advantages	Limitations	Applications	References
6.	Thermo-responsive Support Ink	PluroInk™	Poloxamer 407 (Pluronic F-127)	Reversible phase transition, temperature-sensitive gelation, and embedded printing support	Enables complex geometry formation, removable after printing	Not a permanent scaffold, bio-inert	Support bath for indirect scaffold shaping and orthopedic bioprinting	[74].
7.	Synthetic PEG-Calcium Phosphate Bioink	OsteoInk™	Calcium phosphate, diacrylate, and polyethylene glycol	Mechanical qualities that are adjustable, light-curable, and synthetic	High reproducibility, supports mineral deposition	requires biofunctionalization and lacks natural biological signals."	Bone graft substitutes, craniofacial or dental scaffold printing	[74]
8.	Alginate-Hydroxyapatite Composite Bioink	AlginInk® + nHA	Alginate blended with nano-hydroxyapatite	Ionically crosslinked, osteoconductive, easy to extrude	Simple formulation, tunable stiffness, low-cost	Poor natural cell binding, requires modification	Bone filler constructs, low-load scaffolds, injectable formulation	[75].
9.	Fibrin-Hydroxyapatite Composite Bioink	FibriBone™	Fibrinogen with dispersed nano-hydroxyapatite	biodegradable, mimics the milieu of blood clots, and starts angiogenesis	Natural healing mimicry, supports bone matrix deposition	Soft matrix, lacks load-bearing capacity	Fracture repair, early-stage bone healing, periosteal reconstruction	[76].
10.	Hyaluronic Acid–Collagen Cartilage Bioink	HyStem®-C	Hyaluronic acid + collagen peptides + thiol-reactive crosslinkers	Hydrophilic, mimics cartilage ECM, retains chondrocyte phenotype	Promotes cartilage ECM expression, injectable, low cytotoxicity	Weak mechanical strength, not ideal for large bone loads	Cartilage tissue engineering, osteochondral repair	[76].

gives bone its remarkable mechanical resilience. The layered nature of cortical bone gives it mechanical resilience, which serves as a framework for designing biomaterials and serves as a blueprint for the development of biomimetic structures.

5.7.2 Topologically Optimized Designs for Load-bearing

In orthopedics, topologically optimized designs utilize computational techniques to create robust, lightweight implants for load-bearing applications. They improve mechanical performance, reduce weight, improve osseointegration, and minimize stress-shielding – all of which are critical for joint replacements, spinal cages, and femoral stems by mimicking stress distribution and eliminating unused material. Maximum stiffness with the lowest material volume is achieved through topology optimization. Bone plates containing 30% and 70% volume fractions were processed using the Abaqus Topology Optimization Module (ATOM). Enhancing bone loading, decreasing implant weight and improving biomechanical performance structural integrity, and geometry to site-specific requirements are all made possible by topology optimization. Designs for pelvic prosthesis, mandibular fracture plates, and femur plates have been influenced by topology optimization. Importantly, Al-Tamimi [82] proved that multi-load case optimization of locking compression plates yielded lower stiffness designs that decreased stress-shielding without loss of strength, while Smit et al. [83] proved that patient-specific, strain-constrained spinal fusion cages decreased implant subsidence risk by ~91% in normal bone and 54% in osteopenic bone relative to traditional cages. However, during optimization, few studies consider the physiological forces – compression, bending, and torsion – that are essential to bone repair. This emphasizes the necessity for next-generation orthopedic implants to have load-informed, patient-specific, topically optimized design [84].

5.7.3 Generative Design and AI in Scaffold Architecture

Orthopedic scaffold architecture has evolved due to generative design and AI, enabling the rapid creation of implants optimized for each patient. To alleviate material consumption and optimize mechanical strength and biological compatibility, these advanced computational methods assess a wide range of design options [85]. By anticipating ideal pore size and shape, evaluating medical imaging data, and simulating scaffold function under physiological conditions, AI enhances this process. This method promotes enhanced vascularization and osseointegration through the enabling of the development of complex lattice structures that resemble the microarchitecture of normal bone. In addition to solving the problems associated with the treatment of critical-size bone defects, predictive modeling through AI speeds up scaffold production and preclinical testing [86]. Orthopedic scaffolds become more precise, mechanically functional, and regenerative in potential by combining AI with generative design, ending up with improved patient outcomes as well as faster rehabilitation.

5.8 Future Trends: 4D Bioprinting

Conventional 3D printing is improved by four-dimensional (4D) bioprinting, in which intelligent materials are employed that respond dynamically to external stimuli like light, temperature, pH, humidity, or magnetism. 4D is a favorable technology that has great potential for the fabrication of other 4D-printed products; a few examples in medicine have been depicted in Figure 5.6 [87]. This technique, introduced in 2013, renders printed structures ideal for tissue engineering and regenerative medicine as it enables them to transform in shape or function with time.

These materials, also referred to as active origami systems or shape-morphing materials, are printed layer by layer with technologies such as stereolithography (SLA), FDM, inkjet printing (IJP), DLP, selective laser sintering (SLS), micro-extrusion, and DIW [88]. Based on biocompatible and biodegradable materials, 4D bioprinting allows the formation of complex, highly accurate structures; however, the response and application of the material should be thoughtfully contemplated in selecting a printer [89]. The remarkable form recovery, biocompatibility, and ease of processing of shape-memory polymers (SMPs) have led to their widespread application in 4D bioprinting. Stimuli-responsive 4D-printed scaffolds can benefit from the great sensitivity of some biopolymers, such as cellulose and lignin, to humidity. By altering their shape in response to stimuli, 4D-printed scaffolds in bone regeneration can adapt to irregular flaws and improve grafting results. Self-folding structures are now commonly created using photo-cross-linkable hydrogels and SMPs to create micro-scaled hollow tubules with improved cell distribution.

4D-printed polymer materials for biomedical applications must meet 3D bioprinting requirements and respond to various stimuli. Single-stimulus sensitivity limits the complex transformations needed for in vivo use, which is a common limitation of most existing materials. It is essential to utilize advanced multi-responsive SMPs (shape-memory polymers) and hydrogels enhanced with nanomaterials such as ceramics, graphene, and MNPs (magnetic nanoparticles). Design prediction limitations necessitate empirical modeling. Innovative bioinks with properties like rigidity, cell adhesion, and dynamic behavior are also required, alongside a cost-effective, state-of-the-art bioprinter. Integrating vascular tissues and replicating their complexity remains difficult. SWOT (strengths, weaknesses, opportunities, and threats) analysis and TRL (technology readiness level) assessment are crucial for biomedical applications, given the restricted commercialization, despite recent advances [89].

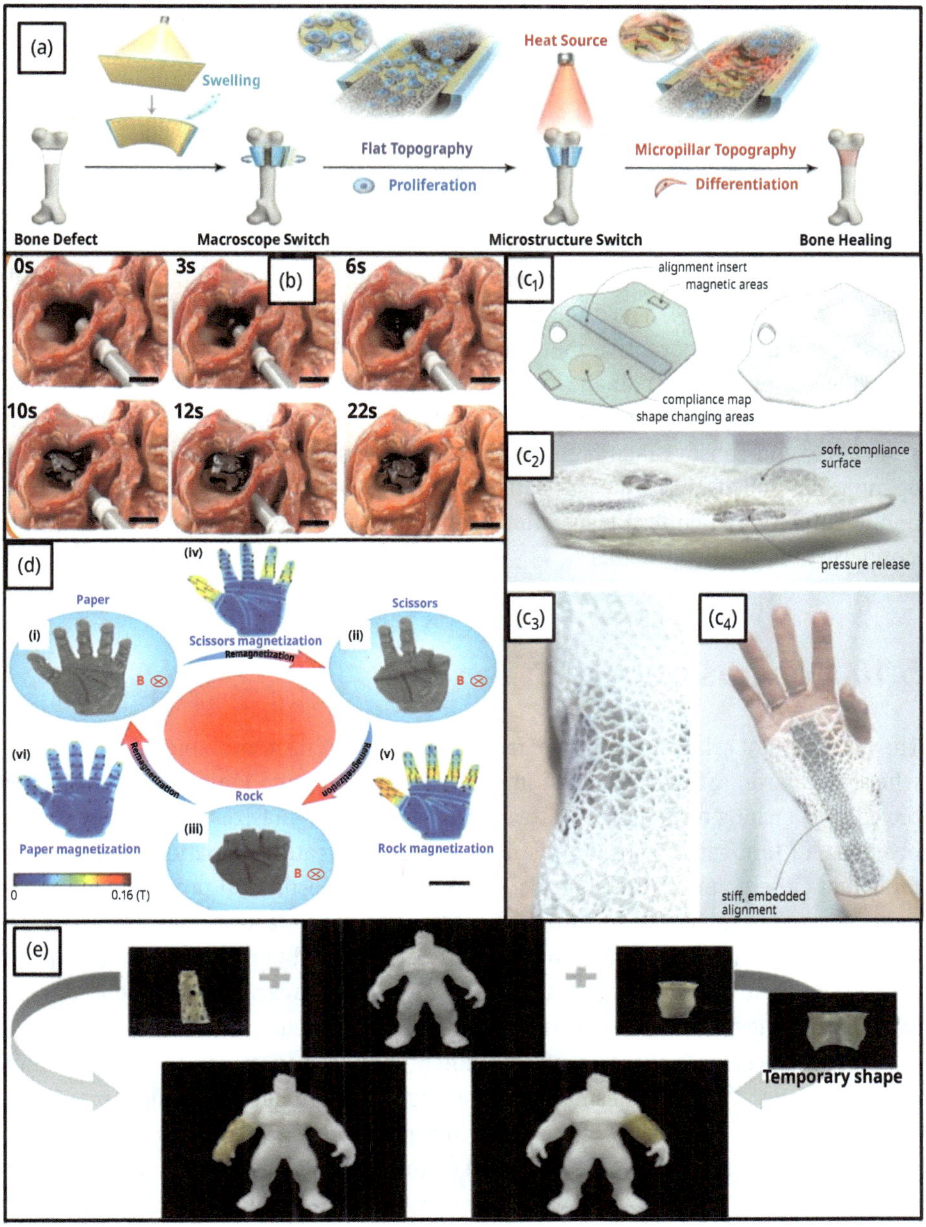

Figure 5.6: Examples of 4D-printed parts in biomedical applications; (a) bilayer membrane for bone repair; (b) in vitro study of transcatheter LAA closure; (c1–c4) multipurpose orthotic splint: design model, pressure distribution, mesostructured features, and worn splint; (d) bionic hand transforming gestures – paper, scissors, rock; (e) PLA/PCL filaments for adaptable elbow protectors. Adapted with permission from ref. [87]. Copyright 2022 Published by Elsevier B.V.

5.9 Outlook for Scalable, Cost-Effective Biomanufacturing

Tissue engineering has long been a key component of biomedical engineering and regenerative medicine. In vitro preclinical research models and tissue substitutes [90] can be established through the specific interaction of cells, carrier material, and growth stimuli. In 1999, Anthony Atala was successful in creating a human bladder and implanting it into a patient. Nevertheless, conventional techniques rely on molds and are labor-intensive, have limited geometric freedom, and are neither scalable nor standardizable. An alternative that shows promise is 3D-bioprinting, which uses digital models to produce personalized tissues like skin, liver, or bones in a reproducible, automated, and scalable manner. The fusion of robotic automation, AI-based quality assurance, and sensors facilitates real-time monitoring and regulatory compliance, opening the door for ATMP certification and industrial-scale biomanufacturing. Economic viability and clinical translation are improved by this shift from handicraft to standardized manufacture [91].

5.10 Conclusion

The treatment of critical-sized bone defects remains a critical problem in orthopedics, where standard grafting and metal implants fall short due to limited supply, reduced bioactivity, or long-term adverse effects. This chapter emphasizes that 3D bioprinting provides an innovative solution by allowing the fabrication of patient-specific scaffolds that closely mimic the biological, chemical, and mechanical properties of native bone. Advances in bioink formulation, composite biomaterials, and AM processes have facilitated the development of scaffolds with tailored porosity, mechanical properties, and controlled biodegradation, as well as the integration of osteoinductive drugs, pro-angiogenic factors, and multifunctional therapeutic agents.

Despite recent advances, issues of limited vascularization, material degradation mismatch, and regulatory obstacles still restrict the more general clinical use. Nonetheless, the convergence of biomimetic designs, topology optimization, AI-based modeling, and innovative 4D bioprinting technologies holds the potential to transcend many of these challenges. Through the synergistic integration of biological signals with engineering accuracy, 3D bioprinting is moving increasingly toward scalable, economically viable, and clinically applicable solutions for severe bone defect repair. Ongoing interdisciplinary cooperation will be essential to move these innovations from bench to bedside, eventually delivering individualized therapies that enhance healing, restore function, and improve patient outcomes.

References

[1] Roddy, E., DeBaun, M. R., Daoud-Gray, A., Yang, Y. P. & Gardner, M. J. (2018). Treatment of critical-sized bone defects: Clinical and tissue engineering perspectives. European Journal of Orthopaedic Surgery & Traumatology, 28, 351–362. https://doi.org/10.1007/s00590-017-2063-0.

[2] Becker, W., Urist, M., Becker, B. E., Jackson, W., Party, D. A., Bartold, M., Vincenzzi, G., De Georges, D. & Niederwanger, M. (1996). Clinical and histologic observations of sites implanted with intraoral autologous bone grafts or allografts. 15 human case reports. Journal of Periodontology, 67, 1025–1033. https://doi.org/10.1902/jop.1996.67.10.1025.

[3] Davis, R., Singh, A., Jackson, M. J., Coelho, R. T., Prakash, D., Charalambous, C. P., Ahmed, W., Da Silva, L. R. R. & Lawrence, A. A. (2022). A comprehensive review on metallic implant biomaterials and their subtractive manufacturing. The International Journal of Advanced Manufacturing Technology, 120, 1473–1530. https://doi.org/10.1007/s00170-022-08770-8.

[4] Ellermann, E., Meyer, N., Cameron, R. E. & Best, S. M. (2023). In vitro angiogenesis in response to biomaterial properties for bone tissue engineering: A review of the state of the art. Regenerative Biomaterials, 10. https://doi.org/10.1093/rb/rbad027.

[5] Mandrycky, C., Wang, Z., Kim, K. & Kim, D.-H. (2016). 3D bioprinting for engineering complex tissues. Biotechnology Advances, 34, 422–434. https://doi.org/10.1016/j.biotechadv.2015.12.011.

[6] Ramesh, S., Deep, A., Tamayol, A., Kamaraj, A., Mahajan, C. & Madihally, S. (2024). Advancing 3D bioprinting through machine learning and artificial intelligence. Bioprinting, 38, e00331. https://doi.org/10.1016/j.bprint.2024.e00331.

[7] Yazdanpanah, Z., Johnston, J. D., Cooper, D. M. L. & Chen, X. (2022). 3D bioprinted scaffolds for bone tissue engineering: State-of-the-art and emerging technologies. Front Bioeng Biotechnol, 10. https://doi.org/10.3389/fbioe.2022.824156.

[8] Jakus, A. E., Rutz, A. L., Jordan, S. W., Kannan, A., Mitchell, S. M., Yun, C., Koube, K. D., Yoo, S. C., Whiteley, H. E., Richter, C.-P., Galiano, R. D., Hsu, W. K., Stock, S. R., Hsu, E. L. & Shah, R. N. (2016). Hyperelastic "bone": A highly versatile, growth factor–free, osteoregenerative, scalable, and surgically friendly biomaterial. Science Translational Medicine, 8. https://doi.org/10.1126/scitranslmed.aaf7704.

[9] Temple, J. P., Hutton, D. L., Hung, B. P., Huri, P. Y., Cook, C. A., Kondragunta, R., Jia, X. & Grayson, W. L. (2014). Engineering anatomically shaped vascularized bone grafts with hASCs and 3D-printed PCL scaffolds. Journal of Biomedical Materials Research Part A. https://doi.org/10.1002/jbm.a.35107.

[10] Levato, R., Visser, J., Planell, J. A., Engel, E., Malda, J. & Mateos-Timoneda, M. A. (2014). Biofabrication of tissue constructs by 3D bioprinting of cell-laden microcarriers. Biofabrication, 6, 035020. https://doi.org/10.1088/1758-5082/6/3/035020.

[11] Dubey, A., Vahabi, H. & Kumaravel, V. (2023). Antimicrobial and biodegradable 3D printed scaffolds for orthopedic infections. ACS Biomaterials Science & Engineering, 9, 4020–4044. https://doi.org/10.1021/acsbiomaterials.3c00115.

[12] Wei, S., Ma, J.-X., Xu, L., Gu, X.-S. & Ma, X.-L. (2020). Biodegradable materials for bone defect repair. Military Medical Research, 7(54), https://doi.org/10.1186/s40779-020-00280-6.

[13] Brown, A., Zaky, S., Ray, H. & Sfeir, C. (2015). Porous magnesium/PLGA composite scaffolds for enhanced bone regeneration following tooth extraction. Acta Biomater, 11, 543–553. https://doi.org/10.1016/j.actbio.2014.09.008.

[14] Heidarian, P., Kouzani, A. Z., Kaynak, A., Paulino, M. & Nasri-Nasrabadi, B. (2019). Dynamic hydrogels and polymers as inks for three-dimensional printing. ACS Biomaterials Science & Engineering, 5, 2688–2707. https://doi.org/10.1021/acsbiomaterials.9b00047.

[15] Gao, F., Ruan, C. & Liu, W. (2019). High-strength hydrogel-based bioinks. Materials Chemistry Frontiers, 3, 1736–1746. https://doi.org/10.1039/C9QM00373H.

[16] Shuai, C., Yu, L., Yang, W., Peng, S., Zhong, Y. & Feng, P. (2020). Phosphonic acid coupling agent modification of HAP nanoparticles: Interfacial effects in PLLA/HAP bone scaffold. Polymers (Basel), 12, 199. https://doi.org/10.3390/polym12010199.

[17] Fousová, M., Kubásek, J., Vojtěch, D., Fojt, J. & Čapek, J. (2017). 3D printed porous stainless steel for potential use in medicine. IOP Conference Series: Materials Science and Engineering, 179, 012025. https://doi.org/10.1088/1757-899X/179/1/012025.

[18] Zhang, C., Zhang, L., Liu, L., Lv, L., Gao, L., Liu, N., Wang, X. & Ye, J. (2020). Mechanical behavior of a titanium alloy scaffold mimicking trabecular structure. Journal of Orthopaedic Surgery and Research, 15, 40. https://doi.org/10.1186/s13018-019-1489-y.

[19] Arjunan, A., Demetriou, M., Baroutaji, A. & Wang, C. (2020). Mechanical performance of highly permeable laser melted Ti6Al4V bone scaffolds. The Journal of the Mechanical Behavior of Biomedical Materials, 102, 103517. https://doi.org/10.1016/j.jmbbm.2019.103517.

[20] Qing, Y., Li, K., Li, D. & Qin, Y. (2020). Antibacterial effects of silver incorporated zeolite coatings on 3D printed porous stainless steels. Materials Science and Engineering: C, 108, 110430. https://doi.org/10.1016/j.msec.2019.110430.

[21] Drummer, D., Cifuentes-Cuéllar, S. & Rietzel, D. (2012). Suitability of PLA/TCP for fused deposition modeling. Rapid Prototyping Journal, 18, 500–507. https://doi.org/10.1108/13552541211272045.

[22] Deng, L., Wang, Y., Peng, Y., Wu, Y., Ding, Y., Jiang, Y., Shen, Z. & Fu, Q. (2015). Osteoblast-derived microvesicles: A novel mechanism for communication between osteoblasts and osteoclasts. Bone, 79, 37–42. https://doi.org/10.1016/j.bone.2015.05.022.

[23] Kuhlmann, J., Bartsch, I., Willbold, E., Schuchardt, S., Holz, O., Hort, N., Höche, D., Heineman, W. R. & Witte, F. (2013). Fast escape of hydrogen from gas cavities around corroding magnesium implants. Acta Biomater, 9, 8714–8721. https://doi.org/10.1016/j.actbio.2012.10.008.

[24] McCoy, R. J. & O'Brien, F. J. (2010). Influence of shear stress in perfusion bioreactor cultures for the development of three-dimensional bone tissue constructs: A review. Tissue Engineering Part B: Reviews, 16, 587–601. https://doi.org/10.1089/ten.teb.2010.0370.

[25] Chen, G., Taylor, P. A., Shin, Y. W., Reynolds, R. C. & Cox, R. W. (2017). Untangling the relatedness among correlations, part II: Inter-subject correlation group analysis through linear mixed-effects modeling. Neuroimage, 147, 825–840. https://doi.org/10.1016/J.NEUROIMAGE.2016.08.029.

[26] Wang, Z., Sun, Y. & Li, C. (2024). Advances in 3D printing technology for preparing bone tissue engineering scaffolds from biodegradable materials. Front Bioeng Biotechnol, 12. https://doi.org/10.3389/fbioe.2024.1483547.

[27] Cong, B. & Zhang, H. (2025). Innovative 3D printing technologies and advanced materials revolutionizing orthopedic surgery: Current applications and future directions. Front Bioeng Biotechnol, 13. https://doi.org/10.3389/fbioe.2025.1542179.

[28] Rodrigues, I. C. P., Orrantia Clark, L. C., Kuang, X., Sanchez Flores, R., Lopes, É. S. N., Gabriel, L. P. & Zhang, Y. S. (2024). Multimaterial coextrusion (bio)printing of composite polymer biomaterial ink and hydrogel bioink for tissue fabrication. Composites Part B: Engineering, 275, 111337. https://doi.org/10.1016/j.compositesb.2024.111337.

[29] Kang, H.-W., Lee, S. J., Ko, I. K., Kengla, C., Yoo, J. J. & Atala, A. (2016). A 3D bioprinting system to produce human-scale tissue constructs with structural integrity. Nature Biotechnology, 34, 312–319. https://doi.org/10.1038/nbt.3413.

[30] Schuurman, W., Khristov, V., Pot, M. W., Van Weeren, P. R., Dhert, W. J. A. & Malda, J. (2011). Bioprinting of hybrid tissue constructs with tailorable mechanical properties. Biofabrication, 3, 021001. https://doi.org/10.1088/1758-5082/3/2/021001.

[31] Salamanca, E., Choy, C. S., Aung, L. M., Tsao, T.-C., Wang, P.-H., Lin, W.-A., Wu, Y.-F. & Chang, W.-J. (2023). 3D-printed PLA scaffold with fibronectin enhances in vitro osteogenesis. Polymers (Basel), 15, 2619. https://doi.org/10.3390/polym15122619.

[32] Li, S., Liu, Z., Gao, X., Cheng, L., Xu, Z., Li, L., Diao, Y., Chen, L., Liu, Y. & Sun, J. (2024). Preparation and properties of a 3D printed nHA/PLA bone tissue engineering scaffold loaded with a β-CD–CHX combined dECM hydrogel. RSC Advances, 14, 9848–9859. https://doi.org/10.1039/D4RA00261J.
[33] Mi, L., Li, F., Xu, D., Liu, J., Li, J., Zhong, L., Liu, Y. & Bai, N. (2024). Performance of 3D printed porous polyetheretherketone composite scaffolds combined with nano-hydroxyapatite/carbon fiber in bone tissue engineering: A biological evaluation. Front Bioeng Biotechnol, 12. https://doi.org/10.3389/fbioe.2024.1343294.
[34] Ouyang, L., Chen, M., Wang, D., Lu, T., Wang, H., Meng, F., Yang, Y., Ma, J., Yeung, K. W. K. & Liu, X. (2019). Nano textured PEEK surface for enhanced osseointegration. ACS Biomaterials Science & Engineering, 5, 1279–1289. https://doi.org/10.1021/acsbiomaterials.8b01425.
[35] Kurtz, S. M. & Devine, J. N. (2007). PEEK biomaterials in trauma, orthopedic, and spinal implants. Biomaterials, 28, 4845–4869. https://doi.org/10.1016/j.biomaterials.2007.07.013.
[36] Feng, P., Jia, J., Liu, M., Peng, S., Zhao, Z. & Shuai, C. (2021). Degradation mechanisms and acceleration strategies of poly (lactic acid) scaffold for bone regeneration. Materials & Design, 210, 110066. https://doi.org/10.1016/j.matdes.2021.110066.
[37] Mahmud, M. A. P., Zolfagharian, A., Gharaie, S., Kaynak, A., Farjana, S. H., Ellis, A. V., Chen, J. & Kouzani, A. Z. (2021). 3D-printed triboelectric nanogenerators: State of the art, applications, and challenges. Advanced Energy and Sustainability Research, 2. https://doi.org/10.1002/aesr.202000045.
[38] Oh, S.-H. & Park, K. (2024). Direct slicing of microcellular structures for digital light processing (DLP) additive manufacturing. Rapid Prototyping Journal, 30, 633–642. https://doi.org/10.1108/RPJ-08-2023-0289.
[39] Tao, J., Zhu, S., Liao, X., Wang, Y., Zhou, N., Li, Z., Wan, H., Tang, Y., Yang, S., Du, T., Yang, Y., Song, J. & Liu, R. (2022). DLP-based bioprinting of void-forming hydrogels for enhanced stem-cell-mediated bone regeneration. Mater Today Bio, 17, 100487. https://doi.org/10.1016/j.mtbio.2022.100487.
[40] Hussain, M. I., Xia, M., Ren, X., Ge, C., Jamil, M. & Gupta, M. K. (2024). Digital light processing 3D printing of ceramic materials: A review on basic concept, challenges, and applications. The International Journal of Advanced Manufacturing Technology, 130, 2241–2267. https://doi.org/10.1007/s00170-023-12847-3.
[41] Wegmüller, L., Halbeisen, F., Sharma, N., Kühl, S. & Thieringer, F. M. (2021). Consumer vs. high-end 3D printers for guided implant surgery – an in vitro accuracy assessment study of different 3D printing technologies. Journal of Clinical Medicine, 10, 4894. https://doi.org/10.3390/jcm10214894.
[42] Mahmud, M. A. P., Zolfagharian, A., Gharaie, S., Kaynak, A., Farjana, S. H., Ellis, A. V., Chen, J. & Kouzani, A. Z. (2021). 3D-printed triboelectric nanogenerators: State of the art, applications, and challenges. Advanced Energy and Sustainability Research, 2. https://doi.org/10.1002/aesr.202000045.
[43] Maguire, A., Pottackal, N., Saadi, M. A. S. R., Rahman, M. M. & Ajayan, P. M. (2020). Additive manufacturing of polymer-based structures by extrusion technologies. Oxford Open Materials Science, 1. https://doi.org/10.1093/oxfmat/itaa004.
[44] Gibson, I., Rosen, D. W. & Stucker, B. (2010). Additive Manufacturing Technologies. Boston, MA: Springer US.
[45] Vidal, L., Kampleitner, C., Brennan, M. Á., Hoornaert, A. & Layrolle, P. (2020). Reconstruction of large skeletal defects: Current clinical therapeutic strategies and future directions using 3D printing. Front Bioeng Biotechnol, 8. https://doi.org/10.3389/fbioe.2020.00061.
[46] Li, X. & Chen, Y. (2021). Vat-photopolymerization-based ceramic manufacturing. Journal of Materials Engineering and Performance, 30, 4819–4836. https://doi.org/10.1007/s11665-021-05920-z.
[47] Owen, R., Sherborne, C., Paterson, T., Green, N. H., Reilly, G. C. & Claeyssens, F. (2016). Emulsion templated scaffolds with tunable mechanical properties for bone tissue engineering. The Journal of

the Mechanical Behavior of Biomedical Materials, 54, 159–172. https://doi.org/10.1016/j.jmbbm.2015.09.019.
[48] Mayfield, C. K., Ayad, M., Lechtholz-Zey, E., Chen, Y. & Lieberman, J. R. (2022). 3D-printing for critical sized bone defects: Current concepts and future directions. Bioengineering, 9, 680. https://doi.org/10.3390/bioengineering9110680.
[49] Liu, M., Wang, Y., Liu, X., Wei, Q., Bao, C. & Zhang, K. (2023). Comprehensive review on fabricating bioactive ceramic bone scaffold using vat photopolymerization. ACS Biomaterials Science & Engineering, 9, 3032–3057. https://doi.org/10.1021/acsbiomaterials.3c00051.
[50] Lee, J. W., Kang, K. S., Lee, S. H., Kim, J.-Y., Lee, B.-K. & Cho, D.-W. (2011). Bone regeneration using a microstereolithography-produced customized poly(propylene fumarate)/diethyl fumarate photopolymer 3D scaffold incorporating BMP-2 loaded PLGA microspheres. Biomaterials, 32, 744–752. https://doi.org/10.1016/j.biomaterials.2010.09.035.
[51] Husna, A., Ashrafi, S., Tomal, A. A., Tuli, N. T. & Bin Rashid, A. (2024). Recent advancements in stereolithography (SLA) and their optimization of process parameters for sustainable manufacturing. Hybrid Advances, 7. https://doi.org/10.1016/j.hybadv.2024.100307.
[52] Ghobadi, F., Mohammadi, M., Kalantarzadeh, R., Lotfi, E., Borhan, S., Pal, N., Chauhan, S., Salehi, G. & Simorgh, S. (2025). Advanced 3D-printed multiphasic scaffold with optimal PRP dosage for chondrogenesis of BM-MSCs in osteochondral tissue engineering.
[53] Gao, L., Li, Y., Liu, G., Lin, X., Tan, Y., Liu, J., Li, R. & Zhang, C. (2025). Mechanical properties and biocompatibility characterization of 3D printed collagen type II/silk fibroin/hyaluronic acid scaffold. Journal of Biomaterials Science, Polymer Edition, 36, 564–586. https://doi.org/10.1080/09205063.2024.2411797.
[54] Kavya, K. C., Jayakumar, R., Nair, S. & Chennazhi, K. P. (2013). Fabrication and characterization of chitosan/gelatin/nSiO2 composite scaffold for bone tissue engineering. International Journal of Biological Macromolecules, 59, 255–263. https://doi.org/10.1016/j.ijbiomac.2013.04.023.
[55] Singh, D., Tripathi, A., Zo, S., Singh, D. & Han, S. S. (2014). Synthesis of composite gelatin-hyaluronic acid-alginate porous scaffold and evaluation for in vitro stem cell growth and in vivo tissue integration. Colloids and Surfaces B: Biointerfaces, 116, 502–509. https://doi.org/10.1016/j.colsurfb.2014.01.049.
[56] Stichler, S., Böck, T., Paxton, N., Bertlein, S., Levato, R., Schill, V., Smolan, W., Malda, J., Teßmar, J., Blunk, T. & Groll, J. (2017). Double printing of hyaluronic acid/poly(glycidol) hybrid hydrogels with poly(ε -caprolactone) for MSC chondrogenesis. Biofabrication, 9, 044108. https://doi.org/10.1088/1758-5090/aa8cb7.
[57] Wen, J., Song, M., Zeng, Y. & Dong, X. (2023). Effect of different HA/β-TCP coated 3D printed bioceramic scaffolds on repairing large bone defects in rabbits. Journal of Orthopaedic Surgery, 31. https://doi.org/10.1177/10225536231222121.
[58] Shen, D., Li, Y., Shi, J., Zhang, T., Nie, -J.-J., Chen, D., Xia, D. & Zheng, Y. (2025). Biodegradable Zn-Li-Mn alloy to achieve optimal strength and ductility for bone implants. Acta Biomater, 199, 483–499. https://doi.org/10.1016/j.actbio.2025.04.056.
[59] Kawai, T. (2025). Preclinical evaluation and advancements in vascularized bone tissue engineering. Biomimetics, 10, 412. https://doi.org/10.3390/biomimetics10070412.
[60] Synofzik, J., Heene, S., Jonczyk, R. & Blume, C. (2024). Ink-structing the future of vascular tissue engineering: A review of the physiological bioink design. Bio-Design and Manufacturing, 7, 181–205. https://doi.org/10.1007/s42242-024-00270-w.
[61] Lang, Z., Chen, T., Zhu, S., Wu, X., Wu, Y., Miao, X., Wang, Q., Zhao, L., Zhu, Z. & Xu, R. X. (2024). Construction of vascular grafts based on tissue-engineered scaffolds. Mater Today Bio, 29, 101336. https://doi.org/10.1016/j.mtbio.2024.101336.
[62] Qavi, I., Halder, S. & Tan, G. (2025). Optimization of printability of bioinks with multi-response optimization (MRO) and artificial neural networks (ANN). Progress in Additive Manufacturing, 10, 3573–3598. https://doi.org/10.1007/s40964-024-00828-1.

[63] Huang, X., Huang, Z. & LI, W. (2014). Highly efficient release of simvastatin from simvastatin-loaded calcium sulphate scaffolds enhances segmental bone regeneration in rabbits. Molecular Medicine Reports, 9, 2152–2158. https://doi.org/10.3892/mmr.2014.2101.

[64] Rather, H. A., Varghese, J. F., Dhimmar, B., Yadav, U. C. S. & Vasita, R. (2022). Polycaprolactone-collagen nanofibers loaded with dexamethasone and simvastatin as an osteoinductive and immunocompatible scaffold for bone regeneration applications. Biomaterials and Biosystems, 8, 100064. https://doi.org/10.1016/j.bbiosy.2022.100064.

[65] Zhang, J., Liu, C., Li, X., Liu, Z. & Zhang, Z. (2023). Application of photo-crosslinkable gelatin methacryloyl in wound healing. Front Bioeng Biotechnol, 11. https://doi.org/10.3389/fbioe.2023.1303709.

[66] Researchers develop modified glue gun that can print bone – device 3D prints synthetic grafts directly onto patients' living tissue during surgery | Tom's Hardware, https://www.tomshardware.com/3d-printing/researchers-develop-modified-glue-gun-that-can-print-bone-device-3d-prints-synthetic-grafts-directly-onto-patients-living-tissue-during-surgery

[67] Chaudhari, V. S., Kushram, P. & Bose, S. (2024). Drug delivery strategies through 3D-printed calcium phosphate. Trends in Biotechnology, 42, 1396–1409. https://doi.org/10.1016/j.tibtech.2024.05.006.

[68] Waidi, Y. O., Debnath, S., Datta, S. & Chatterjee, K. (2024). 3D-printed silk proteins for bone tissue regeneration and associated immunomodulation. Biomacromolecules, 25, 5512–5540. https://doi.org/10.1021/acs.biomac.4c00540.

[69] Wang, Z., Sun, Y. & Li, C. (2024). Advances in 3D printing technology for preparing bone tissue engineering scaffolds from biodegradable materials. Front Bioeng Biotechnol, 12. https://doi.org/10.3389/fbioe.2024.1483547.

[70] Chiticaru, E. A. & Ioniță, M. (2024). Commercially available bioinks and state-of-the-art lab-made formulations for bone tissue engineering: A comprehensive review. Mater Today Bio, 29, 101341. https://doi.org/10.1016/j.mtbio.2024.101341.

[71] Seok, J. M., Ahn, M., Kim, D., Lee, J.-S., Lee, D., Choi, M.-J., Yeo, S. J., Lee, J. H., Lee, K., Kim, B. S. & Park, S. A. (2024). Decellularized matrix bioink with gelatin methacrylate for simultaneous improvements in printability and biofunctionality. International Journal of Biological Macromolecules, 262, 130194. https://doi.org/10.1016/j.ijbiomac.2024.130194.

[72] Chakraborty, J., Mu, X., Pramanick, A., Kaplan, D. L. & Ghosh, S. (2022). Recent advances in bioprinting using silk protein-based bioinks. Biomaterials, 287, 121672. https://doi.org/10.1016/j.biomaterials.2022.121672.

[73] Kim, Y. S., Majid, M., Melchiorri, A. J. & Mikos, A. G. (2019). Applications of decellularized extracellular matrix in bone and cartilage tissue engineering. Bioengineering & Translational Medicine, 4, 83–95. https://doi.org/10.1002/btm2.10110.

[74] Liu, X., Feng, B., Tagliaferri, S., Constantinou, A. P., Porter, A. E., Mattevi, C. & Georgiou, T. K. (2025). Graphene inks for printing based on thermoresponsive ABC triblock terpolymer gels. RSC Applied Polymers, 3, 973–989. https://doi.org/10.1039/D5LP00071H.

[75] Thakur, K. K., Lekurwale, R., Bansode, S. & Pansare, R. (2024). Optimization and characterization of 3D bioprintable alginate and hydroxyapatite based biomaterial ink. Journal of the Institution of Engineers (India): Series C, 105, 1531–1543. https://doi.org/10.1007/s40032-024-01112-5.

[76] Lan, X., Ma, Z., Dimitrov, A., Kunze, M., Mulet-Sierra, A., Ansari, K., Osswald, M., Seikaly, H., Boluk, Y. & Adesida, A. B. (2024). Double crosslinked hyaluronic acid and collagen as a potential bioink for cartilage tissue engineering. International Journal of Biological Macromolecules, 273, 132819. https://doi.org/10.1016/j.ijbiomac.2024.132819.

[77] Ghazlan, A., Ngo, T., Nguyen, T., Linforth, S. & Van Le, T. (2020). Uncovering a high-performance bio-mimetic cellular structure from trabecular bone. Scientific Reports, 10, 14247. https://doi.org/10.1038/s41598-020-70536-7.

[78] Kivell, T. L. (2016). A review of trabecular bone functional adaptation: What have we learned from trabecular analyses in extant hominoids and what can we apply to fossils? Journal of Anatomy, 228, 569–594. https://doi.org/10.1111/joa.12446.
[79] Zhao, F., Xiong, Y., Ito, K., Van Rietbergen, B. & Hofmann, S. (2021). Porous geometry guided micro-mechanical environment within scaffolds for cell mechanobiology study in bone tissue engineering. Front Bioeng Biotechnol, 9, 736489. https://doi.org/10.3389/FBIOE.2021.736489/BIBTEX.
[80] Fernandes, M. C., Aizenberg, J., Weaver, J. C. & Bertoldi, K. (2021). Mechanically robust lattices inspired by deep-sea glass sponges. Nature Materials, 20, 237–241. https://doi.org/10.1038/s41563-020-0798-1.
[81] Ledda, M., Merco, M., Sciortino, A., Scatena, E., Convertino, A., Lisi, A. & Del Gaudio, C. (2022). Biological response to bioinspired microporous 3D-printed scaffolds for bone tissue engineering. International Journal of Molecular Sciences, 23, 5383. https://doi.org/10.3390/ijms23105383.
[82] Al-Tamimi, A. A. (2024). 3D topology optimization and mesh dependency for redesigning locking compression plates aiming to reduce stress shielding. International Journal of Bioprinting, 7, 339. https://doi.org/10.18063/ijb.v7i3.339.
[83] Tayebi, M., Bizari, D. & Hassanzade, Z. (2020). Investigation of mechanical properties and biocorrosion behavior of in situ and ex situ Mg composite for orthopedic implants. Materials Science and Engineering: C, 113, 110974. https://doi.org/10.1016/j.msec.2020.110974.
[84] Al-Tamimi, A. A., Quental, C., Folgado, J., Peach, C. & Bartolo, P. (2020). Stress analysis in a bone fracture fixed with topology-optimised plates. Biomechanics and Modeling in Mechanobiology, 19, 693–699. https://doi.org/10.1007/s10237-019-01240-3.
[85] Omigbodun, F. T. & Oladapo, B. I. (2025). AI-optimized lattice structures for biomechanics scaffold design. Biomimetics, 10(88), https://doi.org/10.3390/biomimetics10020088.
[86] Chen, H., Han, Q., Wang, C., Liu, Y., Chen, B. & Wang, J. (2020). Porous scaffold design for additive manufacturing in orthopedics: A review. Front Bioeng Biotechnol, 8. https://doi.org/10.3389/fbioe.2020.00609.
[87] Khalid, M. Y., Imran, R., Arif, Z. U., Akram, N., Arshad, H., Al Rashid, A. & García Márquez, F. P. (2021). Developments in chemical treatments, manufacturing techniques and potential applications of natural-fibers-based biodegradable composites. Coatings, 11, 293. https://doi.org/10.3390/coatings11030293.
[88] Tie, D., Liu, H., Guan, R., Holt-Torres, P., Liu, Y., Wang, Y. & Hort, N. (2020). In vivo assessment of biodegradable magnesium alloy ureteral stents in a pig model. Acta Biomater, 116, 415–425. https://doi.org/10.1016/j.actbio.2020.09.023.
[89] Naveau, A., Smirani, R., Catros, S., De Oliveira, H., Fricain, J.-C. & Devillard, R. (2017). A bibliometric study to assess bioprinting evolution. Applied Sciences, 7, 1331. https://doi.org/10.3390/app7121331.
[90] Nerem, R. M. & Sambanis, A. (1995). Tissue engineering: From biology to biological substitutes. Tissue Engineering, 1, 3–13. https://doi.org/10.1089/ten.1995.1.3.
[91] Lindner, N. & Blaeser, A. (2022). Scalable biofabrication: A perspective on the current state and future potentials of process automation in 3D-bioprinting applications. Front Bioeng Biotechnol, 10. https://doi.org/10.3389/fbioe.2022.855042.
[92] Zhao, Y., Wu, Q., Zhao, C., Zhou, H. & Wu, L. (2024). Progress of structural scaffold biomaterials for bone tissue defect repair: A cutting-edge review. Composite Structures, 349, 118542.
[93] Lee JW, Kang KS, Lee SH, Kim JY, Lee BK, Cho DW. Bone regeneration using a microstereolithograph y-produced customized poly (propylene fumarate) /diethyl fumarate photopolymer 3D scaffold incorporating BMP-2 loaded PLGA microspheres. Biomaterials. 2011 Jan;32(3):744–52. doi: 10.1016/j.biomaterials.2010.09.035. Epub 2010 Oct 8. PMID: 20933279.
[94] Bose, S., Roy, M., Bandyopadhyay, A.: Recent advances in bone tissue engineering scaffolds. Trends Biotechnol. 30, 546–554 (2012). https://doi.org/10.1016/j.tibtech.2012.07.005

Ahsan Riaz Khan*, Navdeep Singh Grewal, Zhang Hai-Jun

Chapter 6
Innovative Design in 3D Bioprinting Toward the Digital Revolution

Abstract: 3D bioprinting has ushered in a new era of innovation, merging the realms of biology, engineering, and digital technology to redefine the future of healthcare and manufacturing. This chapter explores the transformative role of innovative design in 3D bioprinting as a driving force behind the ongoing digital revolution. By integrating advanced computational tools, artificial intelligence (AI), and cutting-edge fabrication techniques, 3D bioprinting is poised to revolutionize personalized medicine, tissue engineering, and regenerative therapies.

This transformation lies in the synergy between digital design and bioprinting technologies. Computational modeling and simulation enable the precise design of complex, patient-specific structures, while AI-driven algorithms optimize the material selection, printing parameters, and scaffold architectures. These advancements are further enhanced by integrating multi-material and 4D bioprinting, which allow for the creation of dynamic, functional tissues that can adapt and evolve over time. Such innovations are pushing the boundaries of what is possible in tissue engineering and paving the way for the development of smart implants and biohybrid devices.

Moreover, the convergence of 3D bioprinting with digital technologies such as the Internet of Things (IoT), virtual reality (VR), and digital twins creates a seamless ecosystem for innovation. For instance, VR-based design platforms enable researchers to visualize and manipulate 3D-bioprinted structures in real time, while IoT-connected bioprinters facilitate remote monitoring and control of the printing process. These integrations are accelerating the transition toward personalized and on-demand healthcare solutions, where treatments are tailored to the unique needs of each patient.

***Corresponding author: Ahsan Riaz Khan**, School of Medical Informational Engineering, Shandong University of Traditional Chinese Medicine, Jinan 250355, China; National United Engineering Laboratory for Biomedical Material Modification, Branden Industrial Park, Qihe Economic and Development Zone, Dezhou City, Shandong 251100, China, e-mail: ahsan_tareen@outlook.com
Navdeep Singh Grewal, University of South Bohemia, Branisovska 1760, 37005 Ceske Budejovice, Czech Republic; Department of Mechanical Engineering, Guru Kashi University, Talwandi Sabo 151302, India
Zhang Hai-Jun, Department of Interventional and Vascular Surgery, Shanghai Tenth People's Hospital, Tongji University School of Medicine, Shanghai 200072, China; National United Engineering Laboratory for Biomedical Material Modification, Branden Industrial Park, Qihe Economic and Development Zone, Dezhou City, Shandong 251100, China

 | https://doi.org/10.1515/9783111719993-006

Despite these advancements, challenges such as scalability, regulatory hurdles, and ethical considerations remain. This chapter also highlights the potential of 3D bioprinting to address global healthcare challenges, from organ shortages to the development of cost-effective medical devices. By embracing the principles of innovative design and digital transformation, 3D bioprinting is not only reshaping the future of medicine but also contributing to a broader digital revolution that transcends disciplinary boundaries.

Keywords: 3D bioprinting, innovative design, digital revolution, tissue engineering, artificial intelligence (AI)

6.1 Introduction

6.1.1 Overview of 3D Bioprinting

6.1.1.1 Definition and significance of 3D bioprinting

3D bioprinting is a relatively new term that employs innovative technology and traditional 3D printing techniques to develop complex biological organs and tissues utilizing biomaterials, living cells, and growth factors. The method uses a computer-generated design to make layer-by-layer structures using the precise deposition of bioinks, materials made from bioactive components. The printed tissues are utilized for various medical testing, such as regenerative medicine or drug testing [1].

The emergence of 3D bioprinting technology has opened up new opportunities in regenerative medicine by providing a medium to develop personalized models according to patient requirements and conditions, enabling scientists to replicate human tissues with precision. Bioprinting can be extensively applied in the field of medicine. It could be used to create customized tissue models for studying diseases, creating scaffolds for tissues, and testing drugs.

Researchers and scientists are actively involved in maximizing the potential of 3D bioprinting to print fully functional organs that could significantly elevate the shortage of transplantable organs and offer customized solutions for patients with organ failure conditions [2]. Further, the 3D-printed models of tissues can help biomedical educators improve their surgical training by practicing realistic and patient-specific anatomical replicas.

6.1.2 Evolution from Traditional Manufacturing to Additive Manufacturing in Healthcare

This innovative technology marks a significant departure from conventional manufacturing techniques used in healthcare. Historically, traditionally, healthcare indus-

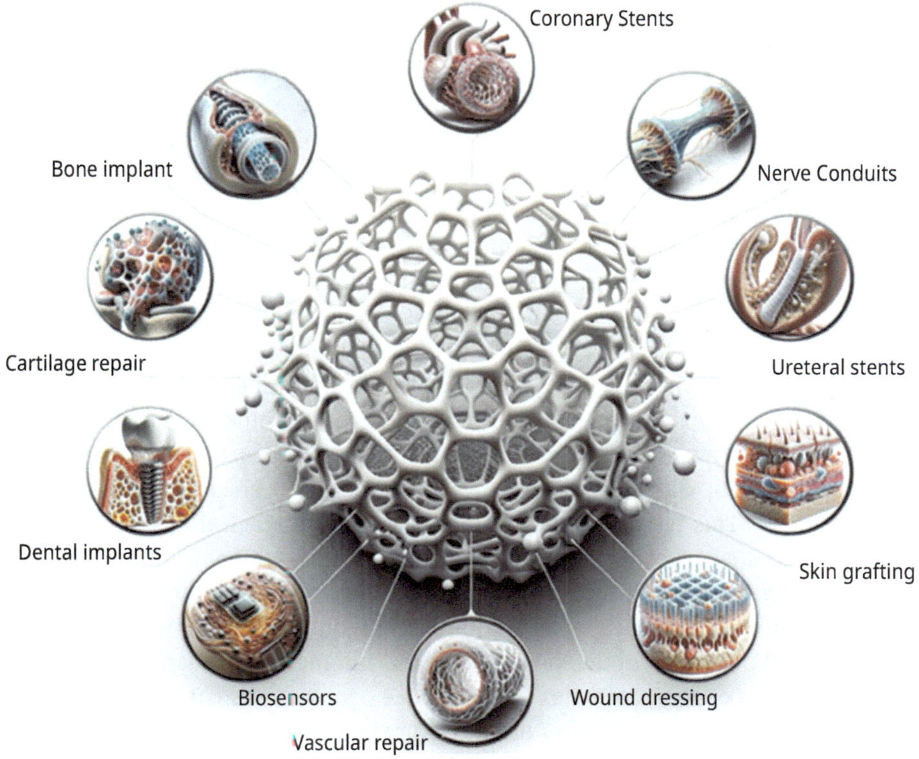

Figure 6.1: Implications of 3D bioprinting in various biomedical areas.

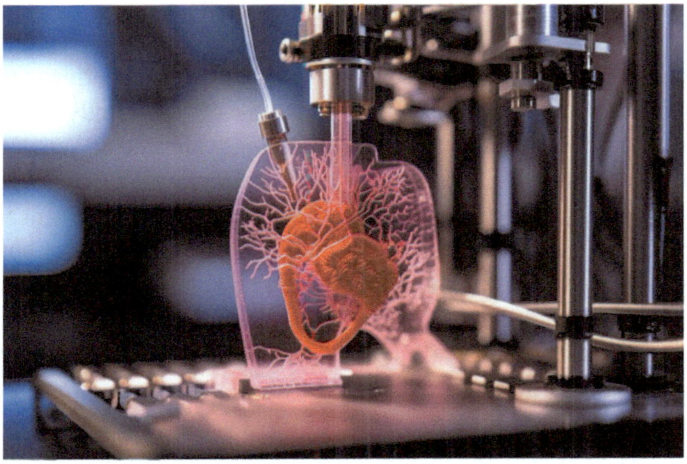

Figure 6.2: Visual representation of 3D bioprinting of organs.

try employs modeling methods such as molding, casting, and machining [3]. While effective, these methods demonstrate several limitations in producing complex and customized structure. Conventionally, these methods require rigid material and to work with and use significant time, labor and cost to produce a single implant or device. Additionally, traditional scaffold manufacturing is incapable of creating intricate design features necessary to produce complex biological systems such as vascular networks within organs and microstructures of tissues. This issue was significantly addressed with the introduction of additive manufacturing or 3D printing. Additive manufacturing has revolutionized the manufacturing processes in healthcare by offering layer-by-layer constructions of structures enabling to replicate complex designs [4]. Furthermore, these methods offer benefits like ability to develop complex structure with precision, short production time, and less waste material. These technologies are already being utilized to produce surgical tools, prosthetics, and implant; traditionally, healthcare industry employs modeling methods such as molding, casting and machining [5]. 3D bioprinting, however, is one step ahead of these additive manufacturing. This technique utilizes living cells and biological material to create human tissue structures [6]. This dynamic shift from traditional to 3D bioprinting method especially in healthcare has opened up the possibility to manufacture human tissue structures that are capable of interacting with human body. Achieving this milestone will be critical in the field of medicine and medical academia as it will enable researchers examine complex in vitro tissue behavior and can provide accurate models to understand morphology of human organs and tissues, diseases, and growing tissues for clinical applications as shown in Figure 6.1.

6.1.3 The Digital Revolution and Its Impact on Bioprinting

The rapid advancements of digital technologies have reshaped the 3D bioprinting processes enhancing its efficacy, capacity, and precision. They have significantly influenced industries globally and the healthcare is no exception. Advancements such as Internet of Things (IoT), artificial intelligence (AI), big data, and virtual a reality have paved the way for advance bio manufacturing solutions. These technological advancements have not only improved the efficacy and precision of bioprinting processes but also facilitated the biomedical experts to create highly complex, personalized, and functional tissues and organs [7].

Among these innovations, virtual reality (VR) plays a critical part. VR significantly facilitates the design phase of bioprinting by offering immersive visualization tools. It helps researchers to study and observe intricate structures by enabling them to interact with 3D models of tissues and organs. Observing the near-to-real 3D models greatly enhances their ability to design prints and facilitates them in identifying issues before actual physical printing [8]. In this way, the overall precision of bioproducts increases, and the chances of error are reduced. Complementing VR, the IoT facilitates real-time feedback and monitoring during the printing process. IoT enables researchers to put sensors in bioprinting systems that collect data on material properties, humidity, and temperature. This data is then transmitted and remotely analyzed to ensure control and maintain the precision of the bioprinting environment, enabling adjustments to be made in real. The IoT integration in bioprinting also augments the reproducibility, consistency, and quality of printing tissues for clinical applications [8]. Central to these digital technologies is the AI that provides robust predictive modeling and data analysis tools [9]. Further, the machine learning (ML) algorithm facilitates the optimization of the printing process and adjusts variables like layer height, cell behavior, and print speed, all based on AI data-driven insights [10]. The quality and predictability of bioprinting outcomes are also significantly enhanced using AI systems, as they can suggest the best materials for desired tissue outcomes.

Further, digital technologies offer interdisciplinary and collaborative approaches to healthcare innovation. Digital transformation has enabled the healthcare industry to utilize highly specific and customized patient solutions, which previously relied on "one-size-fits-all" approach [11]. Today with the help of digital technologies, healthcare professionals are able to design treatments tailored specifically based on patient's medical needs and unique anatomy. Digital technologies, when combined with medical professionals, bioprinting specialists, and engineers, foster a collaborative environment and result in the development of advance medical treatments. Digital platforms enable the medical teams to effectively research, design, and share data among themselves and facilitate the integration of latest advancements in patient care and bioprinting [12].

The current chapter aims to explore and investigate the nexus between digital designing and 3D bioprinting. The role and significance of advanced imaging techniques and computational tools in enhancing the fabrication of complex biological constructs are explored. Further, the chapter dwells on recent innovations in 3D bioprinting, including printing technologies, design strategies, and material development. The chapter also provides insights into potential solutions by examining the challenges faced in 3D bioprinting, including precision, scalability, and clinical translation issues. Discussion related to ML integration, personalized medicine, and multi-material printing is also provided to inspire further research.

6.2 Fundamentals of 3D Bioprinting

3D bioprinting involves precisely fabricating biological constructs layer by layer while maintaining control over biomaterials, cells, and biomolecules. The procedure relies on the basic principle of mimicking tissues and organs' natural architecture and functions by depositing "bioinks" through an advanced software-controlled bioprinter to develop three-dimensional and complex living tissues and organs [13].

6.2.1 Key Components: Bioinks, Printers, and Software

The key components of 3D bioprinting are bioprinters, bioinks, and printing software. Bioprinters are the hardware platform that executes the printing process. These highly advanced machines comprise precise deposition systems and mechanical, pneumatic, or laser-based dispensing units. They are capable of creating various cell densities and viscosities with precision [14]. They are categorized based on their printing modalities, such as laser-assisted, extrusion, or inkjet systems, offering unique speed resolution and cell viability. Software, like computer-aided design (CAD) models, is usually used in these printers to develop digital blueprints for printing. This sophisticated software enables researchers to control print parameters, manage toolpaths, and optimize and simulate printing strategies [14]. Further, advanced software works with computational modeling that maintains structural integrity enhances fidelity and adapts designs according to patient needs. The central element, however, is the bioinks. These are cell-based biomaterials designed and formulated to provide a microenvironment that supports proliferation, viability, and differentiation during and after printing. Bioinks are commonly composed of cells, hydrogels, growth factors, and other bioactive molecules, offering biocompatibility, mechanical stability, and printability to enable successful biomimicry of extracellular matrix (ECM) [15].

6.2.2 Types of Bioprinting Techniques (Extrusion-Based, Inkjet, Laser-Assisted, etc.)

Figure 6.3 3D bioprinting is done through different techniques, each with a unique bioink deposition mechanism. Among these, extrusion-based bioprinting is widely employed. This technique uses piston, pneumatic or screw-driven systems, to excrete bioink with the help of nozzle enabling the printer to print high cell densities and viscous materials, resulting in stable mechanical constructs [16]. However, a primary limitation is the amount of stress it imposes on cells, causing them to reduce their viability. Despite this, the balance of speed and moderate resolution makes it appropriate for developing large tissue organs such as kidneys, liver, and musculoskeletal tissues. Another popular method is inkjet bioprinting, which is well suited for creating skin and vascular tissue models. It works by depositing low-viscosity bioink droplets for printing ejected by piezoelectric, thermal, or electromagnetic pulses. The process occurs in a non-contact manner and results in high resolution. The method works with high processing speed, which helps achieve good cell viability [17]. Although inkjet printing offers precise placement of biomolecules or cells in defined patterns, it often encounters issues like nozzle clogging and viscosity constraints.

Contrary to this, laser-assisted bioprinting (LAB) does not utilize nozzles and creates a high-pressure bubble to deposit propelled droplets with high-pressure bubbles through pulsed laser beams, thus eliminating the problem of clogging. Laser used for printing has the excitation near ultraviolet (UV) range of 300–400 nm, or at UV range of 193–248 nm [18]. LAB is a highly effective method capable of supporting and achieving micrometer scale resolutions and printing with high cell viscosities and densities, resulting in excellent cell viability (up to 95%). Because of its precision, it is well suited for delicate tissue development such as liver lobule, skin, and bone [19].

Meanwhile, another method, stereolithography (SLA), employs photopolymerization and deposit bioinks through UV or laser light. The high beams solidify biomaterials into a hydrogel in layer-by-layer formation, resulting in smooth surface finishes and high resolution. While exposure to UV lights can potentially damage the cells, SLA remains highly effective in fabricating intricate scaffolds with mechanical structures [20]. Other techniques, such as plotting, are used for developing versatile tissue fabrication. It utilizes UV or chemical curing effective for developing multi-material extrusion and layered stacking of cells. Different printing techniques are shown in Figure 6.3.

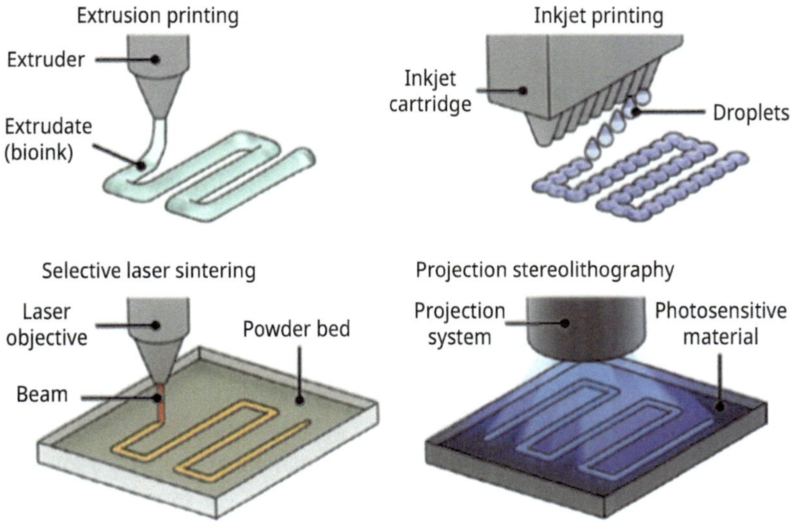

Figure 6.3: Comparison of four 3D printing techniques: extrusion printing: bioink is extruded layer by layer; inkjet printing: deposits droplets of material onto a substrate; selective laser sintering: laser fuses powder particles to form structures; and projection stereolithography: uses light to solidify photosensitive material layer by layer. Each method offers unique advantages for different material and resolution needs [20].

6.2.3 Materials for Bioprinting

The selection of appropriate materials, commonly known as bioinks, for bioprinting is critical for its success. These materials serve as a fundamental building block to develop complex tissue constructs. Bioinks are explicitly designed to replicate an ECM environment that supports cell viability, proliferation, adhesion, and differentiation

Table 6.1: Comparison of features like resolution, printing speed, cellular integrity, materials, and curing methods of different bioprinting techniques.

Feature	Laser-based	Inkjet printing	Extrusion printing	Stereolithography process
Detail resolution	~20–100 μm	~30 μm	~100 μm	~5–100 μm
Printing rate	Slow	Rapid	Moderate	Rapid
Finish quality	Excellent	Top-notch	Fair	Good
Cellular integrity	–	Preserved	Preserved	Preserved
Materials used	Biocompatible materials	Hydrogels, living cells	Ceramics, polymers, metals, and hydrogels	Photocurable polymers
Curing methods	Thermal ionic photopolymerization	Ionic pH-based thermal process	Photopolymerization and ionic pH curing	Photopolymerization

while maintaining biocompatibility and mechanical integrity [21]. They are classified into natural and synthetic types, offering unique advantages in tissue engineering. Natural bioinks are obtained from biological sources such as gelatin, collagen, hyaluronic acid, fibrin, and alginate. These materials are preferred because of their inherent bioactivity and biocompatibility. Their high compatibility with ECM facilitates the interactions of cell matrixes necessary for tissue regeneration [22]. However, their limited mechanical strength and batch-to-batch variability limit their application in load bearing tissues. In contrary, synthetic bioinks such as polyethylene glycol, polyglycolic acid, polycaprolactone, and polylactic acid offer good mechanical properties and exhibit controlled degradation rates. These synthetic polymers are reproducible and allow tailored customization of specific tissues requirements like softness for cartilage and stiffness for bone regeneration and soft tissues. The Table 6.1 shows the comparison of features like resolution, printing speed and others of different bioprinting techniques.

Furthermore, they incorporate bioactive molecules like cell adhesion peptides such as RGD growth factors (e.g., TGF-β, BMPs, and VEGF) to improve the cellular response. This significantly enhances the maturation of tissues post-printing.

Composite and multi-material bioinks have emerged to meet the demand for complex and intricate tissue models and implants. Multi-material printing enables the deposition of different bioinks simultaneously, each engineered to replicate a specific tissue environment in a single construct. These multilateral bioinks support the fabrication of heterogeneous tissues with varied mechanical properties, cell types, and biochemical signals [42]. Composite bioinks, on the other hand, use natural and synthetic

Table 6.2: Summary of various hydrogels, their testing methods, determined properties, and degradation rates, highlighting the differences in their performance and durability.

Hydrogel	Testing method	Determined properties	Degradation rate	Source
Alginate	Compression test	Compressive modulus and compressive strength	Approximately 54.67% over 7 days	[23–25]
Chitosan	Tensile and compression tests	Tensile strength and compressive strength	Complete degradation observed by week 4	[26, 27]
Gelatin	Rheological and tensile tests	Loss modulus, storage modulus, and tensile strength	Nearly 80% mass loss over 3 weeks	[28, 29]
Agarose	Rheological, compression, and tensile tests	Loss modulus, storage modulus, tensile strength, and compressive strength	Size conserved over 21 days in cell-laden gels	[30, 31]
Collagen	Rheological and tensile tests	Loss modulus, storage modulus, tensile strength, ultimate strain, resilience, and toughness	Complete degradation observed at 6 weeks	[32, 33]
Polyethylene glycol (PEG)	Rheological and confined compression tests	Loss modulus, storage modulus, loss tangent, and elastic modulus	Approximately 30% mass loss over 14 days	[34]
Polyethylene oxide (PEO)	Tensile test	Elastic modulus and tensile strength	Specific degradation rates not detailed in the provided sources	[35, 36]
Polyvinyl alcohol (PVA)	Tensile test	Elongation percentage, elastic modulus, tensile strength, and toughness	Degradation rates vary; specific data not detailed in the provided sources	[37, 38]
Polycaprolactone (PCL)	Tensile test	Tensile strength, yield strength, elastic modulus, and elongation percentage	Degradation rates vary; specific data not detailed in the provided sources	[39]
Polylactic acid (PLA)	Tensile, bending, shear, and impact tests	Yield strength, elastic modulus, elongation percentage, flexural strength, flexural modulus, shear strength, and impact strength	Approximately 20% mass loss over 30 days in DMEM + FBS	[40, 41]

polymers along with nanomaterials to increase biological functionality and mechanical strength. For instance, polymerics and hydroxyapatite in tissue engineering create composites that mimic the mineralized bone matrix while maintaining its scaffold flexibility [43]. Advancements in bioprinting techniques, such as light-based bioprinting, expand bioink versatility, enabling them to fabricate high-resolution constructs through photocurable bioinks that can be easily tuned to increase biological and mechanical performance [44].

The successful clinical translation, biocompatibility, and functionality of bioprinted tissues and implants depend upon their designs. Designing them requires patient-specific data, integration, and computational models. Computational models are key players in predicting mechanical behavior and improving printed constructs' functional optimization and vascularization patterns. They help achieve rational design of scaffolds, enabling adequate diffusion of oxygen and nutrients necessary for tissue maturation and cell survival [45]. Further, the integration of AI approaches and ML facilitates analyzing large datasets, improves printing parameters, and refines bioink formulations, thus resulting in improved functionality and fidelity of bioconstructs. Additionally, ML and AI approaches are being incorporated to analyze large datasets, refine bioink formulations, and improve printing parameters, thereby enhancing construct fidelity and functionality [46]. The incorporation of patient-specific data obtained from medical imaging modalities like CT scans or MRI enables the development of personalized bioconstructs tailored to individual's pathological and anatomical features. The personalization enhances implant integration and fit resulting in better clinical outcomes. For example, scaffold printed from imaging data can easily replicate the complex defect geometries offering maximum biocompatibility and mechanical support [47]. Similarly, patient-specific tumor models developed through 3D bioprinting allow efficient drug testing, personalized medicine strategies, and accurate disease modeling. The use of such design considerations in biomaterials and bioprinting helps overcoming the gap between the theoretical research and clinical application of the medical solutions.

6.3 Innovative Design Strategies in 3D Bioprinting

The technological advancements in 3D bioprinting have optimized innovative design strategies in 3D bioprinting. By combining AI, ML and computational models, researchers are able to develop biomimetic tissue constructs with unprecedented precision and functionality. The innovative techniques and methods are primarily supported by computational designs and optimization enabling the development of patient-specific and complex tissues along with overcoming the shortcoming of the conventional trial and error methods.

6.3.1 Computational Design and Optimization

AI and ML algorithms have become integral tools for optimizing bioprinting parameters and materials, significantly enhancing print fidelity, mechanical properties, and biological outcomes. ML models excel at analyzing multifactorial experimental data to predict optimal printing conditions – such as extrusion temperature, printing speed, and layer thickness – and to balance trade-offs between mechanical strength and biocompatibility [48]. For example, recent studies employing design of experiments (DoE) combined with random forest regression and genetic algorithms have demonstrated the ability to optimize fused deposition modeling (FDM) parameters for improved mechanical performance with remarkable accuracy, surpassing traditional statistical methods [49].

Beyond parameter tuning, AI-powered generative design algorithms are transforming scaffold architecture by enabling the creation of highly complex and biomimetic structures. Generative AI models, such as generative adversarial networks and variational autoencoders, facilitate the autonomous design of bioinspired scaffolds by learning from natural tissue architectures and predicting novel structural configurations optimized for mechanical resilience, porosity, and cell viability [50]. These AI models operate across multiple scales, integrating nanoscale material properties with macroscale tissue demands, and offer an unprecedented capacity to design hierarchical and multifunctional scaffolds that closely mimic natural extracellular matrices.

The synergy between generative AI and 3D bioprinting accelerates biomaterial discovery and design by efficiently exploring vast chemical and structural spaces, thereby reducing the need for costly and time-consuming physical experiments [51]. AI-driven inverse design approaches allow researchers to specify desired scaffold properties – such as stiffness gradients or growth factor distributions – and generate candidate architectures that meet these criteria. This design paradigm is especially critical for fabricating tissues with complex cellular heterogeneity and mechanical gradients, such as osteochondral interfaces or vascularized organs [52].

Moreover, integrating patient-specific data from medical imaging (e.g., MRI and CT scans) with computational modeling enhances the personalization of bioprinting. ML algorithms can translate anatomical and physiological data into optimized digital blueprints for implants or tissue grafts tailored to individual patients, improving implant fit, biological integration, and clinical outcomes [48]. This patient-centric design approach enables precision medicine applications by allowing for custom bioprinted tissues that address unique defect geometries and pathological conditions.

Despite these advances, challenges remain in data quality, model interpretability, and real-time process control. Large, high-quality datasets are essential to train robust AI models, but such datasets are scarce in bioprinting. Additionally, ML models must be tightly integrated with bioprinting hardware and software for real-time monitoring and adaptive control, enabling the dynamic correction of printing errors and ensuring construct fidelity. Advances in multimodal AI systems that combine imaging, material, and biological data hold promise for overcoming these limitations and fostering autonomous bioprinting workflows.

6.3.2 Multi-material and 4D Bioprinting

Recent advances have significantly broadened the scope and capabilities of bioprinting through multi-material printing and emergence of 4D bioprinting. These advancements have transformed the tissue engineering field as they not only allow the replication of native biological system but also support dynamic evolution to replicate the natural tissue function and remodeling. Especially, in an additive manufacturing, multi-material represents a major breakthrough in biomedical application. The application of layering and co-printing biomaterials with varied degradation rates, stiffness, and bioactivities enables the development-graded structures that faithfully replicate the natural transition among tissue types such as bone-tendon junctions and bone-cartilage interface [42]. Gradation is critical for biological function, mechanical stability facilitating proliferation, cell adhesion, and differentiation within the scaffold.

Some notable advance multi-material techniques include FDM. This method uses multiple nozzles or co-axial extrusion for simultaneous deposition of flexible and stiff polymers and enhances energy absorption and mechanical properties [21]. It is ideal for load bearing scaffolds or prosthetic design. Another advance method is the PolyJet printing that utilizes photopolymer resins cured with UV light in layer-by-layer fashion. This technique offers precise control over material mixing, allowing the fabrication of intricate internal structures with complex material distribution. Bioprinting on the other hand is a technique that employs specialized extrusion method to deposit bioinks made up from living cells and hydrogel with growth factors, thereby, recreating the microenvironment. The application of these advance methods includes fabrication of soft tissues constructs, vascularized organs, and multifunctional scaffolds with musculoskeletal interfaces and mechanical gradients. The basic methods are demonstrated in Figure 6.4. The biological constructs demonstrate excellent fidelity in replicating native ECM and promote successful tissue integration and regeneration. However, challenges remain in achieving optimal biocompatibility during and after printing process to maintain cell viability and enable scalability for clinical application.

6.3.3 Introduction to 4D Bioprinting: Time-Responsive and Dynamic Structures

While 3D bioprinting results in static and redefined architecture constricts, 4D bioprinting introduces a fourth dimension in printing processes. This technology brings

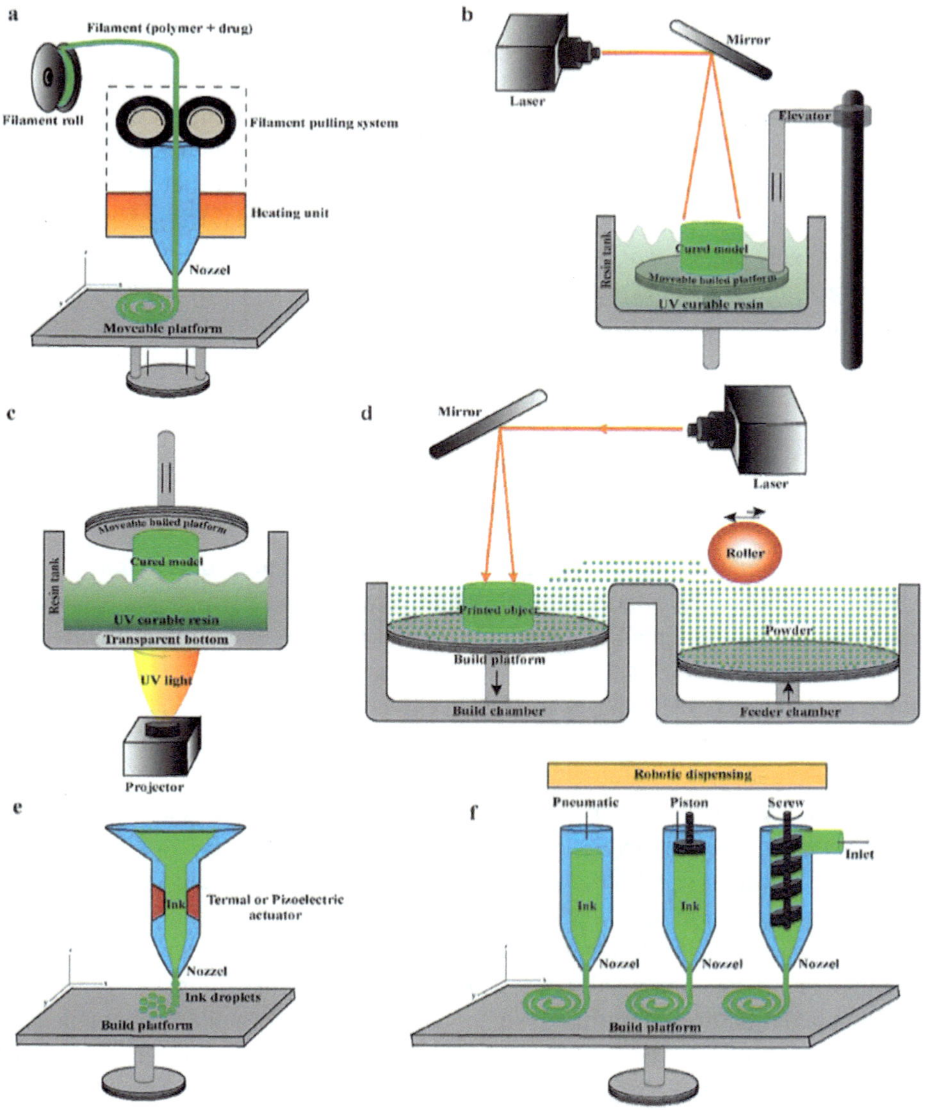

Figure 6.4: (a) Fused deposition modeling (FDM): thermoplastic filament is melted and deposited layer by layer via a heated nozzle. (b) Stereolithography (SLA): a laser beam selectively cures photosensitive resin layer-wise. (c) Digital light processing (DLP): UV light from a projector solidifies patterned resin simultaneously across an entire layer. (d) Selective laser sintering (SLS): laser sinters powder particles layer by layer without support structures. (e) Inkjet printing: thermal or piezoelectric actuation ejects bioink droplets to form constructs. (f) Direct ink writing (DIW): viscoelastic inks are extruded through nozzles under robotic control for high-resolution builds [53].

revolution in bioprinting by using smart and stimuli-responsive materials and enables the printed constructs to undertake dynamic transformation after production. It allows the bioconstructs to change shape, functions, and properties over time in response to their environmental conditions [54]. 4D bioprinting is the basically the extension of 3D bioprinting. In 4D bioprinting stimuli-responsive biomaterials such as biocomposites, hydrogel, and shape memory polymers are used that are capable to react and change their properties to the external environmental triggers such as PH humidity, temperature, biochemical signals, or magnetic field. These responses can be a contraction, bending, expansion, contraction, or changes in mechanical stiffness. What important is that the functional or shape changes not only happen in response to degradation but also rely on programmable and reversible transformation [55]. A graphical abstract of the 4D-bioprinting platform is shown in Figure 6.5.

6.3.3.1 Fabrication Techniques

The transformation from conventional 3D printing techniques to 4D bioprinting involves integration of biomaterials that can be programmed for dynamic responsiveness and can be fabricated into complex architectures. Some of the 4D fabrication techniques include FDM that utilizes shape memory polymer composites that enable the scaffold to alter their shapes in response to heat or magnetic field [65]. SLA and photopolymerization are another emerging techniques that employ photosensitive smart hydrogel capable of stimulus-responsive behavior all while maintaining high resolution. Some other methods include chemical cross-linking and thermal gelation for developing dynamic bioinks [65].

The application of 4D bioprinting in regenerative medicine and tissue engineering remains limited but holds transformative potential by creating living tissues and implants capable to adapt to their biological environment. This significantly improves the implants functionality and integration. For instance, smart implants can morph post-implantation to conform precisely to anatomical space. Similarly, dynamic scaffolds can modulate porosity or stiffness in response to different cell activities and healing stages [66]. 4D bioprinting also facilitates the advance drug delivery systems in the bioprinted tissues and organs enabling them to receive therapeutics in case of demand triggered by local tissue conditions. Soft robotics represents another promising application. It uses biological motion and enables safe interaction with living tissues. Vascular stents are printed through 4D technology integrating shape memory features, which allows them to expand in narrow blood vessels after implantation. Further, magnetic nanoparticles composites are used to fabricate shape shifting bone scaffolds that can be activated remotely to assist tissue regenerations [67].

Despite its transformative potential, 4D bioprinting faces challenges in developing biocompatible, multi-stimuli smart materials that can integrate diverse behavior within single construct. Further, smart materials demonstrate limitations in retaining

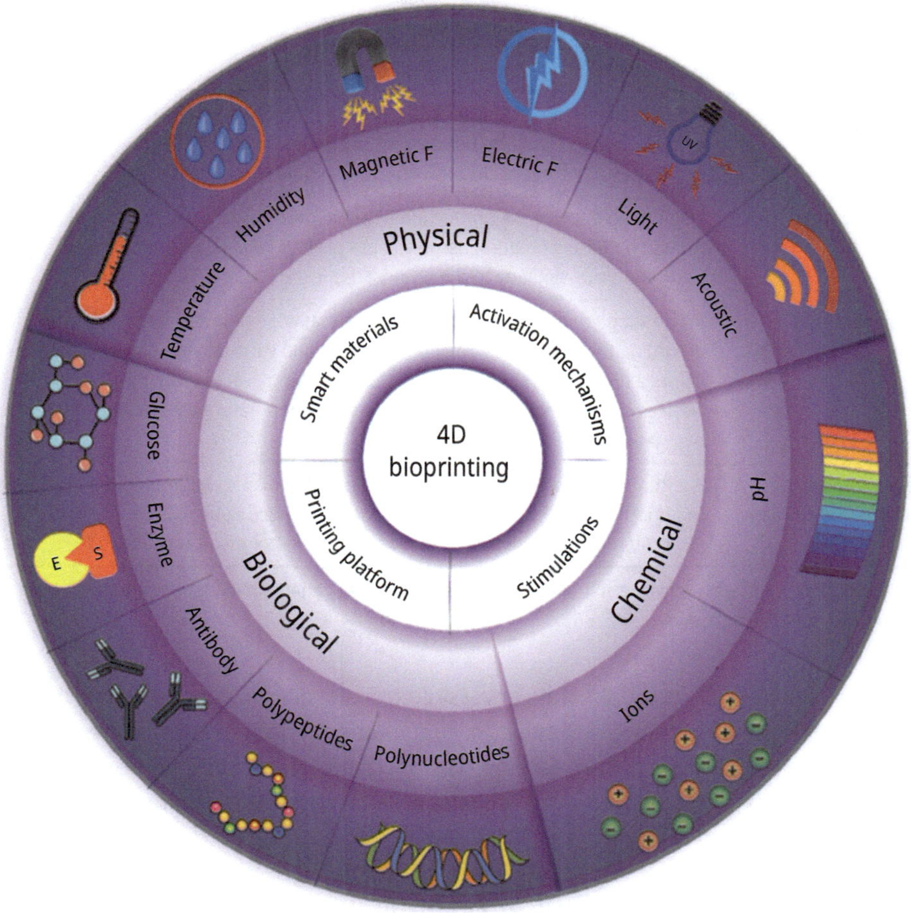

Figure 6.5: 4D printing components and materials. The various stimuli used to fabricate 4D-printed materials such as temperature, humidity, magnetic, and electric forces.

Table 6.3: Various applications of 4D printing in healthcare, showcasing advancements such as smart surgical tools, tissue grafts, and multi-material implants.

Application	Description	References
Surgical tools	Development of smart surgical instruments with precise control for complex procedures. Instruments can be adapted to different surgical situations and anatomical structures and offer improved precision. Minimizes tissue damage, enhances surgical outcomes, and shortens recovery time for patients.	[56, 57]

Table 6.3 (continued)

Application	Description	References
4D printing of heart and kidney	These tissues exhibit high flexibility, allowing for printing based on genetic compatibility. The use of smart materials for future heart and kidney applications through 4D printing holds great potential.	[58]
Tissue grafts	4D printing enables the production of tissue grafts that mimic the growth patterns of natural tissues. These grafts integrate with the body and grow similarly to the original tissue.	[59, 60]
Smart stents	4D printing enables the creation of stents that adjust their shape according to the patient's body temperature and varying conditions. Offers a high-speed solution, critical for life-saving procedures. Devices can undergo changes in response to temperature variations over time.	[61, 62]
Smart multi-material printing	A cutting-edge method for producing medical implants with multiple materials using 4D printing and a layer-by-layer technique. Offers customization in the design of implants for different medical needs.	[63, 64]

Each application offers innovative solutions that enhance precision, adaptability, and customization for improved medical outcomes.

precise control, cell variability, and reversible transformation. However, the integration of advance bioprinting technologies, computational designs, and convergence of materials science ushers a future where tissue substitutes not only mimic static structure but also dynamically respond and mature, closely resembling natural tissues.

6.3.4 Integration with Digital Technologies

6.3.4.1 Role of IoT in Real-Time Monitoring and Control of Bioprinters

Building on the integration of digital technologies in bioprinting, the IoT has become fundamental in refining control over process through real-time monitoring. As discussed, IoT integrates sensors to collect critical data related to temperature, mechanical movement, bioink viscosity, and humidity. The constant feedback helps engineers and biomedical experts to make necessary adjustments to printing parameters thus, maintaining optimal conditions throughout fabrication. This authority to control reduces variability and error critical while working with bioactive materials and delicate living cells [68]. Further, the mechanical and environmental monitoring facilitated with IoT systems enables tracking printer usage patterns and bioink supply inks resulting in efficient resource management and timely replenishment [69]. Further, the use of cloud-based platforms facilitates the analysis and aggregation of large datasets obtained from multiple printing processes. The cloud computing allows the knowledge sharing among specialists and facilitates the continuous improvement during the printing process [70]. Data-driven approaches also help in quality assurance and traceability to ensure that clinical application is according to regulatory compliance. Additionally, the integration of IoT enables remote management and supervision of different bioprinting units at the same time. This facilitates scalability and collaboration among different production sites. Another important aspect is the predictive analytics supported with the data collected through IoT. Predictive analytics help in anticipating potential system failure and maintenance needs thus reducing downtime and improves reliability [71]. The transformation of bioprinters into interconnected smart devices supports precise and automated biomanufacturing environment crucial for the production of clinical grade production.

6.3.4.2 Use of VR and AR for Visualizing and Manipulating 3D-Bioprinted Models

The use of VR and augmented reality (AR) has significantly extended the capabilities and application of 3D bioprinting models. VR provides a three-dimensional view and digital space that help researchers explore and observe complex tissues in detail. The fully digitalized environment provides a holistic perspective to understand the spatial relationship within the printing models. The detailed analysis of constructs helps to identify and fix errors before actual costly printing. VR, on the other hand, supports a dynamic environment that can simulate physiological conditions, allowing the observation of how printed tissues and organs will react and respond to biochemical stimuli or mechanical stress, enabling a deeper understanding of the durability and functionality of implants [72]. The introduction of AR further enhances the application of VR models, and they allow real-world demonstration and hands-on manipulation of digitally printed models. Biomedical engineers and surgeons can interact with bioprinted tissues in this digitally simulated environment to improve designs, precision, and personalization of implants and constructs. AR has also been used not only for designing and customizing but also in training by showing anatomical images on physical models, and it has even been tested on real patients. The understanding of tissue and organ functionality in real-life environments significantly improves surgical outcomes. The gap between digital modeling and physical realization can be successfully bridged through AR and VR technologies through model adjustments like scaling and orientation. The processes are usually automatic, thereby excluding chances of errors and enhancing the overall quality and performance of bioprinting processes [73]. VR and AR are both key players in driving 3D bioprinting innovations and translational outcomes.

6.4 Applications of Innovative Design in 3D Bioprinting

6.4.1 Personalized Medicine

3D bioprinting has been extensively applied in personalized medicine. The innovative designs and modeling processes has revolutionized the healthcare industry by introducing devices and medical treatments designed specifically to meet the patient's genetic, anatomical and psychological requirements. The efficacy of medical interventions has been boosted significantly through personalized medicine, making them a driving force in medical innovation. 3D bioprinting has been widely used for personalized medicine.

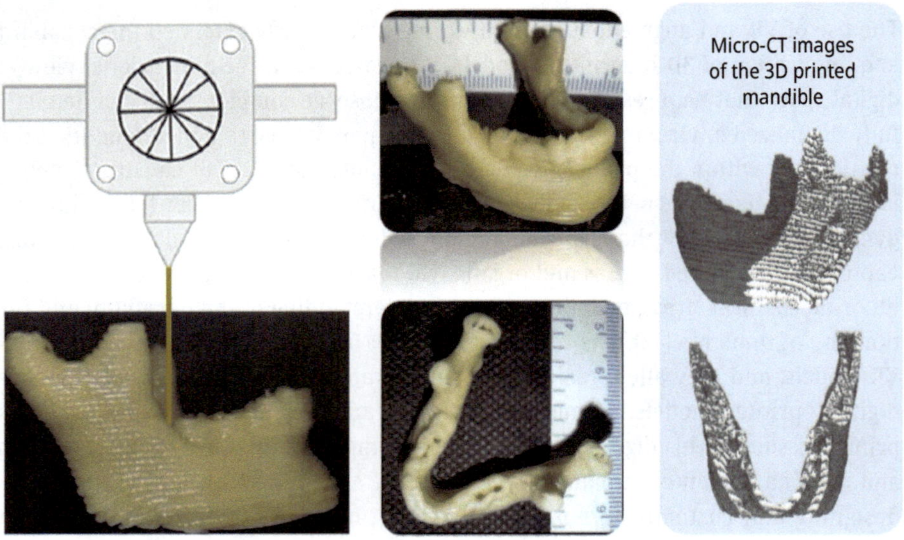

Figure 6.6: Schematics of the use of 3D-printed composites for dental implants [72].

3D-printed tissue constructs, patient-specific implants, and prosthetics are designed and developed based on computational data obtained from imaging techniques such as CT and MRI scans. CAD and advanced biomaterials lead the production of prosthetics and implants that perfectly fit with the patient's body and demonstrate high biological integrity with the patient's tissues. They have been proven to offer optimal results when compared to traditional manufacturing methods [74]. For instance, Bojedla et al. [75] utilized 3D bioprinting to develop dental implants (see Figure 6.6). They utilize titanium, lithium disilicate, and zirconia to produce highly customized implants. These materials had previously demonstrated high biocompatibility and mechanical stability in patient-specific implants. The 3D-bioprinted dental implants have led to a substantial increase in implant success rates, with studies reporting a 90% success rate, particularly in upper molar implants, due to their anatomical fit and enhanced osseointegration [76]. The researchers further enhance the efficacy of implants by integrating AI with 3D printing, thereby increasing structural characteristics such as porosity and stiffness to align with the patient's bone physiology and density. The AI integration augmented both biological integration and mechanical stability.

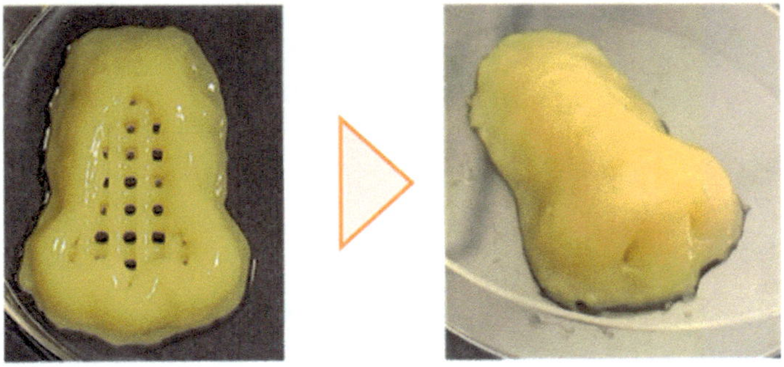

Figure 6.7: First layers of the nose-shaped structure (left) and final construct (right) [63].

In addition to prosthetics and implants, 3D bioprinting has also demonstrated tremendous potential in the field of regenerative medicine. 3D-bioprinted tissues and constructs can successfully mimic the natural function and architecture of human tissues and without the risk of nozzle clogging seen in the case of the NFC4FP formulation. Furthermore, bioinks composed of living cells, along with biocompatible hydrogels, enable the detailed layering of cells, similar to human tissues, thereby enhancing the biological integrity of tissues. For instance, Carvalho et al. [77] utilize nanocomposite bioinks combining nanocellulose fibers and polysaccharides, such as fucopol, to develop 3D-printed skin tissues. These skin tissues demonstrated excellent mechanical stability and cell viability, making them suitable for skin regeneration and wound healing applications. Intricate structures, such a nose-shaped construct represented in Figure 6.6, were printed using the ink NFC3FP. This ink was chosen because of the adequate balance between rheological and mechanical properties, enabling the printing of more complex structures with higher shape fidelity than with the ink NFC2FP Similarly, Chen et al. [78] developed 3D-printed scaffolds for a female reproductive system that can support tissue repair and cell proliferation. The main steps of 3D-printed reproductive organs and their application are shown in Figure 6.7. The purpose was to address the challenges faced when dealing with tissue loss during a disease or surgery. The developed bioprinted scaffolds overcome the limitations generally faced during stem cell therapies and transplantation, promoting functional regeneration.

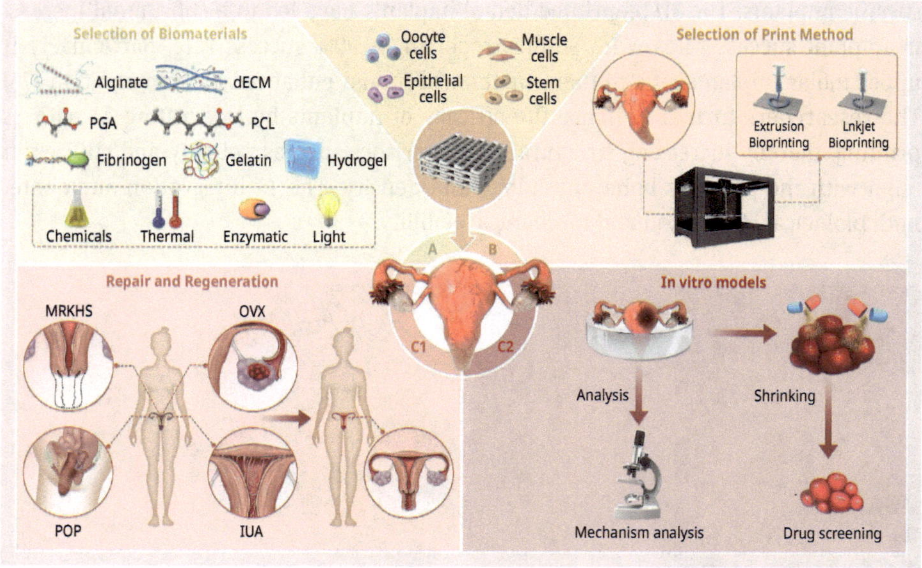

Figure 6.8: The process of 3D bioprinting in the context of female reproductive system research. The figure highlights the selection of biomaterials (like alginate, gelatin, and hydrogel), print methods (extrusion and inkjet bioprinting), and the creation of in vitro models for tissue regeneration and tumor studies. It emphasizes applications in repairing reproductive conditions (e.g., MRKHS, POP) and drug screening using high-resolution, multi-material tumor models [79].

The application of personalized tissue constructs is also tested in oncology. Biomedical engineers develop 3D-bioprinted tumor models that can replicate the tumor model with high fidelity. These patient-specific models enhance the design of targeted therapies and drug screening, thus improving treatment effectiveness and reducing side effects. The integration of innovative technology results in the development of personalized cancer vaccines and drug testing combinations explicitly designed for patient's tumor profiles. The tumor models have been proven to accelerate drug development and enhance clinical outcomes [80]. A summary of recent studies on the application in cancer treatment is shown in Table 6.3. Recent studies on 3D-bioprinted scaffolds were also successfully utilized for bone regeneration in craniomaxillofacial disorders. Their preclinical models have demonstrated effective restoration of functional and osteogenic properties [81]

Although personalized medicine driven by AI technologies and 3D bioprinting is demonstrating promising solutions in tissue engineering and implant development, several challenges remain. The primary challenge is to develop bioinks using materials that strike a balance between printability, mechanical strength, and biocompatibility with the host's biological system [88]. The long-lasting functions and safety requirements need further research. Currently, 3D bioprinting has become a standard component of personalized healthcare, offering effective, efficient, and customized in-

Table 6.4: Various bioprinted models and scaffolds developed for cancer research, focusing on their bioprinting techniques, targeted cancer types, and therapeutic implications.

Bioprinted model/ scaffold	Primary bioprinting technique	Targeted cancer type	Key contribution/therapeutic implication	Original reference
3D-bioprinted tumor model	Extrusion-based bioprinting	Breast cancer	Maintained native breast cancer cell morphologies when exposed to bioink, enabling high-fidelity studies.	[82]
3D-bioprinted organoid	Extrusion-based bioprinting	Breast cancer	Provided a robust process for creating 3D cancer models suitable for high-throughput screening, preserving original tumor shape, histology, and gene expression.	[83]
3D-printed, implantable ALG/ CuS nanoparticle scaffold	Extrusion-based bioprinting	Breast cancer	Demonstrated complementary photothermal, photodynamic, and chemo-dynamic therapeutic effects in both in vivo and in vitro models.	[84]
3D-bioprinted nanoengineered hydrogel scaffold	Extrusion-based bioprinting	Osteosarcoma	Exhibited excellent anti-osteosarcoma activity with remarkably regulated release of encapsulated medicines (approx. 49%) specifically at pH 6.5, enabling targeted delivery.	[85]
Cu/AG hydrogel scaffold	Extrusion-based bioprinting	Thyroid cancer	Demonstrated effective photothermal effects leading to thyroid cancer cell inhibition, coupled with good in vitro release kinetics for therapeutic agents.	[86]
3D-bioprinted vascularized breast tumor model	Aspiration-based bioprinting	Breast cancer	Paved the way for developing reliable, accurately constructed, and physiologically accurate tumor models for personalized anti-cancer treatments.	[87]

terventions for a wide range of medical applications. However, the accessibility and high cost pose significant barriers to its widespread application. Ethical and regulatory frameworks must evolve in tandem with these technologies to address issues related to data privacy, standardization, and clinical translation. AI-driven design and 3D-bioprinted implants have already demonstrated success in skin tissue engineering, dental implants, cancer therapy, and reproductive system repair. The Table 6.4 shows the various bioprinted models and scaffolds developed for cancer research. The ongoing advancements and stem cell technology will further optimize their potential in broader clinical implementations [74].

6.4.2 Tissue Engineering and Regenerative Medicine

6.4.2.1 Bioprinting of Skin, Cartilage, Bone, and Vascular Networks

3D bioprinting has also emerged as a powerful engineering tool in regenerative medicine, as it allows control over the biomaterials required to fabricate living tissues and the spatial arrangement of cells. It is widely applied for the development of skin tissues that address the requirements for burn treatments, wound healing and reconstructive surgery [89]. Figure 6.8 shows the different examples of 3D-bioprinted tissues including heart, skin, blood vessels, etc. Recent advances have focused on the development of nanocomposite hydrogel bioinks. Hydrogel is commonly preferred for creating bioinks because of its ability to encapsulate viable cells and its similarity to the native ECM. They are developed by combining FucoPol- and fucose-rich bacterial polysaccharides, along with nanocellulose, for optimal biocompatibility, mechanical stability, and rheological properties [89, 90]. Hydrogel-based bioinks were used to successfully print melanoma and keratinocyte cells, demonstrating cell viability of more than 88% for at least 21 days. Their success demonstrates that they can be utilized to develop functional skin tissues with suitable biomedical applications [91]. Another key focus of 3D bioprinting is the cartilage regeneration. Despite limited self-healing properties of cartilage, patient-specific 3D-bioprinted scaffolds facilitate chondrocyte growth and differentiation. Collagen, alginate, and gelatin are typically used materials for cartilage bioprinting. They are often combined with synthetic polymers to enhance the mechanical properties. 3D-printed scaffolds successfully mimic the biometric environment of native cartilage facilitating tissue integration and maturation post-implantation. Table 6.4 demonstrates different scaffolds developed with varied combination of bioinks, their characteristics and medical application. 3D bioprinting integrated with innovative methods results in precise deposition of multiple growth types factors and cell types, refabricating the specific zonal characteristics of cartilage tissues to improve functional outcomes [92].

Bioprinting technologies have also significantly enhanced bone tissue engineering. It enables the development of bone implants and scaffolds with sufficient bioactivity to support osteogenesis, as well as mechanical strength and porosity for vascularization. Recently developed composite scaffolds combine polymeric hydrogels with ceramic materials, such as bioactive glass or hydroxyapatite, to create a favorable environment for bone-forming cells and provide structural integrity. 3D-printed patient-specific bone implants have resulted in successful craniomaxillofacial reconstruction by replicating the defective bone geometry and promoting bone growth in preclinical models [94]. The integration of growth factors and living cells in bone scaffolds promoted integration and vascularization with host tissue, which is necessary for the function and survival of engineered bone.

The application of 3D bioprinting in tissue vascularization remains challenging. Despite significant advancements in 3D bioprinting techniques that promote vascular-

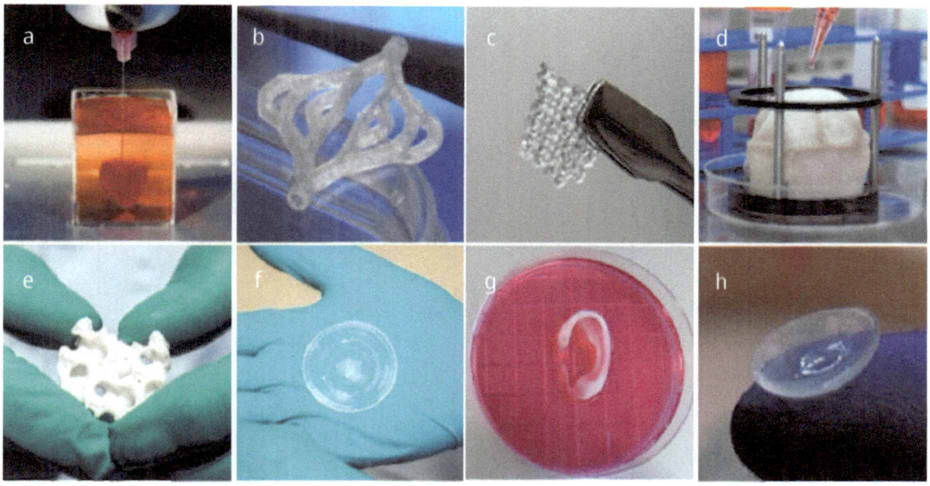

Figure 6.9: Examples of 3D-bioprinted tissues. (a) Heart tissue: bioprinted heart-like structure using specialized bioink for cardiac tissue. (b) Blood vessels: the creation of complex vascular structures, crucial for tissue integration and nutrient supply. (c) Ovarian cells: 3D printing of ovarian cells, focusing on fertility and tissue regeneration applications. (d) Bladder: printed bladder tissue, showcasing advancements in organ regeneration and transplantation. (e) Bone tissue: 3D-printed bone scaffold, aiding in bone repair and regeneration. (f) Skin tissue: printed skin layers, used for wound healing and skin graft applications. (g) Ear: bioprinted ear shape, often used in reconstructive surgery and tissue engineering for ear regeneration. (h) Cornea: bioprinted corneal tissue, providing innovative approaches to eye-related regenerative medicine [93].

ization in thick and complex tissues with limited nutrient transport and oxygen diffusion, this remains a challenge for biomedical engineers and researchers [95]. Significant improvement has been achieved so far, as 3D-printed and fabricated vascular networks have demonstrated promising results in promoting the integration of engineered tissues, thereby enhancing cell viability and perfusion. To achieve successful vascularization, scientists are using techniques like embedded bioprinting, in which sacrificial bioinks are used to print and later removed to create hollow channels that can be endothelialized to create blood vessel analogues [96]. Vascularized constructs that can replicate the natural microvasculature are typically developed using bioinks containing pericytes, endothelial cells, and supportive ECM components. These innovations led to the development of organ-on-a-chip models and play a fundamental role in the progression of functional bioprinting [97].

6.4.2.2 Challenges and Breakthroughs in Organ Bioprinting

Despite rapid advancement and innovation in 3D bioprinting techniques, the clinical translation of organ printing still remains challenging. The core issue is to replicate

Table 6.5: Summary of hybrid scaffold types used for tissue engineering, detailing their constituent materials, fabrication methods, mechanical properties, bioactivity highlights, incorporated factors, biodegradation periods, and target applications.

Scaffold ID	Constituent materials	Fabrication method	Average pore size (μm)	Mechanical features	Bioactivity highlights	Incorporated factors	Biodegradation period (months)	Target application
S-01	PLA combined with HA	Fused filament fabrication	310–480	Compression resistance: ~5 MPa	Encourages bone cell expansion	BMP-2	~6 to 11	Skeletal tissue repair
S-02	PCL with GelMA	SLA 3D printing	110–290	Elastic stiffness: ~48 MPa	Promotes formation of blood vessels	VEGF, TGF-β1	~13 to 17	Cartilage restoration
S-03	PLGA blended with collagen	Laser sintering	190–420	Tensile durability: ~9.5 MPa	Enhances cell binding and development	FGF-2	~4 to 6	Soft tissue regeneration
S-04	PEGDA with HAp	Digital light projection	260–340	Flexural strength: ~14 MPa	Exhibits strong cellular compatibility	IGF-1	~3 to 5	Dental prosthetics
S-05	Silk protein + bioactive glass	Inkjet 3D printing	140–260	Shear resistance: ~21 MPa	Facilitates osteogenic lineage commitment	BMP-7	~8 to 10	Bone reconstruction
S-06	Chitosan mixed with β-TCP	Extrusion bioprinting	210–490	Compression modulus: ~6 MPa	Exhibits antibacterial effects, aids cartilage	PDGF, TGF-β3	~3 to 6	Cartilage and bone regrowth
S-07	Alginate combined with GelMA	Micro-extrusion printing	95–205	Young's modulus: ~1.5 MPa	Promotes vessel formation and compatibility	VEGF, bFGF	~1 to 3	Vascular tissue synthesis

S-08	PEEK integrated with CNTs	Melt extrusion	410–590	Elasticity: ~6–9 MPa	Mechanical strength aids bone tissue support	BMP-2, IGF-1	<2 years	Structural orthopedic implants
S-09	HA with PLGA	Electrospinning	55–145	Compression strength: ~3 MPa	Enhances dermal recovery and fibroblast activity	EGF, PDGF	~2 to 4	Skin healing scaffold
S-10	PVA fused with hydroxyapatite	Direct ink deposition	160–340	Tensile performance: ~78 MPa	Encourages bone connectivity and growth	BMP-4	~6 to 8	Repair of bone discontinuities

Each scaffold is tailored to promote specific tissue regeneration, from skeletal repair to skin healing, by incorporating growth factors and ensuring optimal mechanical and biological performance.

the high complex, heterogeneous, and hierarchical assembly of body organs. The organ development requires precise arrangement of multiple cell types with specific spatial patterns along with supportive nerves, vasculature and ECM components. The reproducibility and resolution required for fabricating complex structures remain problematic. Further creating bioinks with suitable printing, biocompatibility, and mechanical strength for diverse tissues is still under research and currently many formulations failed to mimic the native cellular microenvironment or to facilitate long term functionality [74, 78]. Vascularization of large bioprinted organs is another challenge in 3D bioprinting. These bioprinted organs should survive after implantation. 3D bioprinting enables the development of microvascular networks but ensuring proper function and integration with the host circulation system remains a significant challenge. The integration of stem cell technology and angiogenic factors aims to address these hurdles [98]; however, the complete solution to address the complexity of organ-level perfusion is still far from fully solved Figure 6.9.

Additionally, the host response to printed implants and tissues, as well as immunogenicity, requires careful consideration. The use of autologous cells minimizes the risk of rejection [99], but maintaining their phenotype and achieving sufficient cell numbers can be challenging. Furthermore, developing high-quality 3D-bioprinted organs of the relevant size while ensuring regulatory compliance is a critical challenge in their clinical translation. The required technical expertise and high cost also limit its accessibility [97]. The table 6.5 shows summary of hybrid scaffold type used for tissue engineering. Despite these challenges, significant breakthroughs continue to emerge. The integration of AI in process optimization, innovations in multi-material bioprinting, and the utilization of advanced biomaterials, such as nanocomposites and smart hydrogels, have significantly enhanced tissue functionality and print fidelity. For instance, recent advancements in the bioprinting of liver tissues and miniature kidneys with functional units represent significant progress toward the fabrication of complete organs [100]. Technological and innovative advancements, along with interdisciplinary collaborations and bioreactor systems for tissue maturation, are offering a promising future for printed, fully functional, transplantable organs [97].

6.4.3 Beyond Healthcare: Industrial and Environmental Applications

Other than healthcare, the application of bioprinting is rapidly expanding its influence on industrial and environmental domains. Industries like biofabrication, food production, and ecological remedies are widely adopting bioprinting methods and techniques in their manufacturing processes [101]. In food production, extrusion-based technologies are being utilized to create cell-laden bioinks. These bioinks are composed of plant proteins, animal cells, and other biomaterials to develop food-like meat analogues. These innovations are in response to environmental pressure caused by traditional livestock farming. Livestock farming significantly contributes to greenhouse gas emissions [102].

Additionally, the concerns regarding land and water use are expected to intensify, with different projects estimated to increase the urban population by 68% by the end of 2050 [103]. 3D bioprinting enables the development of food items with precise arrangement of cells and nutrients that replicate the nutrition and texture of natural tissues. It also offers scalable and sustainable alternatives capable of meeting the growing demands of urban centers while reducing environmental impact.

Bioprinting also extends to environmental remediation. It enables the development of functional and bioactive materials that can detoxify polluted air, soil, and water. 3D printing techniques facilitate the fabrication of customized scaffolds, membranes, and photocatalytic devices that can act as catalytic agents for pollutant breakouts and can immobilize microbial communities. Unlike traditional manufacturing, 3D-printed constructs maximize the surface area, thus increasing the degradation of contaminants and minimizing material waste [104]. The environmentally focused bioprinting addresses the sustainability issues and offers a site-specific and flexible approach for mitigating pollution and supporting efficient resource management and a cleaner ecosystem [105].

3D bioprinting has also provided opportunities to achieve sustainability in the construction industry. The industry is responsible for 40% of solid waste, 38% of total greenhouse gas emissions, and 12% of potable water use. With the help of additive manufacturing and digital fabrication, the industry is capable of producing complex concrete geometries that result in reduced resource consumption, waste materials, and embodied energy [106, 107]. Unlike traditional top-down casting methods, the bottom-up approach of 3D bioprinting allows for the efficient use of raw materials and greater design freedom, thereby minimizing the carbon footprint of construction projects [108, 109]. The integration of bioprinting principles with advanced construction techniques results in the development of materials and bio-based composites that surpass functionality, offering durability, strength, and environmental responsiveness. The utilization of advanced fabrication methods in construction demonstrates the potential to achieve sustainable growth in infrastructure and housing while promoting ecofriendly and innovative construction practices.

6.5 Challenges and Limitations

Despite its promising results and promising future prospects, 3D bioprinting is not free from challenges. Some the main challenges are discussed below.

6.5.1 Technical Challenges

The central technical issue in 3D bioprinting is scaling laboratory models of bioprinted constructs to clinically required volumes and sizes. The majority of 3D printing techniques can successfully develop detailed small constructs. However, when scaling, issues such as insufficient vascularization and limited nutrient diffusion arise, resulting in the death of cells in core regions [110]. Acquiring vascular networks necessary for developing thick, multi-cellular tissues with adequate spatial organization in large-scale constructs is quite tricky. The most common challenges of vascular tissue engineering are show in Figure 6.10. The image highlights challenges like replicating the intricate architecture of blood vessel and mimicking of fine structures that require precise engineering requirements. The incorporation of multi-materials to ensure that they work in harmony is also difficult. The printed tissues should also be cell-friendly to avoid rejection and promote cell growth and function. Lastly, durability is a significant challenge, as the tissue must withstand mechanical stresses, such as blood flow, without degradation over time, ensuring long-term functionality. The printing speed also impacts scalability, as prolonged printing durations can reduce cell viability [111]. Biomedical experts are combining hydrogels with mechanical scaffolds and sacrificial materials to develop vasculature. The results appear promising, but they have not yet been clinically approved [91].

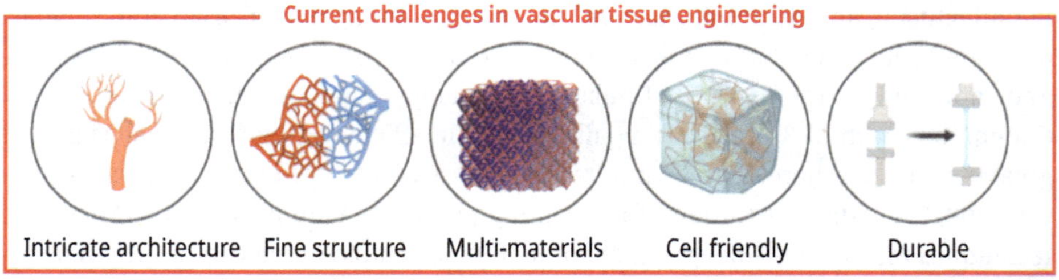

Figure 6.10: Challenges in vascular tissue engineering.

Further acquiring appropriate resolution is necessary as it determines how closely the bioprinted constructs mimic the native microarchitecture. Bioprinting methods that utilize photopolymerization and laser-assisted techniques can achieve high resolution, but they require photopolymerizable bioinks that can potentially damage cells [112]. Generally, extrusion-based bioprinting achieves a resolution of over 50 μm but is limited in replicating capillaries or complex ECM environments [113]. Inkjet bioprinting, another bioprinting method, offers moderate resolution; however, the bioinks used in this method demonstrate issues with evaporation and inappropriate viscosity ranges, which affect uniform cell distribution [110]. Balancing biocompatibility, resolution, and cell viability remains a significant technical challenge [114]. Reproducibility is another technical requirement for the successful clinical translation of bioprinted constructs, which is often challenged by variations in printing parameters and biological variability. The varied printing speed, printing pressure, bioink properties, and environmental factors result in inconsistent cellular behavior and architecture of the developed construct [115]. The multifaced evaluation parameters of 3D bioprinting are shown in Figure 6.11. The validity of these 3D-bioprinted constructs is also questioned due to the lack of quality control metrics and standardized protocols across laboratories [116]. The development of robust bioinks and rigorous standards is necessary for reliable manufacturing. Establishing rigorous standards and robust bioinks is essential for reliable manufacturing [117].

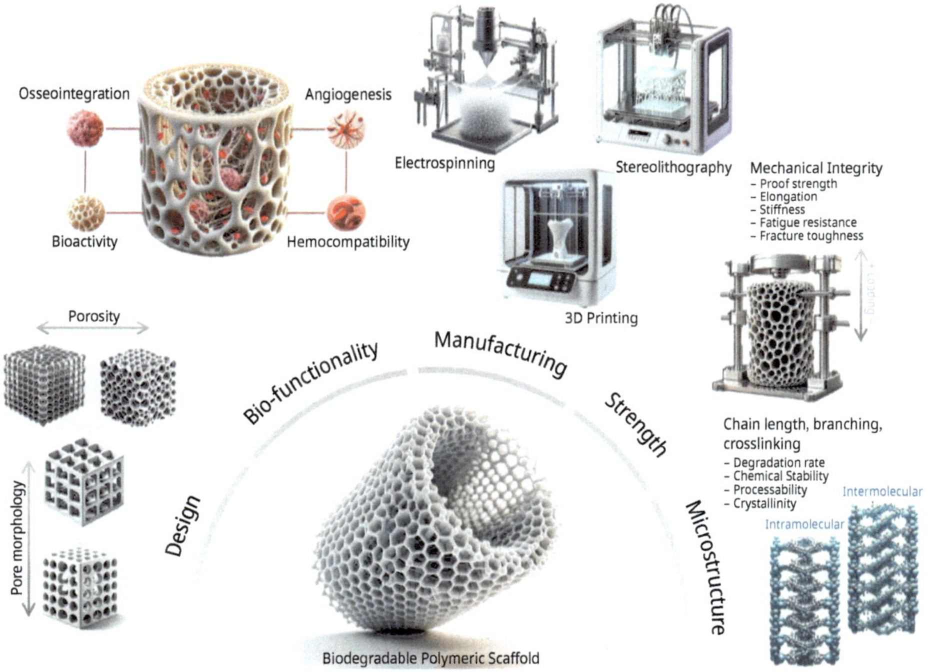

Figure 6.11: Multifaceted evaluation parameters, including design, functionality, manufacturing, mechanical integrity, and microstructure for 3D implant scaffolds.

In addition to technical challenges, the bioinks used for 3D printing also demonstrate several limitations. They should provide a nurturing environment for the cells while maintaining mechanical strength and print fidelity. Natural bioinks are typically biocompatible but often lack the necessary mechanical strength and degrade rapidly. Synthetic bioinks, on the other hand, exhibit tunability but demonstrate limited bioactivity, which is essential for functionality [118]. The key issue is the trade-off between cell viability and viscosity. As the viscosity improves, it puts stress on the cells, causing damage [119]. Printing techniques also demonstrate limitations. For instance, extrusion printing is versatile but offers low resolution and puts sheer stress on the cells. Inkjet printing offers moderate resolution, but the bioinks used in it result in low viscosity, and its efficacy is also affected by droplet evaporation. On the other hand, laser-assisted printing and photopolymerization offer high to excellent resolution and exert low mechanical stress. However, their extreme cost and potential cytotoxicity and UV exposure pose limitations in their clinical applications [120]. Scientist come up with hybrid printing techniques that combine different approaches such as using UV lights, multi-nozzles, and multi-feedstock at the same time. These techniques offer potential solutions but add complexity [116].

6.5.2 Regulatory and Ethical Considerations

Beyond technical challenges, the adherence to regulatory frameworks significantly limits the clinical adoption of 3D-bioprinted implants and tissue constructs. The traditional drug discovery and its clinical translation took almost 10–15 years (see Figure 6.12). This diagram illustrates the long processes of developing vaccine and diagnostic devices depicting the integration of 3D bioprinting in large-scale manufacturing and clinical trials. The recent advancement and innovations in bioprinting are not yet covered in current regulations resulting in uncertainty regarding quality control standards, safety, and efficacy [116]. The issue lies in defining the manufacturing standards, safety assessment, and validation protocols because of the complexity of biological variability and personalized requirements of the construct. Further, the current regulations do not cover bioprinted constructs like scaffold degradation and live cell incorporation as they differ from the traditional medical devices or drugs [121]. Most of the jurisdiction's regulatory frameworks for bioprinting are non-existent making it difficult to approve different processes and increase timeline and cost for clinical trials Figure 6.12.

The ethical issues surrounding bioprinting of organs and protection of intellectual property is a major concern in the field of bioprinting. People often raise questions on the moral status of bioprinter organs and accuse interfering with God's power while creating human tissues [121] The consent, sourcing of cells, and ownership rights of bioprinter constructs raise ethical debate. The common IP concerns include the ownership of bioink formulations and bioprinting technologies especially because of the interdisciplinary and collaborative nature of the field. Open science principles are necessary for patent protection as their absence may lead limited access and prolonged innovation [116].

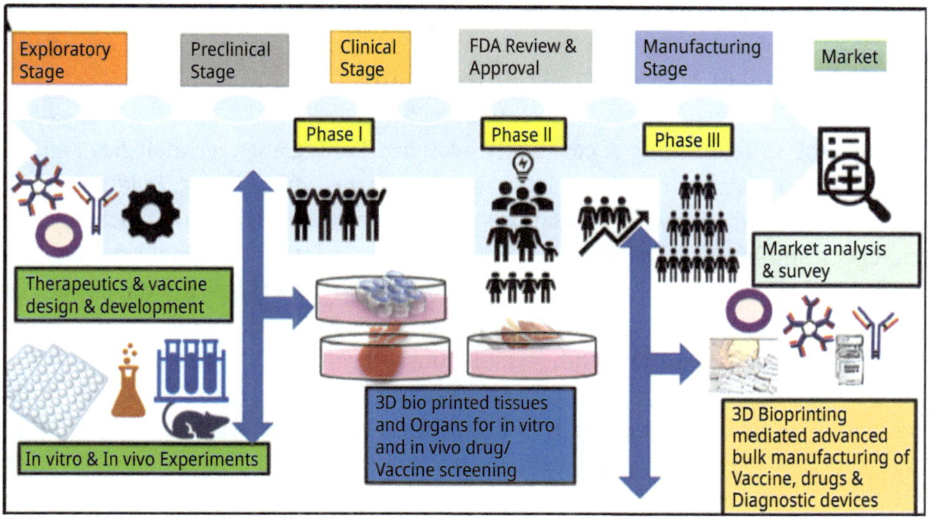

Figure 6.12: Traditional drug discovery timeline including the exploration and developing of vaccines, therapeutics and vaccines. The figure depicts the long time taking process of testing and approval before the drug or vaccine actually reaches the market.

6.5.3 Economic and Accessibility Issues

The associated high cost also limits the widespread adoption of 3D bioprinting. High-quality and high-resolution printers are often quite expensive and can be challenging to cover within the research budgets of most universities [122]. Additionally, advanced formulated bioinks with nanomaterial further add to the production cost. Financial constraints also limit clinical translation, as the process of validation, regulatory compliance, and scale-up manufacturing require significant investments. The high cost of bioprinting has limited its use in wealthy regions, exacerbating global health disparities [123]. It is, therefore, crucial to develop strategies that make bioprinting accessible to researchers worldwide. Subsidies and government grants should be provided for developing user-friendly bioprinters, advanced bioink formulation, and capacity building in the lower-income sector.

Furthermore, inclusive policy-making, international collaboration, and technology transfer should be promoted to prevent a digital divide in advanced regenerative therapies. The development of equitable and open regulatory frameworks with ethical guidelines is necessary. The full potential of bioprinting on a broad scale can only be achieved by addressing the cost and accessibility issues.

6.6 Future Directions and Opportunities

6.6.1 Emerging Trends in 3D Bioprinting

The field of 3D bioprinting is constantly evolving. Cutting-edge technologies and advanced bioink formulations have led to new trends in 3D bioprinting. Traditional bioinks, developed from hydrogels and polymeric materials, have been replaced by biomaterials and living cells, which are necessary for printing functional tissues. The advanced bioinks overcome the limitations of basic hydrogel-based bioinks, such as the need for biological cues, and can mimic complex tissue environments. Advanced bioprinting techniques and bioink formulations are capable of replicating the ECM of various tissues, including the liver, bone, skin, and cartilage. These bioinks are incorporated with biological cues, such as biochemical signals, growth factors, and adhesion peptides, to enhance proliferation, cell viability, and differentiation after printing. The innovations in multi-material bioinks have enabled the printing of complex tissues comprising heterogeneous cell populations and precise spacing.

Advancements and new trends have also emerged in bioprinting techniques. The traditional ink-jet and extrusion methods have been transformed into volumetric and laser-assisted printing, which is capable of printing high-resolution cells and tissues rapidly and with improved fidelity. 4D bioprinting further enhances the process by introducing a time factor, allowing the printed constructs to modify their functionality and shape in response to external environmental conditions, such as temperature and pH, as well as biochemical signals. These robust innovations have transformed bioprinters into intelligent machines capable of printing tissues and constructs that can replicate and remodel natural tissues, resulting in enhanced integrity and function post-implantation. The innovative trends and advances are driving 3D bioprinting to be able to create complex, functional, and biomimetic constructs and tissues that will be capable of addressing limitations related to simplistic and static printed structures.

6.6.2 Integration of Bioprinting with Other Emerging Technologies (e.g., Nanotechnology, CRISPR)

In tissue engineering and regenerative medicine, advances such as nanotechnology and genome editing (CRISPR) are opening new avenues in the field of 3D bioprinting. Through nanotechnology, scientists can manipulate materials at the nanoscale to enhance the bioink properties and scaffold structure and maintain control over cell behavior. Nanoparticles are capable of delivering drugs and growth factors within printed tissues, offering mechanical reinforcement to scaffolds. CRISPR technology enables precise genetic modification, adding another transformative layer to the cells used in bioprinting. The modified cells can be programmed to enhance regenerative capacity, resist immune rejection or express therapeutic proteins. The synergy facilitates the fabrication of genetically tailored organs and tissues that can surpass immunological expectations, thereby enhancing transplant results. Furthermore, the combination of microfluids and bioprinting techniques, along with the availability of organ-on-chip platforms, offers sophisticated in vitro models for drug screening and disease studies, supporting translational research. The fusion of multidisciplines promises a bright future for the fabrication of genetic and personalized tissues, thus improving the efficacy of treatment and patient outcomes.

6.6.3 Role of Digital Transformation in Shaping the Future

As discussed above, digital technologies like AI, ML, and digital twin technologies have tremendously revolutionized the 3D bioprinting. Digital twin technology is an emerging innovation that is used to stimulate, monitor, optimize, and analyze physical bioprinting systems or tissues. This enables the real-time control over bioprinting processes through optimization and stimulation. They also offer continuous feedback loops that help predict cell behavior mechanical performance and tissue maturation ensuring precise adjustments of printing parameters before actual printing process.

ML and AI algorithms are used to identify complex patterns and correlations through analyzing large dataset generated during bioprinting experiments. The analyzed data provide insights on effect of printing speed, bioink formulations, nozzle performance, and environmental conditions. This information significantly enhances the viability and reproducibility of the construct. Further, AI can detect flaws or deviations in real time ensuring quality control thus reducing errors and waste. The AI-driven loop control systems can adapt bioprinting processes to varying environmental factors or bioink properties. This improves scalability, reliability, and precision of bioprinted tissues making technology closer to manufacture clinical grade constructs.

The digital vision of 3D bioprinting is to establish a fully digitalized bioprinting ecosystem that will cover all aspects of printing process including designing, simulating, manufacturing and post-printing processes. The ecosystem will be supported with AI, big data analysis, cloud computing and robotics to form automated and integrated platforms that can produce patient-specific tissues and constructs on demand. The automated system driven with AI and cloud computing will facilitate the prototyping.

Such a system would enable rapid prototyping of tissues tailored to individual patients' anatomical and genetic profiles, accelerating personalized medicine. Moreover, it would facilitate regulatory compliance by maintaining detailed digital records of the production process, enhancing traceability and quality assurance.

6.6.4 Societal and Global Impact

The integration of 3D bioprinting with remote diagnostics and telemedicine will enable clinicians to design and order bioprinted implants or tissues facilitating the democratic access to regenerative therapies around the globe. This digital future also promises cost reductions and increased accessibility, fostering widespread adoption in healthcare and research [39]. One of the most compelling promises of 3D bioprinting lies in its potential to address pressing global healthcare challenges, notably the chronic shortage of donor organs for transplantation. Currently, there are millions of people who are waiting for organ transplant due to limited and suitable donors. Bioprinting is offering large-scale and customized solution for organ shortage where tissues and organs are generated from patient's own cells thus minimizing the risk of body rejection and need for immunosuppressive drugs. Other than addressing the organ shortage issue, bioprinting can also play a role for pandemic preparation by developing tissue models for drug screening and vaccines production. The developed tissues can simulate the infection process enabling researchers to study and test therapeutic agents in a virtual model which is more ethical than testing on animals. Advancements in in vivo bioprinting techniques can facilitate the real-time tissue repair and wound healing during emergencies and can promote resilience of healthcare system. Moreover, bioprinted skin, cartilage, and vascular grafts can provide immediate solutions in trauma care or chronic disease management, improving patient outcomes and reducing healthcare burdens globally [124]

3D bioprinting aligns with multiple United Nations Sustainable Development Goals (SDGs) by fostering innovation in healthcare, promoting equitable access to medical treatments, and encouraging sustainable manufacturing practices. By reducing dependency on donor organs, the technology supports SDG 3 (Good Health and Well-being) through improved access to life-saving treatments. Furthermore, bioprinting's additive manufacturing nature reduces material waste compared to traditional subtractive methods, contributing to SDG 12 (Responsible Consumption and Production). Its potential to fabricate tissues with fewer animal experiments also supports ethical scientific practices and SDG 15 (Life on Land) [125].

In the longer term, bioprinting could advance SDG 9 (Industry, Innovation, and Infrastructure) by driving high-tech industry growth, creating skilled jobs, and stimulating biomedical research globally. Widespread adoption in low- and middle-income countries could reduce health disparities, fostering inclusive development and resilience in healthcare systems worldwide.

Emerging trends in 3D bioprinting emphasize enhanced bioink development, printing innovations like 4D bioprinting, and integration with nanotechnology and CRISPR to create personalized, functional tissues. Digital transformation through AI, ML, and digital twins is reshaping bioprinting toward fully digital, automated, and scalable manufacturing ecosystems. Societally, bioprinting addresses critical global healthcare challenges such as organ shortages and pandemic responses, while supporting sustainable development through responsible, innovative manufacturing and equitable access to therapies. Together, these future directions promise to transform regenerative medicine, personalized healthcare, and global health outcomes.

6.7 Conclusion

6.7.1 Summary of Key Insights

The field of 3D bioprinting represents a remarkable convergence of biology, engineering, and digital technologies, driving a profound transformation in healthcare and related industries. This chapter has outlined the innovative design strategies that underpin recent advances in 3D bioprinting and emphasized the crucial role of digital technologies in propelling the field forward.

Innovative design strategies, particularly those enabled by computational tools, AI, and ML, have revolutionized the precision, complexity, and functionality of bioprinted constructs. The integration of AI-powered generative design and optimization algorithms allows researchers to transcend the traditional trial-and-error approach, enabling the creation of highly biomimetic tissue scaffolds with complex architectures, graded mechanical properties, and cellular heterogeneity. These advances have facilitated the development of patient-specific implants and tissue constructs tailored precisely to individual anatomical and physiological needs. Multi-material bioprinting and the emerging frontier of 4D bioprinting have further expanded design possibilities by enabling the fabrication of dynamic, stimuli-responsive constructs capable of adapting over time to environmental cues and biological processes.

At the core of these design innovations lies the synergy between digital technologies and bioprinting hardware. Digital tools such as VR and AR platforms enhance the visualization, manipulation, and iterative refinement of bioprinted structures before fabrication, reducing errors and accelerating development. The IoT facilitates real-time monitoring and adaptive control during the printing process, ensuring environmental conditions and printing parameters remain optimal for cell viability and construct fidelity. AI-driven predictive analytics and closed-loop control systems promise autonomous, adaptive bioprinting workflows that dynamically respond to variability in bioinks and operational conditions.

The chapter also highlighted the expanding applications of 3D bioprinting, ranging from personalized medicine – including custom implants, prosthetics, and tumor models – to regenerative medicine, where skin, cartilage, bone, and vascularized tissues are being engineered with increasing complexity and biological functionality. Beyond healthcare, 3D bioprinting shows promise in environmental remediation, sustainable food production through lab-grown meat analogues, and ecofriendly construction materials, underscoring its transformative potential across multiple sectors. Despite these exciting developments, the chapter underscored the technical, regulatory, ethical, and economic challenges that must be overcome to fully realize the clinical and industrial potential of 3D bioprinting. Issues such as scalability, vascularization of large tissue constructs, bioink formulation trade-offs between printability and biocompatibility, and the lack of standardized manufacturing protocols pose ongoing hurdles. Regulatory frameworks have yet to catch up with the rapid pace of innovation, creating uncertainty around quality control, safety, and intellectual property. High costs and limited accessibility continue to restrict widespread adoption, highlighting the need for inclusive policy and global collaboration.

Looking forward, emerging trends such as advanced multi-material bioinks, laser-assisted and volumetric printing methods, integration with nanotechnology and CRISPR gene editing, and the rise of digital twins to simulate and optimize bioprinting processes signal a promising trajectory. These innovations collectively promise more sophisticated, functional, and personalized bioprinted tissues that can dynamically interact with their biological environment. The digital transformation of bioprinting workflows from design to manufacturing to clinical application holds the key to scaling production, ensuring reproducibility and enabling on-demand fabrication tailored to individual patient needs.

6.7.2 Final Thoughts

3D bioprinting is just the beginning of a new era that can transform and redefine healthcare industry. The development of living tissues and organs that are fully capable of enabling blood circulation, drug delivery, and regeneration offers unique opportunities to address global issues of regenerative therapies, complex disease modeling, and organ shortage. The precisely engineered and personalized implants and constructs can successfully restore the lost function. Furthermore, digital advancements and integration of cutting-edge technologies are not only enhancing the designs and manufacturing capabilities but also accelerating innovations, encouraging interdisciplinary collaboration, and speeding successful lab discovery to clinical translation. However, this transformative evolution requires constant effort form all the stakeholders. Researchers must continue pushing the boundaries of materials science, biological engineering, and computational modeling to overcome current limitations in bioprinting resolution, scalability, and biological integration. Policymakers need to establish clear, adaptive regulatory pathways that safeguard safety without stifling innovation, addressing ethical concerns and promoting equitable access. Industry players should invest in scalable manufacturing solutions, cost reduction strategies, and collaborative platforms that foster open innovation and technology transfer.

The integration of AI, IoT, and VR/AR has significantly revolutionized the 3D bioprinting. The ongoing advancements present unique opportunities to fully digitalize the biomanufacturing system that can produce high functional personalized tissues on demand. Further, government subsidies and policies can facilitate the democratic access to advance regenerative therapies and can bridge the health disparities and improve outcomes.

Moreover, as 3D bioprinting expands beyond healthcare into sustainable food production, environmental remediation, and green construction, it can contribute meaningfully to global sustainability goals, reducing waste, lowering emissions, and promoting responsible resource use.

In conclusion, the future of 3D bioprinting is bright, but it requires holistic and coordinated approaches that integrate innovative design, digital transformation, ethical frameworks, and inclusive policies. This chapter calls on researchers, policymakers, industry leaders, and funding bodies to unite in fostering an ecosystem that supports rapid yet responsible advancement of 3D bioprinting technologies. By doing so, we can harness the full potential of this revolutionary technology to improve health, sustainability, and quality of life on a global scale.

References

[1] Santoni, S., Gugliandolo, S. G., Sponchioni, M., Moscatelli, D. & Colosimo, B. M. (Jan. 2022). 3D bioprinting: current status and trends – a guide to the literature and industrial practice. Bio-Design and Manufacturing, 5(1), 14–42. doi: 10.1007/s42242-021-00165-0.

[2] Ma, Y., Deng, B., He, R. & Huang, P. (Feb. 2024). Advancements of 3D bioprinting in regenerative medicine: exploring cell sources for organ fabrication. Heliyon, 10(3), doi: 10.1016/j.heliyon.2024.e24593.

[3] Singh, A. B., Khandelwal, C. & Dangayach, G. S. (Aug. 2024). Revolutionizing healthcare materials: innovations in processing, advancements, and challenges for enhanced medical device integration and performance. Journal of Micromanufacturing, 25165984241256234. doi: 10.1177/25165984241256234.

[4] Mahmood, A., Akram, T., Chen, H. & Chen, S. (Jan. 2022). On the evolution of additive manufacturing (3D/4D printing) technologies: materials, applications, and challenges. Polymers, 14(21, Art. no. 21), doi: 10.3390/polym14214698.

[5] Rothbauer, M. et al. (Feb. 2022). Recent advances in additive manufacturing and 3D bioprinting for organs-on-a-chip and microphysiological systems. Frontiers in Bioengineering and Biotechnology, 10, doi: 10.3389/fbioe.2022.837087.

[6] Alheib, O., da Silva, L. P., Youn, Y. H., Kwon, I. K., Reis, R. L. & Correlo, V. M. (2021). Chapter 19 – 3D bioprinting: a step forward in creating engineered human tissues and organs. In: Pou, J., Riveiro, A. & Davim, J. P. (eds). Additive Manufacturing, in Handbooks in Advanced Manufacturing. Elsevier, 599–633. doi: 10.1016/B978-0-12-818411-0.00016-1.

[7] Rashid, A. B., Uddin, A. S. M. N., Azrin, F. A., Saad, K. S. K. & Hoque, M. E. (May 2023). 3D bioprinting in the era of 4th industrial revolution – insights, advanced applications, and future prospects. Rapid Prototyping Journal, 29(8), 1620–1639. doi: 10.1108/RPJ-02-2023-0041.

[8] Urlings, J., de Jong, G., Maal, T. & Henssen, D. (Aug. 2023). Views on augmented reality, virtual reality, and 3D printing in modern medicine and education: a qualitative exploration of expert opinion. Journal of Digital Imaging, 36(4), 1930–1939. doi: 10.1007/s10278-023-00833-w.

[9] Chen, H., Zhang, B. & Huang, J. (Jul. 2024). Recent advances and applications of artificial intelligence in 3D bioprinting. Biophysics Reviews, 5(3), 031301. doi: 10.1063/5.0190208.

[10] Ramesh, S., Deep, A., Tamayol, A., Kamaraj, A., Mahajan, C. & Madihally, S. (Apr. 2024). Advancing 3D bioprinting through machine learning and artificial intelligence. Bioprinting, 38, e00331. doi: 10.1016/j.bprint.2024.e00331.

[11] Bicudo, E. & Faulkner, A. & Li, P. (Mar. 2021). Digital readiness in 3D bioprinting: software, governance and hospitals' proto-clinical interfaces. Regenerative Medicine, 16(3), 237–252. doi: 10.2217/rme-2020-0132.

[12] Bhardwaj, N., Sood, M. & Gill, S. S. (Jan. 2024). 3D-bioprinting and AI-empowered anatomical structure designing: a review. Current Medical Imaging, 20(1), e15734056259274. doi: 10.2174/0115734056259274231019061329.

[13] Vieira, J. L., Carneiro, D. C., Soares, M. B. P. & Barbosa, J. D. V. (Jul. 2021). Fundamentals of 3D bioprinting technology. Journal of Bioengineering, Technologies and Health, 4(2, Art. no. 2), doi: 10.34178/jbth.v4i2.162.

[14] Tashman, J. W., Shiwarski, D. J. & Feinberg, A. W. (Dec. 2022). Development of a high-performance open-source 3D bioprinter. Scientific Reports, 12(1), 22652. doi: 10.1038/s41598-022-26809-4.

[15] Decante, G., Costa, J. B., Silva-Correia, J., Collins, M. N., Reis, R. L. & Oliveira, J. M. (Apr. 2021). Engineering bioinks for 3D bioprinting. Biofabrication, 13(3), 032001. doi: 10.1088/1758-5090/abec2c.

[16] Xiaorui, L. et al. (Dec. 2022). Biomaterial inks for extrusion-based 3D bioprinting: property, classification, modification, and selection. International Journal of Bioprinting, 9(2), 649. doi: 10.18063/ijb.v9i2.649.

[17] Park, J. A., Lee, Y. & Jung, S. (Aug. 2023). Inkjet-based bioprinting for tissue engineering. Organoid, 3, doi: 10.51335/organoid.2023.3.e12.

[18] Ventura, R. D. (Jun. 2021). An overview of laser-assisted bioprinting (LAB) in tissue engineering applications. Medical Lasers; Engineering, Basic Research, and Clinical Application, 10(2), 76–81. doi: 10.25289/ML.2021.10.2.76.

[19] Dou, C., Perez, V., Qu, J., Tsin, A., Xu, B. & Li, J. (2021). A state-of-the-art review of laser-assisted bioprinting and its future research trends. ChemBioEng Reviews, 8(5), 517–534. doi: 10.1002/cben.202000037.

[20] Kafle, A., Luis, E., Silwal, R., Pan, H. M., Shrestha, P. L. & Bastola, A. K. (Jan. 2021). 3D/4D printing of polymers: fused deposition modelling (FDM), selective laser sintering (SLS), and stereolithography (SLA). Polymers, 13(18, Art. no. 18), doi: 10.3390/polym13183101.

[21] Yilmaz, B., Rashid, A. A., Mou, Y. A., Evis, Z. & Koç, M. (Aug. 2021). Bioprinting: a review of processes, materials and applications. Bioprinting, 23, e00148. doi: 10.1016/j.bprint.2021.e00148.

[22] Chen, X. B. et al. (Oct. 2023). Biomaterials/bioinks and extrusion bioprinting. Bioactive Materials, 28, 511–536. doi: 10.1016/j.bioactmat.2023.06.006.

[23] Li, Z. et al. (May 2018). Tuning alginate-gelatin bioink properties by varying solvent and their impact on stem cell behavior. Scientific Reports, 8(1), 8020. doi: 10.1038/s41598-018-26407-3.

[24] Sarker, M., Izadifar, M., Schreyer, D. & Chen, X. (Jul. 2018). Influence of ionic crosslinkers (Ca2+/Ba2+/Zn2+) on the mechanical and biological properties of 3D bioplotted hydrogel scaffolds. Journal of Biomaterials Science, Polymer Edition, 29(10), 1126–1154. doi: 10.1080/09205063.2018.1433420.

[25] You, F., Xia, W. & Chen, X. (Apr. 2017). 3D printing of porous alginate/gelatin hydrogel scaffolds and their mechanical property characterization. International Journal of Polymeric Materials and Polymeric Biomaterials, 66(6), 299–306. doi: 10.1080/00914037.2016.1201830.

[26] Bakhsheshi-Rad, H. R. et al. (Feb. 2020). In vitro and in vivo evaluation of chitosan-alginate/gentamicin wound dressing nanofibrous with high antibacterial performance. Polymer Testing, 82, 106298. doi: 10.1016/j.polymertesting.2019.106298.

[27] Harish Prashanth, K. V. & Tharanathan, R. N. (Jan. 2006). Crosslinked chitosan – preparation and characterization. Carbohydrate Research, 341(1), 169–173. doi: 10.1016/j.carres.2005.10.016.

[28] Campiglio, C. E., Contessi Negrini, N., Farè, S. & Draghi, L. (Jan. 2019). Cross-linking strategies for electrospun gelatin scaffolds. Materials, 12(15, Art. no. 15), doi: 10.3390/ma12152476.

[29] Pottathara, Y. B. et al. (Jun. 2022). Solidification of gelatine hydrogels by using a cryoplatform and its validation through CFD approaches. Gels, 8(6, Art. no. 6), doi: 10.3390/gels8060368.

[30] Zucca, P., Fernandez-Lafuente, R. & Sanjust, E. (Nov. 2016). Agarose and its derivatives as supports for enzyme immobilization. Molecules, 21(11, Art. no. 11), doi: 10.3390/molecules21111577.

[31] Awadhiya, A., Kumar, D. & Verma, V. (Oct. 2016). Crosslinking of agarose bioplastic using citric acid. Carbohydrate Polymers, 151, 60–67. doi: 10.1016/j.carbpol.2016.05.040.

[32] Doyle, A. D. (2016). Generation of 3D collagen gels with controlled diverse architectures. Current Protocols in Cell Biology, 72(1), 10.20.1–10.20.16. doi: 10.1002/cpcb.9.

[33] Brinkman, W. T., Nagapudi, K., Thomas, B. S. & Chaikof, E. L. (Jul. 2003). Photo-cross-linking of type I collagen gels in the presence of smooth muscle cells: Mechanical properties, cell viability, and function. Biomacromolecules, 4(4), 890–895. doi: 10.1021/bm0257412.

[34] Lee, S., Tong, X. & Yang, F. (Feb. 2016). Effects of the poly(ethylene glycol) hydrogel crosslinking mechanism on protein release. Biomaterials Science, 4(3), 405–411. doi: 10.1039/C5BM00256G.

[35] Haryanto, D. S., Huh, P. H. & Kim, S. C. (2016). Hyperbranched poly(glycidol)/poly(ethylene oxide) crosslinked hydrogel for tissue engineering scaffold using e-beams. Journal of Biomedical Materials Research Part A, 104(1), 48–56. doi: 10.1002/jbm.a.35539.

[36] Fan, J. et al. (Aug. 2016). High protein content keratin/poly (ethylene oxide) nanofibers crosslinked in oxygen atmosphere and its cell culture. Materials & Design, 104, 60–67. doi: 10.1016/j.matdes.2016.05.022.

[37] Minhas, M. U., Ahmad, M., Ali, L. & Sohail, M. (May 2013). Synthesis of chemically cross-linked polyvinyl alcohol-co-poly (methacrylic acid) hydrogels by copolymerization; a potential graft-polymeric carrier for oral delivery of 5-fluorouracil. DARU Journal of Pharmaceutical Sciences, 21(1), 44. doi: 10.1186/2008-2231-21-44.

[38] Yokoyama, F., Masada, I., Shimamura, K., Ikawa, T. & Monobe, K. (Jul. 1986). Morphology and structure of highly elastic poly(vinyl alcohol) hydrogel prepared by repeated freezing-and-melting. Colloid and Polymer Science, 264(7), 595–601. doi: 10.1007/BF01412597.

[39] He, Y., Wildman, R. D., Tuck, C. J., Christie, S. D. R. & Edmondson, S. (Feb. 2016). An investigation of the behavior of solvent based polycaprolactone ink for material jetting. Scientific Reports, 6(1), 20852. doi: 10.1038/srep20852.

[40] Sonchaeng, U., Auras, R., Selke, S., Rubino, M. & Lim, L.-T. (Feb. 2020). In-situ changes of thermo-mechanical properties of poly(lactic acid) film immersed in alcohol solutions. Polymer Testing, 82, 106320. doi: 10.1016/j.polymertesting.2019.106320.

[41] Bednarek, M., Borska, K. & Kubisa, P. (Jan. 2020). Crosslinking of polylactide by high energy irradiation and photo-curing. Molecules, 25(21, Art. no. 21), doi: 10.3390/molecules25214919.

[42] Rafiee, M., Farahani, R. D. & Therriault, D. (2020). Multi-material 3D and 4D printing: a survey. Advanced Science, 7(12), 1902307. doi: 10.1002/advs.201902307.

[43] Ma, J., Qi, C., Liu, Z., Meng, S. & Kong, T. (Sep. 2024). Instability-driven 3D bioprinting for engineering composite bio-inks. Engineered Regeneration, 5(3), 350–360. doi: 10.1016/j.engreg.2023.12.004.

[44] Mirshafiei, M., Rashedi, H., Yazdian, F., Rahdar, A. & Baino, F. (Apr. 2024). Advancements in tissue and organ 3D bioprinting: current techniques, applications, and future perspectives. Materials & Design, 240, 112853. doi: 10.1016/j.matdes.2024.112853.

[45] Kumar, V., Mistri, A., Jain, V. & Ghosh, M. (2024). Computational engineering for 3D bioprinting. In: Saha, P., Thomas, S., Kim, J., Ghosh, M. (eds). 3D Bioprinting from Lab to Industry. John Wiley & Sons, Ltd, 301–322. doi: 10.1002/9781119894407.ch10.

[46] Neagu, A. (Apr. 2017). Role of computer simulation to predict the outcome of 3D bioprinting. Journal of 3D Printing in Medicine, 1(2), 103–121. doi: 10.2217/3dp-2016-0008.

[47] Sahai, N. & Gogoi, M. (Jan. 2020). 3D tissue scaffold library development form medical images for bioprinting application. Materials Today: Proceedings, 26, 399–404. doi: 10.1016/j.matpr.2019.12.063.

[48] Shin, J., Lee, Y., Li, Z., Hu, J., Park, S. S. & Kim, K. (Mar. 2022). Optimized 3D bioprinting technology based on machine learning: a review of recent trends and advances. Micromachines, 13(3, Art. no. 3), doi: 10.3390/mi13030363.

[49] Panico, A., Corvi, A., Collini, L. & Sciancalepore, C. (May 2025). Multi objective optimization of FDM 3D printing parameters set via design of experiments and machine learning algorithms. Scientific Reports, 15(1), 16753. doi: 10.1038/s41598-025-01016-z.

[50] Pugliese, R., Badini, S., Frontoni, E. & Regondi, S. (May 2025). Generative artificial intelligence for advancing discovery and design in biomateriomics. Intelligent Computing, 4, 0117. doi: 10.34133/icomputing.0117.

[51] Zhang, Z., Zhou, X., Fang, Y., Xiong, Z. & Zhang, T. (Mar. 2025). AI-driven 3D bioprinting for regenerative medicine: from bench to bedside. Bioactive Materials, 45, 201–230. doi: 10.1016/j.bioactmat.2024.11.021.

[52] Bhardwaj, N., Sood, M. & Gill, S. S. (Jan. 2024). 3D-bioprinting and AI-empowered anatomical structure designing: a review. Current Medical Imaging, 20(1), e15734056259274. doi: 10.2174/0115734056259274231019061329.

[53] Abolhassani, S., Fattahi, R., Safshekan, F., Saremi, J. & Hasanzadeh, E. (Feb. 2025). Advances in 4D bioprinting: the next frontier in regenerative medicine and tissue engineering applications. Advanced Healthcare Materials, 14(4), e2403065. doi: 10.1002/adhm.202403065.

[54] Ashammakhi, N. et al. (2018). Advances and future perspectives in 4D bioprinting. Biotechnology Journal, 13(12), 1800148. doi: 10.1002/biot.201800148.

[55] Yang, Q., Gao, B. & Xu, F. (2020). Recent advances in 4D bioprinting. Biotechnology Journal, 15(1), 1900086. doi: 10.1002/biot.201900086.

[56] Ock, J. et al. (May 2023). An interactive and realistic phantom for cricothyroidotomy simulation of a patient with obesity through a reusable design using 3D-printing and Arduino. Computer Methods and Programs in Biomedicine, 233, 107478. doi: 10.1016/j.cmpb.2023.107478.

[57] Ambagaspitiya, S. S., Appuhamillage, G. A. & Dassanayake, R. S. (May 2024). Impact of vitamin D on ultraviolet-induced photoaging and skin diseases. Exploration of Medicine, 5(3, Art. no. 3), doi: 10.37349/emed.2024.00225.

[58] Kabirian, F., Mela, P. & Heying, R. (2022). 4D printing applications in the development of smart cardiovascular implants. Frontiers in Bioengineering and Biotechnology, 10, 873453. doi: 10.3389/fbioe.2022.873453.

[59] Zhou, L., Min, T., Bian, X., Dong, Y., Zhang, P. & Wen, Y. Rational design of intelligent and multifunctional dressing to promote acute/chronic wound healing. ACS Applied Bio Materials, Aug. 2022. doi: 10.1021/acsabm.2c00500.

[60] Choudhury, S. et al. (Jun. 2024). Design-encoded dual shape-morphing and shape-memory in 4D printed polymer parts toward cellularized vascular grafts. Journal of Materials Chemistry B, 12(23), 5678–5689. doi: 10.1039/D4TB00437J.

[61] Goudie, C., Gill, A., Shanahan, J., Furey, A. & Dubrowski, A. (Jan. 2019). Development of an anatomical silicone model for simulation-based medical training of obstetric anal sphincter injury repair in Bangladesh. Cureus, 11(1), e3991. doi: 10.7759/cureus.3991.

[62] Li, Y. et al. (May 2025). Ultrasensitive piezoelectric-like film with designed cross-scale pores. Science Advances, 11(19), eadt4003. doi: 10.1126/sciadv.adt4003.

[63] Yin, M.-J., Yin, Z., Zhang, Y., Zheng, Q. & Zhang, A. P. (Apr. 2019). Micropatterned elastic ionic polyacrylamide hydrogel for low-voltage capacitive and organic thin-film transistor pressure sensors. Nano Energy, 58, 96–104. doi: 10.1016/j.nanoen.2019.01.032.

[64] Manikandan, N. & Rajesh, P. K. (Feb. 2024). A constitutive model for predicting the time-dependent behavior of multi-material 4D printed structures. Progress in Additive Manufacturing, 9(1), 27–35. doi: 10.1007/s40964-023-00408-9.

[65] Aberoumand, M., Rahmatabadi, D., Aminzadeh, A. & Moradi, M. (2021). 4D printing by fused deposition modeling (FDM). In: Dave, H. K. & Davim, J. P. (eds). Fused Deposition Modeling Based 3D Printing, Cham: Springer International Publishing,377–402. 10.1007/978-3-030-68024-4_20

[66] Kennedy, S. M., Sekar, M. & Vasanthanathan, A. & A. K. 4D bioprinting for personalized medicine, innovations in implant fabrication and regenerative therapies. Polymer-Plastics Technology and Materials, 0(0), 1–26. doi: 10.1080/25740881.2025.2483763.

[67] Pourmasoumi, P. et al. (Jan. 2023). A review on the recent progress, opportunities, and challenges of 4D printing and bioprinting in regenerative medicine. Journal of Biomaterials Science, Polymer Edition, 34(1), 108–146. doi: 10.1080/09205063.2022.2110480.

[68] Dewang, Y., Khan, A., Sharma, V. & Mohan, S. R. (2025). Role of IOT in additive manufacturing. In: Mallaiah, M., Thapliyal, S. & Chandra Bose, S. (eds). Recent Advances in Additive Manufacturing, Volume 1. Singapore: Springer Nature, 315–325. 10.1007/978-981-97-6016-9_25

[69] Kanthimathi, T., Rathika, N., Fathima, A. J., S, R. K., Srinivasan, S. & R, T. (Jan. 2024). Robotic 3D printing for customized industrial components: IoT and AI-enabled innovation. In: *2024 14th International Conference on Cloud Computing, Data Science & Engineering (Confluence)*, 509–513. doi: 10.1109/Confluence60223.2024.10463472.

[70] Gangadevi, E., Shri, M. L., Dhanaraj, R. K. & Balusamy, B. (2024). Computational Intelligence in Bioprinting: Challenges and Future Directions. John Wiley & Sons.

[71] Kazhymurat, T., Shehab, E. & Ali, M. H. (Apr. 2022). IoT-based real-time 3D printing monitoring system. In: *2022 International Conference on Smart Information Systems and Technologies (SIST)*, 1–5. doi: 10.1109/SIST54437.2022.9945778.

[72] González-López, P. et al. (Feb. 2024). The integration of 3D virtual reality and 3D printing technology as innovative approaches to preoperative planning in neuro-oncology. Journal of Personalized Medicine, 14(2, Art. no. 2), doi: 10.3390/jpm14020187.

[73] Urlings, J., De Jong, G., Maal, T. & Henssen, D. (Aug. 2023). Views on augmented reality, virtual reality, and 3D printing in modern medicine and education: a qualitative exploration of expert opinion. Journal of Digital Imaging, 36(4), 1930–1939. doi: 10.1007/s10278-023-00833-w.

[74] Parihar, A. et al. (Jun. 2022). 3D printing: advancement in biogenerative engineering to combat shortage of organs and bioapplicable materials. Regenerative Engineering and Translational Medicine, 8(2), 173–199. doi: 10.1007/s40883-021-00219-w.

[75] Bojedla, S. S. R. et al. (Sep. 2022). Three-dimensional printing of customized scaffolds with polycaprolactone–silk fibroin composites and integration of gingival tissue-derived stem cells for personalized bone therapy. ACS Applied Bio Materials, 5(9), 4465–4479. doi: 10.1021/acsabm.2c00560.

[76] Xu, H. et al. (May 2024). 3D bioprinting advanced biomaterials for craniofacial and dental tissue engineering – a review. Materials & Design, 241, 112886. doi: 10.1016/j.matdes.2024.112886.

[77] Carvalho, J. P. F. et al. (Mar. 2025). All-cellulose hydrogel-based bioinks for the versatile 3D bioprinting of different cell lines. Biomacromolecules, 26(3), 1761–1770. doi: 10.1021/acs.biomac.4c01546.

[78] Chen, S. et al. (Apr. 2025). 3D bioprinting technology innovation in female reproductive system. Materials Today Bio, 31, 101551. doi: 10.1016/j.mtbio.2025.101551.

[79] Chen, S. et al. (Apr. 2025). 3D bioprinting technology innovation in female reproductive system. Materials Today Bio, 31, 101551. doi: 10.1016/j.mtbio.2025.101551.

[80] Behera, S. A., Nanda, B. & Achary, P. G. R. (Nov. 2024). Recent advancements and challenges in 3D bioprinting for cancer applications. Bioprinting, 43, e00357. doi: 10.1016/j.bprint.2024.e00357.

[81] Yang, Z. et al. (Apr. 2023). Research landscape of 3D printing in bone regeneration and bone repair: a bibliometric and visualized analysis from 2012 to 2022. International Journal of Bioprinting, 9(4), 737. doi: 10.18063/ijb.737.

[82] Shi, W. et al. (2023). Embedded bioprinting of breast tumor cells and organoids using low-concentration collagen-based bioinks. Advanced Healthcare Materials, 12(26), 2300905. doi: 10.1002/adhm.202300905.

[83] Tebon, P. J. et al. (Jun. 2023). Drug screening at single-organoid resolution via bioprinting and interferometry. Nature Communications, 14(1), 3168. doi: 10.1038/s41467-023-38832-8.

[84] Colak, B., Cihan, M. C. & Ertas, Y. N. (Sep. 2023). 3D-printed, implantable alginate/CuS nanoparticle scaffolds for local tumor treatment via synergistic photothermal, photodynamic, and chemodynamic therapy. ACS Applied Nano Materials, 6(17), 16076–16085. doi: 10.1021/acsanm.3c03433.

[85] Dutta, S. D., Ganguly, K., Hexiu, J., Randhawa, A., Moniruzzaman, M. & Lim, K.-T. (2023). A 3D bioprinted nanoengineered hydrogel with photoactivated drug delivery for tumor apoptosis and simultaneous bone regeneration via macrophage immunomodulation. Macromolecular Bioscience, 23(9), 2300096. doi: 10.1002/mabi.202300096.

[86] Wei, H. et al. (Oct. 2023). 3D-printed scaffold harboring copper ions combined with near-infrared irradiation for local therapy of cancer. iScience, 26(10), doi: 10.1016/j.isci.2023.108076.

[87] Dey, M. et al. (2022). Chemotherapeutics and CAR-T cell-based immunotherapeutics screening on a 3D bioprinted vascularized breast tumor model. Advanced Functional Materials, 32(52), 2203966. doi: 10.1002/adfm.202203966.

[88] Lam, E. H. Y., Yu, F., Zhu, S. & Wang, Z. (Jan. 2023). 3D bioprinting for next-generation personalized medicine. International Journal of Molecular Sciences, 24(7, Art. no. 7). doi: 10.3390/ijms24076357.

[89] Gupta, S. & Bit, A. (Jun. 2022). 3D bioprinting in tissue engineering and regenerative medicine. Cell and Tissue Banking, 23(2), 199–212. doi: 10.1007/s10561-021-09936-6.

[90] Fang, W. et al. (May 2023). Hydrogels for 3D bioprinting in tissue engineering and regenerative medicine: current progress and challenges. International Journal of Bioprinting, 9(5), 759. doi: 10.18063/ijb.759.

[91] Carvalho, J. P. F. et al. (Mar. 2025). All-cellulose hydrogel-based bioinks for the versatile 3D bioprinting of different cell lines. Biomacromolecules, 26(3), 1761–1770. doi: 10.1021/acs.biomac.4c01546.

[92] Noor, A. F. H. M. & Johari, N. H. (2022). Brief review on recent technology in particle image velocimetry studies on hemodynamics in carotid artery. In: Hassan, M. H. A., Ahmad (A) Manap, Z., Baharom, M. Z., Johari, N. H., Jamaludin, U. K., Jalil, M. H., Mat Sahat, I. & Omar, M. N. (eds). Human-Centered Technology for a Better Tomorrow. Singapore: Springer, 267–277. 10.1007/978-981-16-4115-2_21

[93] Saini, G., Segaran, N., Mayer, J. L., Saini, A., Albadawi, H. & Oklu, R. (Oct. 2021). Applications of 3D bioprinting in tissue engineering and regenerative medicine. Journal of Clinical Medicine, 10(21), 4966. doi: 10.3390/jcm10214966.

[94] Liang, X. et al. (May 2025). Three-dimensional printing resin-based dental provisional crowns and bridges: recent progress in properties, applications, and perspectives. Materials (Basel), 18(10), 2202. doi: 10.3390/ma18102202.

[95] Joshi, A., Choudhury, S., Gugulothu, S. B., Visweswariah, S. S. & Chatterjee, K. (Jul. 2022). Strategies to promote vascularization in 3D printed tissue scaffolds: trends and challenges. Biomacromolecules, 23(7), 2730–2751. doi: 10.1021/acs.biomac.2c00423.

[96] Richards, D., Jia, J., Yost, M., Markwald, R. & Mei, Y. (Jan. 2017). 3D bioprinting for vascularized tissue fabrication. Annals of Biomedical Engineering, 45(1), 132–147. doi: 10.1007/s10439-016-1653-z.

[97] Behera, S. A., Nanda, B. & Achary, P. G. R. (Nov. 2024). Recent advancements and challenges in 3D bioprinting for cancer applications. Bioprinting, 43, e00357. doi: 10.1016/j.bprint.2024.e00357.

[98] Ong, C. S. et al. (Jan. 2018). 3D bioprinting using stem cells. Pediatric Research, 83(1), 223–231. doi: 10.1038/pr.2017.252.
[99] Jovic, T. H., Combellack, E. J., Jessop, Z. M. & Whitaker, I. S. (Nov. 2020). 3D bioprinting and the future of surgery. Frontiers in Surgery, 7, doi: 10.3389/fsurg.2020.609836.
[100] Panda, S. et al. (Sep. 2022). A focused review on three-dimensional bioprinting technology for artificial organ fabrication. Biomaterials Science, 10(18), 5054–5080. doi: 10.1039/D2BM00797E.
[101] Santoni, S., Gugliandolo, S. G., Sponchioni, M., Moscatelli, D. & Colosimo, B. M. (Jan. 2022). 3D bioprinting: current status and trends – a guide to the literature and industrial practice. Bio-Design and Manufacturing, 5(1), 14–42. doi: 10.1007/s42242-021-00165-0.
[102] Gurel, M. et al. (Oct. 2024). A narrative review: 3D bioprinting of cultured muscle meat and seafood products and its potential for the food industry. Trends in Food Science & Technology, 152, 104670. doi: 10.1016/j.tifs.2024.104670.
[103] Khan, S. A., Koç, M. & Al-Ghamdi, S. G. (Jun. 2021). Sustainability assessment, potentials and challenges of 3D printed concrete structures: a systematic review for built environmental applications. Journal of Cleaner Production, 303, 127027. doi: 10.1016/j.jclepro.2021.127027.
[104] Nadagouda, M. N., Ginn, M. & Rastogi, V. (Jun. 2020). A review of 3D printing techniques for environmental applications. Current Opinion in Chemical Engineering, 28, 173–178. doi: 10.1016/j.coche.2020.08.002.
[105] Kishore, A., Singh, C. & Kaur*, G. Sharma, N., Sharma, R., Dakal, T. (2025). Bio-nanomaterials: an introduction. In: Bio-Nanomaterials in Environmental Remediation. John Wiley & Sons, Ltd, 1–46. doi: 10.1002/9783527848546.ch1.
[106] Rane, N. (Sep. 28, 2023). 3D, 4D, and 5D printing in architecture, engineering, and construction (AEC) industry: applications, challenges, and future scope. In: Gangadevi, E., Lawanya Shri, M., Dhanaraj, R. K., Balusamy, B. (eds). Social Science Research Network, Rochester, NY, 1, 4609912. doi: 10.2139/ssrn.4609912.
[107] Kaswan, K. S., Dhatterwal, J. S., Prakash, O., Balusamy, B. & Mon, F. A. (2024). Research trends in intelligence-based bioprinting for construction engineering applications. In: Computational Intelligence in Bioprinting. John Wiley & Sons, Ltd, 175–191. doi: 10.1002/9781394204878.ch9.
[108] Jipa, A. et al. (Nov. 2018). 3d-printed formwork for prefabricated concrete slabs. Presented at the 1st International Conference on 3D Construction Printing (3Dcp), ETH Zurich, Digital Building Technologies (ITA). doi: 10.3929/ethz-b-000507651.
[109] Panda, B., Unluer, C. & Tan, M. J. (Nov. 2018). Investigation of the rheology and strength of geopolymer mixtures for extrusion-based 3D printing. Cement and Concrete Composites, 94, 307–314. doi: 10.1016/j.cemconcomp.2018.10.002.
[110] Mathur, V., Agarwal, P., Kasturi, M., Srinivasan, V., Seetharam, R. N. & Vasanthan, K. S. (Jan. 2025). Innovative bioinks for 3D bioprinting: exploring technological potential and regulatory challenges. Journal of Tissue Engineering, 16, 20417314241308022. doi: 10.1177/20417314241308022.
[111] Lu, C. et al. (Apr. 2025). Advancing tissue engineering through vascularized cell spheroids: building blocks of the future. Biomaterials Science, 13(8), 1901–1922. doi: 10.1039/D4BM01206B.
[112] Mei, X. et al. (Feb. 2025). Integrating microfluidic and bioprinting technologies: advanced strategies for tissue vascularization. Lab on a Chip, 25(5), 764–786. doi: 10.1039/D4LC00280F.
[113] Ozbolat, I. T. & Hospodiuk, M. (Jan. 2016). Current advances and future perspectives in extrusion-based bioprinting. Biomaterials, 76, 321–343. doi: 10.1016/j.biomaterials.2015.10.076.
[114] Zhang, B. et al. (Mar. 2018). 3D bioprinting: an emerging technology full of opportunities and challenges. Bio-Design and Manufacturing, 1(1), 2–13. doi: 10.1007/s42242-018-0004-3.
[115] Chen, X. B. et al. (Oct. 2023). Biomaterials / bioinks and extrusion bioprinting. Bioactive Materials, 28, 511–536. doi: 10.1016/j.bioactmat.2023.06.006.

[116] Mathur, V., Agarwal, P., Kasturi, M., Srinivasan, V., Seetharam, R. N. & Vasanthan, K. S. (May 2025). Innovative bioinks for 3D bioprinting: exploring technological potential and regulatory challenges. Journal of Tissue Engineering, 16, 20417314241308022. doi: 10.1177/20417314241308022.

[117] Sekar, M. P. et al. (Jan. 2021). Current standards and ethical landscape of engineered tissues – 3D bioprinting perspective. Journal of Tissue Engineering, 12, 20417314211027677. doi: 10.1177/20417314211027677.

[118] Kačarević, Ž. P. et al. (Nov. 2018). An introduction to 3D bioprinting: possibilities, challenges and future aspects. Materials, 11(11, Art. no. 11), doi: 10.3390/ma11112199.

[119] Donderwinkel, I., van Hest, J. C. M. & Cameron, N. R. (Aug. 2017). Bio-inks for 3D bioprinting: recent advances and future prospects. Polymer Chemistry, 8(31), 4451–4471. doi: 10.1039/C7PY00826K.

[120] Patra, S. & Young, V. (Jun. 2016). A review of 3D printing techniques and the future in biofabrication of bioprinted tissue. Cell Biochemistry and Biophysics, 74(2), 93–98. doi: 10.1007/s12013-016-0730-0.

[121] Rizzo, M. L. et al. (Jun. 10, 2025). 3D printing and 3D bioprinting technology in medicine: ethical and legal issues. La Clinica Terapeutica, 174(1, Art. no. 1). doi: 10.7417/CT.2023.2501.

[122] Patuzzo, S., Goracci, G., Gasperini, L. & Ciliberti, R. (Apr. 2018). 3D bioprinting technology: scientific aspects and ethical issues. Science and Engineering Ethics, 24(2), 335–348. doi: 10.1007/s11948-017-9918-y.

[123] Li, P., Faulkner, A. & Medcalf, N. (Jan. 2020). 3D bioprinting in a 2d regulatory landscape: gaps, uncertainties, and problems. Law, Innovation and Technology, 12(1), 1–29. doi: 10.1080/17579961.2020.1727054.

[124] Campbell, T., Williams, C., Ivanova, O. & Garrett, B., "Could 3D printing change the world?: Technologies, potential, and implications of additive manufacturing," Atlantic Council, 2011. Accessed: Jun. 15, 2025. [Online]. Available: https://www.jstor.org/stable/resrep03564

[125] Gebler, M., Schoot Uiterkamp, A. J. M. & Visser, C. (Nov. 2014). A global sustainability perspective on 3D printing technologies. Energy Policy, 74, 158–167. doi: 10.1016/j.enpol.2014.08.033.

Saswata Mitra, Anwesha Mukherjee, Bodhisatwa Das*

Chapter 7 Biomanufacturing and Bioprinting of Vasculatures

Abstract: In native tissues, vascular networks supply oxygen and nutrients, remove metabolic waste, and ensure proper tissue function. Incorporating vasculatures in 3D-bioprinted structures is essential to ensure graft viability and appropriate functionality. Furthermore, bioprinted vasculatures can be used as functional vascular grafts, in vitro disease models, and organ-on-chip systems. Advances in 3D bioprinting technologies allow the fabrication of complex tissue structures with precise spatial control. Functional vasculatures can be fabricated by synergizing biomaterial properties with biomanufacturing techniques. Bioinks formulated using natural biomaterials such as collagen, gelatin, decellularized extracellular matrix, silk fibroin, elastin, and fibronectin can effectively mimic the natural extracellular matrix of blood vessels. Bioprinted vasculatures also must be able to withstand burst pressure, tensile, shear, and compressive forces like native vessels for appropriate functionality and compliance matching. Bioinks can be laden with angiogenic growth factors to aid in cell differentiation and endothelialization. Several bioprinting approaches, such as extrusion-based, inkjet-based, and digital light processing, can be employed to manufacture complex geometries and hierarchical structures. However, limitations arise while bioprinting hollow structures with high shape fidelity and complex geometry. Freeform reversible embedding of suspended hydrogels bioprinting approaches are currently being explored to print hollow structures with high precision within a sacrificial support matrix, which allows overcoming geometric constraints. Additionally, sacrificial molding and coaxial extrusion can be employed to generate hierarchical vascular networks. Furthermore, strategies for vascular maturation, including endothelial-pericyte co-culturing, angiogenic gradients, and bioreactor systems, are analyzed. Finally, the integration of emerging technologies in conjunction with innovative biomaterials is expected to accelerate the biomanufacturing of clinically viable vascular grafts, bridging the gaps in translational biomaterial research.

Keywords: Biomanufacturing, bioprinting, tissue engineering, blood vessels, vasculatures

---

***Corresponding author: Bodhisatwa Das,** Department of Biomedical Engineering, Indian Institute of Technology Ropar, Rupnagar, Punjab, India, e-mail: bodhisatwa.das@iitrpr.ac.in
Saswata Mitra, Anwesha Mukherjee, Department of Biomedical Engineering, Indian Institute of Technology Ropar, Punjab, India

 | https://doi.org/10.1515/9783111719993-007

7.1 Introduction

Tissue-engineered artificial organs have garnered significant interest in recent decades, particularly for organ transplantations and models for drug screening. One of the crucial parameters to ensure the functional viability of engineered tissues is the incorporation of vasculature into the models. The vascular system transports nutrients, gases, bioactive molecules, and toxic substances, thereby playing a crucial role in maintaining cellular functions. The diffusion limit of nutrients and oxygen is 100–200 μm in physiological conditions. Thus, beyond that distance, cells will experience significant distress due to the lack of oxygen and nutrients, eventually leading to cell death and tissue necrosis. In this context, the diffusion limit without vasculature becomes a critical factor in determining the size of viable and functional tissue, highlighting the necessity of blood vessels in ensuring tissue growth and sustenance [1]. Hence, large tissue models without functional vasculature often exhibit poor viability, significantly limiting the size and viability of engineered tissues. In addition to the development of organ models for drug screening and tissue engineering, bioengineered blood vessels can be a sustainable alternative for graft therapies, where vessels are transplanted to diseased or damaged sites to restore blood flow in the body. Transplantable blood vessels are required for several clinical conditions. Coronary artery disease affects 315 million people globally, and peripheral artery disease affects an estimated 113 million people, thus highlighting the importance of transplantable blood vessels in clinical perspectives. Autologous grafts are currently the gold standard for blood vessel transplantation. However, shortages in autologous grafts due to preexisting medical conditions and the unavailability of sufficient healthy vessels pose a significant challenge. Allogenic or xenogenic grafts pose severe risks of rejection, inflammation, blood compatibility challenges, infection, vessel integration, and subsequent graft failure. Thus, engineered blood vessels are of significant importance from a clinical perspective. Synthetic blood vessels are typically fabricated using biocompatible materials. However, poor integration, lack of biomimetic properties, mechanical failure, and challenging blood-material interactions often lead to graft failure due to bleeding risks, thrombus formation, low blood pressure in vessels of smaller diameter, and fibrosis [2]. As such, it is significantly challenging to produce artificial blood vessels that can match the gold standard [3].

Traditional tissue-engineering approaches involve fabricating a scaffold and seeding cells on it, then allowing it to mature to achieve a sufficient number of cells to be functionally viable before implantation. However, the process is slow, laborious, time-intensive, and clinically difficult to translate. Moreover, non-uniform cell distribution, lack of spatiotemporal control on cell distribution on scaffolds, and improper cell-material interactions act as significant hurdles. 3D bioprinting has emerged as a potential alternative to fabricating bioengineered tissue constructs and addressing these challenges [4]. Furthermore, it provides flexibility in design, offering opportunities for fabricating patient-specific grafts. Patient-specific grafts are incorporated with the individual's own cells, lowering the possibility of immune rejection and graft failure. Furthermore, they can be tailored to specific geometries as per the clinical requirement. This advantage can significantly improve patient outcomes in several applications. In addition to fabricating macroscale vasculature, a significant research gap persists in fabricating blood vessels while developing tissue models and artificial organs. As mentioned earlier, vascularization is essential for ensuring oxygen and nutrient transport and the removal of cellular waste by-products. Inadequate vascularization significantly impacts tissue viability, size, and functionality [1]. Thus, integrating vasculature in tissue models is essential to engineering functionally viable constructs. The advances in 3D bioprinting technologies have enabled the fabrication of functionally viable blood vessels with diameters ranging from macroscale to microscale [5]. Thus, 3D bioprinting can be used to generate blood vessels with capillary-sized diameters, which makes the vasculature suitable for mass transport, ensuring the viability of fabricated tissue constructs [6]. Significant research is being carried out to fabricate vasculature using different strategies involving bioprinting technologies, biomaterials, bioinks, and innovative materials. Most of these studies aim to overcome challenges involving synthetic blood vessels, particularly those related to the endothelial layer [4]. Blood compatibility with the endothelial layer is essential for ensuring the functional viability of the vasculature. The endothelium, which is comprised of endothelial cells, is highly crucial in maintaining vascular homeostasis through the regulation of vascular tone, cell adhesion, inflammation, and coagulation. It influences blood flow and pressure, responses to inflammation and damage, coagulation and thrombosis, and metabolic regulation. It helps in preventing unwanted hemostasis by preventing platelet activation, thrombogenesis, and fibrinolysis [2]. The endothelium also prevents the smooth muscle cells from migrating into the inner lumen and thus prevents conditions such as restenosis. Therefore, fabricating a healthy and functional endothelial layer is crucial to ensure proper blood flow and to eliminate blood vessel patency [7]. An understanding of blood vessel architecture and composition is thus essential for printing blood vessels. Since the functionality of the blood vessels is dependent on the hierarchical organization of different layers that comprise the vessel, understanding native composition is necessary to achieve successful 3D bioprinting of blood vessels.

7.2 Composition of Blood Vessels

Blood vessels are composed of three distinct layers: the inner lumen, which is the endothelium or tunica intima; the medial layer, which is tunica media; and the outermost layer, which is tunica adventitia. The tunica intima is comprised primarily of three major parts: the endothelial layer, which is made up of one layer of simple squamous epithelial cells; the basal lamina, which is made up of collagen type IV and laminin; and the subendothelial layer, which is primarily composed of loose connective tissue. The endothelial layer is the thinnest among all three, functioning as a nonthrombogenic barrier, providing protection against infection and inflammation. In arteries and arterioles, the subendothelial layer consists of a fenestrated acellular elastic lamella known as the internal elastic membrane, which provides structural support, prevents cell migration, and aids in the diffusion of molecules across the layers. The tunica intima is encompassed by the tunica media, which is formed by collagen types I and III, along with circumferentially arranged smooth muscle cells. It also consists of elastin and proteoglycans, along with reticular fibers that are present between layers of smooth muscle cells. The tunica media is relatively thinner in veins than in arteries. In arteries, it covers the space in between the internal and external elastic membranes. The external elastic membrane, present in arteries, is composed of fenestrated elastic fibers that separate the tunica media from the tunica adventitia. The tunica adventitia, which is the outermost layer of blood vessels, is formed by collagen and elastic fibers along with fibroblast cells. It provides mechanical support and plays a crucial role in anchoring the blood vessels to the surrounding tissues. Based on the blood vessel type and size, these layers vary. The arteries and veins have similar anatomy and can be distinguished by the thickness, cellular, and extracellular matrix compositions. In contrast, capillaries have small diameters and comprise only the endothelial layer and the basal lamina. The diameter of capillaries is sufficiently large only to allow one single red blood cell to pass through at one time. The tunica media and adventitia layers are entirely absent in capillaries, unlike arteries and veins [7].

The endothelial layer in blood vessels prevents thrombosis and aids in vascular homeostasis. It thus provides a semipermeable barrier for the selective transport of molecules between the circulating blood, blood vessels, and the tissues surrounding them. A healthy endothelium also controls platelet activation and aggregation, leukocyte attachment, and the proliferation and migration of smooth muscle cells. Hence, it plays a significant role in preventing embolus formation, thrombosis, and restenosis due to the ingrowth of smooth muscle cells [2]. On the other hand, smooth muscle cells influence the mechanical properties of the blood vessels by producing extracellular matrix components such as collagen, elastin, and proteoglycans. This, in turn, maintains the compliance and elastic properties of the blood vessels. Thus, to successfully bioprint vasculatures, the organization of the different layers is crucial and should be consistent with the requirements of various types of blood vessels.

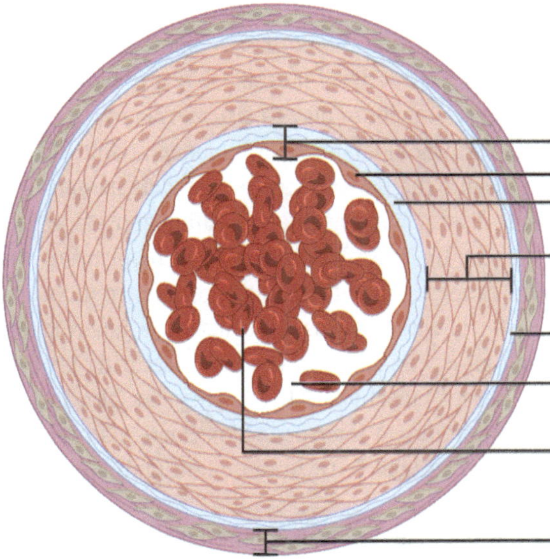

Figure 7.1: Basic architecture of a blood vessel.

7.3 Bioink Design for Bioprinting Vasculatures

Bioprinting vasculatures requires the synthesis of bioinks with appropriate biocompatibility, hemocompatibility, rheology, and mechanical properties to mimic native blood vessels. Bioinks, comprising biomaterials, cells, and growth factors, play a pivotal role in mimicking the native blood vessel microenvironment, thereby facilitating cell proliferation and providing mechanical integrity. Appropriate interaction between blood and bioink is the key prerequisite in 3D biofabrication of vasculatures [8]. Additionally, the biocompatibility, printability, structural integrity, mechanical compliance, degradability, and porosity are among the key parameters to consider when fabricating bioinks for vascular tissue bioprinting [9].

7.4 Choice of Biomaterial

The evaluation of the biological properties of biomaterials is critical to determine the successful fabrication of blood vessels. Biomaterials effectively form the extracellular matrix component of bioinks, which is essential in the context of biofabrication. This artificial matrix allows the embedded cells to attach, proliferate, and form new tissue. Furthermore, the biomaterial of choice largely determines the immunogenicity of the fabricated constructs and host response upon implantation. Thus, the choice of biomaterial is extremely pivotal to ensure appropriate blood–biomaterial and tissue–biomaterial interactions to prevent thrombosis and subsequent graft failure. Furthermore, the biomaterial should support endothelialization since the endothelium plays a crucial role in maintaining the functionality of the blood vessels. Natural biomaterials are biodegradable, resorb while new tissue forms, can effectively mimic the native extracellular matrix, and provide a suitable matrix for embedded cells to attach and proliferate. Although natural biomaterials have superior biological attributes, their use is constrained in bioprinting due to their poor mechanical and rheological properties. Synthetic biomaterials are more stable in physiological conditions, degrade slowly while new tissue forms, have superior mechanical and rheological properties, and allow tunability in the manufacturing process while lacking cell adhesion sites and inherent bioactivity [10, 11]. They can also invoke the host immune response upon implantation due to their poor biomimetic nature. Furthermore, poor blood-material interaction can lead to thrombosis, inflammation, and subsequent failure.

Collagen, a protein-based polymer, is often selected for bioink fabrication for vascular tissue engineering due to its abundance in the extracellular matrix of blood vessels. Being a significant component, collagen provides a biomimetic nature, low immunogenicity, and cell-binding sites in bioink. Collagen fibers are also resistant to strain deformation up to a specific limit, which makes collagen suitable for fabricating blood vessels. However, collagen scaffolds can be stiff and have limited elasticity, which is an essential mechanical property required for blood vessel fabrication. Fibrin has emerged as a suitable natural polymer in place of collagen for fabricating blood vessels due to its excellent biocompatibility and hemocompatibility. Since it can be obtained from patient-derived blood, it demonstrates minimal inflammatory response upon implantation. Fibrin binds to key proteins such as fibronectin and Vascular endothelial growth factor (VEGF), directing cell fate [11]. One study has reported that smooth muscle cells secrete more elastin in fibrin gel than collagen gel, demonstrating the bioactive properties of fibrin and its suitability for vascular tissue engineering [11]. Gelatin, a derivative of collagen, is widely used in tissue engineering due to its economic value and biological properties [12]. Gelatin is often modified with the addition of methacrylate groups to form gelatin methacrylate (GelMA), which is a popular choice in bioprinting due to its biomimetic nature, biocompatibility, and photosensitivity through which it can be readily cross-linked without employing any chemical cross-linkers. More recently, composite materials composed of natural as well as synthetic biopolymers have been used to fabricate blood vessels [13]. Furthermore, nanomaterials have also been used in bioink formulations as fillers to improve rheological, mechanical, and biological properties of fabricated blood vessels. With new bioink formulations involving composite materials, several research groups have reported the fabrication of functional vascular constructs (Table 7.1).

Table 7.1: Biomaterials for blood vessel biofabrication.

Biomaterials	Advantages	Limitations	Compatible cell lines	Relevance in vascular tissue engineering
Gelatin/GelMA	Biomimetic, biocompatible, cost-effective, modifiable, and supports cell adhesion	Thermally unstable, reduced mechanical stability unless cross-linked	HUVECs, MSCs, epithelial progenitor cells (EPCs), and NIH-3T3 fibroblasts	Suitable for vascular bioprinting due to tunability and cytocompatibility [14]
Fibrin	Biocompatible, hemocompatible, and binds fibronectin and VEGF	Rapid degradation and weak mechanical strength	HUVECs and ECs	Bioactive and hemocompatible; suitable for vascular graft coatings and early constructs [11]
Collagen	ECM protein, with low immunogenicity, and provides cell-binding sites	Limited elasticity, stiffness, and batch-to-batch variability	HUVECs, MSCs, and SMCs	Mimics vascular ECM; often combined with elastin or fibrin for compliance [15]
Hyaluronic acid (HA)	Highly biocompatible, high water absorption, and promotes cell migration and proliferation	Poor mechanical strength and rapid degradation	HUVECs and MSCs	Excellent for angiogenic cues; blended with stronger polymers [11]
dECM (decellularized ECM)	Highest biomimetic property, promotes cell adhesion and proliferation, and has a certain antithrombotic effect	Poor mechanical strength, slow gelation, complex preparation process	HUVECs, MSCs, iPSCs	Gold-standard biomimetic bioink [16]; ideal for vascular constructs [11]
Pluronic F127	Thermoresponsive, printable, and easy gelation	Rapid degradation and weak mechanical strength	MSCs (as carrier)	Used as sacrificial bioink for creating vascular channels [11]
Synthetic polymers (PCL, PLA, PEG, PGA, PLGA, and **PU)**	Tunable degradation and high mechanical strength	Poor bioactivity, immune risk, and no inherent cell adhesion	HUVECs, MSCs, SMCs (after functionalization)	Provide structural/mechanical support; usually blended with natural polymers [17]

Table 7.1 (continued)

Biomaterials	Advantages	Limitations	Compatible cell lines	Relevance in vascular tissue engineering
Composite materials (natural + synthetic)	Combine bioactivity + mechanical tunability, and customizable degradation	Complex fabrication, higher cost	HUVECs, MSCs, SMCs, and EPCs	Balances printability, stability, and biological function
Nanomaterial-based bioinks (graphene oxide, nanocellulose, silica, and hydroxyapatite NPs)	Improve rheology, mechanics, bioactivity, and conductivity	Potential cytotoxicity	HUVECs, MSCs, EPCs, and SMCs (depending on nanomaterial type)	Enhance vascular construct fidelity, angiogenesis [18], and support cellular organization [10]

7.5 Cell Types

The primary cells required to fabricate the layers of blood vessels are endothelial cells and smooth muscle cells. Endothelial cells form the tunica intima and are crucial for angiogenesis and vascularization [17]. Appropriate stimuli provided to endothelial cells can aid in their activation, upon which they become tip or stalk cells, and migrate following the principles of chemotaxis along concentration gradients of growth factors. In bioprinted scaffolds, the primary sources of endothelial cells are human umbilical vein endothelial cells (HUVECs and human dermal microvascular endothelial cells (HDMECs) [13, 19]. Here, smooth muscle cells make up the tunica media and are enveloped by a basement membrane that restricts the proliferation and migration of these cells. Similar to endothelial cells, smooth muscle cells can be harvested from human umbilical vein (HUVSMCs) as well as coronary arteries and the aorta [14]. The precise control of smooth muscle cells in an engineered blood vessel in terms of arrangement and distribution can guide the physiological properties of the blood vessel construct [20, 21]. In addition, bioprinted blood vessels can be co-cultured with pericytes. Pericytes stabilize blood vessels and control angiogenesis through several processes [22]. They anchor to leaky endothelial sprouts through the recruitment via growth factors such as platelet-derived growth factor (PDGF), modulate endothelial cell behavior by secreting growth factors like transforming growth factor beta (TGF-β) and angiopoietin-1 (Ang-1), and interact with the extracellular matrix to guide endothelial cell migration. Stem cells can also be potentially used to fabricate functionally viable blood vessels [23]. Pluripotent stem cells can be directed to differentiate into endothelial cells. At the same time, embryonic stem cells have also been reported to differentiate into endothelial cells, which, upon transplantation in the body, can increase capillary density and integrate with preexisting microvasculature [24].

7.6 Incorporation of Bioactive Molecules

Several growth factors and small molecules are involved in vascularization and directly influence the formation of blood vessels [23]. The incorporation of such bioactive molecules in conjunction with specific types of cells in bioinks designed for vascular structure fabrication can aid the cells to proliferate, differentiate, and form functional vascular conduits. VEGF is reported to stimulate the proliferation of endothelial cells and aid in vascularization by stimulating endothelial cells to migrate, proliferate, and form tubes [25, [26]. One research reported a gelatin methacrylate (GelMA)-laponite bioink integrated with VEGF that demonstrated potent angiogenic ability in an in ovo CAM study [27]. Fibroblast growth factors (bFGF and FGF-2) are also angiogenic growth factors that aid in the differentiation and proliferation of endothelial cells. PDGF is reported to stimulate the proliferation of vascular smooth muscle cells and pericytes, which is key to stabilizing nascent blood vessels during vascularization. TGF-β plays a dual role in vascularization, stimulating the proliferation, migration, and differentiation of endothelial cells at low concentrations, while inhibiting them at high concentrations. Ang-1 is known to stabilize nascent blood vessels by recruiting pericytes, while insulin-like growth factor-1 promotes the proliferation of endothelial cells and shields the cells from oxidative stress. Anticoagulants like heparin can also be used in conjunction with growth factors since they can improve blood–material interaction by preventing any unwanted platelet adhesion and subsequent clot formation, while also promoting the growth of endothelial cells. One study reported the fabrication of a polyurethane-based blood vessel functionalized with heparin and gelatin [12]. Apart from growth factors and small molecules, ions such as lithium, magnesium, copper, and silicon can upregulate angiogenic genes in a dose-dependent manner. Low doses of lithium promote vascularization and reportedly stabilize vascular barriers. Magnesium can enhance angiogenesis, as reported by a recent study, which demonstrated that the presence of magnesium silicate enhanced vascular network formation in a CAM study [28]. Silicon can promote endothelial cell migration and tube formation and stimulate the production of VEGF and endothelial nitric oxide synthase, which facilitates angiogenesis through the production of nitric oxide. Nitric oxide, notable for its role in vasodilation, enhances the survival and proliferation of endothelial cells. Copper ions act as cofactors for VEGF and FGF, which in turn stimulate angiogenesis.

7.7 Biofabrication Strategies to Bioprint Blood Vessels

Bioprinting allows precise control over scaffold architecture and porosity, while being able to generate constructs rapidly with high precision over their geometries. 3D bioprinting primarily involves three primary techniques: laser-assisted, inkjet-based, and extrusion-based [14]. Other methods, such as stereolithography or syringe molding, although not widely used, have been explored for fabricating blood vessels with varying success. Each technique has its unique set of advantages and disadvantages, which must be taken into consideration in the context of bioprinting blood vessels.

7.8 Laser-Assisted Bioprinting

Laser-assisted bioprinting strategy involves laser-induced forward transfer (LIFT), a technique for transferring cells to a printing base by the application of a pulsed laser. Essentially, there are three components in this bioprinting setup: a pulsed laser source, a donor layer containing cells and biomaterials, and a substrate on which the cells and biomaterials are deposited. Pulsed laser strikes the donor layer, vaporizing it and forming bubbles. The bubble formation generates shockwaves that propel the cell-material layer to form droplets and move toward the substrate, i.e., the receiving stage. In this way, high-resolution patterned structures with vessel-like geometries can be fabricated [7]. The overall performance of laser bioprinting and patterning is influenced by several factors, including the laser energy, laser pulse frequency, viscosity of the material that is deposited, and deposition speed. One study demonstrated the successful patterning of endothelial cells in an alginate matrix through laser-assisted bioprinting. High-resolution structures can be fabricated using the LIFT technique, which can be used to fabricate thin capillaries with excellent precision. A polyester urethane urea-based cardiac patch was successfully patterned with mesenchymal stem cells and endothelial cells to fabricate functional cardiac patches [14]. Similar strategies can be employed to design hollow blood vessels lined with endothelial and smooth muscle cells. One study demonstrated biological laser printing of HUVEC and HUVSMC [29]. HUVECs were first patterned and cultured, allowing the formation of the lumen, bordering which HUVSMCs were deposited. The smooth muscle cells restricted the migration of endothelial cells, resulting in a vessel with designated geometry. However, laser-based bioprinting suffers from several drawbacks, including cell stress due to the application of laser shock, slow fabrication time, and random assembly of cells within the cell-biomaterial precursor solution.

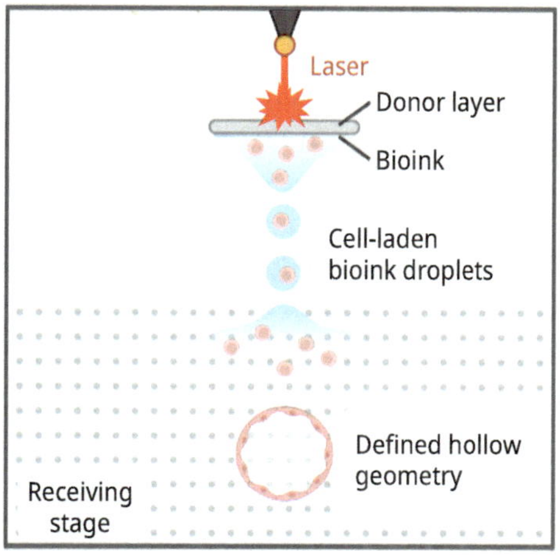

Figure 7.2: Schematic representation of laser-assisted bioprinting to fabricate vascular structures.

7.9 Inkjet-Based Bioprinting

Inkjet-based bioprinting involves the fabrication of structures by dispensing droplets of bioink onto a substrate through a nozzle using thermal or piezoelectric strategies. This non-contact, high-throughput droplet-based deposition strategy is employed for depositing inks in predetermined specific positions. The requirements for inkjet bioprinting include bioinks, biopapers, models for printing, and specified printing parameters. Bioprinting of vasculatures through inkjet printing mainly involves the patterning of vasculatures onto the biopaper as microchannels for blood flow [30]. For example, a thermal inkjet bioprinter has been used to fabricate microchannels using endothelial cells and fibrin as a biomaterial, which resulted in the formation of a vasculature lining that is like the endothelial layer present in native blood vessels. Another group investigated the same strategy using type 1 collagen and rat smooth muscle cells. An inkjet strategy was used to pattern acellular bioink onto a substrate coated with agarose [14]. Following the fabrication of microvasculature, it was seeded with rat smooth muscle cells, which selectively bound to the collagen-based structure, while agarose prevented any nonspecific cell adhesion [15]. These strategies have resulted in the fabrication of precise and accurate biomimetic vasculatures that can be employed for organ-on-a-chip models effectively. Inkjet-based bioprinting can also be employed to pattern substrates with specific bioactive molecules that can enhance endothelialization. One study has demonstrated the use of peptides to promote cell adhesion and cell migration. The use of the CGRDS peptide for enhancing cell adhesion and CWQPPRARI to improve the migration of cells was reported. The surfaces that were fabricated with the peptides demonstrated enhanced endothelialization compared to unmodified surfaces.

Inkjet bioprinting is not limited to two-dimensional biofabrication; it can be employed to generate hollow, vasculature-mimicking structures by depositing subsequent layers of droplets. One example is the deposition of spheroids, the fusion of which results in blood vessel-like structures. A study demonstrated the fabrication of vasculature using alginate that resulted in vessels with approximately 90 µm diameters. Droplets of sodium alginate were stacked to generate hollow structures that were able to withstand pressures similar to physiological conditions. Another study reported the fabrication of polyurethane-based constructs that could be used for cardiovascular implants. Multicellular constructs can also be fabricated using inkjet-based bioprinting approaches [7]. One group reported the fabrication of an inkjet-based construct consisting of three different types of cells – smooth muscle cells, human amniotic-fluid derived stem cells, and bovine aortic endothelial cells. A collagen-alginate composite was used as a substrate for printing. Cells suspended in calcium chloride solution were deposited onto the biopolymer composite matrix, and cross-linking of alginate ensured that the cells were positioned in specified locations. After printing one layer, the substrate was immersed in fresh uncross-linked substrate to provide a new interface for the subsequent layer and ensure proper fusion with the previous layer. The fabricated structure demonstrated adequate in vivo vascularization upon implantation [19].

Since inkjet bioprinting is a non-contact fabrication strategy, it can be employed for direct in situ bioprinting, in which the cell-laden bioinks can be directly deposited on the injured tissue. However, inkjet-based strategies can affect cell viability due to harsh parameters used for deposition. This can negatively affect the viability of the constructs by compromising cells [2]. Moreover, due to the small orifice diameter of

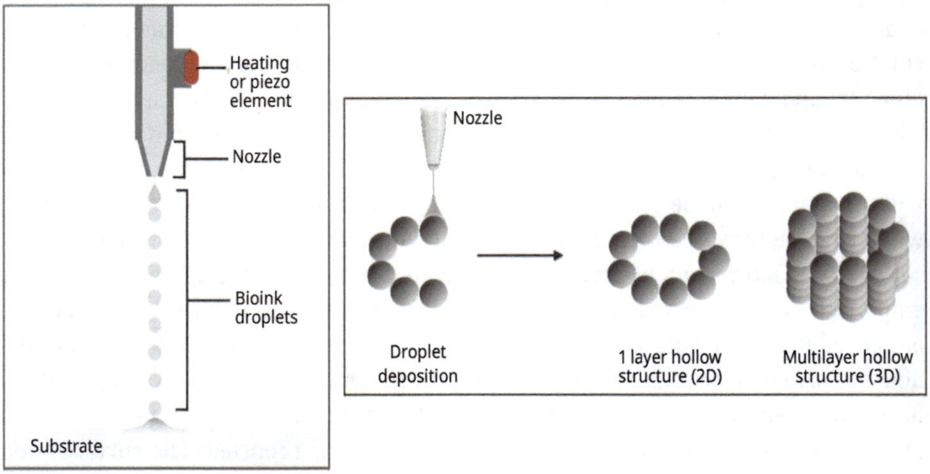

Figure 7.3: Illustration demonstrating an inkjet-based bioprinting strategy to fabricate hollow blood vessel conduits.

the nozzles, cells tend to aggregate, and thus, maintaining high cell density and uniformity can be challenging. Furthermore, if the droplets are unable to fuse, they can generate leaky vasculatures, which can be catastrophic in physiological contexts. Such vessels can rupture, causing the construct to fail. These parameters and limitations are to be studied extensively to fabricate functional vascular constructs.

7.10 Extrusion-Based Bioprinting

The primary concept behind extrusion-based bioprinting is to deposit continuous layers of bioink through nozzles using pneumatic systems. The bioinks used could be both acellular and cellular and are typically made of biocompatible materials able to mimic the native tissue microstructure. A pneumatic fluid dispensing system controlled by motors on three axes is used for printing, enabling precise deposition of bioink to fabricate three-dimensional (3D) structures. The post-printing cell viability is largely dependent on nozzle diameters, flow rate, viscosity of the bioink, pressure during deposition, and biomaterial concentration in the bioink [14]. As such, hollow structures up to a certain height can be fabricated, which is mostly governed by the rheological properties of the bioinks. High shape fidelity bioinks are ideal for printing hollow structures since they are more likely to suffer from minimal collapse when printing tall and hollow constructs [11]. However, very high viscosity can result in significant cell death during printing, lowering cell viability and cell density in the printed construct. One approach to address this issue is to use multi-printhead systems to fabricate acellular filaments to provide support for the cell-laden bioink, which can be printed as a vascular structure mimicking the lumen of the blood vessel [2]. Another approach is to fabricate core/shell structures and then removing the sacrificial core to obtain a hollow vasculature. One group has reported the fabrication of polyvinyl alcohol (PVA) filaments using extrusion printing. The PVA strands were then successively dipped in a mixture of polydimethylsiloxane (PDMS) and curing agent. Once the structure was completely coated with PDMS, the PVA core was removed by sonicating in a hydrogen peroxide solution to obtain hollow filaments.

Freeform reversible embedding of suspended hydrogel (FRESH), a modified strategy of extrusion bioprinting, involves printing 3D structures in a sacrificial support bath. The support bath is usually comprised of thermoreversible materials such as gelatin or agarose, such that after cross-linking of the printed structures, the support bath can be removed via heating [31]. It must also have a viscosity high enough to provide structural support during printing, without exerting any mechanical resistance as the nozzle moves across positions. FRESH printing is particularly suitable for fabricating complex vasculature systems. One study reported the use of a gelatin slurry bath to print a bioink composed of sodium alginate, fibrinogen, and collagen-based bioinks [32]. The key parameter to consider in this form of bioprinting is that the bioinks should be able to cross-link rapidly upon deposition without spreading. Another study reported the fabrication of heart components using an acidified collagen solution in a support bath consisting of gelatin microparticles. Recombinant VEGF and fibronectin were used to promote rapid vascularization [25]. Microvasculatures of resolution as fine as 10 μm could be fabricated using this approach.

A significant drawback in using extrusion-based bioprinting is its resolution. Thicker vessels are easier to fabricate; however, printing capillary-sized vasculatures can be challenging [24]. Additionally, the choice of biopolymers with appropriate printability is limited. Hydrogels fabricated through extrusion-based printing via subsequent layer deposition can also have structural artifacts and inconsistencies, which can result in in vivo failure of the blood vessels.

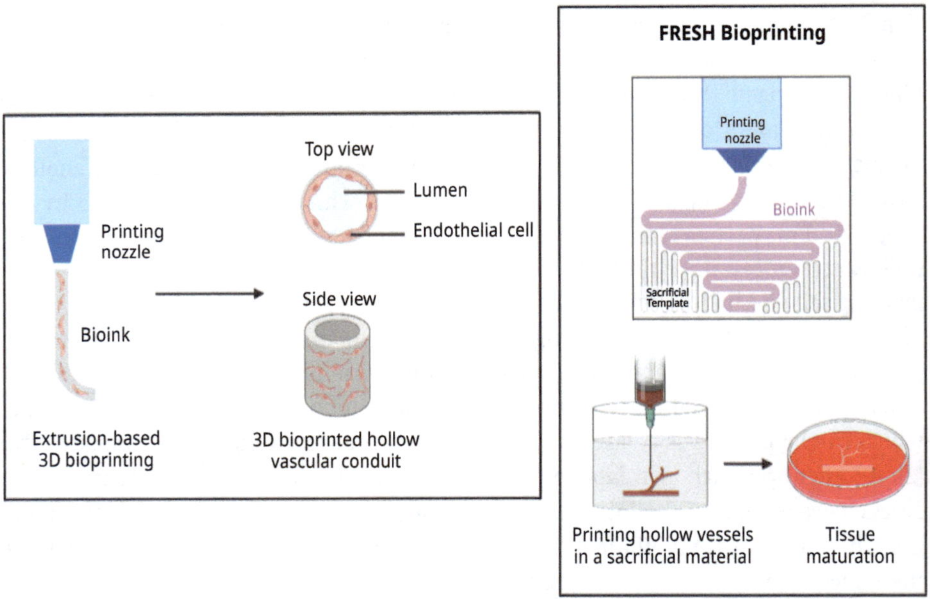

Figure 7.4: Basic illustration demonstrating extrusion-based bioprinting for fabricating hollow structures (left). Illustration demonstrating freeform reversible embedding of suspended hydrogel (FRESH) bioprinting to fabricate complex hollow vessel-like architecture (right).

7.11 Digital Light Processing (DLP) or Stereolithography

Digital light processing (DLP) is a process that uses a photocurable resin for fabricating 3D constructs. A reservoir is used to hold the resin, below which there is a light source that irradiates the resin with ultraviolet or visible light. The resin is cured layer by layer to generate a 3D structure by photopolymerization of the resin. DLP-based printing can fabricate structures with high resolution at the scale of micrometers but has been limited to printing acellular structures [7].

The choice of biomaterial is crucial for fabricating vasculatures using DLP methods. The material should be photosensitive and capable of polymerizing upon exposure to light. They should also be biocompatible, possess suitable mechanical properties after cross-linking, and be able to integrate correctly with native tissue. Materials such as gelatin methacrylate (GelMA) are particularly ideal due to their biomimetic nature and ability to be cross-linked upon exposure to light in the presence of photoinitators. Other synthetic biomaterials, such as urethane acrylate (UA), have also been explored. One research group has reported the use of UA in combination with 2-hydroxyethyl acrylate for fabricating biomimetic scaffolds, which are similar to native vasculatures, using a DLP-based approach. DLP can also be used to fabricate capillary-like channels through patterning. One group has reported that patterned substrates can be seeded with endothelial cells to form capillary-mimicking networks.

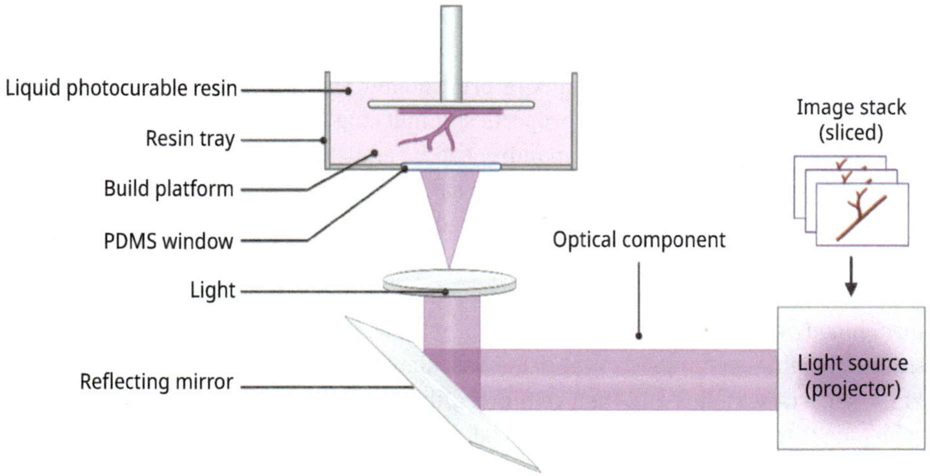

Figure 7.5: Schematic illustration of a basic digital light processing (DLP) setup for bioprinting blood vessels.

7.12 Syringe Molding

The basic principle in syringe molding-based approaches for fabricating blood vessels is the use of a coaxial nozzle to create hollow vascularized structures. The outer nozzle holds a biopolymer, such as sodium alginate, and a cross-linker solution, such as calcium chloride, is passed through the inner nozzle. Upon injection, the two solutions interact, allowing cross-linking of the outer polymer shell, leaving behind a hollow core [7]. However, this requires optimization of appropriate polymer and cross-linker concentrations so that the fabricated hollow structures are mechanically stable.

7.13 Hybrid Strategies (Perfusion, Two-Photon, LIFT, Self-Assembly)

Hybrid strategies to bioprint vascular structures usually combine multiple strategies and materials to fabricate functional tissue grafts. One group reported the technique of "organ weaving" by using coaxial-nozzle-assisted extrusion bioprinting to fabricate multilevel fluid channels using alginate bioink printed along a rotating rod, which served as the template. Partial hollow alginate filaments fused to form a central macro-channel. The first layer was incorporated with smooth muscle cells, while the next layer contained fibroblasts [11]. After the rod was removed, the inner layer was seeded with endothelial cells to form multilevel multicell constructs that hold applications in organ-on-a-chip models to replicate the microenvironment of blood vessels better. A similar strategy was used in another study where carbon nanotubes were blended with gelatin-alginate bioink to print hollow structures mimicking blood vessels with enhanced mechanical properties, mimicking those of a native blood vessel [33]. The diameter of the central mandrel can be adjusted to fabricate vessels of varying diameters, but the restriction in length can pose some limitations [7].

In a separate study, one group developed scaffold-free, perfusable vascular grafts using multicellular spheroids. Agarose rods were printed as a mold to support the subsequent deposition of spheroid layers, which fused upon subsequent culturing to form blood vessel conduits. Another group combined electrospinning and fused deposition modeling techniques to fabricate vasculatures. The group electrospun tubular PLLA/heparin scaffolds and then reinforced the scaffold with a single coil of polycaprolactone through fused deposition modeling. The inner PLLA/heparin layer provided a microenvironment suitable for endothelialization. A hybrid approach combining two-photon polymerization (2PP) and laser-induced forward transfer (LIFT) also demonstrated potential to fabricate functional blood vessels. Acrylated PEG was cross-linked through 2PP to form hexagonal porous PEGDA rings, and LIFT was used to guide the seeding of smooth muscle cells and endothelial cells [34, 35].

7.14 Conclusion and Future Perspectives

Significant strides have been made in the field of bioprinting to manufacture clinically relevant tissue constructs. Bioprinted blood vessels can play a key role in tissue engineering, as well as organ-on-chip models, by generating patient-specific grafts to understand disease progression better, identify appropriate treatment strategies, and provide a functional alternative to autologous grafts. However, in terms of blood vessels, current research is limited. Significant restrictions based on dimensions, mechanical similarity to native tissues, dynamic culture conditions, resolution, and scalability limit the use of the currently reported bioprinted blood vessels in clinical contexts [11]. One of the significant barriers is designing suitable bioinks that can effectively mimic native vessel properties and provide an appropriate microenvironment for cells to attach, proliferate, and differentiate to form functional blood vessels. Another challenge lies in the maturation of these bioprinted constructs. Current strategy dictates culturing printed constructs in static conditions till maturation before implantation. However, appropriate dynamic culture conditions to provide biomechanical cues are crucial in cell differentiation, rapid tissue maturation, and tissue functionalization. Engineered blood vessels must also allow vascular anastomosis for successful transplantation. To date, autologous grafts remain the gold standard. Vascularization will likely remain one of the predominant challenges in tissue engineering, necessitating extensive research in bioink formulation, printing modification, and bioreactor design. Regardless, as technology evolves, emerging strategies can significantly impact the aspects of fabrication in a positive direction.

References

[1] Rouwkema, J., Koopman, B. F. J. M., Blitterswijk, C. A. V., Dhert, W. J. A., & Malda, J. (2009). Supply of nutrients to cells in engineered tissues. Biotechnology and Genetic Engineering Reviews, 26, 163–178. https://doi.org/10.5661/bger-26-163.

[2] Liu, Y., Huang, T., Yap, N. A., Lim, K., & Ju, L. A. (2024). Harnessing the power of bioprinting for the development of next-generation models of thrombosis. Bioactive Materials, 42, 328–344. https://doi.org/10.1016/j.bioactmat.2024.08.040.

[3] Ng, H. Y., Lee, K.-X. A., Kuo, C.-N., & Shen, Y.-F. (2024). Bioprinting of artificial blood vessels. IJB, 4, 140. https://doi.org/10.18063/ijb.v4i2.140.

[4] Kolesky, D. B., Truby, R. L., Gladman, A. S., Busbee, T. A., Homan, K. A., & Lewis, J. A. (2014). 3D bioprinting of vascularized, heterogeneous cell-laden tissue constructs. Advanced Materials, 26, 3124–3130. https://doi.org/10.1002/adma.201305506.

[5] Zhu, J., Wang, Y., Zhong, L., Pan, F., & Wang, J. (2021). Advances in tissue engineering of vasculature through three-dimensional bioprinting. Developmental Dynamics, 250, 1717–1738. https://doi.org/10.1002/dvdy.385.

[6] Wang, L., Shen, M., Tang, Z., Tan, J., Li, K., & Ma, H. (2025). 3D printed magnesium silicate/β-tricalcium phosphate scaffolds promote coupled osteogenesis and angiogenesis. Frontiers in Bioengineering and Biotechnology, 12, 1518145. https://doi.org/10.3389/fbioe.2024.1518145.

[7] Melchiorri, A. J., & Fisher, J. P. Bioprinting of blood vessels. In: Essentials of 3D Biofabrication and Translation. 2015 (pp. 337–350). Elsevier. https://doi.org/10.1016/B978-0-12-800972-7.00020-7.

[8] Hou, Y.-C., Cui, X., Qin, Z., Su, C., Zhang, G., Tang, J.-N., Li, J.-A., & Zhang, J.-Y. (2023). Three-dimensional bioprinting of artificial blood vessel: process, bioinks, and challenges. IJB, 9, 740. https://doi.org/10.18063/ijb.740.

[9] Khalighi, S., & Saadatmand, M. (2021). Bioprinting a thick and cell-laden partially oxidized alginate-gelatin scaffold with embedded micro-channels as future soft tissue platform. International Journal of Biological Macromolecules, 193, 2153–2164. https://doi.org/10.1016/j.ijbiomac.2021.11.046.

[10] Ravi, S., & Chaikof, E. L. (2010). Biomaterials for vascular tissue engineering. Regenerative Medicine, 5, 107–120. https://doi.org/10.2217/rme.09.77.

[11] Solis, D. M., & Czekanski, A. (2022). 3D and 4D additive manufacturing techniques for vascular-like structures – a review. Bioprinting, 25, e00182. https://doi.org/10.1016/j.bprint.2021.e00182.

[12] Zhang, J., Guo, J., Zhang, J., Li, D., Zhong, M., Gu, Y., Yan, X., & Huang, P. (2025). Heparin and gelatin co-functionalized polyurethane artificial blood vessel for improving anticoagulation and biocompatibility. Bioengineering, 12, 304. https://doi.org/10.3390/bioengineering12030304.

[13] Zhu, W., Qu, X., Zhu, J., Ma, X., Patel, S., Liu, J., Wang, P., Lai, C. S. E., Gou, M., Xu, Y., Zhang, K., & Chen, S. (2017). Direct 3D bioprinting of prevascularized tissue constructs with complex microarchitecture. Biomaterials, 124, 106–115. https://doi.org/10.1016/j.biomaterials.2017.01.042.

[14] Kong, Z., & Wang, X. (2023). Bioprinting technologies and bioinks for vascular model establishment. IJMS, 24, 891. https://doi.org/10.3390/ijms24010891.

[15] Bosch-Rué, È., Díez-Tercero, L., Delgado, L. M., & Pérez, R. A. (2022). Biofabrication of collagen tissue-engineered blood vessels with direct co-axial extrusion. IJMS, 23, 5618. https://doi.org/10.3390/ijms23105618.

[16] Kobayashi, M., Kadota, J., Hashimoto, Y., Fujisato, T., Nakamura, N., Kimura, T., & Kishida, A. (2020). Elastic modulus of ECM hydrogels derived from decellularized tissue affects capillary network formation in endothelial cells. IJMS, 21, 6304. https://doi.org/10.3390/ijms21176304.

[17] Yan, Y., Wang, X., Pan, Y., Liu, H., Cheng, J., Xiong, Z., Lin, F., Wu, R., Zhang, R., & Lu, Q. (2005). Fabrication of viable tissue-engineered constructs with 3D cell-assembly technique. Biomaterials, 26, 5864–5871. https://doi.org/10.1016/j.biomaterials.2005.02.027.

[18] Dermanaki Farahani, R., & Dubé, M. (2018). Printing polymer nanocomposites and composites in three dimensions. Advanced Engineering Materials, 20, 1700539. https://doi.org/10.1002/adem.201700539.

[19] Zheng, F., Derby, B., & Wong, J. (2021). Fabrication of microvascular constructs using high resolution electrohydrodynamic inkjet printing. Biofabrication, 13, 035006. https://doi.org/10.1088/1758-5090/abd158.

[20] Figueiredo, L., Le Visage, C., Weiss, P., & Yang, J. (2020). Quantifying oxygen levels in 3D bioprinted cell-laden thick constructs with perfusable microchannel networks. Polymers, 12, 1260. https://doi.org/10.3390/polym12061260.

[21] Gao, G., Lee, J. H., Jang, J., Lee, D. H., Kong, J.-S., Kim, B. S., Choi, Y.-J., Jang, W. B., Hong, Y. J., Kwon, S.-M., & Cho, D.-W. (2017). Tissue engineered bio-blood-vessels constructed using a tissue-specific bioink and 3D coaxial cell printing technique: a novel therapy for ischemic disease. Advanced Functional Materials, 27, 1700798. https://doi.org/10.1002/adfm.201700798.

[22] Rouwkema, J., & Khademhosseini, A. (2016). Vascularization and angiogenesis in tissue engineering: beyond creating static networks. Trends in Biotechnology, 34, 733–745. https://doi.org/10.1016/j.tibtech.2016.03.002.

[23] Laowpanitchakorn, P., Zeng, J., Piantino, M., Uchida, K., Katsuyama, M., & Matsusaki, M. (2024). Biofabrication of engineered blood vessels for biomedical applications. Science and Technology of Advanced Materials, 25, 2330339. https://doi.org/10.1080/14686996.2024.2330339.

[24] Fleischer, S., Tavakol, D. N., & Vunjak-Novakovic, G. (2020). From arteries to capillaries: approaches to engineering human vasculature. Advanced Functional Materials, 30, 1910811. https://doi.org/10.1002/adfm.201910811.

[25] Chiu, L. L. Y., & Radisic, M. (2010). Scaffolds with covalently immobilized VEGF and qngiopoietin-1 for vascularization of engineered tissues. Biomaterials, 31, 226–241. https://doi.org/10.1016/j.biomaterials.2009.09.039.

[26] Lee, S. J., Kim, M. E., Nah, H., Seok, J. M., Jeong, M. H., Park, K., Kwon, I. K., Lee, J. S., & Park, S. A. (2019). Vascular endothelial growth factor immobilized on mussel-inspired three-dimensional bilayered scaffold for artificial vascular graft application: in vitro and in vivo evaluations. Journal of Colloid and Interface Science, 537, 333–344. https://doi.org/10.1016/j.jcis.2018.11.039.

[27] Cidonio, G., Alcala-Orozco, C. R., Lim, K. S., Glinka, M., Mutreja, I., Kim, Y.-H., Dawson, J. I., Woodfield, T. B. F., & Oreffo, R. O. C. (2019). Osteogenic and angiogenic tissue formation in high fidelity nanocomposite laponite-gelatin bioinks. Biofabrication, 11, 035027. https://doi.org/10.1088/1758-5090/ab19fd.

[28] Su, H., Li, Q., Li, D., Li, H., Feng, Q., Cao, X., & Dong, H. (2022). A versatile strategy to construct free-standing multi-furcated vessels and a complicated vascular network in heterogeneous porous scaffolds *via* combination of 3D printing and stimuli-responsive hydrogels. Materials Horizons, 9, 2393–2407. https://doi.org/10.1039/D2MH00314G.

[29] Henrich, J. (2004). Inequity aversion in capuchins? Nature, 428, 139–139. https://doi.org/10.1038/428139a.

[30] Chang, J., & Sun, X. (2023). Laser-induced forward transfer based laser bioprinting in biomedical applications. Frontiers in Bioengineering and Biotechnology, 11, 1255782. https://doi.org/10.3389/fbioe.2023.1255782.

[31] Andreazza, R., Morales, A., Pieniz, S., & Labidi, J. (1026). Gelatin-based hydrogels: potential biomaterials for remediation. Polymers, 15, 2023, https://doi.org/10.3390/polym15041026.

[32] Pan, T., Song, W., Cao, X., & Wang, Y. (2016). 3D bioplotting of gelatin/alginate scaffolds for tissue engineering: influence of crosslinking degree and pore architecture on physicochemical properties. Journal of Materials Science & Technology, 32, 889–900. https://doi.org/10.1016/j.jmst.2016.01.007.

[33] Dranseikiene, D., Schrüfer, S., Schubert, D. W., Reakasame, S., & Boccaccini, A. R. (2020). Cell-laden alginate dialdehyde–gelatin hydrogels formed in 3D printed sacrificial gel. Journal of Materials Science: Materials in Medicine, 31, 31. https://doi.org/10.1007/s10856-020-06369-7.

[34] Xue, D., Wang, Y., Zhang, J., Mei, D., Wang, Y., & Chen, S. (2018). Projection-based 3D printing of cell patterning scaffolds with multiscale channels. ACS Applied Materials & Interfaces, 10, 19428–19435. https://doi.org/10.1021/acsami.8b03867.

[35] Zhang, J., Wehrle, E., Adamek, P., Paul, G. R., Qin, X.-H., Rubert, M., & Müller, R. (2020). Optimization of mechanical stiffness and cell density of 3D bioprinted cell-laden scaffolds improves extracellular matrix mineralization and cellular organization for bone tissue engineering. Acta Biomaterialia, 114, 307–322. https://doi.org/10.1016/j.actbio.2020.07.016.

Menaga S., Abira R., Pratima Parulekar, and Sushma Kumari*

Chapter 8
Bioprinting of Skin

Abstract: Skin, being the primary barrier of our body, has multiple functions, including protecting against the entry of pathogens, guarding the internal organs, maintaining body temperature, and excreting waste through sweat glands. Being the foremost barrier, the skin is the first site prone to external injuries. Repairing damaged tissues is always a challenging research gap in the biomedical field. Many skin substitutes are available for skin tissue repair. However, there is still a need to develop a skin substitute for full-thickness wounds, diabetic wounds, and burns that supports the complex skin architecture and facilitates faster healing of these wounds. To overcome this gap, three-dimensional (3D) bioprinting of skin has been evolving rapidly due to its superior performance in bioclinical applications, which will enable faster rejuvenation of damaged tissues with structural support. 3D bioprinting is a patient-specific type of rapid prototyping technique that utilizes varied biopolymers as supporting materials, along with cells such as fibroblasts, keratinocytes, endothelial cells, immune cells, and stem cells to repair damaged tissue by mimicking the native extracellular matrix (ECM) of the skin.

Keywords: 3D bioprinting, skin substitute, wound healing, extracellular matrix, keratinocytes, fibroblasts, bioink, regenerative medicine

8.1 Introduction

Skin, being the primary physical barrier, acts as a response system and constitutes the first safeguard against external harsh environments. The skin is a secretory organ com-

---

Acknowledgment: S.K. would like to acknowledge the financial support from the Department of Science and Technology, New Delhi, for the INSPIRE Faculty Fellowship (Faculty Registration No. IFA21-MS 179).

***Corresponding author: Sushma Kumari**, Centre for Biomaterials, Cellular and Molecular Theranostics (CBCMT), Vellore Institute of Technology (VIT), Vellore, Tamil Nadu, India, e-mail: sushma.kumari@vit.ac.in
Menaga S, Centre for Biomaterials, Cellular and Molecular Theranostics (CBCMT), Vellore Institute of Technology (VIT), Vellore, Tamil Nadu, India; School of Biosciences and Technology (SBST), Vellore Institute of Technology (VIT), Vellore, Tamil Nadu, India
Abira R, School of Biosciences and Technology (SBST), Vellore Institute of Technology (VIT), Vellore, Tamil Nadu, India
Pratima Parulekar, Centre for Biomaterials, Cellular and Molecular Theranostics (CBCMT), Vellore Institute of Technology (VIT), Vellore, Tamil Nadu, India

 | https://doi.org/10.1515/9783111719993-008

posed of an intricate network of interconnecting structures that function to regulate body temperature, sensitivity, energy storage, water storage, absorption, regeneration, expression, and protection against various external environments, accounting for approximately 16% of a person's body weight [1]. They are composed of three layers, including the hypodermis (the bottom layer), dermis (the middle layer), and epidermis (the upper layer), and each layer plays a distinct function in skin regeneration [2].

Anatomy of the skin is structured as the epidermis (outermost layer), which comprises keratinocytes, Langerhans cells, melanocytes, and Merkel cells. They do not constitute blood vessels but serve to protect against the extrinsic environment, supporting proliferation cycles, pigment production, integrity, and replenishment. This layer constitutes approximately 90% of the keratinocytes generated from stem cells. It differentiates over 3–6 weeks, converting into corneocytes and forming the outermost epidermal layer, known as the stratum corneum, followed by the stratum granulosum, stratum spinosum, stratum lucidum, and stratum basale. The stratum corneum plays a pivotal function in protecting skin against microbial invasion and dehydration. There is an anchoring junction intermediate to the epidermis and dermis called the dermo-epidermal junction, which constitutes the extracellular matrix (ECM), basal lamina, filaments, and anchoring fibrils that keep the epidermis and dermis layers intact in the skin regeneration process [3]. Following the epidermis layer is the dermis layer (middle layer), which functions as a home for glands, hair follicles, blood vessels, immune cells, nerves, and other structures. The dermis layer accounts for 90% of the skin's mass and contains an abundant ECM, as well as endothelial cells, Schwann cells, and various connective tissues. This layer further encompasses papillary dermis and reticular dermis, populated with collagen, fibroblast and other neural and vascular tissues for keeping the layer intact by elasticity, keeping the body temperature in control, sensation, waste removal, repairing, remodeling, defending against invading pathogens, and giving mechanical support to the skin [4]. The hypodermis (bottom layer), the deepest layer of skin, consists of connective tissues and fat. It functions as a protective layer, serves as a guard for internal organs, and acts as a storage area, protecting against violent trauma. The cells present in this layer, such as macrophages, facilitate phagocytosis, which helps wounds heal faster and exhibits an adaptive immune response. These layers collectively serve as a protective function, ranging from simple to complex structures, and have been a protective layer for both internal and external environments [5, 6].

8.2 Types of Wounds and Their Function in Wound Healing

The outermost layer of the human body, the skin, is the first area to be affected by an external harsh environment and trauma. Typically, the skin is affected by accidents such as cuts, burns, pressure, surgery, or medical traumas, including diabetes. We classify wounds as acute and chronic wounds based on the duration and sequence of events in the healing process [7]. Acute wounds are caused by radiation, external temperature changes, punctures, abrasions, lacerations, and incisions, which typically heal within two months by restoring their original function and anatomical integrity. In contrast, chronic wounds stall and take longer (more than 6 months) to recover. Chronic wounds are pressure ulcers, diabetic ulcers, autoimmune diseases, and some surgical wounds. Physiological conditions such as low levels of mitogenic activity, growth factors, a lack of angiogenesis, and higher secretion of matrix metalloproteinases (MMPs), reactive oxygen species (ROS), cytokines, and proteases hinder the healing process in chronic wound healing [8]. As the skin has a high regenerative capacity, it typically heals on its own for most people. Typically, for people without medical complications, there should be no hindrance to the healing process, and the wound usually heals on its own within two months. However, individuals with diabetes, low immune response, obesity, or other medical complications may experience delayed wound healing and persistent bacterial infections, which can take more than eight months to resolve [9].

Wound healing undergoes a four-stage process (Figure 8.1), including hemostasis, inflammation, proliferation, and remodeling [10]. In routine wound healing, hemostasis is the first stage, which responds to the affected area by supplying platelets and fibrin to clot the blood at the site. These further promote the synthesis of inflammatory cytokines, such as those produced by macrophages, neutrophils, and fibroblasts, in the affected area, which helps remove debris and defend against bacterial invasions. Furthermore, the inflammatory cells and cytokines enter the proliferative stage, where the help of fibroblast cells remodels the affected tissues. Oxygen and nutrients are carried to the affected area through new blood vessels, facilitating faster wound healing. In the final stage, MMPs facilitate remodeling, during which collagen maturation and tissue granulation occur, and the wound is healed with a newly developed epidermis, thereby maintaining tissue integrity through hemostasis. These four stages should happen sequentially, and any disturbance delays the wound healing process or may prevent it from recovering. To overcome delayed and scar-free healing in medically complicated individuals, various techniques and products have been used to treat chronic wounds. Several strategies, including skin grafts, skin flaps, bandages, hyperbaric oxygen therapy, negative pressure therapy, ultrasound therapy, exosome-based therapies, and electromagnetic therapies, were employed to treat the wound [10, 11].

8.3 Importance of Skin Bioprinting

Many skin injuries cause irritation, pain, and discomfort to patients. Skin abrasion can damage the epidermis and dermis layers, but it is capable of natural healing to restore functionality. However, deeper wounds are unable to regenerate the full skin

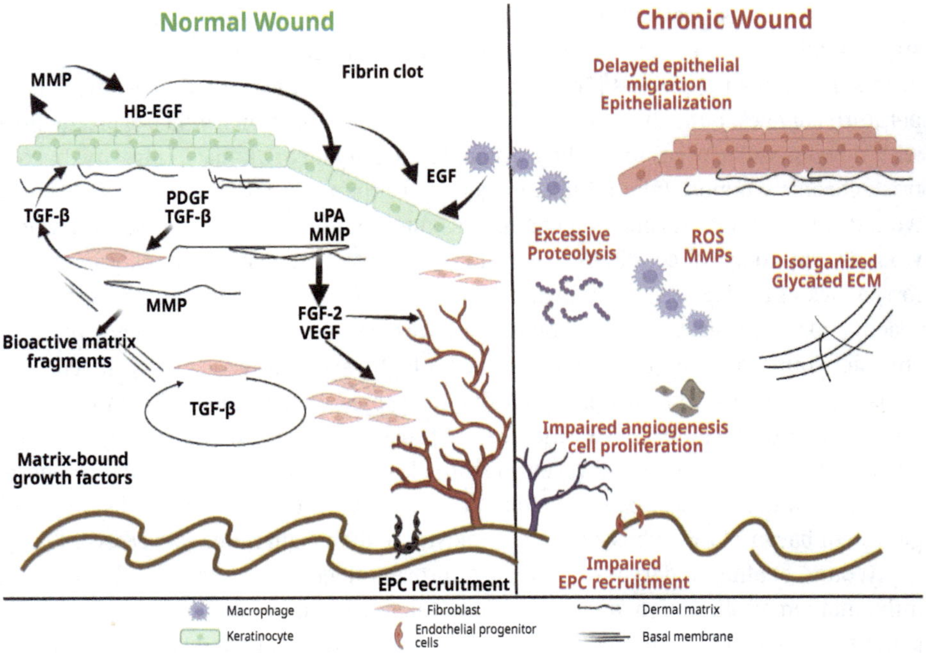

Figure 8.1: Schematic comparison between normal and chronic wound healing. Chronic wounds are characterized by delayed keratinocyte migration and re-epithelialization, excessive proteolytic activity, elevated reactive oxygen species (ROS) mediated tissue damage, impaired endothelial progenitor cell (EPC) recruitment, reduced angiogenesis, and compromised cellular proliferation during the regenerative phase [10].

due to the formation of scars [12]. Even though skin injuries do not cause significant deaths, chronic wounds like deep burns, diabetic ulcers, pressure ulcers, venous ulcers compromise a patient's quality of life and lead to psychological depression [13].

Chronic wounds affect millions of people (approximately 8.2 million) due to delayed wound healing and pose a threat both economically and socially, as well as to people's lifespan. For instance, chronic diabetic foot ulcer (DFU) has a mortality rate of around 30.5%, which is the 5-year mortality rate for cancer patients worldwide. Approximately $12 billion has been spent annually on treating this type of wound, and it is expected to increase 10-fold in another decade, which has been described as a "silent epidemic" [14, 15].

Global statistics of burn patients are in millions, among which about 10% patients have almost their total body surface covered with burn wounds, and a high mortality rate is observed in such patients [13]. People who survive from large-scale chronic wounds are a burden on the economy (billion US dollars per year) as well as on the medical field. Surgical wounds, such as incisions, are surgical cuts into the patient's body, while removing tissue from the body causes an excision wound [16]. They require more attention for healing carefully, as it is affected by risk factors such as infection, delayed healing, and scarring.

Furthermore, skin regeneration is challenging due to a prolonged inflammatory phase, impaired cell function, and reduced growth factor levels, resulting in fibrotic scar formation [12]. Commonly, wounds are cleansed and covered with a wound dressing. Traditionally used gauze, bandages, lint, and plasters for treating wounds are not effective in fully repairing skin. Dressings such as Biobrane, Alloderm, and Integra help maintain the wound's moisture content and support its healing process. These treatment methods are associated with pain [17] and poor functional regeneration. Negative pressure wound closure therapy (NPWT) is performed by attaching a sealed, open-cell foam or gauze dressing pump to create a vacuum at the wound site. The mechanism of macro- and micro-deformation reduces wound inflammation and restores tissue through NPWT [18]. Hyperbaric oxygen tanks create optimal conditions at the wound bed, increasing oxygen supply. Despite the availability of various treatments, complicated wounds cannot be cured fully and may lead to amputation of the body part. Therefore, there is a need for efficient therapies that can completely regenerate the affected skin.

Grafting can be the best choice for treating large-scale, full-thickness wounds. Autologous grafts, where skin tissue is extracted from the patient, are counted as the gold standard for the complete regeneration of skin tissue. Allogenic grafts refer to skin tissue from another human donor that can be used to replace the wound site. The availability of donors and the hazard of secondary wounds at the donor site are the biggest challenges in using these treatments [19]. The grafts from allogenic as well as xenogeneic sources have a limitation of immune rejection within the patient's body, delayed healing, being unfriendly to the skin, requiring surgical interventions, and being unaffordable. Therefore, the requirement for abundantly available and reliable skin regeneration treatments necessitates the attention of researchers.

In addition to disease conditions, there is a huge demand for artificial models for skin in the pharmaceutical and cosmetic industries to replace animal testing. Furthermore, skin care products, cosmetics, topical agents, and Light-emitting diode light for acne therapy are continuously monitored and tested on animals before commercialization [20]. The efficacy of drugs or cosmetic ingredients, as well as their adverse effects, such as irritation or corrosion, and effectiveness over time have traditionally been studied using animal models. Therefore, in vitro skin models serve as substitutes for preclinical studies on animals. Notably, an artificial implant that mimics natural skin structure can address the limitations of currently available treatments by providing a controlled microenvironment, which can contribute to effective healing without the risk of immune rejection.

Considering the scarcity of unmet therapeutics for chronic wound healing applications and the lack of in vitro models for testing drugs and cosmetics, new methods, techniques, and alternative approaches are emerging in the research community [21].

8.3.1 Conventional and Innovative Approaches for Wound Healing

Conventional approach: In this approach, wound management is achieved through surgeries, the use of bandages, skin grafts, skin flaps, and wound dressing materials combined with pharmacological agents and non-surgical procedures. Debridement helps in the healing process by accelerating the ECM remodeling. Patient-derived full-thickness skin autograft was used in significant tissue loss, which helps in healing deeper wounds, allograft (skin from a different person) can be stored and used for burn wounds, along with non-surgical therapies like utilizing bandages, gauzes, hydrogel scaffolds, foams, lotions, creams, sprays, and nanoparticles to balance the moisture and protection against bacterial invasions with re-epithelialization. However, all these conventional methods have significant disadvantages, including graft rejection, bacterial infections, restricted donor availability, limited contractions during healing, pain, itchiness, lack of specificity to individual patients, low exudate removal, frequent dressing changes, risk of disease transmission, and scarring [22].

Innovative strategy: To overcome the conventional method flaws, in recent decades, many innovative approaches have been developed for wound healing like smart dressings, growth factor-based therapies, bioengineered skin substitutes, 3D-printed scaffolds, 3D-bioprinted skins, platelet-rich plasma (PRP) therapy and ECM- based therapies due to their advantage of personalized medicine, effectiveness, benefit to the risk and heals the wound faster compared to conventional methods. New techniques and products are being developed to address the current research gap in chronic wound healing, such as stem cell-based therapies, polymer-based films, 3D printing, 3D bioprinting, and engineered soft tissue products, which are gaining center stage in the research community.

3D printing is a technique first developed by Charles W. Hull in the 1980s, called initially stereolithography. Investigators have utilized the three-dimensional printing technique in various fields, including pharmaceuticals, cosmetics, food technology, aerospace engineering, biomedical fields (such as implants), and architectural and automotive design. 3D printing has been extensively explored in the biomedical field, as it can mimic the natural environment and involves complex structures made with biocompatible polymers tailored to specific patients. In the biomedical field, 3D printing involves three distinct processes: pre-printing, printing, and post-printing. This process follows the selection of biomaterials, inks, and optimization of pressure, speed, and infill density during printing, followed by cell maturation [12,23]. This innovative additive manufacturing technique empowers the fabrication of tissue-mimicking scaffolds, and the products can be developed as "patient-specific." Some of the advantages of 3D printing include patient-specificity, fast fabrication, precise incorporation of multiple cells during 3D printing, and fabrication of porous scaffolds to stimulate angiogenesis and vascularization. Furthermore, 3D-printed scaffolds mimic the native mechanical properties of skin by utilizing skin-friendly biomaterials [3].

8.4 3D Bioprinting in Skin Tissue Engineering: Bridging the Gap in Chronic Wound Healing

Additive manufacturing facilitates the fabrication of scaffolds using layer-by-layer printing technology. 3D bioprinting modifies this technology to make functional implants using cells or biological material while printing. The advantage of incorporating cells along with scaffold material during printing is the controlled, uniform distribution throughout the tissue. Key features, including high manufacturing throughput, high reproducibility, and short production times, make 3D bioprinting a promising method for fabricating artificial skin compared to traditional manufacturing techniques [24]. Commercially available skin reconstructs are helping to reduce pain and improve treatment at the injury site. Furthermore, extensive research on 3D-bioprinted skin holds promise for fabricating reliable grafts for skin tissue engineering.

Various types of 3D printers are available, depending on the raw material utilized and their intended application. It follows a sequential layering deposition technique to fabricate 3D scaffolds. The major types of 3D printers for skin substitutes are extrusion, inkjet, laser-assisted, and digital light processing (DLP)-based 3D bioprinting. Extrusion-based printing is a type of printing where the desired biomaterial ink is prepared, and with pneumatic pressure, the nozzle continuously exudes the ink on the substrate layer by layer to form 3D structures. In inkjet-based printing, the material is exuded in a droplet fashion using thermal or piezoelectric actuation. In laser-assisted bioprinting, a laser pulse generates a microbubble intermediate between the absorber layer and the donor film to deposit bioink droplets containing cells onto the receiving substrate. In DLP-based 3D printing, ultraviolet (UV) and visible light triggers the ink to cross-link, allowing for the printing of 3D structures with precise and higher resolution [25–27]. Extrusion-based 3D printers are typically used for fabricating tissue engineering and regenerative medicine-based skin substitutes, as they can print complex structures in a shorter time with high printing speeds and allow the printing of a wide range of materials. This technique will help bridge the gap in the wound care system by fabricating a realistic, tissue-mimicking complex structure and a drug-testing 3D-printed animal model. When the cells are incorporated into the fabricated ink and printed, the process is referred to as 3D bioprinting. Bioinks are essentially a combination of biomaterials, desired cells, growth factors, and bioactive compounds [28, 29].

Skin bioprinting is a 3D bioprinting technique developed to reconstruct natural, tissue-mimicking tissue with an artificially developed printer. In the conventional method, scaffolds are produced, and then cells are seeded and allowed to mature. In contrast, the newly developed 3D bioprinting technology involves depositing cells along with the ink, which facilitates precise cell positioning. Furthermore, skin bioprinting employs two distinct approaches: in situ bioprinting and in vitro bioprinting (Figure 8.2).

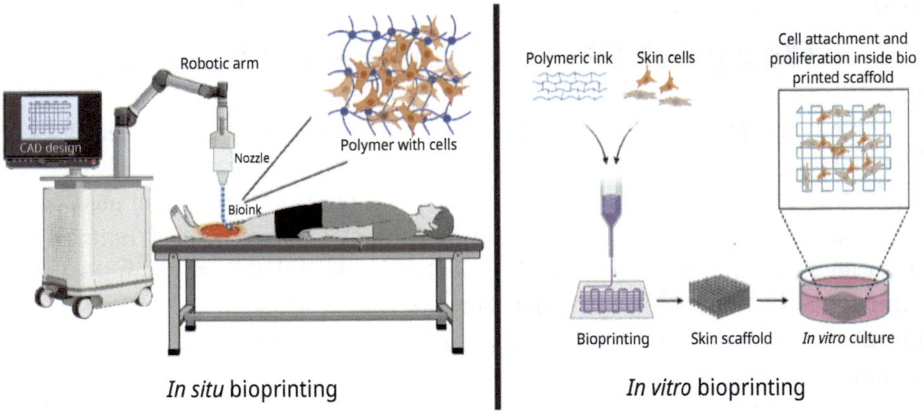

Figure 8.2: Schematic representation of bioprinting strategies, where in situ bioprinting involves direct deposition of cell-laden bioinks at the defect site for on-site tissue regeneration, while in vitro bioprinting entails fabrication of tissue constructs under controlled laboratory conditions, followed by maturation and subsequent implantation into the target site.

In situ bioprinting enables the fabrication of 3D scaffolds using ink containing cells, which are directly printed onto the affected area and allowed to mature. This type of bioprinting can be applied to burn wounds, offering a wide range of advantages, including ease of handling, time saving, hassle-free procedures, and eliminating the need for transportation of fabricated scaffolds. Additionally, it eliminates the need for packaging materials, preventing contamination and preserving the integrity of the biomaterial. In contrast, in vitro bioprinting involves embedding cells into the fabricated ink, allowing them to differentiate, mature, and then transport them to the affected area [30–32]. In this bioprinting, various types of biocompatible ink were prepared using natural biopolymers, such as collagen, alginate, gelatin, carrageenan, xanthan gum, guar gum, chitosan, and fibrin, to mimic and enhance the healing properties, as some of their chemical structures resemble those of natural glycosaminoglycans [33–35]. Along with the biopolymers, cells are also incorporated to promote and aid in wound healing. The outer layer (epidermis) comprises a diverse range of cells, including keratinocytes, melanocytes, Merkel cells, antigen-presenting cells, Langerhans cells, and intercellular fluids. In this layer, 90% of the overall population of cells comprise keratinocyte cells, which provide a primary healing and improve the transport of water. While melanocytes are pigmentation cells, Langerhans cells support both innate and acquired immunity. In skin bioprinting, the incorporation of cells plays a crucial role in the regeneration and healing process. In some studies, keratinocytes and fibroblasts incorporated into the ink facilitate complete re-epithelialization in deeper wounds within an 8-week timeframe, as these cells can enhance the healing properties in both the dermis and epidermis layers [36]. In another study, 3D bioprinting was used to target the wound area, utilizing stem cells derived from amniotic fluid, fibrin, and collagen with a thrombin solution. This approach effectively healed full-thickness wounds through re-epithelialization, facilitated by the impact of cytokines and growth factors present in the stem cells [37,38]. A combination of fibroblasts and keratinocyte cells has been widely used in skin substitute bioprinting, as they contain essential components such as platelet-derived growth factors, transforming growth factors, and cytokines that promote cellular differentiation and accelerate wound healing by mimicking the natural ECM. Recent studies have reported that 3D-bioprinted skin substitutes, which resemble the native structure and incorporate human plasma, fibroblasts, and keratinocytes, successfully regenerate not only the glands present in the skin layer but also melanocytes and keratinocytes in the burn wound area [39]. The most crucial cell line to be incorporated into skin bioprinting is melanocytes, which mimic natural pigmentation and protect against light. Research studies on 3D bioprinting with these cells have shown improved pigmentation [40]. Regenerating the vascular and lymphatic networks is a very risky process, and research is still ongoing; however, these are the main characteristics that need to be developed to transport oxygen, nutrients, and remove debris from the infected site [41–45].

8.5 Steps in 3D Bioprinting, Workflow, and Therapeutic Advantages of 3D-Bioprinted Skin Substitutes

In skin bioprinting, three main processes are followed: pre-printing, bioprinting, and skin maturation. In the pre-printing stage, the proper bioink, comprising biocompatible materials and cells, must be selected. Cells from primary, secondary, or stem cells must be isolated, expanded, and differentiated before being used as bioink. The biomaterials need to be sterilized to ensure they remain sterile for 3D bioprinting. The desired structure to be printed should be designed using computer-aided design (CAD) and computer-aided manufacturing (CAM) software, which utilizes graphics from clinical images, such as magnetic resonance imaging or computed tomography scans. The CAD-CAM file needs to be converted to a stereolithography (STL) file format to enable accurate 3D bioprinting. In the following process, the STL slicing and thickness determine the resolution of the 3D printing structure, which is dependent on the 3D printer. The designed structure of the STL file is inserted into the 3D printer, where the printer reads the file, and the printing process begins with the layer-by-layer deposition of the bioink on the substrate to create 3D models. The final stage of 3D skin printing is the maturation stage. The cells incorporated into the 3D model will be maintained within the bioreactor for maturation, proliferation, and differentiation before transplantation. When the 3D-bioprinted skin substitute is ready, it is transplanted to the site of injury. The 3D-bioprinted substitutes have proven to enhance the wound healing process. Some researchers have 3D-bioprinted two-layered skin substitutes of 5 mm thickness using gelatin and fibrinogen and reported that they revealed the native skin complex structure after 26 days of culture [28]. In a pioneering study, a full-thickness wound was grafted with a bioprinted scaffold containing keratinocytes, fibroblasts, and human plasma. They demonstrated that it mimicked natural human skin, exhibiting prominent epidermal and dermal layers both in vitro and in vivo [46]. In a subsequent innovative study, the transwell method was developed, combining extrusion and inkjet printing. Collagen and poly-ε-caprolactone (PCL) have been utilized, exhibiting a favorable biological process that breaks the stereotype, characterized by lower costs, high efficiency, and reduced time. Prominent layers were seen in the bioprinted scaffold. This technique has advanced significantly, offering innovation, and researchers have begun to explore it for fabricating skin substitutes and equivalents to aid in healing chronic wounds [43]. This technique nowadays has become an alternative approach for healing chronic wounds due to the following applications [11, 41, 47]:

1. An automated model that will be faster than the manual method.
2. 3D printing allows precise deposition of cells with higher reproducibility and flexibility.
3. The cells and biomaterials incorporated in 3D bioprinting will induce vascularization and angiogenesis and promote pigmentation, supporting a scar-free, faster-healing method than conventional methods.
4. Bioprinting can be patient-specific and tailored to the size of the wound in each patient, which is not possible with conventional methods.
5. The fabricated scaffold will mimic the complex native skin architecture with a homogenous cell suspension.
6. Personalized skin substitutes and therapies can be achieved through large-scale 3D bioprinting with precision and homogeneity.

8.6 Bioinks for Skin 3D Bioprinting

The material selection for bioink plays an essential role in the success of bioprinting, as well as the efficacy of the skin graft. There is a necessity to verify the biocompatibility of the materials used to prepare the bioink, as the implant should not exhibit cytotoxicity or immune rejection after grafting at the wound site.

8.6.1 Natural Bioinks for Skin Tissue Engineering

Bioink composed of decellularized ECM (dECM) exhibits characteristics similar to those of the natural skin environment, enabling cell migration, development, differentiation, and proliferation, which ultimately leads to the regeneration of skin tissue [2].

Although dECM can provide an exact cellular microenvironment, the time and resources required for the decellularization process pose a barrier to its implementation for clinical applications. Natural polymers, such as collagen, gelatin, dextran, alginate, hyaluronic acid, and chitosan, can serve as good alternatives to dECM, offering excellent biocompatibility and similar properties [24].

Collagen is the most abundant protein in the human body, as well as in the human skin ECM, which provides excellent biocompatibility and attachment sites for cell growth and proliferation. The property of forming a hydrogel through self-crosslinking at temperatures ranging from 20 to 37 °C is vital for the clinical application of skin tissue engineering [48]. Bioinks prepared from collagen, incorporating fibroblasts and keratinocytes, offer a morphology and similarity to the biology of human skin tissue. Collagens derived from animal sources are used in tissue engineering, including bovine collagen, avian collagen, rat tail collagen, ovine collagen, duck foot collagen, and porcine collagen, as well as human collagen from skin biopsies. However, low mechanical stability, high cost, and poor solubility are barriers to achieving the desired properties of a skin construct. Gelatin is a collagen derivative used for biofabrication due to its low immunogenicity, good biocompatibility, and biodegradation similar to that of collagen [2]. As pure gelatin has poor thermal stability, crosslinked gelatin will address the stability issue. Substituting the amine group from gelatin with a methacryloyl group by adding methacrylic acid to synthesize gelatin methacrylamide, which can be self-crosslinked under UV light to form a 3D structure. It has been observed that methacrylated gelatin (GelMA) shows upregulation of keratinocytes and fibroblast cells, which are helpful in skin tissue engineering [2].

A dimeric glycoprotein containing the RGD (Arg-Gly-Asp) motif, known as fibronectin, exhibits a biocompatible nature by providing attachment sites for fibroblasts. Fibrin-based dermal matrix exhibits compatibility with fibroblasts; however, an increase in concentration has adverse effects on cells due to its dense structure and modified mechanical properties. Similarly, chitosan also exhibits properties similar to those of natural ECM, with a non-toxic and hydrophilic nature. Glycosaminoglycans (GAGs) are hydrophilic polysaccharide chains that carry a negative charge. Hyaluronic acid is one of the large GAGs that upregulates cytokinin production at skin injury and promotes angiogenesis. GAGs also encourage the migration of fibroblasts, which helps in wound healing. Alginate is a natural, seaweed-derived polysaccharide widely used in bioprinting applications due to its rapid crosslinking and high biocompatibility. Hyaluronic acid is a linear polysaccharide present in connective tissues that targets cell migration and signaling in wound healing [17].

8.6.2 Synthetic Bioinks for Skin Tissue Engineering

Synthetic polymers provide strength and elasticity to enhance the mechanical properties of the skin implant [49]. Commonly used synthetic polymers include polyurethane

(PU), polylactic-co-glycolic acid (PLGA), polyglycolide (PGA), poly(vinyl alcohol) (PVA), polyethylene glycol (PEG), poly(lactic acid) (PLA), PCL, polycarbonates, polyorthoesters, and polyanhydrides. We can tailor the mechanical characteristics by altering the polymer's structure, enabling us to design degradation kinetics tailored to the specific application. Polyphosphazenes are a diverse range of synthetic polymers used in the production of tissue-engineered skin [2]. PEG easily reacts with various functional groups, like acrylates and amines [50]. Bioinks made of PEG are rich in mechanical integrity and biocompatibility. PVA has a hydrophilic nature, which enhances the graft's ability to retain water and is mechanically flexible. Tegaderm and OpSite, which are commercially available, are popular examples of PU-based dressing materials. Dermagraft, a dressing used for treating DFUs, is fabricated using a knitted PGA/PLA mesh that is provided with allogenic fibroblasts [51]. A synthetic bioprinted scaffold composed of PLGA exhibits excellent cell spread and upregulated collagen expression, confirming ECM formation similar to native tissue [52].

8.6.3 Hybrid Boinks for Skin Tissue Engineering

Natural polymers provide an ECM microenvironment but exhibit weak mechanical properties, while synthetic materials offer mechanical stiffness to the skin construct but lack biocompatibility. Therefore, composite materials play a key role in overcoming the limitations of both natural and synthetic materials by combining them. For example, researchers developed a microfabricated adipose ECM composite bioink, along with GelMA and methacrylated hyaluronic acid (GelMA-HAMA), using photocrosslinking [19]. This multilayer skin implant replicates full-thickness skin architecture, comprising one layer of Human Umbilical Vein Endothelial Cell, two layers of fibroblasts, and one layer of keratinocytes, thereby mimicking the native epidermal, dermal, and vascular functions of skin tissue.

8.6.4 Conductive Composite Bioiks for Skin Tissue Engineering

Polyaniline (PANI), polythiophene, and polypyrrole (PPy) are examples of conducting polymers that exhibit electrical conductivities in the middle range, between those of conductors and insulators, ranging from about 10^{-6} to 10^{-1} S/cm [53]. An alginate-PANI hydrogel has been applied as a supercapacitor in wearable skin biosensors [54]. PPy-based hydrogels can be used to make flexible electrodes for real-time analysis through skin grafts [55]. Conducting polymers combined with bioactive and biocompatible materials have the potential to enhance bioprinting applications for skin tissue engineering by reducing toxicity.

8.6.5 Expected Parameters of 3D Skin Substitutes

Bioprinting targets to directly deliver cells to replace lost cells at the injury site or integrate progenitor cells, which attach and form skin tissue after differentiation. Mesenchymal stem cells (MSCs) extracted from adult bone marrow have the ability to facilitate wound repair due to their potential to differentiate into keratinocytes, endothelial cells, and skin appendage cells [20]. Autologous MSCs have the capacity to heal various types of cutaneous wounds, including excisional wounds, burns, and radiation-induced wounds, due to the cytokine production, differentiation potential, and immunomodulatory effects. Thus, MSCs immobilized in a hydrogel and applied to a wound play a crucial role as an intermediary layer in split-thickness grafting.

Additionally, bioink must exhibit properties such as good biocompatibility, fidelity, and printability. The structure of the skin implant should remain intact throughout the healing process. 3D-bioprinted skin should demonstrate gradual biodegradation without toxic byproducts and should be substituted by natural tissue over time after being implanted at the wound site. Reconstructed skin should exhibit excellent porosity to mimic the microstructure of natural skin and possess excellent biocompatibility, allowing the incorporated cells to regenerate the tissue without exhibiting cytotoxicity. The skin construct should provide mechanical stability and structural rigidity, along with uniform pores and interconnected channels, for cell migration and nutrient transport. The fiber network within native human skin determines the tensile strength, which ranges from 5 to 30 MPa, and Young's Modulus ranges between 4.6 and 20 MPa [56]. Skin reconstruction should exhibit high water content and hydrophilicity to mimic the properties of natural tissue closely. By optimizing all parameters, we can achieve a high success rate in skin regeneration using 3D-bioprinted skin constructs.

8.7 Commercial 3D Skin Products

Traditionally constructed, the first dermal construct was developed by incorporating fibroblasts into a collagen hydrogel inside a cell culture insert [57]. Then, culturing keratinocytes along with this dermal construct containing fibroblasts in a submerged condition resulted in mature skin with highly stratified layers. Other research on the fabrication of skin-like tissue construct using drop-on-demand bioprinting manufactured by 20 layers of NIH3T3 mouse fibroblast and Human immortalized Keratinocyte Cell line, each in collagen hydrogel on Matridem® sheet [58]. Bioink prepared using stem cells could be a novel approach to target wound healing. So, a variety of stem cells, like bone marrow-derived MSCs (BMSCs), epidermal stem cells (ESCs), adipose-derived stem cells (ASCs), hair follicle stem cells, induced pluripotent stem cells (iPSCs), sweat gland-derived stem cells, have been utilized along with polymeric hydrogels for skin reconstruction [51].

Advanced skin models, including full-thickness skin reconstruction, hair induction, and vascularized models, are being utilized for drug screening as well as clinical implants [49]. The largest cosmetic company, L'Oreal, is a major manufacturer of tissue-engineered skin. Their product Episkin (Skinethic) and other reconstructed skin models are being used as in vitro alternatives for human skin [20]. Epi-model 24, Keraskin™, and Epiderm™ are the 3D-bioprinted skin models by companies worldwide used for skin itching testing and drug screening [49]. Major companies such as Johnson & Johnson, Procter & Gamble, L'Oréal, Unilever, GlaxoSmithKline, and Novartis, have collaborated on the advancement of alternative in vitro models for animal testing. Tissue-engineered skins, such as Dermagraf, PELNAC, Integra, OrCel, Apligraft, Transcyte, Hyalomatrix, Theraskin, and GRAFIX-Prime (viable cryopreserved placental membrane), are available for clinical treatments [51, 59]. Matriderm is used to create bilayered skin grafts with HaCaT and NIH3T3 cells, which were printed using a laser-assisted bioprinter, showing cell adhesion [58]. Commercially available autologous skin cell suspension spray, named RECELL, delivers cells through flat sheet-like scaffolds [20]. In another product, autologous cells are suspended in a spray solution and sprayed onto the wound. In this, more than 64% keratinocytes, along with a considerable number of fibroblasts and viable melanocytes, were mixed. The application of RECELL is designed to significantly reduce the requirement for skin donors for acute burn patients, by up to 40 times. Epidermal substitutes have provision for surface area to facilitate effective engraftment [60]. Epicel, Laserskin, Epidex, Bioseed-S, Myskin, and Cryoskin are grafts with epidermal cells loaded inside [51].

A wide range of clinical skin products have not passed trials due to clinical inefficiency, high manufacturing costs, and time-consuming cell expansion [20]. Most skin bioprinting studies have been conducted without considering skin pigmentation. Necessary melanin-producing units, known as melanocytes, are responsible for skin pigmentation. Non-uniform skin pigmentation is a significant challenge in skin tissue engineering, which is addressed by a two-step skin construct bioprinting technique. The pigmented skin structure was bioprinted by adding fibroblasts with collagen for the dermis layer, and further keratinocytes and melanocytes were printed along with the dermal surface after 4 days of culture [57]. Using 3D bioprinting, it is possible to achieve functional and structural characteristics specific to each layer of the epidermis, dermis, and hypodermis [51].

Sweat gland restoration has been proven using 3D-bioprinted tissue, which facilitates specific cell differentiation, and confirmed by its application to burn wounds on mice's paws [60]. Lipid vesicles and sebaceous gland markers are observed on the surface when human sebocytes are cultured in a multilayered skin construct [61]. Stem cells from hair follicles can be stimulated to induce hair growth in human skin constructs. Human hair papilla cells were bioprinted in conjunction with HUVECs and fibroblasts to achieve successful graft survival and hair growth in mice [62].

8.8 Cell-Based Commercial Skin Templates

8.8.1 Placental Membranes

Placental membranes are inherently rich in biologically active elements such as epithelial cells, neonatal fibroblasts, and MSCs, all of which contribute substantially to wound healing. Among these, MSCs are particularly valuable due to their ability to secrete bioactive factors that enhance the migration and proliferation of critical cells involved in tissue repair. They also produce growth factors, such as hepatocyte growth factor and vascular endothelial growth factor (VEGF), which are crucial for promoting angiogenesis and reducing the formation of scar tissue. Furthermore, MSCs possess the potential to develop into multiple cell lineages and release regenerative cytokines, making MSC-based therapies a compelling alternative to conventional wound treatment strategies [38]. A commercially available product that utilizes placental tissue is *Grafix*, a cryopreserved placental allograft intended for use in the treatment of both acute and chronic wounds, including DFUs, surgical wounds, burns, and rare genetic skin conditions such as epidermolysis bullosa. *Grafix* maintains the natural structural integrity of the placental membrane and provides a three-dimensional ECM containing viable epithelial cells, fibroblasts, and MSCs. The fibroblasts present in the graft actively secrete proteins and growth factors that support ECM development, promote re-epithelialization, and assist in wound contraction. Clinical research has shown that *Grafix* significantly enhances healing in chronic, non-healing wounds, establishing it as a promising solution in the field of advanced wound management [63].

8.8.2 Cultured Epithelial Sheets

Advancements in tissue engineering resulted in the development of cultured epithelial autografts (CEAs), which are used to promote wound healing and skin regeneration [22]. These grafts are typically composed of keratinocytes sourced either from the patient (autologous) or from a donor (allogeneic), making them particularly valuable for treating extensive burns and chronic skin ulcers. In cases where burns affect more than half of the body's surface area, donor skin becomes scarce, and CEAs provide a practical solution for covering and repairing large wounds. The foundation for CEA technology was established by Green and Rheinwald, who successfully isolated and cultivated human keratinocytes in a laboratory setting [64]. They further enhanced the culture process by incorporating irradiated mouse fibroblasts (3T3 cells), which supported the growth of human epidermal cells. Their pioneering work in the 1970s and 1980s laid the groundwork for the widespread medical use of CEAs in burn and reconstructive surgeries across the globe. Despite their clinical relevance, CEAs face several limitations. Challenges such as variable success in graft integration, susceptibility to infections, and less-than-ideal cosmetic and functional outcomes hinder their broader use. These issues primarily arise from the absence of a structurally and biologically functional dermal layer within the grafts [65].

8.8.3 Dermal and Epidermal Framework

The dermis, the thickest layer of human skin, measures about 1 mm in depth and possesses a mechanical strength (Young's modulus) ranging from 88 to 300 kPa. While it is less rigid than the outer epidermis, it is considerably stiffer than the underlying subcutaneous fat, which has a modulus around 34 kPa [66]. For effective dermal repair, scaffolds must be designed with mechanical characteristics and biological signals that closely mimic the native dermal tissue, ensuring compatibility in terms of elasticity and structural integrity. One example of a clinically applied dermal substitute is Dermagraft, developed by Smith and Nephew. This product consists of allogeneic human fibroblasts embedded in a biodegradable polyglactin scaffold. It is supplied as a single-use, frozen sheet and is primarily used to treat chronic, full-thickness DFUs and other deep skin wounds that do not involve deeper tissues such as muscles or bones. To produce Dermagraft, fibroblasts sourced from neonatal foreskin are cultured onto the polyglactin mesh, which gradually degrades within 20–30 days through hydrolysis. During this time, the cells multiply and secrete essential biological components, such as collagen, growth factors, and cytokines, thereby forming a living, three-dimensional dermal construct [67]. Clinical research has shown that Dermagraft is effective in promoting the healing of complex and slow-to-recover wounds. In one study focused on patients with leg ulcers, those treated with Dermagraft showed a significantly faster healing rate compared to those who received standard compression therapy alone. Despite its benefits, Dermagraft does have some limitations. It lacks essential cellular components, including immune cells, blood vessels, and skin appendages such as hair follicles. Moreover, it often requires repeated applications, carries potential risks due to the use of donor-derived cells, and involves substantial treatment costs.

The epidermis is the outermost layer of the skin, measuring about 0.1 mm in thickness and exhibiting the highest mechanical strength among the skin layers, with a Young's modulus around 1 MPa. Engineering substitutes for this layer primarily focuses on developing stratified layers of keratinocytes that can replicate its essential barrier functions, which are critical for protecting the body and ensuring survival. To achieve this, a variety of scaffold materials have been employed, all designed to provide a supportive framework for cell attachment and migration. These scaffolds also facilitate the release of signaling molecules, such as chemokines and growth factors, which are crucial for promoting the movement of epidermal cells, enhancing dermal regeneration, and encouraging the formation of new blood vessels [66]. One notable example of an engineered epidermal substitute is Apligraf, developed by Organogenesis. It is a bilayer skin equivalent composed of a bovine-derived collagen base populated with human fibroblasts, topped with a layer of human keratinocytes. This structure closely resembles natural skin and is approved by the Food and Drug Administration (FDA) for treating both partial- and full-thickness wounds. It is especially effective in managing chronic wounds, including DFU and injuries that penetrate the dermis without affecting deeper anatomical structures like muscles or bones. Apligraf enriches the wound environment by supplying vital ECM components and biological factors, including platelet-derived growth factor and various cytokines and interleukins. However, it lacks immune-related cells such as antigen-presenting cells, endothelial cells, and other immune effectors. Clinical evaluations have shown no signs of immune rejection and no adverse responses to the keratinocytes or fibroblasts in the construct, as documented. Still, the donor-derived cells within the graft typically do not persist beyond one to two months after application. In a clinical trial involving over 100 patients following excisional surgery, Apligraf showed excellent biocompatibility with no evidence of rejection. Nonetheless, the structural presence of the graft significantly diminished after the first month, highlighting its role as a temporary yet effective solution for stimulating wound healing [68].

8.8.4 Hybrid Skin Constructs: Dermal–Epidermal Integration

Composite grafts are engineered constructs that replicate both the dermal and epidermal layers of the skin, thereby closely imitating the anatomy and physiology of natural human skin. Composite grafts often combine an allogeneic dermal matrix with autologous keratinocytes, facilitating rapid epithelial regeneration while reducing the risk of immune rejection. A key advantage of these grafts is their ability to be applied in a single step, unlike some traditional dermal substitutes that require multiple applications. Alloskin, developed by AlloSource, is a composite graft derived from cadaveric tissue and is intended for temporary use in treating various acute and chronic skin injuries. Notably, cellular DNA from this graft is not detected in the wound site 14–21 days post-application, reinforcing its role as a temporary cover [69]. Another example is OrCel, created by Ortec International. This product is engineered by embedding neonatal keratinocytes (NHEKs) and fibroblasts (NHDFs) into a porous collagen sponge derived from bovine tissue, with a non-porous collagen gel layer. Fibroblasts are first seeded into the sponge to form the dermal layer, followed by the addition of keratinocytes to establish an epidermal surface. This dual-layered construct secretes essential growth factors, including VEGF, PDGF, FGF-1, KGF-1, and TGF-α, which support cell proliferation, migration, and tissue regeneration. OrCel has received FDA approval for clinical use in specific cases, such as reconstructive hand surgery in patients with epidermolysis bullosa and for treating donor sites. Clinical evaluations have confirmed the safety and therapeutic effectiveness of this treatment. In a study involving patients with severe burns, OrCel was shown to promote faster healing and reduce scarring more effectively than standard dressings, such as Biobrane-L.

These findings highlight its potential as an advanced treatment option for enhancing skin repair and improving wound outcomes [70].

8.8.5 Next-Generation Bioengineered Skin Substitutes

Next-generation bioengineered skin substitutes aim to replicate the architecture and functionality of natural skin, serving as effective alternatives to conventional skin grafts in cases of severe skin loss. An overview of next-generation skin substitutes is given in Figure 8.3. These substitutes are typically composed of synthetic or natural biomaterials and are often combined with cells or growth factors to support tissue repair and facilitate better integration. Unlike traditional grafts, they offer advantages such as ready availability and minimized damage to donor sites.

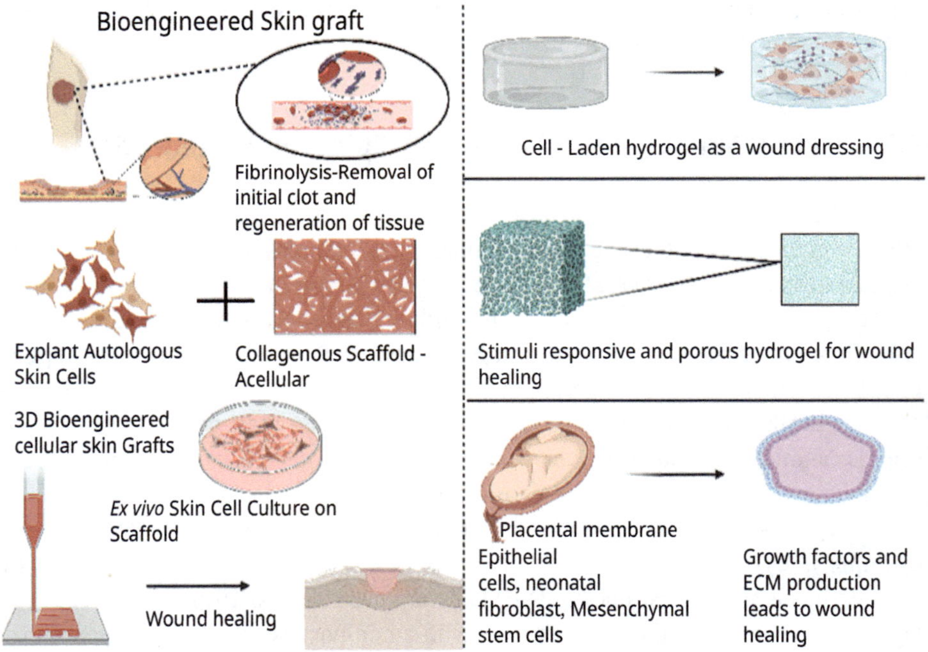

Figure 8.3: Schematic illustration of advanced skin replacement strategies, including bioengineered skin grafts, cell-laden hydrogels used as wound dressings, stimuli-responsive and porous hydrogel systems, and placental membrane-based cellular constructs for enhanced regeneration and accelerated wound healing.

8.8.5.1 Bioengineered Dermo-epidermal Skin Substitutes (Under Development)

Addressing extensive, deep skin injuries remains a significant challenge in clinical practice. Currently, standard treatments for such wounds encompass split- and full-thickness autografts, skin flaps, expansion procedures, and the use of dermal substitutes. However, these methods are often limited by the availability of healthy donor skin, especially in patients with widespread damage. As a result, tissue-engineered skin substitutes have emerged as a promising alternative for treating severe full-thickness wounds. To overcome these limitations, research groups worldwide, including the Tissue Biology Research Unit at the University of Zurich, have been developing dermo-epidermal skin substitutes that replicate both the dermal and epidermal layers of native skin. These substitutes aim to closely replicate the anatomy and physiology of human skin, which is expected to improve both the cosmetic and functional outcomes of wound healing. Significantly, incorporating a dermal layer enhances the mechanical integrity of the graft and promotes interactions between mesenchymal and epithelial cells [71]. Further efforts have been made to enhance the mechanical robustness of these constructs, thereby facilitating their surgical application. For this purpose, a plastically compressed hydrogel based on type I collagen was designed as a dermal scaffold. While uncompressed collagen matrices are delicate and prone to folding under manipulation, the compression technique enhances their stability, making them easier to handle during implantation. This dermal component has been effectively utilized to create large-format skin constructs (up to 7.5 × 7.5 cm), which have been successfully tested in preclinical animal models, including pigs.

One such product, DenovoSkin, which is derived from a patient's own cells, has progressed to clinical testing. A phase I clinical trial involving 10 pediatric patients was completed at the University Children's Hospital in Zurich. Following its success, a phase II trial was launched across multiple burn and reconstructive surgery centers in Switzerland and other European countries. Despite these advancements, a key obstacle remains: the limited vascularization of these grafts post-implantation, which compromises their long-term survival and effectiveness, particularly in chronic, non-healing wounds. To address this issue, researchers have experimented with the in vitro formation of capillary-like networks within the skin substitutes. This was achieved using endothelial and mesenchymal progenitor cells derived from the stromal vascular fraction of human adipose tissue. Adipose tissue serves as a favorable cell source due to its abundance and accessibility. This vascularization strategy not only improved the viability of the grafts but has also shown promise in other tissue engineering contexts, such as the formation of uniform bone constructs, where an enhanced vascular supply is critical for tissue integration and function [72].

8.8.5.2 Cell-Laden Hydrogels as Wound Dressings

In recent years, research interest has been directed in designing hydrogels to act as skin substitutes that can encapsulate cells and biologically active molecules. These engineered hydrogels are designed to support interactions between cells and their surrounding environment, thereby facilitating tissue repair. Hydrogels are among the most widely used scaffolds in skin regeneration due to their favorable characteristics. Their water-rich three-dimensional networks support cell growth and are biodegradable, making them ideal for tissue repair applications. Most hydrogels also exhibit excellent biocompatibility, which minimizes the risk of immune rejection or inflammation after implantation. Additionally, their mechanical features, such as elasticity, self-healing ability, and stiffness, can be adjusted by modifying polymer compositions, incorporating nanoparticles, or altering concentration ratios. Their structure closely resembles the body's natural tissue environment, promoting cellular interactions and integration with the host tissue. Commercially available cell-laden hydrogel wound dressings, such as TransCyte (produced by Advanced BioHealing, Inc.), are already in clinical use. This dressing contains human neonatal fibroblasts cultured on a nylon mesh scaffold known as Biobrane, topped with a silicone membrane to control moisture loss from the wound. TransCyte is placed directly over the wound and secured in place using adhesive strips or, in some cases, surgical staples. The general procedure for creating a cell-laden hydrogel starts with isolating cells from a patient, which are then cultured within a hydrogel matrix. This scaffold supports cell proliferation and skin tissue formation, which can be re-applied to the patient's wound. These hydrogels are often produced by mixing cells with a liquid pre-polymer solution and subsequent crosslinking using thermal, ionic, or light-based processes. Careful control of temperature, light exposure, and photoinitiator types is crucial for preserving cell viability during this step [73].

8.8.5.3 Porous and Stimuli-Responsive Hydrogels

Hydrogels can be tailored into different structures, including porous and stimuli-responsive types. Porous hydrogels, which contain interconnected networks or foams, are designed to allow cell infiltration and protein diffusion, key to mimicking the native tissue structure. Pore size is crucial: pores that are too small may block cell migration, ECM formation, and blood vessel growth. Therefore, designing a scaffold requires attention to characteristics like pore size, distribution, wall texture, and interconnectivity. Ideal pore sizes vary by cell type and application; for example, fibroblast growth is supported by pores of 5–15 μm, hepatocytes by 20 μm, and skin regeneration by pores of 20–125 μm. Stimuli-responsive scaffolds are another innovative approach. These hydrogels are formulated from materials that react to specific internal or external cues, such as heat or light, triggering the release of cells and bioactive molecules at the wound site. Typically, a polymer that responds to stimuli is combined with cells, then applied to the injury via spraying or injection. Upon exposure to a stimulus, the material transitions into a gel, forming a 3D structure that encapsulates the cells. For instance, Eke et al. developed a UV-light-sensitive hydrogel using GelMA and HAMA. This gel, infused with ADSCs, supported vascularization in chronic wounds. The photo-initiator and cells were added to the pre-gel solution before UV-induced cross-linking. By varying the ratio of GelMA to HAMA, researchers were able to tune the hydrogel's mechanical properties. Although its elasticity (6 kPa) was below the level of natural skin, it was easy to handle in lab and clinical environments. In vitro tests confirmed that ADSCs proliferated effectively within the gel, and in vivo experiments showed enhanced blood vessel formation compared to cell-free versions [74]. In another study, Yanez et al. used 3D bioprinting to incorporate vascular structures into a layered skin graft composed of NHEKs and NHDFs embedded in a fibrin-collagen hydrogel. Endothelial cells mixed with thrombin were printed onto a pre-formed fibroblast-laden collagen layer containing fibrinogen. This was then covered with a keratinocyte-containing collagen layer to create a bilayered graft. The printed constructs were implanted in full-thickness skin wounds in mice. Healing occurred significantly faster within 14–16 days compared to untreated wounds (21 days) and wounds treated with Apligraf (28 days). Histological analysis revealed newly formed skin layers and blood vessels, attributed to the angiogenic activity of endothelial and keratinocyte cells [75]. In an additional study, Hakimi et al. created a handheld bioprinter capable of forming customized skin tissue layers directly on the wound. This device uses bioinks containing dermal and epidermal cells within alginate (crosslinked by ions), fibrin (enzyme-crosslinked), and blends of collagen type I and hyaluronic acid [76]. Similarly, Liu et al. formulated a temperature-sensitive hydrogel made of alginate and gelatin for 3D bioprinting. This hydrogel encapsulated amniotic epithelial cells and MSCs from Wharton's jelly. By modifying the alginate-to-gelatin ratio, they were able to optimize the bioink's flow and stability to meet the demands of extrusion-based printing [77].

8.8.5.4 Injectable and Dual-Responsive Hydrogels

Injectable hydrogels offer the advantage of conforming precisely to wound shapes, providing a close fit with the damaged tissue. Several advanced hydrogels have been developed to be stimulus-responsive to specific triggers in the wound environment. For instance, a dual-responsive hydrogel loaded with antibiotics and anti-inflammatory drugs was developed using modified hyaluronic acid and alginate. This system responded to low pH and high levels of ROS, releasing over 80% of the therapeutic agents within 24 h and showing vigorous antibacterial activity to support healing in infected wounds. Another approach involves combining chitosan-based hydrogels with exosomes to enhance immune modulation and tissue repair. These hydrogels function by promoting the polarization of macrophages toward a healing-supportive phenotype and enhancing the formation of new blood vessels, resulting in improved outcomes in diabetic wound models [78]. Researchers have also developed hydrogels that integrate silver nanoparticles within a dopamine-modified gelatin matrix, embedded in a guar gum scaffold. This system is tailored to treat infections caused by bacteria and address tissue damage associated with high oxidative stress levels [55]. Despite their advantages, traditional hydrogels often suffer from poor strength, limited elasticity, and inadequate adhesion. Their stability under harsh conditions is also limited, which affects their mechanical integrity and conductivity. These challenges could be addressed by utilizing reversible covalent bonds and designing double-network structures, which enhance durability and self-healing capacity [79].

8.9 Technological Innovations in Skin Substitutes

8.9.1 Oxygen-Releasing Structures

Oxygen plays a vital role in maintaining the health, functionality, and behavior of mammalian cells. It influences cellular activity by regulating metabolic processes, which are essential for tissue growth and repair. Apart from being a key element for sustaining life, oxygen also serves as a signaling molecule in various metabolic pathways. In conditions where oxygen is scarce, tissues can undergo necrosis, and cells may experience programmed death. In chronic wounds, impaired blood flow often restricts the delivery of oxygen, hampering the movement of immune cells and the growth of new blood vessels. However, passive oxygen diffusion is limited to a short distance, typically between 100 and 200 μm. To overcome this barrier, oxygen-releasing materials have been engineered to deliver targeted and controlled oxygen to affected areas. These materials come in both organic and inorganic forms [80]. Organic-based systems include those utilizing hemoglobin or oxygen-producing microorganisms such as microalgae or photosynthetic bacteria. Inorganic oxygen-releasing agents include compounds like calcium peroxide (CPO), magnesium peroxide, sodium carbonate, and hydrogen peroxide. One innovative approach involved incorporating microalgae into a dermal scaffold to promote photosynthesis, resulting in increased oxygen availability and enhanced vascular growth after application in living tissue (Figure 8.4a). This approach stimulated angiogenesis and the recruitment of vascular-related cells, aiding tissue regeneration. Another strategy involved the use of microneedle patches infused with materials capable of carrying and releasing oxygen in a controlled manner. These microneedles contained substances responsive to light and heat, enabling the release of oxygen upon exposure to near-infrared light. The treatment proved effective in accelerating wound healing, particularly in diabetic skin injury models, by improving oxygen supply directly at the wound site [80]. Abdullah et al. utilized calcium peroxide nanoparticles incorporated into composite polymers such as polycaprolactone and poly(glycerol sebacate) for oxygen delivery, resulting in enhanced cellular metabolic activity and alleviation of hypoxic conditions in chronic wound areas [81]. In another approach, sodium alginate–GelMA copolymer microfibre scaffolds were directly printed onto mouse wounds. These scaffolds, containing Chlorella microalgae cells, facilitated sustained oxygen release at the wound site and promoted healing under light exposure [82].

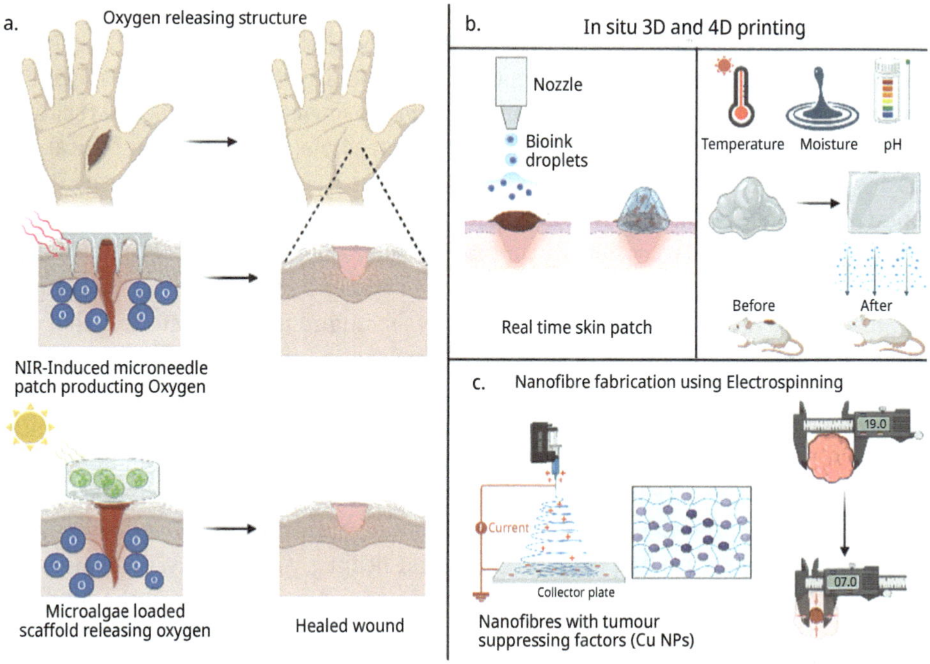

Figure 8.4: Technological innovations in skin substitutes: a) oxygen-releasing structures, b) in situ 3D and 4D printing, and c) nanofibres using an electrospinning device.

Additionally, collagen-based cryogels containing CPO demonstrated enhanced blood glucose regulation in diabetic mouse models receiving islet implants. Beyond islet transplantation, oxygen-delivering systems have also been explored for their potential to improve the survival of various therapeutic implants used in muscle, cardiac, bone, and skin repair. Zhang et al. developed controllable oxygen-delivery microneedles incorporating black phosphorus quantum dots for treating full-thickness wounds in a diabetic model [83]. Similarly, Wenjing Zai et al. designed oxygen-releasing sutures for deep wound healing, capable of delivering over 100-fold higher oxygen levels to 15 mm-deep skin wounds in a model system [84].

8.9.2 In Situ 3D And 4D Bioprinting

In situ 3D printing refers to the direct application of bioprinting technology at the site of tissue damage or organ defects, enabling on-the-spot tissue construction or repair. With recent innovations, compact and portable skin printers have been introduced, enabling skin regeneration treatments to be performed directly on wounds [85]. For instance, one approach involves using extrusion-based bioprinting techniques to create structures containing dermal fibroblasts and epidermal stem cells, enhanced with PRP [86]. PRP serves as a personalized source of growth factors derived from the patient, promoting healing. This method has been successfully tested in full-thickness skin injuries in animal models. Another advancement includes the development of lightweight, handheld skin printers capable of producing cellular patches in real time [87]. These portable devices open the door for immediate intervention in critical scenarios such as burns, combat injuries, and accidents. Despite these promising developments, further evaluation is essential to ensure that these technologies meet stringent clinical standards for sterility and safety before being used in routine medical applications. 4D printing, on the other hand, builds upon traditional 3D printing by incorporating time as a dynamic factor. This technique utilizes materials that can alter their shape, function, or properties in response to specific stimuli, such as heat, light, magnetic fields, or biological cues like temperature, stress, or moisture (Figure 8.4b). These responsive materials enable the creation of innovative medical devices and implants that can adapt to the body's conditions over time. In biomedical applications, 4D printing holds significant potential. It may enable the fabrication of wearable devices and implants that conform to the body and adapt to physiological changes, thereby supporting diagnostics, wound healing, and tissue regeneration. As this technology advances, it is expected to play a transformative role in the future of personalized and adaptive medicine [88].

8.9.3 Electrospinning-Based Skin Scaffolds

The electrospinning technique enables the fabrication of scaffolds or wound dressings with customizable three-dimensional fibrous architectures and porosity. A wide range of materials, including fibrinogen, collagen, gelatin, chitosan, PU, PLA, and PCL, have been utilized in this method, either individually or in various combinations. Additionally, electrospun nanofibers can be functionalized with drugs (Figure 8.4c) or biologically active molecules to achieve controlled release profiles and multifunctional properties, including antibacterial effects. The standard electrospinning apparatus comprises four primary components: a high-voltage power supply, a fluid delivery system, a spinneret, and a collector. By fine-tuning the processing parameters and selecting appropriate raw materials, it is possible to control the morphology and diameter of the resulting nanofibers. This enables the creation of fibrous structures with tailored pore sizes and porosity, closely resembling the ECM of natural tissues [89]. He et al. developed an electroactive nanofibrous membrane by electrospinning solutions of PCL and quaternized chitosan-graft-PANI. The resulting wound dressing exhibited multiple beneficial properties, including antibacterial, antioxidant, and electroactive functions. In a full-thickness wound model in mice, the electrospun membrane significantly enhanced collagen deposition, granulation tissue thickness, and angiogenesis compared to the commercial wound dressing Tegaderm Film [90]. Xingxing Liu and collaborators developed a PCL nanofiber–alginate hydrogel interpenetrating network scaffold designed to function as a synthetic skin substitute. This advanced scaffold demonstrates excellent performance in critical wound-healing parameters, including high water absorption capacity and a water vapor transmission rate exceeding 6,000 g/m^2/day, ensuring optimal moisture balance at the wound site. It also possesses notable mechanical flexibility and stretchability, essential for adapting to dynamic skin movements. To enhance its functionality, the scaffold was modified with amino-terminated hyperbranched polyamide, imparting dual antibacterial activity and ROS scavenging capabilities, both of which are vital for reducing the risk of infection and inflammation. Additionally, the scaffold supports deep three-dimensional cellular infiltration of fibroblasts, extending beyond 100 μm, which promotes tissue regeneration. Given these combined properties, this multifunctional scaffold shows strong potential as a promising skin.

8.10 Conclusion and Future Perspectives

The advancement of 3D bioprinting technologies has revolutionized the development of engineered skin substitutes, providing novel solutions to the challenges of wound healing, particularly in cases of chronic and complex wounds. Bioprinted skin constructs, incorporating a variety of bioinks, cell types, and layered architectures, closely mimic native skin structure and function. This enables not only accelerated healing but also the regeneration of critical skin components, including pigmentation, vasculature, and appendages. Clinical evidence supports the effectiveness of these constructs in restoring skin integrity with minimal scarring and improved aesthetic outcomes. In situ bioprinting approaches further enhance clinical applicability by allowing real-time printing of patient-specific grafts directly at the wound site, thereby reducing contamination risks and improving integration. The integration of smart and stimuli-responsive materials also opens new avenues in personalized wound care, diagnostics, and therapy.

To bridge the gap between laboratory innovation and clinical application, several key challenges must be addressed. First, long-term validation of bioprinted skin grafts in large animal models and human trials is crucial to confirm their safety, efficacy, and functional integration. Second, there is a need for the development of next-generation bioinks with enhanced mechanical, rheological, and bioactive properties to support complex tissue functions while maintaining print fidelity and cell viability. Third, strategies must be refined to include fully functional skin appendages such as sweat glands, sebaceous glands, and vascular and neural networks, ensuring complete skin regeneration. The differentiation of functional cell types from iPSCs, ESCs, and other progenitors offers promising avenues in this direction. Fourth, improvements in printer resolution, reproducibility, and speed are needed to meet clinical demands and ensure cost-effectiveness. In parallel, regulatory standardization is urgently required. Currently, there are no universal guidelines for bioprinting processes, bioink formulations, or quality control measures. Regulatory frameworks, such as those of the FDA, must evolve to account for the complexity of living, patient-specific implants. Additionally, interdisciplinary collaboration among material scientists, biomedical engineers, clinicians, and regulatory experts will be essential for translating bioprinting technologies into standardized, clinically viable therapies. Emerging technologies such as artificial intelligence (AI) and machine learning (ML) hold transformative potential in optimizing bioprinting workflows, predictive modeling of skin architecture based on patient-specific anatomical data, and simulation of wound healing kinetics. ML algorithms can analyze large datasets to predict optimal printing parameters, monitor real-time printing fidelity, and improve quality control during manufacturing. These tools also enable the rapid screening of bioink compositions, cellular arrangements, and therapeutic responses, accelerating the development of next-generation skin substitutes.

With sustained innovation, collaborative efforts, and robust validation, 3D bioprinting holds the potential to redefine wound management and skin regeneration, shifting from supportive therapies to curative, personalized solutions. As research continues to bridge biological complexity and therapies with technological innovation, 3D-bioprinted skin constructs supported by AI/ML tools and advanced biomanufacturing are poised to redefine the future of wound healing, regenerative medicine, and personalized skin therapy.

Abbreviations

Three-dimensional	3D
Extracellular matrix	ECM
Matrix metalloproteinases	MMPs
Diabetic foot ulcer	DFU
Negative pressure wound closure therapy	NPWT
Glycosaminoglycan	GAG
Digital light processing	DLP
Ultraviolet	UV
Computer-aided design	CAD
Computer-aided manufacturing	CAM
magnetic resonance imaging	MRI
Computed Tomography	CT
Stereolithography	STL
Poly-ε-caprolactone:	PCL
Polyurethane	PU
Polylactic-co-glycolic acid	PLGA

Polyglycolide	PGA
Poly(vinyl alcohol)	PVA
Polyethylene glycol	PEG
Poly(lactic acid)	PLA
Methacrylated gelatin	GelMA
Methacrylated hyaluronic acid	HAMA
Polyaniline	PANI
Polypyrrole	PPy
Mesenchymal stem cells	MSCs
Bone marrow-derived mesenchymal stem cells	BMSCs
Epidermal stem cells	ESCs
Adipose-derived stem cells	ASCs
Induced pluripotent stem cells	iPSCs
Neonatal fibroblasts	NHDFs
Neonatal keratinocytes	NHEKs
Vascular endothelial growth factor	VEGF
Cultured epithelial autografts	CEA
Food and Drug Administration	FDA
Calcium peroxide:	CPO
Platelet-rich plasma	PRP
Synthetic skin substitute	SSS
Reactive oxygen species	ROS
Artificial intelligence	AI
Machine learning	ML

References

[1] Lin, Z., Chen, L., Qi, C., & Wang, G. (2025). Skin microecology and skin barrier repair, wound healing and appendage regeneration. Regenesis Repair Rehabilitation, 1, 1–5. https://doi.org/10.1016/j.rerere.2024.07.001.

[2] Phang, S. J., Basak, S., Teh, H. X., Packirisamy, G., Fauzi, M. B., Kuppusamy, U. R. et al. (2022). Advancements in extracellular matrix-based biomaterials and biofabrication of 3D organotypic skin models. ACS Biomaterials Science & Engineering, 8, 3220–3241. https://doi.org/10.1021/acsbiomaterials.2c00342.

[3] Wei, Q., An, Y., Zhao, X., Li, M., & Zhang, J. (2024). Three-dimensional bioprinting of tissue-engineered skin: biomaterials, fabrication techniques, challenging difficulties, and future directions: a review. International Journal of Biological Macromolecules, 266, 131281. https://doi.org/10.1016/j.ijbiomac.2024.131281.

[4] Javaid, M., & Haleem, A. (2021). 3D bioprinting applications for the printing of skin: a brief study. Sensors International, 2. https://doi.org/10.1016/j.sintl.2021.100123.

[5] Dal Prà, I., Chiarini, A., De Santis, D., Nocini, R., Chang, S., & Armato, U. (2025). The quest for the perfect healing of human skin wounds : promising models. Regenesis Repair Rehabilitation, 1, 66–79. https://doi.org/10.1016/j.rerere.2025.03.003.

[6] Abdo, J. M., Sopko, N. A., & Milner, S. M. (2020). The applied anatomy of human skin: a model for regeneration. Wound Medicine, 28, 100179. https://doi.org/10.1016/j.wndm.2020.100179.

[7] Raziyeva, K., Kim, Y., Zharkinbekov, Z., Kassymbek, K., Jimi, S., & Saparov, A. (2021). Immunology of acute and chronic wound healing. Biomolecules, 11, 1–25. https://doi.org/10.3390/biom11050700.

[8] Cañedo-Dorantes, L., & Cañedo-Ayala, M. (2019 2019). Skin acute wound healing: a comprehensive review. International Journal of Inflammation, https://doi.org/10.1155/2019/3706315.

[9] Almadani, Y. H., Vorstenbosch, J., Davison, P. G., & Murphy, A. M. (2021). Wound healing: a comprehensive review. Seminars in Plastic Surgery, 35, 141–144. https://doi.org/10.1055/s-0041-1731791.

[10] Fuenmayor, P., Huaman, G., Maita, K., Schwemmer, K., Soliman, W., Abdelmoneim, S. et al. (2024). Skin substitutes: filling the gap in the reconstructive algorithm. Trauma Care, 4, 148–166. https://doi.org/10.3390/traumacare4020012.

[11] Zhou, X., Yu, X., You, T., Zhao, B., Dong, L., Huang, C. et al. (2024). 3D printing-based hydrogel dressings for wound healing. Advanced Science, 11, 2404580. https://doi.org/https://doi.org/10.1002/advs.202404580.

[12] Derman, I. D., Rivera, T., Garriga Cerda, L., Singh, Y. P., Saini, S., Abaci, H. E. et al. (2025). Advancements in 3D skin bioprinting: processes, bioinks, applications and sensor integration. International Journal of Extreme Manufacturing, 7, 012009. https://doi.org/10.1088/2631-7990/ad878c.

[13] Maniţă, P. G., García-Orue, I., Santos-Vizcaíno, E., Hernández, R. M., & Igartua, M. (2021). 3D bioprinting of functional skin substitutes for chronic wound treatment: from current achievements to future goals. Pharmaceuticals, 14, 362. https://doi.org/10.2139/ssrn.3751557.

[14] Rehak, L., Giurato, L., Meloni, M., Panunzi, A., Manti, G. M., & Uccioli, L. (2022). The immune-centric revolution in the diabetic foot: monocytes and lymphocytes role in wound healing and tissue regeneration – a narrative review. Journal of Clinical Medicine, 11. https://doi.org/10.3390/jcm11030889.

[15] Thangavel, P., Ramachandran, B., Chakraborty, S., Kannan, R., Lonchin, S., & Muthuvijayan, V. (2017). Accelerated healing of diabetic wounds treated with L-glutamic acid loaded hydrogels through enhanced collagen deposition and angiogenesis: an in vivo study. Scientific Reports, 7, 1–15. https://doi.org/10.1038/s41598-017-10882-1.

[16] Derakhshanfar, A., Moayedi, J., Derakhshanfar, G., & Fard, A. P. (2019). The role of Iranian medicinal plants in experimental surgical skin wound healing: an integrative review. Iranian Journal of Basic Medical Sciences, 22, 590–600. https://doi.org/10.22038/ijbms.2019.32963.7873.

[17] Smandri, A., Nordin, A., Hwei, N. M., Chin, K. Y., Abd Aziz, I., & Fauzi, M. B. (2020). Natural 3D-printed bioinks for skin regeneration and wound healing: a systematic review. Polymers (Basel), 12. https://doi.org/10.3390/polym12081782.

[18] Flynn, K., Mahmoud, N. N., Sharifi, S., Gould, L. J., & Mahmoudi, M. (2023). Chronic wound healing models. ACS Pharmacology & Translational Science, 6, 783–801. https://doi.org/10.1021/acsptsci.3c00030.

[19] Zhang, D., Lai, L., Fu, H., Fu, Q., & Chen, M. (2023). 3D-bioprinted biomimetic multilayer implants comprising microfragmented adipose extracellular matrix and cells improve wound healing in a murine model of full-thickness skin defects. ACS Applied Materials & Interfaces, 15, 29713–29728. https://doi.org/10.1021/acsami.2c21629.

[20] Yu, J. R., Navarro, J., Coburn, J. C., Mahadik, B., Molnar, J., Holmes, J. H. (2019). et al. Current and future perspectives on skin tissue engineering: key features of biomedical research, translational assessment, and clinical application. Advanced Healthcare Materials, 8. https://doi.org/10.1002/adhm.201801471.

[21] Varkey, M., Visscher, D. O., Van Zuijlen, P. P. M., Atala, A., & Yoo, J. J. (2019). Skin bioprinting: the future of burn wound reconstruction?. Burns & Trauma, 7, 1–12. https://doi.org/10.1186/s41038-019-0142-7.

[22] Kolimi, P., Narala, S., Nyavanandi, D., Youssef, A. A. A., & Dudhipala, N. (2022). Innovative treatment strategies to accelerate wound healing: trajectory and recent advancements. Cells, 11. https://doi.org/10.3390/cells11152439.

[23] Chakraborty, A., Alexander, S., Luo, W., Al-Salam, N., Van Oirschot, M., Ranganath, S. H. et al. (2023). Engineering multifunctional adhesive hydrogel patches for biomedical applications. Interdisciplinary Medicine, 1, 1–21. https://doi.org/10.1002/INMD.20230008.

[24] Gao, C., Lu, C., Jian, Z., Zhang, T., Chen, Z., Zhu, Q. et al. (2021). 3D bioprinting for fabricating artificial skin tissue. Colloids and Surfaces B: Biointerfaces, 208, 112041. https://doi.org/10.1016/j.colsurfb.2021.112041.
[25] Choudhury, D., Anand, S., & Naing, M. W. (2018). The arrival of commercial bioprinters – towards 3D bioprinting revolution! International Journal of Bioprinting, 4, 1–20. https://doi.org/10.18063/IJB.v4i2.139.
[26] Hospodiuk, M., Moncal, K. K., Ibrahim, T., & Ozbolat. (2018). Extrusion-based biofabrication in tissue engineering and regenerative medicine. 4601.
[27] Song, Y., Ghafari, Y., Asefnejad, A., & Toghraie, D. (2024). An overview of selective laser sintering 3D printing technology for biomedical and sports device applications: processes, materials, and applications. Optics and Laser Technology, 171, 110459. https://doi.org/10.1016/j.optlastec.2023.110459.
[28] Murphy, S. V., & Atala, A. (2014). 3D bioprinting of tissues and organs. Nature Biotechnology, 32, 773–785. https://doi.org/10.1038/nbt.2958.
[29] Zadpoor, A. A., & Malda, J. (2017). Additive manufacturing of biomaterials, tissues, and organs. Annals of Biomedical Engineering, 45, 1–11. https://doi.org/10.1007/s10439-016-1719-y.
[30] Moroni, L., Burdick, J. A., Highley, C., Lee, S. J., Morimoto, Y., Takeuchi, S. et al. (2018). Biofabrication strategies for 3D in vitro models and regenerative medicine. Nature Reviews Materials, 3, 21–37. https://doi.org/10.1038/s41578-018-0006-y.
[31] Chaudhry, M. S., & Czekanski, A. (2023). In-situ bioprinting of skin – a review. Bioprinting, 31, e00271. https://doi.org/10.1016/j.bprint.2023.e00271.
[32] Devi, M. G., Amutheesan, M., Govindhan, R., & Karthikeyan, B. (2018). A review of three-dimensional printing for biomedical and tissue engineering applications. The Open Biotechnology Journal, 12, 241–255. https://doi.org/10.2174/1874070701812010241.
[33] Bramhe, P., Rarokar, N., Kumbhalkar, R., Saoji, S., & Khedekar, P. (2024). Natural and synthetic polymeric hydrogel: a bioink for 3D bioprinting of tissue models. Journal of Drug Delivery Science and Technology, 101, 106204. https://doi.org/10.1016/j.jddst.2024.106204.
[34] Cai, R., Shan, Y., Du, F., Miao, Z., Zhu, L., Hang, L. et al. (2024). Injectable hydrogels as promising in situ therapeutic platform for cartilage tissue engineering. International Journal of Biological Macromolecules, 261, 129537. https://doi.org/10.1016/j.ijbiomac.2024.129537.
[35] González-Ulloa, G., Jiménez-Rosado, M., Rafii-El-Idrissi Benhnia, M., Romero, A., Ruiz-Mateos, E., Ostos, F. J. (2023). et al. Hybrid polymeric Hydrogel-based biomaterials with potential applications in regenerative medicine. Journal of Molecular Liquids, 384. https://doi.org/10.1016/j.molliq.2023.122224.
[36] Askari, M., Afzali Naniz, M., Kouhi, M., Saberi, A., Zolfagharian, A., & Bodaghi, M. (2021). Recent progress in extrusion 3D bioprinting of hydrogel biomaterials for tissue regeneration: a comprehensive review with focus on advanced fabrication techniques. Biomaterials Science, 9, 535–573. https://doi.org/10.1039/d0bm00973c.
[37] Kolambkar, Y. M., Peister, A., Soker, S., Atala, A., & Guldberg, R. E. (2007). Chondrogenic differentiation of amniotic fluid-derived stem cells. Journal of Molecular Histology, 38, 405–413. https://doi.org/10.1007/s10735-007-9118-1.
[38] Roy, A., Mantay, M., Brannan, C., & Griffiths, S. (2022). Placental tissues as biomaterials in regenerative medicine. BioMed Research International, 26. https://doi.org/10.1155/2022/6751456.
[39] Cubo, N., Garcia, M., Del Cañizo, J. F., Velasco, D., & Jorcano, J. L. (2017). 3D bioprinting of functional human skin: production and in vivo analysis. Biofabrication, 9. https://doi.org/10.1088/1758-5090/9/1/015006.
[40] Coutant, K., Magne, B., Ferland, K., Fuentes-Rodriguez, A., Chancy, O., Mitchell, A. et al. (2024). Melanocytes in regenerative medicine applications and disease modeling. Journal of Translational Medicine, 22, 1–18. https://doi.org/10.1186/s12967-024-05113-x.
[41] Gao, C., Zhang, L., Wang, J., Jin, M., Tang, Q., Chen, Z. et al. (2021). Electrospun nanofibers promote wound healing: theories, techniques, and perspectives. Journal of Materials Chemistry B, 9, 3106–3130. https://doi.org/10.1039/d1tb00067e.

[42] Gounden, V., & Singh, M. (2024). Hydrogels and wound healing: current and future prospects. Gels, 10. https://doi.org/10.3390/gels10010043.

[43] Lihao, Q., Tingting, L., Jiawei, Z., Yifei, B., Zheyu, T., Jingyan, L. et al. (2024). 3D bioprinting of salvianolic acid B-sodium alginate-gelatin skin scaffolds promotes diabetic wound repair via antioxidant, anti-inflammatory, and proangiogenic effects. Biomedicine & Pharmacotherapy, 171, 116168. https://doi.org/10.1016/j.biopha.2024.116168.

[44] Xu, W., Wu, Y., Lu, H., Zhang, X., Zhu, Y., Liu, S. et al. (2023). Injectable hydrogel encapsulated with VEGF-mimetic peptide-loaded nanoliposomes promotes peripheral nerve repair in vivo. Acta Biomaterialia, 160, 225–238. https://doi.org/10.1016/j.actbio.2023.02.004.

[45] Su, W. Y., Chen, Y. C., & Lin, F. H. (2010). Injectable oxidized hyaluronic acid/adipic acid dihydrazide hydrogel for nucleus pulposus regeneration. Acta Biomaterialia, 6, 3044–3055. https://doi.org/10.1016/j.actbio.2010.02.037.

[46] Tanadchangsaeng, N., Pasanaphong, K., Tawonsawatruk, T., Rattanapinyopituk, K., Tangketsarawan, B., Rawiwet, V. et al. (2024). 3D bioprinting of fish skin-based gelatin methacryloyl (GelMA) bio-ink for use as a potential skin substitute. Scientific Reports, 14, 23240. https://doi.org/10.1038/s41598-024-73774-1.

[47] Augustine, R. (2018). Skin bioprinting: a novel approach for creating artificial skin from synthetic and natural building blocks. Progress in Biomaterials, 7, 77–92. https://doi.org/10.1007/s40204-018-0087-0.

[48] Olejnik, A., Semba, J. A., Kulpa, A., Dańczak-Pazdrowska, A., Rybka, J. D., & Gornowicz-Porowska, J. (2022). 3D bioprinting in skin related research: recent achievements and application perspectives. ACS Synthetic Biology, 11, 26–38. https://doi.org/10.1021/acssynbio.1c00547.

[49] Kang, M. S., Jang, J., Jo, H. J., Kim, W. H., Kim, B., Chun, H. J. (2023). et al. Advances and innovations of 3D bioprinting skin. Biomolecules, 13. https://doi.org/10.3390/biom13010055.

[50] El Sayed, M. M. (2023). Production of polymer hydrogel composites and their applications. Journal of Polymers and the Environment, 31, 2855–2879. https://doi.org/10.1007/s10924-023-02796-z.

[51] Bhar, B., Chouhan, D., Pai, N., & Mandal, B. B. (2021). Harnessing multifaceted next-generation technologies for improved skin wound healing. ACS Applied Bio Materials, 4, 7738–7763. https://doi.org/10.1021/acsabm.1c00880.

[52] Vijayavenkataraman, S., Lu, W. F., & Fuh, J. Y. H. (2016). 3D bioprinting of skin: a state-of-the-art review on modelling, materials, and processes. Biofabrication, 8. https://doi.org/10.1088/1758-5090/8/3/032001.

[53] Casella, A., Panitch, A., & Leach, J. K. (2023). Electroconductive agarose hydrogels modulate mesenchymal stromal cell adhesion and spreading through protein adsorption. Journal of Biomedical Materials Research Part A, 1–13. https://doi.org/10.1002/jbm.a.37503.

[54] Shin, W., Choi, H. J., Kang, B., Lee, K., Choi, Y. S., Choi, J. H. et al. (2025). Materials design and characterization of injectable and degradable oxidized alginate PANI:PSS hydrogels for photothermal therapy. Carbohydrate Polymers, 347, 122652. https://doi.org/10.1016/j.carbpol.2024.122652.

[55] Duarte, J., Mascarenhas-Melo, F., Pires, P. C., Veiga, F., & Paiva-Santos, A. C. (2024). Multifunctional hydrogels-based therapies for chronic diabetic wound healing. European Polymer Journal, 211. https://doi.org/10.1016/j.eurpolymj.2024.113026.

[56] Zahouani, H., Pailler-Mattei, C., Sohm, B., Vargiolu, R., Cenizo, V., & Debret, R. (2009). Characterization of the mechanical properties of a dermal equivalent compared with human skin in vivo by indentation and static friction tests. Skin Research and Technology, 15, 68–76. https://doi.org/10.1111/j.1600-0846.2008.00329.x.

[57] Ng, W. L., Qi, J. T. Z., Yeong, W. Y., & Naing, M. W. (2018). Proof-of-concept: 3D bioprinting of pigmented human skin constructs. Biofabrication, 10. https://doi.org/10.1088/1758-5090/aa9e1e.

[58] Koch, L., Deiwick, A., Schlie, S., Michael, S., Gruene, M., Coger, V. et al. (2012). Skin tissue generation by laser cell printing. Biotechnology and Bioengineering, 109, 1855–1863. https://doi.org/10.1002/bit.24455.

[59] Weng, T., Zhang, W., Xia, Y., Wu, P., Yang, M., Jin, R. (2021). et al. 3D bioprinting for skin tissue engineering: current status and perspectives. Journal of Tissue Engineering, 12. https://doi.org/10.1177/20417314211028574.

[60] Pasierb, A., Jezierska, M., Karpuk, A., Czuwara, J., & Rudnicka, L. (2022). 3D skin bioprinting : future potential for skin regeneration. Advances in Dermatology and Allergology, 845–851. https://doi.org/https://doi.org/10.5114/ada.2021.109692.
[61] Barrault, C., Dichamp, I., Garnier, J., Pedretti, N., Juchaux, F., Deguercy, A. et al. (2012). Immortalized sebocytes can spontaneously differentiate into a sebaceous-like phenotype when cultured as a 3D epithelium. Experimental Dermatology, 21, 314–316. https://doi.org/10.1111/j.1600-0625.2012.01463.x.
[62] Abaci, H. E., Coffman, A., Doucet, Y., Chen, J., Jacków, J., Wang, E. et al. (2018). Tissue engineering of human hair follicles using a biomimetic developmental approach. Nature Communications, 9, 1–11. https://doi.org/10.1038/s41467-018-07579-y.
[63] Gibbons, G. W. (2015). Grafix ®, a cryopreserved placental membrane, for the treatment of chronic/stalled wounds. Advances in Wound Care, 4, 534–544. https://doi.org/10.1089/wound.2015.0647.
[64] Rheinwald, J., & Howard, G. (1977). Epidermal growth factor and the multiplication of cultured human epidermal keratinocytes. Nature, 265, 75.
[65] Cortez Ghio, S., Larouche, D., Doucet, E. J., & Germain, L. (2021). The role of cultured autologous bilayered skin substitutes as epithelial stem cell niches after grafting: a systematic review of clinical studies. Burn Open, 5, 56–66. https://doi.org/10.1016/j.burnso.2021.02.002.
[66] Tavakoli, S., & Klar, A. S. (2021). Bioengineered skin substitutes: advances and future trends. Applied Sciences, 11, 1493. https://doi.org/https://doi.org/10.3390/app11041493.
[67] Hart, C. E., Loewen-rodriguez, A., & Lessem, J. (2012). Dermagraft: use in the treatment of chronic wounds. Advances in Wound Care 1, 138–141. https://doi.org/10.1089/wound.2011.0282.
[68] Wang, Z., Qi, F., Luo, H., Xu, G., & Wang, D. (2022). Inflammatory microenvironment of skin wounds. Frontiers in Immunology, 13, 1–17. https://doi.org/10.3389/fimmu.2022.789274.
[69] Snyder, D., Sullivan, N., Margolis, B. D., & Schoelles, K. (2020). Skin substitutes for treating chronic wounds technical brief. In: Technology Assessment Program – Technical Brief. Project ID No. WNDT0818 (pp. 1–175). Rockville, MD: Agency for Healthcare Research and Quality (US).
[70] Still, J., Glat, P., Silverstein, P., Griswold, J., & Mozingo, D. (2003). The use of a collagen sponge/living cell composite material to treat donor sites in burn patients. Burns, 29, 837–841. https://doi.org/10.1016/S0305-4179(03)00164-5.
[71] Sierra-sánchez, Á. (2021). Cellular human tissue-engineered skin substitutes investigated for deep and dif fi cult to heal injuries. Npj Regenerative Medicine, 6. https://doi.org/10.1038/s41536-021-00144-0.
[72] Schiestl, C., Neuhaus, K., Meuli, M., Farkas, M., Hartmann-fritsch, F., Elrod, J. et al. (2024). Long-term outcomes of a cultured autologous dermo-epidermal skin substitute in children : 5-year results of a phase I clinical trial. Journal of Burn Care & Research, 46, 326–334. https://doi.org/10.1093/jbcr/irae150.
[73] Nifontova, G., Safaryan, S., Khristidis, Y., Smirnova, O., Vosough, M., Shpichka, A. (2024). et al. Advancing wound healing by hydrogel- based dressings loaded with cell-conditioned medium: a systematic review. Stem Cell Research & Therapy, 15. https://doi.org/10.1186/s13287-024-03976-x.
[74] Alaa, M., Fallahi, A., El-sokkary, A. M. A., Salehi, S., Akl, M. A., Jafari, A. et al. (2019). Progress in polymer science stimuli-responsive hydrogels for manipulation of cell microenvironment: from chemistry to biofabrication technology. Progress in Polymer Science, 98, 101147. https://doi.org/10.1016/j.progpolymsci.2019.101147.
[75] Yanez, M., Rincon, J., Dones, A., De Maria, C., Gonzales, R., & Boland, T. (2014). In Vivo assessment of printed microvasculature in a bilayer skin graft to treat full-thickness wounds. Tissue Engineering – Part A, 00, 1–10. https://doi.org/10.1089/ten.tea.2013.0561.
[76] Hakimi, N., Cheng, R., Leng, L., Sotoudehfar, M., Ba, P. Q., Bakhtyar, N. et al. (2018). Handheld skin printer: in situ formation of planar biomaterials and tissues. Lab on a Chip, 18, 1440–1451. https://doi.org/10.1039/c7lc01236e.
[77] Li, H., Tan, C., & Li, L. (2018). Review of 3D printable hydrogels and constructs. Master of Design, 159, 20–38. https://doi.org/10.1016/j.matdes.2018.08.023.

[78] Wang, Y., Li, J., Tang, M., Peng, C., Wang, G., Wang, J. et al. (2023). Smart stimuli-responsive hydrogels for drug delivery in periodontitis treatment. Biomedicine & Pharmacotherapy, 162, 114688. https://doi.org/10.1016/j.biopha.2023.114688.
[79] Hu, C., Zhang, F., Long, L., Kong, Q., Luo, R., & Wang, Y. (2020). Dual-responsive injectable hydrogels encapsulating drug-loaded micelles for on-demand antimicrobial activity and accelerated wound healing. Journal of Controlled Release, 324, 204–217. https://doi.org/10.1016/j.jconrel.2020.05.010.
[80] Willemen, N. G. A., Hassan, S., Gurian, M., Li, J., Allijn, I. E., Shin, S. R. et al. (2021). Oxygen-releasing biomaterials: current challenges and future applications. Trends in Biotechnology, 39, 1144–1159. https://doi.org/10.1016/j.tibtech.2021.01.007.
[81] Abdullah, T., Gauthaman, K., Hammad, A.H., et al. (2020). Oxygen-Releasing Antibacterial Nanofibrous Scaffolds for Tissue Engineering Applications. Polymers, 12, 1233. https://doi.org/10.3390/polym12061233
[82] Wang, X., Yang, C., Yu, Y., et al. (2022). In Situ 3D Bioprinting Living Photosynthetic Scaffolds for Autotrophic Wound Healing. Research, 2022. https://doi.org/10.34133/2022/9794745.
[83] Zhang, X., Chen, G., Liu, Y., et al. (2020). Black Phosphorus-Loaded Separable Microneedles as Responsive Oxygen DeliveryCarriers for Wound Healing. ACS nano, 14, 5901–5908. https://dx.doi.org/10.1021/acsnano.0c01059
[84] Zai, W., Yuan, Y., Kang, L., et al. (2023). Oxygen Penetration Through Full-Thickness Skin by Oxygen-Releasing Sutures for Skin Graft Transplantation. Engineering, 29, 83–94. https://doi.org/10.1016/j.eng.2023.05.006.
[85] Mirshafiei, M., Rashedi, H., Yazdian, F., Rahdar, A., & Baino, F. (2024). Advancements in tissue and organ 3D bioprinting: current techniques, applications, and future perspectives. Master of Design, 240, 112853. https://doi.org/10.1016/j.matdes.2024.112853.
[86] Patel, H., Pundkar, A., Shrivastava, S., Chandanwale, R., & Jaiswal, A. M. (2023). A comprehensive review on platelet-rich plasma activation: a key player in accelerating skin wound healing. Cureus, 15. https://doi.org/10.7759/cureus.48943.
[87] Huang, J., Zhou, G., Jiang, Q., & Li, L. (2025). In situ 3D bioprinting: the future of regenerative medicine. Fundamental Research. https://doi.org/10.1016/j.fmre.2025.06.004.
[88] Zhao, M., Wang, J., Zhang, J., Huang, J., Luo, L., Yang, Y. et al. (2022). Functionalizing multi-component bioink with platelet-rich plasma for customized in-situ bilayer bioprinting for wound healing. Materials Today Bio, 16, 100334. https://doi.org/10.1016/j.mtbio.2022.100334.
[89] Zhao, J., Chen, L., Ma, A., Bai, X., Zeng, Y., & Liu, D. (2024). Recent advances in coaxial electrospun nanofibers for wound healing. Materials Today Bio, 29. https://doi.org/https://doi.org/10.1016/j.mtbio.2024.101309.
[90] He, J., Liang, Y., Shi, M., & Guo, B. (2020). Anti-oxidant electroactive and antibacterial nanofibrous wound dressings based on poly(ε-caprolactone)/quaternized chitosan-graft-polyaniline for full-thickness skin wound healing. Chemical Engineering Journal, 385, 123464. https://doi.org/10.1016/j.cej.2019.123464.

N. Vishnu Devi*, M. Vijay*

Chapter 9
Laser-Based Bioprinting

Abstract: Lasers play a key role in facilitating accurate processing and encouraging the creation of new technologies. Multiphoton lithography (MPL) laser-based 3D printing is an excellent illustration of this. By employing computer-aided designs, this method amazingly makes it possible to print real 3D objects at the micro- and nanoscale without the need for masks or heavy equipment. Because of these special qualities, MPL has become a potent production method in a number of interdisciplinary domains. Improvements in resolution and throughput, the creation of new photosensitive materials, and the printing of extremely complex structures on various substrates have all been made possible by the continuous growth in MPL's use. These developments have significantly aided MPL's recent expansion into new fields. The purpose of this perspective piece is to draw attention to these developments and current MPL tendencies. In order to guarantee MPL's continued incorporation into sophisticated additive manufacturing at the micro- and nanoscale, the present difficulties of MPL will be examined. There will also be a discussion of MPL's potential and future prospects as a laser-based 3D printing method. AM, sometimes referred to as 3D printing, is becoming more and more important in the industrial sector. Laser-assisted manufacturing (LAM) and additive manufacturing (AM) technologies are gaining a lot of attention and interest over conventional techniques because of the great flexibility and efficiency of lasers.

This mainly focuses on some of the basic facts and backgrounds of lasers and their applications in 3D printing and manufacturing. Inventions of new laser sources and assisted technology have evolved by leaps and bounds during the past decade. Many industries today depend on such lasers for a variety of production line applications. In the case of the healthcare industry, especially in diagnostic and therapeutic applications, lasers have found tremendous applications. It was found to be a paradigm shift in the making when laser technology was found to go hand in hand with 3D printing or rapid prototyping applications.

Keywords: Laser, bioprinting, laser-assisted manufacturing, 3D printing, stereolithography

***Corresponding authors: N. Vishnu Devi**, Department of Electronics Engineering (VLSI), Velammal College of Engineering and Technology, Viraganoor, Madurai 625 009, Tamil Nadu, India, e-mail: vichu0408@gmail.com

***Corresponding author: M. Vijay**, Department of Electrical and Electronics Engineering, Aditya University, Surampalem, Kakinada 533437, Andhra Pradesh, India, e-mail: vijayeee050@gmail.com

 | https://doi.org/10.1515/9783111719993-009

9.1 Introduction

Stereolithography has been recognized as the premier commercial rapid prototyping technology, now widely referred to as 3D printing. 3D printing is transforming global thought and creativity, recognized as a "disruptive technology" – an innovation that has supplanted traditional technologies and spawned new sectors. Although the roots of 3D printing dated from the nineteenth century, the technology began to gain traction in the 1980s. In 1983, Charles Hull developed a prototype technology known as stereolithography, which forms layers by curing photopolymers using ultraviolet (UV) lasers. He characterized the process as a "method for producing three-dimensional objects by establishing a cross-sectional template of the object to be created." Mr Hull made two substantial contributions that significantly enhanced the viability of 3D technology: He developed the STL file format, which is now commonly recognized for describing 3D images in 3D printing software. He further developed the digital slicing and in-fill techniques that are common in the majority of 3D printing processes. 3D Systems service-level agreement-1 3D printer is the inaugural 3D printer produced for commercial distribution and utilization. This device initiated the swift advancement of additive production, a technique in which material is incrementally added to create a solid object, as opposed to conventional manufacturing, which involves the removal or machining of material. The SLA-1 employs stereolithography, utilizing a meticulously regulated UV laser beam to harden liquid polymers layer by layer. In 1983, Chuck Hull invented stereolithography and established 3D Systems to produce and sell a commercial printer. 3D printers utilizing Hull's invention are currently extensively employed to manufacture intricate components from a diverse range of materials.

Significant milestones in 3D printing are as follows. In 1860, François Willème's photosculpture technique employed cameras positioned around the subject to capture a three-dimensional representation of an object. In 1892, Joseph E. Blanther proposed a layering technique for creating three-dimensional topographical maps. In 1972, Matsubara of Mitsubishi Motors proposed the utilization of photohardened layers of materials, known as photopolymers, which could be stacked to create a casting mold. In 1980, Dr Hideo Kodama of Japan filed the inaugural patent application for expedited prototyping technology. The researcher showed the method for fabricating 3D plastic components by the photohardening of polymers via UV irradiation. In 1984, Chuck Hull submitted a patent application for a stereolithography system (SLA). In 1986, the inaugural patent was granted to Chuck Hull for the "Apparatus for the production of three-dimensional objects via stereolithography." In 1987, 3D Systems released the SLA-1, the inaugural commercial fast prototyping device. In 1989, Carl Deckard was granted a patent for the laser-based selective sintering rapid prototyping technique that utilizes a laser to fuse powder rather than harden plastic, as utilized in SLA technology. In 1991, Stratasys developed the inaugural fused deposition modeling machine, utilizing plastic and an extruder to build material on a print bed. In 1992, a patent for fused deposition modelling was granted to Stratasys. In 1992, DTM manufactured the inaugural selective laser sintering apparatus. In 1994, initial commercialization of colorjet printing (CJP) was done. In 2002, a functional tiny kidney was created using 3D printing technology. Researchers endeavor to generate fully functional, full-scale organs. The inaugural 3D-printed prosthetic limb was manufactured in 2008. The inaugural 3D-printed robotic airplane and automobile chassis were manufactured in 2011.

The principal long-term objective of bioprinting investigation is to fabricate functional organs or tissues suitable for transplantation. In vivo, natural tissues or organs exhibit three-dimensional cellular growth and spatial communication. Historically, constrained by prevailing methods, the majority of cells or tissues were cultivated in two-dimensional structures. The lack of a three-dimensional framework could lead cells to forfeit some biological functions due to limited cellular interactions, ultimately resulting in difficulties in cell migration, proliferation, and organization essential for tissue regeneration [1]. Diverse technologies have been devised to construct three-dimensional biological models, tackling these issues. The technologies include the rotating method, the hanging drop technique, the microfluidic system, the forced-floating method, scaffold utilization, and 3D bioprinting.

Among all the methods, 3D bioprinting has emerged as the most promising technology for fabricating three-dimensional biological structures using biomaterials, demonstrating significant potential in the production of functioning biological tissues, even at its nascent stage [2]. Four principal bioprinting technologies exist: droplet-based bioprinting (DBB) [3], extrusion-based bioprinting (EBB) [4], vat polymerization [5], and laser-based bioprinting (LBB) [6]. This review will concentrate on LAB, given its distinctive design, significant promise, and unique technical hurdles, although all printing principles are applicable in tissue regeneration.

This chapter provides a comprehensive examination of LBB, detailing various modalities, including photopolymerization methods and cell transfer methodologies. A comprehensive analysis is presented to the reader, elucidating the merits and drawbacks of LBB in comparison to other bioprinting techniques, such as EBB and DBB. Recent significant studies are emphasized, and prospects are outlined for the reader.

9.2 Modalities of Laser-Based Bioprinting

LBB procedures can be categorized into two primary submodalities depending on their operational mechanisms: (1) processes utilizing photopolymerization and (2) processes reliant on cell transfer.

9.2.1 Photopolymerization-Based Processes

The process entails directing light into a reservoir containing photocurable materials; this causes the liquid monomers and oligomers to photopolymerize at a target location on the building platform. Stereolithography (SLA) and digital light processing (DLP) are the two components that make up this approach. See other evaluations for further details on the structural orientation and design architecture of these tools. Carbon 3D Inc.'s recently developed resin-bath technique, continuous liquid interface production (CLIP), allows 3D printing at speeds up to 100 times quicker than those of DLP and SLA.

9.2.1.1 Stereolithography (SLA)

In 1986, Chuck Hull proposed the first SLA 3D printer. Using SLA, solid layers are printed one after the other using a device that employs a movable photon source to start the photopolymerization of photocurable resin. The earliest photocurable materials utilized for SLA applications were methyl ethyl hydroquinone/triallyl phosphate to avoid premature polymerization, benzophenone as a photoinitiator, and urethane dimethacrylate (UDMA) mixed with a tiny amount of acrylic acid. There are now a number of photocurable materials that may be used in a variety of fields and have been developed and used in the SLA 3D printing process. It is possible to get high-quality objects with a resolution as fine as 10 µm with SLA. Using a 3D printer based on SLA, complex and high-resolution objects, like a human ear, were created for tissue engineering applications. It is also possible to create 3D things with organic-inorganic hybrid structures, such as formulations that are ferromagnetically sensitive, using the SLA method.

In the SLA process, a bioink solution including cells embedded in a photocurable medium is introduced into a vat with a porous platform attached to an elevating mechanism that regulates the platform's position along the *z*-axis. In order to instantly polymerize the bioink, the substrate in the first layer is positioned in line with the outer layer of the bioink solution and exposed to UV radiation. A three-dimensional polymeric network is produced during photopolymerization by the interaction of monomers or weakly cross-linked polymers, whether they are liquid or solid. The inhalation of a photon by a photoinitiator results in the formation of radicals that react with monomers, hence initiating radical polymerization [7]. The photoreaction concludes when two radicals interact, which transpires in areas subjected to irradiation. The entire layer is scanned according to the toolpath derived from the computer-aided design (CAD) model. Upon the completion of a layer's solidification, the porous table descends by an amount equivalent to the thickness of that layer, facilitating the printing of the subsequent layer. The procedure continues consistently until the whole tissue construct is assembled. The figure 9.1 shows the schematic diagram of laser based bioprinting.

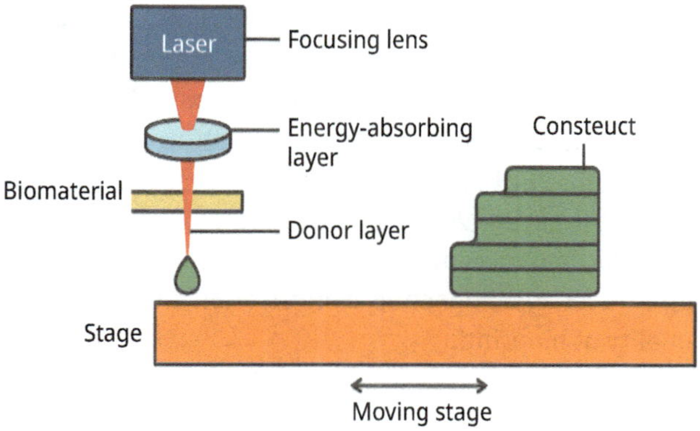

Figure 9.1: Structure and components of LBB.

SLA facilitates the bioprinting of tissue structures varying in dimensions from a few hundred micrometers to several millimeters [8]. A very first demonstration of applying SLA in bioprinting was conducted by [9]. Using SLA-250, a 3D printer, they embedded Chinese hamster ovary cells CHO-B2 in polyethylene oxide and polyethylene glycol dimethacrylate (PEGDMA) hydrogels to create tubular structures. The research demonstrated over 90% cell vitality, with the authors indicating that an increase in photoinitiator concentration inside the hydrogel solution resulted in reduced cell viability by the second day. A comparable methodology was used where 8 utilized a similar 3D printer outfitted with a HeCd laser for the encapsulation of 3T3 fibroblasts into PEGDMA hydrogels. Several channels were bioprinted with cylindrical scaffolds, possibly applicable in the creation of nerve conduits. The same group also showed the production of multimaterial scaffolds in complex geometries using a self-aligning minisetup. In order to promote neovascularization in the chorioallantoic membrane of chick embryos, Kitana et al. [7] used a similar technique, encasing 3T3 fibroblasts in microvascular stamps prepared from PEGDMA hydrogels and polyethylene glycol diacrylate (PEGDA) using a commercial SLA printer. In order to promote neovessel formation within chorioallantoic membranes, the authors showed that adding 12-*O*-tetradecanoylphorbol-13-acetate, a protein kinase C activator, to the printed samples increased the manifestation of several angiogenic factors, such as vascular endothelial growth factor and endothelin-1. The photocurable material in SLA determines the process's resolution and cure rate. It must exhibit certain biological, mechanical, and chemical qualities to facilitate various tissue production applications. In this context, the appropriate selection of photocurable materials, curing agents, solvents, bioreagents, and light absorbers is essential for designing the ideal procedure. A diverse array of photopolymers is used in SLA, including acrylates containing urethane units and various dialkylacrylamides, notably trimethylolpropane triacrylate. To enhance the solidification process and mechanical stability, photoinitiators in conjunction with photocurable hydrogels have been used for tissue constructions due to their low photodissociation energy. Nonetheless, photoinitiators are not often used in bioprinting because of their toxicity, which might adversely affect the cells. The least harmful photoinitiator, Irgacure 2959 (2-hydroxy-1-[4-(2-hydroxyethoxy) phenyl]-2-methyl-1-propanone), exhibits cytotoxicity at doses exceeding 0.5% [11], resulting in only 25% cell viability after one day in an aqueous PEGDMA resin. Alternative research suggests a concentration of less than 0.1% for Irgacure 2959 [12]; however, employing such a low concentration may lead to diminished mechanical properties, excessive swelling, and an increased curing depth, adversely impacting solidification in subsequent layers and compromising the quality of bioprinting.

9.2.1.2 Digital Light Projection (DLP/Dynamic Optical Projection)

Dynamic SLA optical projection is a projection printing technique that works without a physical mask, utilizing a digital micromirror device (DMD), which is commonly found in regular computer projectors. The DLP SLA process diagram is presented in Figure 9.2. Many research groups have examined the implementation of dynamic masks in micro-stereolithography (mSLA) to accelerate the manufacturing process. A liquid crystal display (LCD) was proposed as a dynamic mask to manufacture double-end collector fluidic components and springs [13]. Using LCD projectors in mSLA helps in micropatterning PEGDA and allows the adhesion of endothelial cells (ECs). Due to the constrained optical efficiency of LCD, Chen and his colleagues employed the DMD methodology, which provides superior performance regarding optical fill factors – 85% for DMD compared to 64% for LCD – and light transmission, achieving 71% with DMD versus 21% with LCD [14]. The system functions similarly to a conventional SLA system, using a UV source (365 nm) to polymerize photocurable materials.

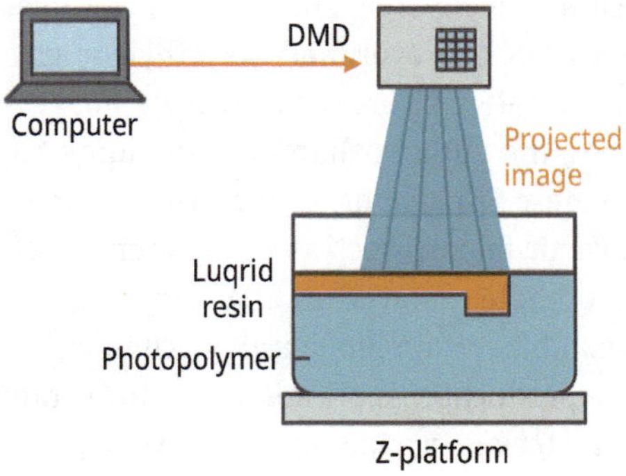

Figure 9.2: Dynamical optical projection SLA.

Unlike the static, inflexible, and expensive masks used in the photolithography process, DMD devices can create digital masks that allow for programmable and interchangeable patterns. A DMD's digital mirrors (or micromirrors), with a 1920 × 1,080 resolution, bounce UV light according to a digitized pattern. Sousa AC et al. [15] created a photomask using a sequence of PowerPoint digital slides. Each chip has a micromirror matrix composed of aluminum-coated mirrors that can tilt 12° in the positive and negative axes (or 12°ove and below the chip surface). Each of the mirrors can be set to spin so that they can be in one of two states: "on" or "off." When a mirror is "off," the UV light is diverted to a light-blocking pixel, creating a dark pixel. A motorized *z*-axis adds a third dimension to the scaffold and can adjust the *z*-axis in traditional layer-by-layer 3D printing. The primary benefit of the DOPsL approach compared to other SLA-based bioprinting methods is its speed, as each layer can be produced simultaneously in seconds, a process that is much more intricate when using serial writing in single-photon polymerization. It facilitates the accurate production of scaffolds with convoluted interior structures. Nonetheless, the primary constraint, in contrast to single- or two-photon polymerization (2PP), is its inadequate resolution stemming from the limitations of the projection lens. Another system's constraint is the significant consumption of photocurable materials, which include costly biological reagents and must be fed into the vat, leading to losses during the loading and unloading processes. In addition, regulating the thickness of individual layers is difficult without incorporating a light-absorbing component into the bioink. The authors described perfluorohexane (C6F14), which is dense (1.685 g/cm^3), inert, and has lower molecular polarity than the photocurable material, as a support material [16].

The authors modified the build platform to use support material. Perfluorohexane was initially added to the vat, allowing space at the top for the photocurable material. The motorized z-stage has been submerged in perfluorohexane to remove the uncured material after the photocurable material had hardened on the vat's surface as a result of laser irradiation. In order to add the next layer, the stage was elevated. This process was repeated until the entire scaffold was constructed. Given that oxygen can act as a strong radical scavenger and can adversely affect polymerization at low initiator levels, the researchers examined the effects of oxygen exclusion. A nitrogen atmosphere was employed that increased the rate of gelation and, as a result, the speed of bioprinting. However, the leaking of the system caused inconsistencies during the curing phase.

Using the DOPsL approach, Chen and co-authors have developed several multiday bioprinted cellular scaffolds. Bioprinting enables the precise observation of the shape of a designed vascular system, including cancer cell migration within that printed vascular network [17]. PEGDA hydrogel encapsulated both HeLa cells and nonmalignant 10 T1/2 fibroblasts, with highly detailed vascular chambers produced. At a narrowed width of the vascular channel, the migration of HeLa cells was significantly reduced. Recently, they showed for the first time the bioprinting of a liver model that includes the use of encapsulated hepatic progenitor cells (iPSC-HPCs) of human pluripotent stem cell origin with supportive cells (human umbilical vein endothelial cells (HUVECs) and adipose-derived stem cells) within double layers of gelatin methacrylate (GelMA). Moreover, they have bioprinted hexagonal structures with HUVECs with labels of green fluorescent protein, which gave evidence of the growth of HUVECs as they progressed in time [18].

9.2.1.3 Two-Photon Polymerization (TPP)

SLA has great resolution along the lateral (*xy*) axes which has proven useful in the manufacturing of microscale structures; however, the same cannot be said of the depth profile resolution. Depth profile resolution of SLA is limited compared to the lateral resolution. SLA resolution also varies with the diameter of the focus spot. Due to diffraction limit, the smallest features that can be manufactured are about half the wave of the applied laser. However, because the technique of SLA has limited capabilities, the best obtainable lateral resolution is in the range of several microns [19, 25]. This has resulted in the development of 2PP such that, in order to improve resolution, it is possible to focus a pair of photons on a single point at the same time, effectively localizing the polymerization region to three dimensions [20]. During 2PP, high resolution of structures beyond the diffraction limit was obtained where the feature size has been reduced by an order of magnitude to less than 50 nm compared to the laser wavelength. As opposed to single-photon polymerization, a single photon with a sufficiently high energy level will excite a fluorophore in multiphoton polymerization, but many more photons are used with a relatively low energy level. Multiphoton absorption is probable with a power that is second to that of the laser and, as a result, necessitates the simultaneous absorption of a large number of photons. Very high peak intensities might be reached using femtosecond pulsed lasers at relatively small average power, making them suitable and widely applied to 2PP. 2PP in bioprinting cannot be used as it has a higher resolution than the normal size of human cells; it has also been employed in tissue engineering, where high-resolution scaffolds have been created. In the beginning, various implementations of the multiphoton approach within biological hydrogels demonstrated spatial patterning of bioactive components within preformed photoactive materials in three dimensions [2]. After allowing physiologically active ingredients in low molecular mass PEGDA or acrylate-PEG-peptide with photoinitiator solution to permeate into PEGDA hydrogel, the physiologically active ingredients embedded in the PEGDA hydrogel were solidified using the multiphoton photopolymerization technique with a digital mask. Additionally, the scientists showed how the HT-1080 cells infiltrated the whole construct's acrylate-PEG-eRGDS-patterned regions. In addition to the above-mentioned hydrogel, a limited number of materials have been exploited in 2PP, such as commercially available ORMOCOMP and SU8 elements that encourage cell growth and expansion as well as facilitate in formation cell-cell junctions. When these commercial materials were utilized, made porous tissue scaffolds, three-dimensional strip-like structures (pulmonary alveoli-like structures), and hollow microneedles to be used in transdermal drug delivery. The primary benefit of this system is that it functions at room temperature, thereby preventing the denaturation of proteins and other bioactive molecules. In addition, costly clean room facilities are not required to apply the technique. This can be combined with the high-definition technology to drive a nanoscale resolution, thus providing the hybrid bioprinting platform with the capability of creating nanosized features to control adhesion and orientation within a three-dimensional setting. An example is shown in Figure 9.3, where a two-step 2PP process produced multiscale constructions consisting of a protein-repellent PEGDA framework and protein-coating Ormocomp cubes to allow cell attachment. Such an environment allowed for the control of cell cultures in 3D with custom adhesion positions.

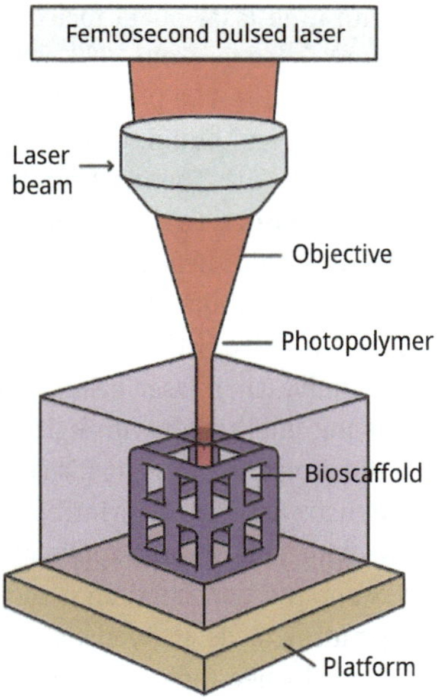

Figure 9.3: Two-step two-photon polymerization process.

The demonstrated bioprinting of live cells with the use of 2PP. Human osteosarcoma MG63 cells were encapsulated by photoinitiators of water-soluble variants (two benzylidene cycloketone-based) (G2CK and P2CK) in 20 percent methacrylamide-derivatized gelatin (gelMOD), thereby making it possible to print Yin-Yang symbols. The results show that approximately only a quarter of cells survived within the voids of the Ying-Yang structures due to serious cellular damage caused by the reactive species produced during 2PP. However, 95% of the cells that were cultured beyond the laser-treated areas survived, and even cells that were entrapped within the pores of the Ying-Yang scaffolds prospered during the 3-week in vitro culture.

9.2.2 Cell-Transfer-Based Processes

In LBB procedures that involve cell transfer, the technique of relocating live cells from a particular location to another, regardless of culture media or viscoelastic hydrogels, which include alginate and Matrigel, is employed to bioprint cells.

9.2.2.1 Laser-Guidance Direct Writing

For bioprinting living cells, LGDW is the oldest LBB technology used. The first cell patterning done in 2D by using laser-induced optical forces was done by Odde and Renn in 1999. To control thousands of particles, Odde and Renn used laser beam focusing and applied the particle control technique by Ashkin and Dziedzic from 1987, who were the first to work on optical forces and particle control issues. The patterning of an array of different organic and inorganic particles, gaseous and liquid, before the deposition of the live cells was depicted by the authors before [21]. The most fundamental aspect of the relationship between light and cells is the refractive index of the cells relative to the surrounding medium; the greater the disparities between the two, the better the interactions will be. That is why the scientists named the method laser-guided direct writing (LGDW) since there is no guiding structure, such as a mask, which is present in the bioprinting process. During that study, when laser beam was weakly focused, cells were added into the media. Following interaction with light, a cell produced a gradient force that instantly drew it in the direction of the light's center, where the intensity was greatest. The authors demonstrated that bioprinting of embryonic chick spinal cord cells took place at 11.4 mm/s with 1 pN of force applied to the cells [22]. The cell was then driven axially in the beam and deposited on a substrate of interest, for example, a coverslip. After bioprinting, cells showed typical characteristics of proliferation and cell spreading, which confirmed their tolerance to the laser irradiation applied. The authors explained the 2D patterning whereby they would vary the orientation by just repositioning the low numerical aperture focusing lens and changing the focal point to a spot near where it previously was before by moving it through the micromanipulator. The cells were deposited with a mean rate of 2.5 cells/min, and clusters or individual cells were printed. This rate is significantly lower than what is accomplished with contemporary LBB techniques like laser-induced forward transfer (LIFT). The major limitation of such a coarse setup was that there was only a low transmission range of about 300 mm, as the beam divergence and the force of the fluid stream exerted overcame the optical force [23]. Utilizing the hollow optical fiber allowed the scientists to simplify the light transmission, which was in the same process of transmission of cells inside the fiber core, in order to support the increased deposition of cells and achieve longer travel distances in the centimeter range. The cells were transported at a mean speed of 53 mm/s along fibers having an inner diameter of 100 mm.

9.2.2.2 Matrix-Assisted Pulsed-Laser Evaporation-Direct Write (MAPLE-DW)

In the late 1990s, MAPLE (matrix-assisted pulsed-laser evaporation) was developed by the US Naval Research Laboratory to implement thin coatings of different types of functional materials, including biomaterials, chemoselective polymers, and other organic materials [24]. When compared to traditional lasers, the laser-guided direct write process offers much more flexibility during fluidic integration operations because of the gradient forces created by the laser pulse, where the cells are captured by the force applied by the pulse and directed to a coverslip. A micromanipulator, three-axis with a low geometric aperture lens, is mounted to deposit cells serially and produce patterns by printing out sequentially. The delivery distance of cells is restricted to 300 mm, and thus, a fused silica hollow optical fiber is used to guide the laser beam and the cells. This fiber is positioned on a spacer of glass coverslips, aligning coaxially with the long axis of the fiber and the axis of the laser beam. Laser-based bioprinting 176 pulsed laser deposition, MAPLE can be utilized to deposit a wide range of organic and polymeric materials, with a lower to higher molecular weight range, with little or no damage to the transition of the condensed substance into the vapor phase gaining [25]. MAPLE acts the same way, except the solubilizing event occurs within a matrix, typically a solvent, for instance, alcohol. This is then frozen to the order of −196 °C to form a laser target. The photon energy that strikes the target when a laser pulse strikes it is transformed into thermal energy and then absorbed by the solvent's organic molecules. The desorption of chemicals in the matrix and their discriminating transfer to the collector depend on a pattern preselected by the user, which is the result of these molecules' increased kinetic energy and appearance of a gaseous state. Consequently, the molecules of volatile solvents with poor adhesion coefficients are sucked clean in the vacuum chamber, resulting in the deposition of a thin layer. Without denaturing the inherent chemical structure or biological function, the MAPLE technique improves direct chemical transfer. According to the research, the temperature of the material that makes the matrix influences the film shape and other characteristics of the film [26]. The correct manifestation of MAPLE technology cannot be applied to the live-cell bioprinting process because the live cells cannot be embedded in the matrix due to the toxicity of the solvent. The hostile nature of live cells to the combination of incompatible materials of cryogenic apparatus, heated substrate, and vacuum chamber provides such an environment. The nature of bioprinting was adapted to incorporate viable cells as well. The cells are initially drawn in bioink solution, and it forms a thin layer beneath a ribbon. Thus, the technique got improved further and evolved into a practical process of bioprinting live cells.

The MAPLE-DW process uses MAPLE technology to coat biomatter and thin film hydrogels onto the quartz back piece (print ribbon). The quartz serves the function of absorbing the laser's wavelength. The ribbon and biomaterial ribbon contact absorb the majority of the laser energy. This counteracts DNA damage caused by the laser's UV rays. To check whether the gelatin-based writing caused double-strand break DNA damage, Corr and coworkers conducted DNA damage tests [27]. Bioprinted fibroblasts revealed strong Hoechst nuclear staining with no colocalization to phosphor-H2AX which shows there were no double-strand DNA breaks in fibroblasts. In MAPLE-DW, it uses different levels of laser powers at the coated material ablation threshold [11]. The laser beam is focused at the boundary of the coated material (sublimated part) and the quartz support, and as a result of rapid localized heating and the high-pressure vapor formation, a bubble of moving plasma is created. The formed bubble rises, and as a result, the coating material is ejected and deposited onto the collecting substrate. Choosing the coating material for rheological properties, thickness, and laser fluence can improve the generation process of plasma bubbles and the jets produced. Only a small number of hydrogels are used as coating materials for LBB, such as alginate [23], and gelatin [24]. Laser parameters bioink will cause a jet to form, which can be either thick or thin, and will then break apart into one or several droplets and be drawn back to the coating. Standard MAPLE-DW systems use a UV pulsed laser that is low-powered and emits a short pulse of about 8 ns. This pulse creates a bubble that aids jet displacement and coating/substrate material exchange. An effective distance of roughly 200–7,000 mm is sufficient to pattern live cells [24]. Figure 9.4 shows the bioprinting and patterning of several cell types that were previously plated onto a ribbon surface coated with a triazene dynamic release layer or Matrigel.

9.2.2.3 Laser-Induced Forward Transfer (LIFT)

LIFT is a version of MAPLE-DW where cells are embedded in a coating material onto a quartz plate. The quartz plate is moved so that the coating material is adjacent to, or in direct contact with, a second substrate; the two substrates must not be separated. The cells remain trapped within the coating material. Unlike MAPLE-DW, LIFT has an energy-absorbing interlayer of an IR-transparent material, essentially a thin layer (10–50 nm) of metals (Ag, Ti, and Au), metal oxides (TiO_2), or photodecomposing volatile polymers (triazene) [28]. The medium layer of light absorption saves well the negative impacts of the strong UV light, therefore increasing the usage of this technology and declining the production of dependence on MAPLE-DW. An apparatus that uses laser can consist of four major parts, in particular: CAD software, laser system, car-

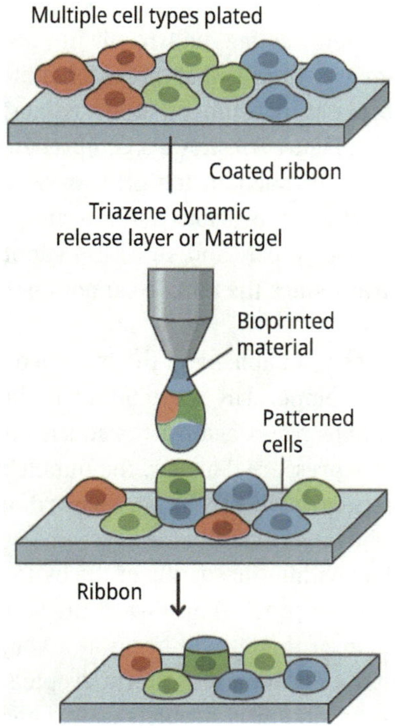

Figure 9.4: Bioprinting and patterning of multiple cell types.

tridge, and substrate, where the design of a cartridge plays a crucial role in the bioprinting of cells effectively. Three main layers are present within the cartridge, meaning that there is a translucent quartz support that holds the entire construction. The quartz substrate has a thin coat of gold, usually applied on the underside. Before incubation, an initial layer of bioink solution is spread beneath the gold layer. One solution could be either spin coating or blade coating where the aim is to obtain a uniform coating of the bioink. The importance of coating is to obtain the desired thickness of the bioink layer since it can affect the size of the bioink droplets. Therefore, coating, as well as its viscoelastic stability, has to be controlled so that files on the LIFT process can be resumed [28]. Meanwhile, due to gravity, cells during the bioprinting process settle at the bottom of the bioink solution which creates patchy effects in the cell printing. With regard to the laser that strikes the clear quartz substrate, it is common that the majority of the laser power gets absorbed by the intermediate layer and is focused at the junction of the absorption layer and the coating. This leads to an increase in temperature which ultimately creates a vapor bubble. The vapor bubble expands as it gets more energy and creates a jet that further extrudes the bioink from the substrate.

LIFT has three prospective regimes. The first of which is the subthreshold regime. This is where the laser is not intense enough and is shown to resemble the shapes of an annulus or coffee ring which is an effect caused by the evaporation of droplets on a surface. Modifying the bioink parameters such as laser fluence and laser pulse energy, which is directed at establishing a specific jetting regime, will result in optimized productive jetting. A characteristic of a high-energy laser is that it sees a bubble bursting. At the same time, the film begins the process of detachment, and it is most noticeable in the indicator locality (point of the laser). Figure 9.5 shows a comprehensive schematic of bubble dynamics and jet production throughout the LIFT process. Regional vaporization of the bioink solution between the subconscious and intermediate layers is being carried out by the nanosecond laser pulse, and since the vapor starts expanding, it can only do so toward the substrate, since the bubble cannot force its way through the quartz support.

The bioink sticking to the intermediate layer stops the bubble and the intermediate layer from pulling apart, and the contact angle is temporarily set to 90° [29]. The contact angle will continue to increase until the bubble grows against the substrate, reaching the vapor pressure equilibrium over the air pressure. Further, the bubble's increased volume results in decreased vapor pressure. However, the tip forward of the advance does not stop because of inertia and the momentum obtained.

Kinetic energy of the vapor is translated into flow within the coating of the bioink that, in turn, causes the moving tip to pull on the entire protrusion toward the substrate, causing the vapor bubble to collapse. Creation of the jet will begin at a very thin tip, which will gradually grow to the point when it decomposes to form droplets. The Rayleigh principle states that the conditions of formation of droplets start when the jet circumference becomes bigger than the perturbation wavelength. For the first time, time-resolved imaging was used by 22, to analyze the kinetics of jet formation and transport hydrogels (without substrate model). Two laser fluences were used in the study: 1.6 J/cm^2 and 2.7 J/cm^2. Protrusion started to develop after 2 ms of laser illumination and continued to extend in the following 5 ms. A jet formation started after 7 ms, and the protrusion was reduced to 10 ms. At 20 ms, the interaction between the flow of hydrogel around the ablation point and collapsing vapor bubble led to the formation of a bulge at the end of the jet [30]. In only 330 ms, the jet then drastically diminished and disintegrated into droplets, before its attractive aspect returned. When the fluence level was quite high (2.7 J/cm^2), the process of jet generation altered significantly. Firstly, the outgrowth was bigger and longer in the earlier stage of jet development. At increased laser fluence, the diameter of the jet was larger than in the case of lowered laser fluence. After a bulge formed in the top portion of the jet in 20 ms, it encircled into a characteristic conic shape. With time, the jet profile shifted; it first broadened at about 330 ms and then narrowed between 20 and 50 ms. Over 670 ms caused the jet to split into a single droplet, which had a much bigger volume than at lower laser fluence. The operation concluded after 690 ms, and the protrusion vanished. The jet was fatter, faster, and had a longer duration when the laser fluence was 2.7 J/cm^2 as opposed to the low fluence of 1.6 J/cm^2.

9.2.2.4 Droplet Impingement onto the Substrate

The LIFT technique uses laser tools to obtain droplets that are placed over a substrate, just like DBB methods. In turn, the tendency of droplets to hit the substrate is necessary because it determines the accuracy of bioprinting and the moldability of three-dimensional objects. There are three main characteristics of droplet impingement observed in LBB hydrogels: splashing, spreading, and rebounding characteristics. In splashing, a droplet will separate into smaller secondary droplets as a result of hitting a substance; in spreading, the droplet spreads out in terms of surface area; and in rebounding, the droplet may bounce back off the surface. Rebound is, however, suppressed with the application of viscoelastic hydrogels (such as alginate) owing to their high viscosity of elongation [30]. The significant value of droplet splashing or spreading is called crucial (We) by Weber, and it is denoted as

$$W_e = \frac{\rho d U^2}{\sigma} \tag{9.1}$$

where ρ is the density of liquid, d the characteristic length of diameter of the droplet, U the velocity, and s the surface tension. The higher the Weber number the more there are chances of splashing, and the lower the Weber number the more spreading comes to be. Along with outside importance of these features to the creation of droplets, the properties of the substrate on the collector like wettability of the surfaces, Zhang, and the roughness of the surfaces as well as viscous forces are very important to the process. Rahman et al. [30] made a novel study focused on the impingement of alginate droplets in case of LBB. The authors have shown that critical Weber numbers of 2%, 4%, 6%, and 8% solutions of alginate are 2,993, 3,331, 5,102, and 13,657, respectively. Respective significant Weber numbers are associated with laser intensities of 1,300, 1,700, 1,900, and 2,500 mJ/cm^2. The group then went on to show bioprinting of 3T3 fibroblasts, whose opening had been blocked by 2% sodium alginate, into a $CaCl_2$ pool creating Y-shaped vascular constructs containing a wall thickness greater than one millimeter, by studying further droplet impingement and its applicability to large-scale tissue fabrication. To conclude, LBB photopolymerization together with cell transfer protocols has interesting advantages and disadvantages in relation to each other.

9.3 Toward Multimaterial and Multidimensional Bioprinting

The majority of the LBB strategies rely on only one type of bioink due to the challenge related to producing multimaterial tissue constructs. Creation of heterocellular patterns is a daunting task owing to the use of one type of bioink in the whole process.

The most common property of natural tissue is its heterocellularity; numerous different types of cells are located in this extremely elaborate structure [11]; the future LBB solutions should resolve this difficulty. In that regard, two primary methodologies were proposed, one regarding SLA and the new regarding LIFT technology. The group of Wicker developed a carousel of the rotating vat system of SLA, which involved the circulation of different materials on a rotating cord by utilizing a commercial machine of 3D systems 250/50 SLA [20]. In this way, various materials were consolidated into a single item. The researchers validated the related technology, where the scaffolds of multimaterial tissues hydrogels were made from PEGDMA or PEGDA and fluorescently labeled dextran. In their paper, a minivat type of machine was made for the cleaning and washing of the printed scaffolds, for the loading and removal of a new photocurable material. Mask-image-projection-based SLA also had similar attempts when a prototype device was made with the first composed of a rotational system with two materials, two brushes, a cleaner, and a dryer; however, the use of that sort of technology in the biomedical field remains unexplored. Wang J et al. (202) proposed a high-resolution location technology, which fits under a carousel holder and has a capacity to support five different ribbons [34]. Ribbons can spin around a holder called a carousel with a motorized system, which provides flexibility for more movement. This process enables the switchable assembly of multiple ribbons of different bioink materials to create heterocellular tissue constructs, on demand. The proposed automation has not taken place in spite of the vision of the authors as a pragmatic approach. Table 9.1 summarizes the LBB approaches and compares their abilities and properties, such as laser spot size, settings, minimum size of printed feature, cell survival, bioink printability, and their facility and limitations.

9.4 Comparison of Laser-Based Other Modalities

The LBB is nozzle free and addresses some of the limitations of the already established bioprinting technologies, such as EBB [31] and the majority of DBB techniques, except for acoustic-based bioprinting [15]. This is one property that negates the issue of damage and perishing of cells due to shear stress. This is more of the case during DBB and EBB, when the nozzle diameter is minimal or when the bioink falls under the high-viscosity range. Concerns about high viscosity are key to direct bioprinting (DBB), as virtually all bioink materials currently available to support EBB cannot be adapted to DBB, but can be applied to LBB. DBB has a bioink substance that has the propensity to block the nozzle or the tube linking the reservoir to the nozzle. This involves cleaning of nozzle tip, bioink fill, and calibration of bioprinting device, which is a cumbersome procedure and can in some cases cause damaged, costly nozzles or cartridge head irreparably. The encapsulation of cells into each single droplet is limited by the intense shear stress and the droplet generation procedure to a minimal

Table 9.1: Comparison of bioprinting processes.

Laser bioprinting process	Laser modality and spot size	Conditions	Smallest feature size	Cell viability	Bioink printability	Strengths	Limitations
Stereolithography (SLA)	UV/visible laser; spot ~ 50–200 μm	Curing in a vat, temperature control	~50 μm	Generally high (>85%)	Photocurable hydrogels only	High throughput; continuous constructs; smooth surfaces	Constrained to photoinks; UV may harm cells; resin scarcity
Dynamic optical projection stereolithography (DOPsL/DLP/CLIP)	Digital projector or scanning laser; similar spot size	Vat-based, projected layers or volumetric	~50 μm or less	High (comparable to SLA)	Photocurable bioresins	Rapid layer curing; high fidelity and structural continuity	Same resin limits; light scattering depth; specialized equipment
Two-photon polymerization (2PP/TPP)	Femtosecond laser; submicron focal spot (<1 μm)	High-intensity focus in inert/controlled atm.	~0.1 μm or less	Very high (>95%)	Limited to photopolymerizable resins	Ultra-high resolution; arbitrary 3D geometries at microscale	Slow build, small volume, expensive systems
Laser-induced forward transfer (LIFT)	Pulsed laser; spot ~10–100 μm	Donor ribbon with metal layer; ambient	~10–20 μm	High (~80–95%)	Wide viscosity range; cell suspensions, hydrogels	Nozzle free; good viability; supports varied bioinks	Complex ribbon prep; lower throughput; costly setups
Absorbing film-assisted LIFT and BioLP	Pulsed laser; similar to LIFT	Thicker metal film (~75–100 nm); donor ribbon	~10–20 μm	High (~85–95%)	Same as LIFT	More stable transfer; minimized heat damage	Same as LIFT

(continued)

Table 9.1 (continued)

Laser bioprinting process	Laser modality and spot size	Conditions	Smallest feature size	Cell viability	Bioink printability	Strengths	Limitations
Matrix-assisted pulsed-laser evaporation-direct write (MAPLE-DW)	UV pulsed laser; ~10–50 µm	UV-transparent ribbon with biofilm; ambient	~20 µm	70–90%	Requires frozen or supported biofilm	Gentle transfer; CAD-controlled; precise single-cell/few-cell patterning	Limited bioink types; elaborate prep; lower speed
Laser-guided direct writing (LGDW)	Continuous IR laser; ~1–5 µm	Focused beam in sterile medium; optical trap	~1 µm	High (>90%)	Cell suspensions only	Single-cell precision; dynamic path control	

amount. In contrast, LBB allows bioprinting more cells, as it does not have the limitations described above. It is particularly beneficial to generating patterns of higher resolutions and more cell densities, which EBB cannot accomplish. The other major advantage of LBB is its higher resolution, which is higher than both DBB and EBB because the latter has a low resolution. The DBB has a dependent resolution of the droplet size, approximately 50 mm that covers one or two cells. In contrast, the LBB allows one to achieve a minimal resolution with a nozzle-less technique down to 10 mm. Although based on crafting a bioprint using a 20-mm nozzle tip that bioprints live-cell targets, DBB cannot do precise positioning of the cells due to the wide output width of the nozzle, which imposes excessive limitations on the effectiveness of manipulating the spacing of the deposited cells. Moreover, unlike the other cell encapsulation methods, in DBB, 186 3D bioprinting, the proportion of cells encapsulated inside each droplet is greatly reliant on the uncontrolled number of cells contained within each droplet on the statistical probability, which is random. Such small resolution ranges are not achievable even under the use of EBB. LBB high-resolution capacity will enable better control of intercellular communication and placement of individual cells. LBB, especially LIFT and MAPLE-DW, has the added benefit of being a non-contact therapy technique that is comparable to DBB. In situ bioprinting of tissues in surgical contexts (such as skin or cranio-maxillofacial surgery) has much promise because to this. It is not possible to physically design the cells within the structure, and damage or faults may be filled in layer by layer. Collisions between printheads and bioprinted structures and other cancelable overbuilds are part of the case with EBB (Ebb Bioprinter). Even with such problems, [7] demonstrated bioprinting nanohydroxyapatite (HA) particles into the calvarial gaps of murine models. With the contactless feature, LBB (laser bioprinter) processes alleviate the out of control challenges of the space between the bioprinter and the receiving substrate. Unlike EBB and DBB, which stand vertically, some forms of LBB,, and MAPLE-DW (matrix-assisted pulsed laser evaporation-direct write) flow in the horizontal direction. Tao et al. [8] demonstrate multiple LIFT studies, where the donor substrate is oriented vertically and the jet is positioned horizontally. This setup is especially suited for the use of stroboscopic imaging, which offers a wide range of imaging systems, and for the analysis of jet structures and the thermodynamics related to the jet. Biolithography is a new field of research that uses direct light processing (DLP) and top-down bioprinting. Although the top-down approach would be more accurate and reduce the surface waves of the photocurable material, there is no evidence that any benefit would be achieved when employing this method in DBB or EBB at this point. This could help to print more complex geometries which require support material due to their need to support their weight, but, when bioprinted using a top-down approach, do not require it.

9.5 Recent Achievements in LBB

Although layered bioprinting (LBB) is older than almost all bioprinting technologies (including EBB and DBB), it is not as advanced as many other technologies. Recently, some of the most notable advancements in the field of LBB have been made. For example, Tripathi et al. [5] illustrated the LIFT bioprinting of MG-63 osteosarcoma cells and layer-by-layer electrospun polycaprolactone bioprinting.

The electrospun layer of sodium alginate was 100 mm thick, and the MG-63 cells were plated onto it three times to create tissue structures that were about 300 mm thick and could be deposited onto the calvarial abnormalities. The cells in the printed scaffolds of tissues greatly proliferated. Even though certain tissue constructions display fibrous tissue formation and capsule surrounding structures with minimal bone integration, the study demonstrated the large-scale production of laser-inkjet-bioprinted constructs and the overcoming of one of the primary limitations of LIFT. Mei et al. [4] cultivated human umbilical vein endothelial cells (HUVECs) and human mesenchymal stem cells using a LIFT technique with polyester urethane urea (PEUU); engineered constructs were implanted into the infarcted zones of LAD ligated rat (infarcted region) hearts. Eight weeks post-implantation, constructs demonstrating patterns generated by the LIFT technique had a higher degree of vascularization compared to the constructs with cells that were randomly bioprinted, and the bioprinted myocardial patch significantly enhanced functional recovery of the myocardium. Besides the primary cells, a scaffold with human cardiac-derived cardiomyocyte progenitor cells (hCMPCs) was also bioprinted [4]. The hCMPCs that were bioprinted showed cardiac-like structures and were positive for the early cardiac markers Nkx2.5, Gata-4, and Mef-2c. In the ex vivo tissue, there was an outpouring of arteries and lymphatic conduits. Fibroblasts were also printed along with cancer cells because they support the migration of the cancer cells. The study established that the potential of the transplantation of cancer cells onto ex vivo tissues in viable form was successful, with proliferation of metastatic MDA-MB-231 cells to a great extent [9]. Remarkably, the vascular network was observed to form new capillaries; bioprinting of cancer cells elicited angiogenic sprouting. The study described above depicts the printing of cells adsorbed onto ex vivo tissues, and this is of great potential to gain insights into the nature of cancer progression and proliferation; however, there is a significant limitation when it comes to bioprinting onto ex vivo tissues in three dimensions. Few cells, such as cancer cells, have the ability to infiltrate stromal tissue and circulate within the blood, including the lymphatic system. In situ bioprinting has the prospect of enhancing the reconstruction of damaged tissue by directly bioprinting the cells into the site of the defect. This article became the first demonstration of bioprinting by LBB in live animal models, but with extremely insignificant bone regeneration.

9.6 Limitations

The LBB devices have high resolution and can pattern live cells precisely, and cells can maintain their pattern in less than 5.6 mm difference along the original pattern during LIFT process. Such accuracy is impossible to achieve with any other bioprinting technology, and LIFT becomes the desired process to bioprint microcellular structures in organs and tissues, including microvasculature. Despite its great resolution, LBB cannot be characterized as perfect. Long production times, cell–laser interaction, costly equipment, and the requirement of photo-cross-linkable bioink materials are impediments to photopolymerization processes. The procedure of cell transfer is faced with various shortcomings, which are cell deformation by heat and laser shocks, constraints in three-dimensional bioprinting, costly laser equipment, and cell drop due to gravitational and stochastic settling in the precursor solution. Regarding the density and uniformity of the loaded cells, SLA has several limitations. Due to an insufficient means of using hydrogels and the cytotoxic properties of photoinitiators, primarily, only simple and weak structures can be created, with the exception of PEGDA, which can create a rigid structure. The elastic modulus in these constructions is frequently lower than 1 kPa, which is reduced to the engineering of soft tissues only. The long time taken to produce scale-up models could cause negative impacts on the cells under prolonged printing times, therefore limiting the inquiries to the production of simple geometries. Due to gravity, the cells will gravitate toward the inner portion of the vat solution, which is another disadvantage of SLA. As a result, there are more cells concentrated at the bottom of the vat and fewer cells at the top. It is particularly problematic when the hydrogels needed must be of low concentration to ensure cell viability. Besides, SLA is also limited in some other ways; the minimum size of a feature is also limited by the laser beam diameter which is around 250 mm. The focusing spot size and diffraction determine the resolution of SLA, and the minimum size is at least half the wavelength of the laser. While these criteria influence the feature size, different photocurable polymers have different resolutions. The resolution that can be obtained, however, is limited to only a few micrometers. The accuracy of the *z*-axis is further limited, which is compensated for by the utilization of the 2PP process; however, this approach has little use in bioprinting, as demonstrated by a recent study. With regard to this, the group of Chichkov combined 2PP with the LIFT method in fabricating high-resolution porous scaffolds made of overlapping rings using polyethylene glycol diacrylate (PEGDA). In the bioprinting process of scaffold production, separately on the donor slide, vascular smooth muscle-like cells (vSMCs) and ovine endothelial cells (ECs) were bioprinted where vSMCs were seeded within the hexagonal boundary and ECs outside the hexagonal boundary. Photopolymerization with UV radiation has certain limitations due to the effects on cells and photosensitive materials and the unsafe nature of photoinitiators applied in bioink solutions. Photoinitiators may selectively generate free radicals that may adversely interact with the cell membranes, proteins, and DNA, thereby restricting their application in the above-mentioned processes. Another completed research also documented the least effect of the Irgacure 2959 photoinitiator across various mammalian cell types and species [16].

The researchers found that cell lines with shorter cell cycles demonstrated higher sensitivity to changes in the cell death phenomenon due to exposure to photoinitiators of the same type and concentrations when compared to other types of cells. Along with the problems associated with three-dimensional bioprinting, one of the primary drawbacks of LIFT and MAPLE-DW for tissue bioprinting is their need for a very high-performance environment. The most popular LIFT and MAPLE-DW methods only produced 2D patterns. A small number of research studies demonstrate the scalable creation of tissue structures using these techniques. In the form of a vat system surrounded by a calcium chloride (CaCl2) pool, Huang and co-authors developed a system whereby an alginate droplet was rapidly cross-linked once it touched the pool and later caused the table to decrease by the thickness of a given layer. It allowed creating vascular structures, but the capability of this procedure depends greatly on the cross-linking speed of hydrogels, as alginate gels form these structures very quickly. Otherwise, limited print speed, droplet consistency, and progression of small droplets into larger tissue constructs are some other serious issues. What is more, a method of cross-linking needs to be successfully incorporated into the bioprinting procedure. When cross-linking is ineffective, rejected droplets would spread easily, and the levels of structural integrity are not sufficient for the development of scaled tissue structures. The inclusion of several components into the bioprinted structure is a significant restriction of LBB. Currently available photopolymerization and cell transfer methods (MAPLE-DW, LIFTDW, and LGDW) are unable to integrate multimaterial bioprinting capabilities. In order to create multimaterial objects, Wicker et al. developed a carousel system that rotates vats filled with various bioinks. However, switching between the various materials takes time and adds additional challenges to the construction process, such as the system's low resolution. The scaffold of the constructed vat is difficult to remove and replace entirely with the photocurable mixture. Eliminating bioink residue is essential when alternating between two materials since it might cause mistakes in the resolution produced. In particular, the procedure of moving to a different vat will need to minimize material contamination since a new layer cannot be constructed until the dust that collects at the scaffold's sides and bottom is cleared. According to [33], 3D bioprinting is accomplished in two steps: First, the building process is cleaned rough, and then the final cleaning is completed. However, since the scaffold is not put together in the initial bioink solution, the carousel approach in LIFT does not need a cleanup procedure. The last and most significant limitation of LBB is that it lacks a sufficient variety of appropriate bioink materials. LIFT and MAPLE-DW approaches are limited, whereas photopolymerization is only applicable to a few hydrogel types, with a reduced choice of bioink photocurable materials available. Therefore, to date, no study has reported the compatibility of other bioink materials other than hydrogels. In particular, the LBB methods have not proven bioink materials that use cell aggregate forms. This is because of the huge size of spheroids and the inability of the spheroids to move within hydrogels, whereas single cells can be isolated easily during bioprinting.

9.7 Applications in Cardiac Tissue Engineering

9.7.1 Cellular Sources

Bioprinted cells need high levels of cell proliferation, along with easy differentiation and maturation into target cells. There should also be easy access to autologous cells, and the cells should exhibit non-antigenicity and infection. The best alternatives for cardiac tissues are natural cardiomyocytes, progenitor cells, and stem cells, such as mesenchymal stem cells (from bone marrow or umbilical cord) and cardiac stem cells. The most important attributes of the collection of stem cells are self-renewal, the ability to differentiate into cardiomyocytes, and the significant levels of proliferation. There is potential to reduce or eliminate immunological graft rejection and thrombogenicity and provide an on-demand gift supply. There are also ethical concerns, immature morphologies, and a lack of transverse tubules. Modified adult cardiomyocytes have decreased contractility and altered metabolic and electrophysiological functions. A report reviewed the use of stem cells for 3D bioprinting with gelatin–fibrin bioink and analyzed the co-culture ratios of the different cardiac cell types (cardiomyocytes, cardiac fibroblasts, and endothelial cells) and showed hetero-cellular coupling among the different cell types using bioprinting. A researcher used hetero-cellular communication between two different cell types (C2C12 myocytes and STO fibroblasts) at the border regions of printed cell sheets within multilayered tissues. The cellular interactions characterized in these studies show promise for the engineering of complex tissues in the future.

9.7.2 Cardiac Tissue and Patches

The heart patches offer the properties that are beneficial when repairing a heart where the damage is clinically significant. They have been applied in repair or replacement of damaged heart tissues and to some extent restart of the heart health [1]. The invention of 3D bioprinting technology has made some recent progress in tissue manufacturing. Rasouli et al. [33] studied development of microvascularization with printing of human vascular endothelial cells and fibrin scaffolding in concurrence [60]. The researchers found printed patterns had a 3D tubular architecture with the directional alignment of cells within channels and the subsequent growth of the cell to form confluent linings. This manuscript revealed the outcome of simultaneous scaffold and cell printing on cell proliferation and development of microvasculature. Cardiomyocytes obtained in neonatal rat onto carbon nanotubes containing photo-crosslinkable gelatin methacrylate hydrogel to produce cardiac patches. The constructs comprised superb mechanical integrity and advanced electrophysiological that pointed out the prospect that carbon nanotube integration could be put to manufacture multifunctional cardiac scaffolds. Subsequent to development, the stem cell patch exhibited significant vascularization and tissue stem matrix production upon in vivo introduction into hearts. The patch demonstrated less cardiac hypertrophy and fibrosis, enhanced restoration of cell migration to the myocardial infarction site, production of neo-muscle and neo-capillaries, and overall better cardiac function. In 2025, Li et al. [11] developed a process for printing thick, vascularized, and perfusable cardiac patches that align with the immunological, cellular, biochemical, and anatomical characteristics of individuals. The reprogramming of patients' omental tissue cells into induced pluripotent stem cells (iPSCs) generated cardiomyocytes and endothelial cells, which were then incorporated into hydrogel as bioink to fabricate a heart and blood arteries. Noor et al. have showed the capacity to create vascularized patches irrespective of patient anatomy by enhancing blood vessel architecture. It also used this work to print cellularized human hearts with natural architecture, implying that creation of personalized tissues and organs is possible. Biofabricating cardiac patches is relatively simple compared to the in vitro tissue engineering of a heart which is more complicated and necessitates the methodological programming of multi-types of cells to create a vascular network on a multiscale level, lymphatic, and neuronal tissues, as well as muscle tissues. Electrical pacing should also be observed in the tissues to get automated contractions. Numerous contemporary investigations have shown encouraging outcomes in cardiac tissue bioprinting. Li et al. [11] showed that a bio-prototyping technique using inkjet technology successfully constructed bioengineered cardiac pseudo-tissues, consisting of contractile cardiac hybrids and a half-heart structure, which exhibited rhythmic cellular responses. Wang et al. [34] conducted a different experiment using cardiomyocyte-laden hydrogel to bioprint cardiac tissue constructs that exhibit spontaneous synchronized contractions in vitro. The progressive growth and maturation of the tissue were shown, with physiological responses to cardiac medicines, indicating potential applications in cardiac tissue engineering and pharmacology. Schlicht et al. [35] conducted a research on heterogeneous multicellular constructions including human umbilical vein endothelial cells and induced pluripotent stem cell-derived cardiomyocytes. Following the incorporation of cells into a highly viscous hydrogel rope composed of alginate and polyethylene glycol–fibrinogen, microfluidic bioprinting technology was used to extrude an iPSC-cardiomyocyte-cardiac tissue. The human umbilical vein endothelial cells added the printed tissue with multiple specified geometries of blood vessel imitating the properties of the natural tissue environment. The 3D bioprinting technologies have proven useful in fabrication of heart tissues with properties similar to the natural tissues environments. An overview of existing bioprinted cardiac structures can be seen in Table 9.2. Cardiac muscles fabricated by tissue engineering could accelerate researches on cardiac physiology and offer in vivo high-throughput drug screening systems. In developing heart tissue/bioprints, the development can lead to a possible advancement in performance and operations of cardiac tissue structures. However, there is a lot of research yet to be done on the limits of printing before further applications of printing in medicine.

Table 9.2: Overview of existing bioprinted cardiac structures.

Study/ year	Bioprinting technique	Bioink used	Printed structure	Application/objective
[16]	Extrusion-based	Alginate/gelatin with patient-specific cardiac cells	Full-thickness human heart with vascularization	Personalized heart transplantation
[27]	Stereolithography	Gelatin methacrylate (GelMA) + cardiomyocytes	3D cardiac patches	Cardiac tissue repair post-myocardial infarction
[26]	Inkjet bioprinting	Alginate with human cardiac progenitor cells	Cardiac patches (2D structures)	Tissue engineering for myocardial therapy
[26]	Coaxial extrusion	Decellularized ECM + human-induced pluripotent stem cells (hiPSCs)	Vascularized cardiac tissue	Functional myocardium regeneration
[36]	Digital light processing (DLP)	GelMA and PEGDA with endothelial and cardiac cells	Vascularized cardiac tissue constructs	Cardiac microtissue modeling
[37]	FRESH	Collagen-based hydrogel with cardiomyocytes	Functional heart tissue	Replication of cardiac architecture for regenerative medicine
[38]	Microfluidic bioprinting	Alginate and PEG-fibrinogen with cardiomyocytes and endothelial cells	Patterned vascularized cardiac tissue	Enhanced contractility and perfusion
[39]	Integrated tissue-organ printer (ITOP)	Decellularized ECM bioink + cells	Cardiac tissue scaffolds with vasculature	Large tissue and organ printing

9.7.3 Full Heart Organoid and Organ

Production of functional heart organs that are similar to natural anatomies is actually the final goal of cardiac tissue engineering. Important progress in this direction is made over recent years. In 2022, Varaprasad and co-authors presented the initial application of bioink alginate materials that were completely customized, non-supplemented to print the hearts that have mechanical properties that are almost identical to those of decellularized rat hearts. Successful bioprinting of five human heart parts including a tri-leaflet heart valve, a neonatal-sized collagen heart, and a model of a human cardiac ventricle was achieved by the group [36] later that same year using the FRESH bioprinting technology. In 2025, Kim et al. generated bioprinted cardiac organoids of macroscale with geometry relevant to the pumping of the heart muscle. Cardiac drugs and pacing were proved to induce rhythmic contraction and prolonged transmission of action potentials in human-chambered muscle pumps. The study by Kupfer has implications on organoid production of this type, in heart medical devices and cell transplants.

9.8 Future Directions

The future outlook requires numerous improvements toward the strength and the effectiveness of the LBB modalities in the final goal of bioprinting functional tissue and organ structures. DLP-based inclusion in the bioprinting industry is also going to be beneficial, as it allows printing large-scale tissue compositions fast; there is no sense of using one UV laser beam sweeping sequentially over the entire region of interest – this is inefficient and time-wasting. This is more injurious to the viability of the cells, as the specific exposure of the cells in monomer solution is of extended period without exposure to oxygen supply. Furthermore, utilization of photoinitiators can also negatively influence the cell viability when the process lasts long. In turn, shorter manufacturing times (in minutes) will improve the bioprinting and tissue engineering procedures greatly. Constant time of photo-cross-linking of each of the layers because of the speedy exposure of hundreds of thousands of micromirrors may result in a longer total time of construction because of the amount of layers required. The number of the layers can be decreased efficiently after one determines the right orientation direction. This, however, can have repercussions with other qualities such as surface quality and mechanical qualities. The majority of the laser-aided bioprinting (LAB) methods, including MAPLE-DW and LIFT, have the main application in the 2D cell patterning and few possibilities to create the 3D structures. This depends on the characteristics of cross-linking and solidification of components in bioink employed in the process. Up to date, these procedures have involved few types of bioinks. These hydrogels are predominately made up of thermally cross-linked varieties such as gelatin and Matrigel type and ionically cross-linked types, such as alginate type. Particularly, with thermally cross-linked hydrogels, constructions are limited to very thin structures, as thermoregulating the thermal surrounding of the volume occupied by the scaffold is difficult. The initial layers will easily be cross-linked when thermally regulation substrates are used, but as the layers increase, it becomes complicated to ensure temperature control. This means more efforts have to be done before realizing successful solidification in three dimensions. Laser-based bioprinting 191 bigger-scale tissue constructs require macroporosity to ensure nutrition and oxygen transport; therefore, LBB modalities, apart from photopolymerization methods, are not so good, because it cannot make it in porous architecture. In that regard, bioprinting the process may incorporate transient or ephemeral hydrogels. As an example, the production of thermally cross-linkable hydrogels can be launched where sodium alginate can be extruded with a secondary ribbon as described above. The cross-linker sodium alginate can be incorporated to the thermally cross-linkable hydrogel and will be cross-linked against alginate when in contact. The temporarily printed alginate can be removed by a decross-linker of alginate thus creating porosity within the 3D structure. Similar design can also be produced by print sacrificial supports made of thermally cross-linking hydrogel at scale in a similar way. The place of substrate may be controlled in z-direction with the help of a movable stage that should be provided with linear motor. Kinetics of the jet and droplet formation change with the variation in distance between substrate and ribbon; therefore, maintenance of the bioprinting spacing must be ensured all through. An important finding that LBB needs to achieve is an expansion of the library of photocurable bioink materials, besides the ones that have already been developed in LIFT. Since LGDW and MAPLE-DW processes have already become a relic in the area of bioprinting, they were replaced with LIFT technique; it is obviously of necessity to find or introduce new materials that guarantee even dispersion in form of bioink solution at the surface of the ribbon and consistent presence of the cells within the bioink coating. These materials should be of high viscoelasticity to avoid the phenomenon of droplet bounces and splashes along with secondary droplets. They also must have high gelation speed to allow printing thick tissue constructs at three dimensions and the extent of biocompatibility must be high allowing the cell to grow and multiply without producing any form of immunogenic response. A combination of various bioink printing methods will timely become a significant boost to the creation of high-resolution tissue building involving many cells in a characteristic arrangement of cells in a tissue-like construct. Although the multi-material printing versatility (various cell types) is developed among photopolymerization techniques, there is currently no research evidence regarding the alternative bioprinting of various cell types based on the cell transfer technique as MAPLE-DW or LIFT cell printing. The proposed carousel mechanism in LIFT has not yet been applied because the switch of ribbon position will significantly influence the bioprinting dynamics of the jet and cause excessive variations in the bioprinting strategy. As a result, instead of moving the ribbon within the carousel system, the utilization of multiple ribbons supported by different mirror arrangements that section the main laser beam one after another, it would be possible to bioprint various bioink materials simultaneously. This architecture requires a translation to move the substrate in alternating tracks in the lateral plane that enables a bioprinting of multiple types of bioink. The strategy enables the combination of multiple bioink substances into a single platform.

9.8.1 AI/ML-Guided Control

The use of artificial intelligence (AI) and machine learning (ML) increasingly implemented in LBB tools has provided significant improvement in real-time procedures control making them able to give dynamic feedback toward defect more minimization and consistency of quality print. During the manufacture process, these systems would continuously measure process data through in situ sensing capabilities such as high-speed optical imaging, temperature capability, and acoustic emission detection. The collected data are analyzed with the help of advanced machine learning algorithms, e.g., convolutional neural networks, support vector machines, random forests, and Gaussian process models in order to detect presence of defects, e.g., droplet misplacement, layer porosity, under- or over-cross-linking, and dislocation of cells. In case of deviations, again instantaneous adjustments in a key process parameter, e.g., laser pulse strength, depth of focus, speed of scanning, and exposure duration, are made to correct deviations and prevent spreading of fault. This feedback loop increases accuracy and consistency of a bioprinting process and maintains high cell viability with structure integrity as well. The control framework based on AI/ML applies to several LBB methods, including LIFT, matrix-assisted pulsed laser evaporation-direct write (MAPLE-DW), stereolithography (SLA), 2PP, and LGDW, which will help the creation of complex, usable tissue constructs with higher reliability or scalability.

9.8.2 Advanced Photoresins

The new developments that have taken place in photoresin formulations have immensely improved the capabilities of LBB, particularly where sensitive biomaterials have to be used. Common photopolymerization processes frequently rely on UV or near-UV light sources as well as cytotoxic photoinitiators, which threatens bioink compatibility and cell health. In solving such concerns, better photoresins such as visible light responsive and non-cytotoxic initiators have been designed so that polymerization may take place through an irradiation of lower intensity that is more appropriate to live cells. The presence of photosensitizers such as eosin Y, camphorquinone, and ruthenium-based compounds, leading to successful cross-linking in the presence of visible light, as well as less harmful cell deaths and oxidative stress, is one of the aspects. Additionally, bioinks loaded with upconversion nanoparticles have emerged as one potential solution to increase the spatial resolution and biocompatibility. These substances convert lower-energy near-infrared light into higher-energy emissions that convert to volumetric curing with reduced photodamage and deeper tissue penetration through photopolymerization. Such developments in photoresin chemistry enable the development of complex, cell-containing structures of high resolution, structural integrity, faster cell growth, and improved cell viability, thus expanding the clinical and translational practice of LBB technologies.

9.8.3 Hybrid Bioprinting Systems

More complex architecture of the native tissue is usually more than such a combination of bioprinting modalities is capable of. To solve this, new hybrid bioprinting approaches are combining LAB with EBB, magnetic, and microgravity-enabled capabilities to create complex and multifunctional tissue constructs. The laser-assisted bioprinting provides high-resolution patterning and accurate cell deposition that are especially applicable in the microregime and fragile cell collections. Nevertheless, due to less capacity of depositing substantial amounts of biomaterial, it has to be accompanied by extrusion-based printing, which offers solid structural support and massive deposition of hydrogel. The addition of magnetic bioprinting allows spatially arranging magnetically responsive cells, nanoparticles, or biomaterials, augmenting vascularization and cell direction in the printed constructs. Moreover, the printing of soft hydrogel structures with high mechanical complexity, i.e., volumetric, can readily collapse due to the gravitational forces acting on them when photosynthesized, but printing in the microgravity regime or simulated microgravity environments removes this problem. Hybrid bioprinting platforms can harness the synergistic control of multiple complementary modalities to obtain new space control, heterogeneity, and functional capability in engineered tissues and organs, expanding bioprinting technologies to biomanufacture tissues and organs, accelerating the development of implants, improving organ-on-chip models, and advancing in vivo disease modeling.

9.8.4 Laser-Based Bioprinting Scaling Strategies

Despite laser bioprinting maintaining exceptional accuracy, the scalability of LBB has become a significant barrier to translation in a clinical and industrial setting. Recent advances have supplied a few scaling solutions to enhance throughput preserving resolution and biological integrity. Parallel beam schemes employ numerous synchronized laser beams to process different regions of the printing surface simultaneously, hence experience enormous improvements to the propagation speed, but still maintain spatial integrity. Roll-to-roll donor ribbon systems have been developed in LIFT and matrix-assisted pulsed laser evaporation (MAPLE-DW) machines to enable high-throughput manufacturing of larger constructs by allowing continual reloading of the bioink-coated substrate, saving downtime associated with exchanging the donor ribbon anew. There are also automated layer matching algorithms, wherein high-precision imaging and feedback control ensure layer-to-layer registration precision, which is critical in maintaining geometric accuracy in complex, layered tissues. It is a combined approach to scaling challenges that are inherent in LBB (interactions between resolution, speed, and the volume of the construct) that promise to promote the ongoing transition to manufacturing-scale bioprinting and the production of therapeutically relevant tissue constructs.

9.9 Summary

LBB has proven to be a successful platform to pattern cells alive because it has better cell-patterning resolution and precision and the fact that it allows a high cell density to be imposed, capabilities which could not be applied to low-resolution EBB or DBB that are restricted by a smaller drop size, thereby allowing lower cell density. Photopolymerization methods, together with LGDW-, LIFT-, and MAPLE-DW-based techniques, have attracted interest in the research community in bioprinting due to the availability and affordability of SLA-based commercial printers as well as their ability to be customized. Despite these advantages, LBB also has disadvantages that can be attributed to being complex and prohibitively expensive to implement, its lack of feasibility in its operative capacity, limited throughput, and limited capacity in making scalable heterogeneous construct of tissues, but the recent developments in the field have indicated that the technology would become more viable in the fabrication of 3D tissue construct in the area of tissue engineering and regenerative medicine in the near future.

References

[1] Gupta, D., Derman, I. D., Xu, C., Huang, Y., & Ozbolat, I. T. (2025 Apr 24). Droplet-based bioprinting. Nature Reviews Methods Primers, 5(1), 25.

[2] He, C. F., Qiao, T. H., Wang, G. H., Sun, Y., & He, Y. (2025 Feb). High-resolution projection-based 3D bioprinting. Nature Reviews Bioengineering, 3(2), 143–158.

[3] Ma, X., Xu, M., Cui, X., Yin, J., & Wu, Q. (2025 Mar). Hybrid 3D bioprinting of sustainable biomaterials for advanced multiscale tissue engineering. Small, 27, 2408947.

[4] Mei, X., Yang, Z., Wang, X., Shi, A., Blanchard, J., Elahi, F., Kang, H., Orive, G., & Zhang, Y. S. (2025). Integrating microfluidic and bioprinting technologies: Advanced strategies for tissue vascularization. Lab on a Chip.

[5] Tripathi, S., Dash, M., Chakraborty, R., Lukman, H. J., Kumar, P., Hassan, S., Mehboob, H., Singh, H., & Nanda, H. S. (2025). Engineering considerations in the design of tissue specific bioink for 3D bioprinting applications. Biomaterials Science, 13(1), 93–129.

[6] Aykora, D., Taşçı, B., Şahin, M. Z., Tekeoğlu, I., Uzun, M., Sarafian, V., & Docheva, D. (2025 Apr 25). Tendon regeneration deserves better: Focused review on In vivo models, artificial intelligence and 3D bioprinting approaches. Frontiers in Bioengineering and Biotechnology, 13, 1580490.

[7] Kitana, W., Apsite, I., & Ionov, L. (2025 Apr). 3D (Bio) printing combined fiber fabrication methods for tissue engineering applications: Possibilities and limitations. Advanced Functional Materials, 14, 2500450.

[8] Tao, H., Zhang, X., Yuan, X., Lian, Z., Xu, J., Shan, D., & Guo, B. (2025 Mar). 3D bioprinting technology in tissue engineering printing method and material selection. BioNanoScience, 15(1), 1–9.

[9] Hernández, J., Santos, N., & Ahumada, M. (2025 May 31). Advances in 3D bioprinting for corneal regeneration. Gels, 11(6), 422.

[10] Karaman, D., Williams, K., Phelps, J., La Boucan, F., Lewandowski, G., O'Grady, K., Yu, B., & Willerth, S. M. (2025 May 26). Microspheres for 3D bioprinting: A review of fabrication methods and applications. Frontiers in Bioengineering and Biotechnology, 13, 1551199.

[11] Li, Y., Cui, H., & Cui, H. (2025 Apr). Precision spatial control of tumor-stroma interactions in cancer models via 3D bioprinting for advanced research and therapy. Advanced Functional Materials, 24, 2503391.

[12] Halper, J. (2025 Jan 15). Narrative review and guide: State of the art and emerging opportunities of bioprinting in tissue regeneration and medical instrumentation. Bioengineering, 12(1), 71.

[13] Kamaraj, M., Moghimi, N., Joshi, A., Rezayof, O., Barer, A., Cao, S., Orkin, R., Alambeigi, F., & John, J. V. (2025 Apr). Recent advances in handheld and robotic bioprinting approach for tissue engineering. Advanced Materials Technologies, 24, 2500206.

[14] Mallya, D., Gadre, M. A., Varadharajan, S., & Vasanthan, K. S. (2025 Feb 14). 3D bioprinting for the construction of drug testing models-development strategies and regulatory concerns. Frontiers in Bioengineering and Biotechnology, 13, 1457872.

[15] Sousa, A. C., Alvites, R., Lopes, B., Sousa, P., Moreira, A., Coelho, A., Santos, J. D., Atayde, L., Alves, N., & Maurício, A. C. (2025 Jan 16). Three-Dimensional Printing/Bioprinting and cellular therapies for regenerative medicine: Current advances. Journal of Functional Biomaterials, 16(1), 28.

[16] Mathur, V., Agarwal, P., Kasturi, M., Srinivasan, V., Seetharam, R. N., & Vasanthan, K. S. (2025 Jan). Innovative bioinks for 3D bioprinting: Exploring technological potential and regulatory challenges. Journal of Tissue Engineering, 16, 20417314241308022.

[17] Dhar, S., Ahmad, F., Deshpande, A., Rana, S. S., Ahmed, A. T., & Priyadarsini, S. (2025 Apr 9). 3-Dimensional printing and bioprinting in neurological sciences: Applications in surgery, imaging, tissue engineering, and pharmacology and therapeutics. Journal of Materials Science: Materials in Medicine, 36(1), 32.

[18] Cha, Y. S., Michaels, A., Wang, J. Z., Niu, Y., Lin, Y., Zhu, L., Zhu, X., Wang, K., Murray, M., & Zhou, F. (2025 May). Recent advances in 3D cell culture models in cancer drug development. Journal of Pharmaceutical Investigation, 14, 1–7.

[19] Balaji Govindaswamy, I. J., Thangaraju, R., Kumarappan, M., & Vasan, S. B. (2025 Jul). Current Approaches in 3D Printed Organ and Tissues Engineering. Challenges and Innovations in 3D Printed Bio-Organs and Their Materials, 8, 1.

[20] Eskandar, K. (2025 May). 3D-bioprinted urethral grafts: Revolutionizing urethral stricture treatment. Arab Journal of Urology, 15, 1–1.

[21] Thirumalaivasan, N., Nangan, S., Verma, D., Shellaiah, M., Ali, S., Rajendran, S., Kanagaraj, K., Pothu, R., Boddula, R., Radwan, A. B., & Al-Qahtani, N. (2025 May 2). Exploring the diverse nanomaterials employed in dental prosthesis and implant techniques: An overview. Nanotechnology Reviews, 14(1), 20250140.

[22] Putra, N. R., & Airlangga, B. Green innovations in natural paper ink: Trends, applications, and future prospects. Nordic Pulp & Paper Research Journal. 2025 May 23.

[23] Maintz, M., Tomooka, Y., Eugster, M., Gerig, N., Sharma, N., Thieringer, F. M., & Rauter, G. (2024 Sep 14). In situ minimally invasive 3D printing for bone and cartilage regeneration-a scoping review. Current Directions in Biomedical Engineering, 10(2), 66–70.

[24] Ramesh, M., Niranjana, K., Bhoopathi, R., & Rajeshkumar, L. (2024 Sep 6). Additive manufacturing (3D printing) technologies for fiber-reinforced polymer composite materials: A review on fabrication methods and process parameters. e-Polymers, 24(1), 20230114.

[25] Blaeser, A. (2024 Jul 26). Evolution of biofabrication and 3D-bioprinting technologies–from market pull to technology push. at-Automatisierungstechnik, 72(7), 645–656.

[26] Mani, M. P., Sadia, M., Jaganathan, S. K., Khudzari, A. Z., Supriyanto, E., Saidin, S., Ramakrishna, S., Ismail, A. F., & Faudzi, A. A. (2022 Mar 28). A review on 3D printing in tissue engineering applications. Journal of Polymer Engineering, 42(3), 243–265.

[27] Cai, R., Gimenez-Camino, N., Xiao, M., Bi, S., & DiVito, K. A. (2023 Feb 2). Technological advances in three-dimensional skin tissue engineering. Reviews on Advanced Materials Science, 62(1), 20220289.

[28] Alex, Y., Shanmugam, R., Salunkhe, S., & Čep, R. (2025 May 26). Advancement of additive manufacturing technology in the development of personalized in vivo and in vitro prosthetic implants. Reviews on Advanced Materials Science, 64(1), 20250109.

[29] Goyal, V., Verma, G. C., & Saxena, P. (2024 Dec). Advancements in 3D printing of functional materials for biomedical applications: Challenges, opportunities, and case studies: A critical review. Progress in Additive Manufacturing, 19, 1–29.

[30] Rahman, M., Dip, T. M., Nur, M. G., Hossain, M. H., Snow, F., Hossain, N. B., Mirabedini, A., Quigley, A., Padhye, R., & Houshyar, S. (2025 May). Nanomaterial-integrated 3D biofabricated structures for advanced biomedical applications. Macromolecular Materials and Engineering, 14, 2500083.

[31] Borthakur, P. P., Das, A., Sahariah, J. J., Pramanik, P., Baruah, E., & Pathak, K. (2025 Apr). Revolutionizing patient care: 3D printing for customized medical devices and therapeutics. Biomedical Materials & Devices, 1, 1–28.

[32] Khosropanah, M. H., Rajabi, M., Behboodi Tanourlouee, S., Azimzadeh, A., Alizadeh Vaghasloo, M., & Hassannejad, Z. (2025 Apr 13). Silk as a promising biomaterial for 3D bioprinting: A comprehensive review of Bombyx mori silk's biomedical applications. International Journal of Polymeric Materials and Polymeric Biomaterials, 74(6), 538–554.

[33] Rasouli, R., Sweeney, C., & Frampton, J. P. (2025 Mar). Heterogeneous and composite bioinks for 3D-bioprinting of complex tissue. Biomedical Materials & Devices, 3(1), 108–126.

[34] Wang, J., Wang, Y., Wang, R., Wang, Q., Wen, M., Wang, J., Sheng, L., Zheng, Y., & Xi, T. (2025 Jan). A review on 3D printing processes in pharmaceutical engineering and tissue engineering: Applications, trends and challenges. Advanced Materials Technologies, 10(2), 2400620.

[35] Schlicht, S., Wesinger, M., Kaufmann, A., Rösel, U., Fischer, D., & Drummer, D. (2025 Mar). Multiscale polyethylene fiber–bacterial nanocellulose composites through combined laser fusion and bacterial in situ synthesis. International Polymer Processing, 19(0).

[36] Gong, J., Qian, Y., Lu, K., Zhu, Z., Siow, L., Zhang, C., Zhou, S., Gu, T., Yin, J., Yu, M., & Wang, H. (2022 Oct 13). Digital light processing (DLP) in tissue engineering: From promise to reality, and perspectives. Biomedical Materials, 17(6), 062004.

[37] Kreimendahl, F., Kniebs, C., Tavares Sobreiro, A. M., Schmitz-Rode, T., Jockenhoevel, S., & Thiebes, A. L. (2021 Jul). FRESH bioprinting technology for tissue engineering–the influence of printing process and bioink composition on cell behavior and vascularization. Journal of Applied Biomaterials & Functional Materials, 19, 22808000211028808.

[38] Colosi, C., Costantini, M., Barbetta, A., & Dentini, M. (2017). Microfluidic Bioprinting of Heterogeneous 3D Tissue Constructs. 3D Cell Culture: Methods and Protocols. 369–380.
[39] Matai, I., Kaur, G., Seyedsalehi, A., McClinton, A., & Laurencin, C. T. (2020 Jan 1). Progress in 3D bioprinting technology for tissue/organ regenerative engineering. Biomaterials, 226, 119536.
[40] Tonk, M., Gupta, V., Dhwaj, A., & Sachdeva, M. (2025 Jan 16). Current developments and advancements of 3-dimensional printing in personalized medication and drug screening. Drug Metabolism and Personalized Therapy, 39(4), 167–182.

Kavita Kumari Thakur*, Ramesh Lekurwale, Tanaya Shyam Salvi

Chapter 10
Extrusion-Based Bioprinting

Abstract: Extrusion-based bioprinting is most widely used 3D bioprinting techniques due to its ability to print bioinks over a broad viscosity range, simple to operate, and high post-printing cell viability. This chapter gives an overview of extrusion-based bioprinting, by covering the fundamental components, working principles, and different types of extrusion mechanism. Different extrusion mechanisms like pneumatic-based, piston-based, and screw-driven systems are discussed along with their operational properties, advantages, limitations, and practical applications in the biomedical field.

The chapter also discusses important parameters such as bioink formulation strategies, rheological optimization, shear stress regulation, crosslinking mechanisms and biocompatibility, mechanical integrity of printed constructs, printability, and post-printing cell viability. Recent advancements in extrusion-based bioprinting are discussed, including multi-material and gradient printing, coaxial nozzle configurations, microfluidic-assisted extrusion, and the use of artificial intelligence for bioink design and process optimization. Finally, the chapter highlights the case studies based on biomedical applications of extrusion-based bioprinting and discusses future research directions, various challenges, and different opportunities toward clinically application of bioprinted tissues.

Keywords: Extrusion-based bioprinting, bioink, extracellular matrix (ECM), viscosity, artificial intelligence (AI)

10.1 Introduction

Over the past two decades, many different bioprinting techniques are emerging. The prominent bioprinting technologies are extrusion-, inkjet-, and light-based bioprinting. Extrusion-based bioprinting (EBB) is a process which provides continuous deposition of bioink filaments through a nozzle. Such an approach enables high cell density and can be used for viscous materials. In inkjet-based bioprinting, droplets of bioink

***Corresponding author: Kavita Kumari Thakur**, Department of Mechanical Engineering, K. J. Somaiya School of Engineering (Formerly Known as K. J. Somaiya College of Engineering), Vidyavihar, Mumbai 400 077, Maharashtra, India, e-mail: kavitakumari.t@somaiya.edu
Ramesh Lekurwale, Department of Mechanical Engineering, K. J. Somaiya School of Engineering (Formerly Known as K. J. Somaiya College of Engineering), Vidyavihar, Mumbai 400 077
Tanaya Shyam Salvi, Research Intern, Department of Mechanical Engineering, K. J. Somaiya School of Engineering (Formerly Known as K. J. Somaiya College of Engineering), Vidyavihar, Mumbai 400 077

 | https://doi.org/10.1515/9783111719993-010

are generated without contact which allows for high speed and precision applicable to low-viscosity materials and fine manipulation of cells. Light-based bioprinting is a technique which uses light to polymerize photosensitive bioresin layers for high-resolution and complex structures [1]. Then, there are new frontiers in advanced bioprinting, such as multi-material, coaxial, and 4D bioprinting, which allow for more complex tissue structures and dynamic functionalities [2]. Each bioprinting technique has certain advantages and limitations in cell viability, cell resolution, material compatibility, and printing speed. It often leads to hybrid approaches to achieve the best possible outcome.

While each technique offers distinct advantages, EBB supports high-viscosity, cell-laden bioinks and enables fabrication of multi-material architectures. EBB is one of the most emerging 3D bioprinting techniques. A nozzle is used with pneumatic, piston, or screw-driven actuation, which allows the printing of tissues with different shapes and complexities. It ensures precise spatial patterning of cells, matrix components, and bioactive factors throughout the bioprinted scaffold. This ability of EBB to handle viscous hydrogels and particulate composites makes EBB more prominent in tissue engineering. It is highly suitable for load-bearing tissues, like bone/cartilage as well as soft tissue or vascularized constructs with high precision [3].

Initial tissue printing has modified approaches in 3D bioprinting and scaffold engineering. Earlier, research focused on acellular constructs designed to mimic the extracellular matrix (ECM). It was designed to make simple hydrogel scaffold without incorporation of cells. This early work provided proof of concept for spatially controlled deposition but lacked cellular complexity. Over the past ten years, EBB has advanced into sophisticated, multi-material, cell-laden manufacturing platform that integrates imaging, computational modeling, and design strategies in order to closely replicate native tissues' heterogeneity and complexity [4, 5]. New developments such as coaxial extrusion systems can be used to print core-shell structure with the deposition of supportive biomaterials and cell-laden hydrogels in a single step. Similarly, multi-cartridge and microfluidic feed systems allow printing of heterogeneous tissue with gradients in mechanical and biological properties [6].

These advances have increased the use of EBB for regenerative medicine, disease modeling, and drug screening. It is essential for any bioprinting process to be reproducible and create physiologically relevant tissues [7]. Despite significant progress, there are still unresolved issues like bioink rheology, printability, cell viability and resolution. Advances in bioink chemistry and formulation are essential which enhance vascularization and functional properties. This leads to further development of tissue constructs which are clinically applicable [8].

EBB is generally included in the category of material-extrusion bioprinters. It can be further categorized according to their mechanisms like pneumatic, piston, and screw systems and feed systems including single- or multi-cartridge, coaxial, and microfluidic printhead [9, 10].

Coaxial nozzle technology now makes it possible to print core-shell structure, where the outer layer is strong and supportive, while the inside of the shell consists of cells and growth factors. This approach is especially useful for printing channels like structures similar to blood vessels in vascular tissue. The microfluidic-based extrusion allows different materials to flow together during printing. This also means that printed structures have different physical and chemical properties in different regions, creating spatially varied designs [11]. Through innovation and new technology, EBB has progressed from producing simple 3D-printed structural scaffolds to making functional tissue and organ level manufacturing areas. This is mainly because EBB can print different materials, cell types, and biological signals all at once, allowing the printing of structures that closely mimic the in vivo organization found inside living tissues. Bioinks made from ECM-based hydrogels are often combined with nanofillers, vascular endothelial growth factors, and supportive polymer framework. These additions help improve the strength and enhance physical properties of tissue [7, 8]. Together, these innovations have made possible the fabrication of constructs that replicates native tissue's stiffness and also respond to biological signals, bridging the gaps between structural scaffolds and physiologically active tissue [5].

As a result, EBB has become a powerful platform not only in regenerative medicine but also in disease modeling and drug screening, where reproducible and physiologically relevant tissue constructs are essential [9]. Its integration with patient-specific imaging data, automation, and advances in whole organ biomanufacturing further enhances its potential [10].

10.2 Core Components and Working Principle of EBB

10.2.1 Core Component of EBB

EBB systems are made up of various key components that work together to ensure precise printing and consistent production of complex tissue structure using bioinks. Every part has an important role in maintaining printing accuracy, keeping the cells alive through the process, and ensuring that final construct has strong structural integrity.

10.2.1.1 Bioink Reservoir/Cartridge

The bioink reservoir or cartridges act like a main container that holds the bioink, which may include cell-filled hydrogels, mixture of polymers or composite suspensions. It helps to keep bioink sterile. These cartridges can be replaced or swapped easily which helps researchers to use more than one type of bioink at the same time. This feature supports the creation of complex and mixed tissue structures. Modern reservoir systems are specifically designed to reduce the chances of contamination and keep cells healthy throughout the printing process. In many cases, the cartridges are made for single use and can be sterilized easily, which helps to prevent cross-contamination between different experiments [4]. In addition, the temperature-controlled cartridges are now widely used to maintain the proper flow and consistency of bioink. This is important when working with temperature-sensitive hydrogels like gelatin, collagen, or pluronic-based materials [8]. In more advanced bioprinting system, multi-cartridge setups make it possible to load and print many bioinks at the same time [5]. This flexibility is used to create tissues which resemble vascularized bone or layered skin models.

Microfluidics cartridges are small, self-containing devices consisting of microscale channels used for a precise handling of small volumes of fluid and their manipulation. These devices are designed for automation and convenience. They combine all functions including mixing, separation, reaction, and analysis into a single disposable unit. Their ability to provide controlled flow of ink is ideal for diagnostics, drug testing, and bioprinting which are characterized by efficiency and reduced sample consumption. This active mixing allows adjustment according to required mechanical strength and biological behavior [11].

Overall, bioink reservoir is not just a container for storage but also a major part of bioprinting system. It directly affects sterility, rheology, and system's ability to print with multiple materials at the same time which improves print accuracy, reliability, and reproducibility in EBB [6].

10.2.1.2 Extrusion Flow Control

There are mainly three types of EBB like pneumatic, piston, or screw driven. Pneumatic systems are adopted widely due to its simplicity, lower cost, and ease of operation. This systems suit flexible laboratory setups and are useful for rapid prototyping. Even with such advantages, this system still lacks accurate flow control, which affects cells uniform distribution and reduces structural integrity of printed structures. Nowadays, to improve this real-time flow rate monitoring with proportional-integral-derivative (PID) feedback control is introduced. This technology adjusts pneumatic pressure continuously during printing, improving flow consistency and overall print quality when compared to traditional constant pressure methods. Even with these upgrades, pneumatic systems are less accurate and precise than other extrusion methods like progressive cavity pumps which offer better volumetric flow control while maintaining cell viability across a wide range of bioink composition [10].

To improve the performance of current bioprinting methods, researchers have developed thermal and mechanical strategies like adaptive nozzle systems and improved thermal management which stabilizes bioink properties and increase dispensing accuracy in pneumatic setups [12]. Although pneumatic extrusion is popular due to its simplicity and flexibility, it still has low precision in flow regulation. The ongoing research is improving the real-time control and exploring alternate extrusion technology to increase reproducibility and printing fidelity [13].

10.2.1.3 Nozzle

The nozzle is an important part of EBB because it controls filament diameter, printing resolution, and the amount of shear stress applied to cells, which affects the cell survival. Bioprinting nozzles are usually 100 to 500 µm in inner diameter. Smaller nozzles (less than 200 µm) approximated to render high resolution but also ascertain higher shear stress on the cells. A medium-sized nozzle (200 to 400 µm) provides the best balance between details and cell viability. The large nozzles (>400 µm) allow printing with viscous bioinks and high cell survival but sacrifice print precision [14, 15]. A small nozzle gives better resolution but causes higher shear stress, which may reduce cell survival, while a large nozzle lowers shear stress but reduces structural accuracy [16]. New nozzle design has improved printing performance, such as coaxial nozzle that prints core-shell structure where the outer shell provides strength and inner core carries cell or growth factors. This allows formation of perusable, blood vessel like channels for vascular tissue engineering [17]. Conical nozzles reduce shear stress by providing a smooth and gradual flow path which increases cell viability and lowers the risk of clogging [18]. Multi-channel and microfluidic nozzles help to print two or more bioinks at the same time, which build tissues with spatial variations in mechanical and biochemical properties, which are useful for complex tissue models. Temperature control nozzle maintains viscosity of material and balances rheological flow and cell survival in EBB [3, 19].

10.2.1.4 XYZ Motion Stage

The XYZ motion stage is the key part of EBB, as it controls movements with micro-level precision, allowing complex structures to be printed layer by layer with accuracy and reproducibility which are essential for fabrication. Integrating them with imaging-based CAD models will further enhance the replication of patient-specific tissue bridging the gap between digital design and physical biofabrication. Stepper motors are widely used to control speed, acceleration, and positioning. They are cost-effective and reliable which makes them suitable for high resolution [1]. There are many upcoming multi-axis and robotic stages with rotational and tilting capabilities, which allow printing on non-planar surfaces and complex curved geometries like vascular networks. Integrating with real-time imaging methods such as optical coherence tomography (OCT), these systems enable feedback control. This feedback helps improve deposition accuracy and structural fidelity. This advancement helps bioprinting move closer to patient-specific imaging data (MRI/CT) into print instructions for personalized models [3].

10.2.1.5 Temperature Control System

Temperature regulation is necessary for EBB to maintain the stability of bioink. Temperature also regulates cell viability, especially for thermosensitive hydrogels like gelatin, collagen, agarose, etc. They undergo sol–gel transitions depending on temperature [8]. Modern bioprinters use print bed and temperature-controlled cartridges to keep bioinks in liquid form during printing to promote gelation or crosslinking immediately after deposition, ensuring structural integrity [20]. In multi-zone temperature control system, regulation of nozzle, cartridge, and print bed happens independently as different bioinks might require different temperatures [21]. Precise thermal management also protects cells from heat damage and prevents clogging. Thermal gradients within printhead influence viscosity, pressure, and shear stress affecting quality and filament morphology of extrusion [22]. Overall temperature regulation is not merely a supportive feature but a core requirement for EBB. It allows use of diverse bioinks and ensures reproducibility across ranging applications.

10.2.1.6 Crosslinking Module

Crosslinking is an important parameter for EBB. Crosslinker is used to solidify the extruded bioink and make it a stable structure. Crosslinking guarantees mechanical strength, shape fidelity, and long-term stability of the bioprinted constructs. Without effective crosslinking, the hydrogel printed may deform or collapse, thus compromising the biological functionality. Above all, thermal crosslinking is mostly used for temperature-sensitive hydrogels. Under the given temperature ranges, these materials transition from sol-gel state and the construct is set after extrusion. The regulation of temperature is more advantageous to soft tissue engineering as low temperature favors cell viability [8].

Crosslinking by ionic interaction allows stabilization of beads through a kind of gelation that is rapid and ion-mediated. For example, alginate bioinks may be crosslinked by calcium chloride, but the stable ionic bond occurs between guluronic acid residues. It is a popular, simple fast method. However, ionic crosslinking may sometimes result in heterogeneous gel formation with limited mechanical properties [23].

Another crosslinking technique is UV crosslinking technique. It is applied to photo-crosslinkable polymers such as GelMA (gelatin methacryloyl), PEGDA (polyethylene glycol diacrylate), and other methacrylated hydrogels. Polymerization occurs upon excitation with UV light by means of photoinitiators, which leads to high-resolution solidification. The two main limitations of this technique are cytotoxicity caused by exposure to UV light and photoinitiators, which can affect the survival of the cell [24]. Recent developments are combining these methods in hybrid crosslinking such as dual ionic and UV crosslinking, and it also shows constructs are strong and biocompatible. Emerging feature improvements also integrate in situ crosslinking modules into the printhead. After extrusion is done, the components can stabilize the structure and minimize deformation of the construction [3].

10.2.2 Working Principle of EBB

EBB consists of four main stages which are CAD model design and slicing, where a 3D digital model is created and converted into printable layers; bioink preparation, where hydrogel-based bioinks with cells are made; printing process, where prepared bioink is printed; and post-processing, where the printed structure is crosslinked using ionic, photo, or thermal methods.

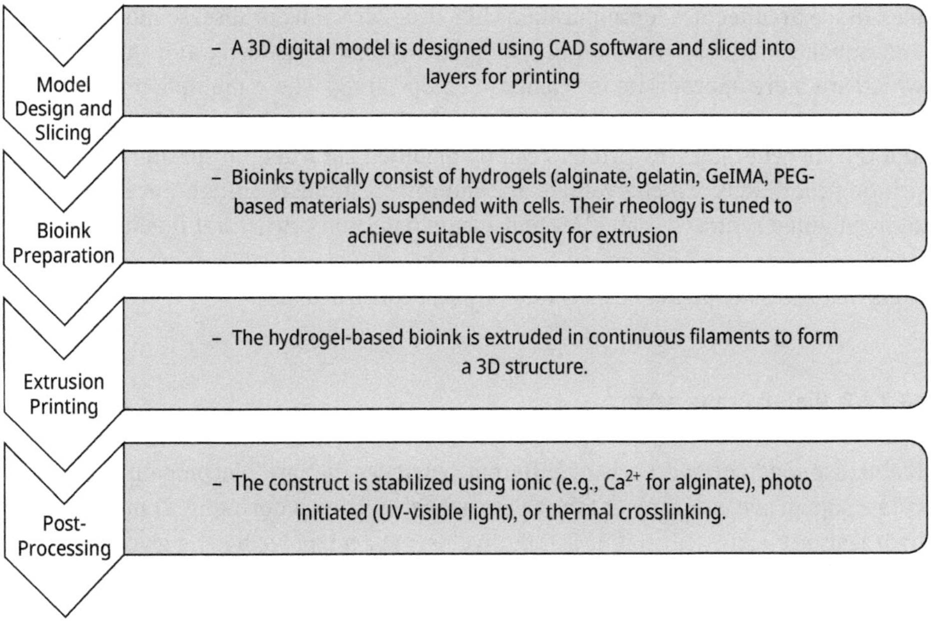

Figure 10.1: Workflow of extrusion-based bioprinting.

Figure 10.1 represents the workflow in EBB. The first step is model design and slicing, where a three-dimensional digital construct is designed using a computer-aided design (CAD) tool and sliced into printable layers. After bioink preparation, the formulation and rheological optimization of cell-laden hydrogel-based bioinks like alginate or gelatin, GelMA, and PEG-based materials is done to achieve adequate viscosity for extrusion. During printing, the hydrogel bioink is deposited as continuous filament through a nozzle, whereby a 3D structure is formed. Finally, post-processing involves stabilization of the printed construct through ionic (e.g., Ca^{2+}-mediated alginate crosslinking), photo-initiated (UV-visible light), or thermal crosslinking to give more integrity to the structure.

10.2.2.1 Model Design and Slicing

3D bioprinting is a technique that starts with designs and slicing. It involves making the structure of the target tissue or organs digitally through CAD software or the reconstruction of that target tissue from MRI or CT scans. The model is then sliced into separate layers by slicing software; it generates a specific G-code for the extrusion paths, speeds, heights, and nozzle pressures that determine the quality of resolution, pattern, pore size, and mechanical properties of the printed scaffold. Multilayer constructs that mimic different cell lineages can be designed and sliced to replicate complex tissue architecture for applications like drug screening or disease modeling. New and advanced slicing and path-planning strategies are growing and taking shape, which are more appropriate for composite bioprinting, where multiple materials and gradients are incorporated with precision [25]. Through open-source slicing software and G-code generators, bioprinters can be modified according to specific bioinks and printing conditions, which evaluate and improve printing conditions, even under resource-limited setup. Overall, CAD and slicing determine structural fidelity and functional performance of bioprinted tissues by providing precise manufacturing instructions that translate digital designs into physical constructs [26].

10.2.2.2 Bioink Preparation

Bioink are made of hydrogels or different polymers that are biocompatible and provide a supportive environment for cell to survive during bioprinting. Commonly used hydrogels are alginate, gelatin, GelMA, hyaluronic acid, polyethylene glycol (PEG) derivatives, and decellularized ECM (dECM) hydrogels. Every material has its own advantages and disadvantages. Alginate allows rapid ionic crosslinking, gelatin helps with cell adhesion, GelMA allows UV crosslinking with required mechanical properties, hyaluronic acid mimics the components that are found in native ECM, PEG derivatives allow for synthetic stability, and dECM hydrogels retain tissue-specific biochemical properties [27].

These hydrogels are usually mixed with living cells along with required biomolecules to make a functional bioinks. The growth factors are then added to this mixture. With proper bioink, the scaffold evolves from a simple structure to an active bioengineered tissue model. Bioinks are very important to regenerate medicine and modeling disease. After correct execution, these growth factors and signaling further activate cell differentiation, which leads to cell proliferation and final tissue maturation. The complex rheological properties of bioinks like viscosity, shear-thinning behavior, and yield stress make smooth extrusion possible without harming the cell. Viscosity should be high enough for the extruded shape to retain its form after printing, yet low enough to allow the ink to flow through the nozzle under applied pressure. Shear-thinning hydrogels are particular advantages as their viscosity decreases under shear stress during extrusion and recovers after deposition, thereby protecting cells while maintaining structural stability [28, 29].

The recent growth in the field has witnessed novel composite and hybrid bioink in the balance between biological functionality and mechanical strength by combining natural and synthetic polymers. For instance, alginate-GelMA blends enable rapid ionic as well as photo-crosslinking, while PEG-collagen composite is improving mechanical strength without changing biocompatibility. This hybrid formula has greater applications in creating complex tissues like osteochondral interfaces and vascularized constructs [3]. Also upcoming bioinks have incorporated nanomaterials and microparticles to improve printability and performance. Nano-clay, graphene oxide, and hydroxyapatite are incorporated into hydrogels for enhancing mechanical strength, electrical conductivity, and osteogenic potential. Ongoing researches are designing bioinks by equally prioritizing rheological properties and biological performance [30, 31].

10.2.2.3 Bioprinting/Material Extrusion

Every time bioink is extruded from a nozzle, EBB employs a controlled pressure or mechanical force to drive the material through a nozzle. After this the nozzle is moved to a spatial pattern of deposition. The process allows precise layer-by-layer assembly and supports fabrication of complex 3D geometries, including anatomically relevant and heterogeneous tissue constructs. Maintaining low shear stress during the extrusion process is very essential for cell viability, screw-assisted extrusion, and shear-thinning hydrogels like GelMA and alginate blends. They help minimize damage to cells while maintaining structural fidelity [5, 31].

Emerging innovations, including progressing cavity pumps and hybrid actuation systems, also improve flow stability, filament uniformity, reproducibility, and overall print resolution. Computational modeling of extrusion dynamics helps to optimize the mechanical stress on cells and improve post-printing viability [14]. Emerging techniques are combining mechanical accuracy with bioink rheology to achieve reproducible, cell-friendly deposition. Future refinements are expected to accelerate the development of highly functional, clinically relevant engineered tissues [4, 32].

10.2.2.4 Post-processing and Crosslinking

Post-processing in EBB basically involves crosslinking, which enhances the mechanical stability and shape fidelity of printed constructs. Common crosslinking methods include polymerization initiated by UV or visible light in methacrylated bioinks like GelMA, ionic crosslinking of alginate-based hydrogels using baths or sprays of calcium or strontium ions, and thermal gelation for temperature responsive materials [33, 34]. More specifically, ionic crosslinkers such as strontium Sr^{2+} have shown good results in higher compressive strength and slower degradation compared to Ca^{2+}, although both maintain good cytocompatibility. Advanced techniques such as the solenoid valve-controlled localized ionic crosslinking, further improve scaffold' stability and reduce the residual crosslinker toxicity, thus enhancing the proliferation of cells [35]. Additional maturation steps include incubation in bioreactor, perfusion-based nutrient exchange, and mechanical or chemical stimulation to promote cell proliferation, ECM formation, and functional tissue development. Emerging enzymatic and dual-step crosslinking techniques provide accurate control over gelation kinetics and bioink rheology, which leads to improvement of printing fidelity and cell viability in complex tissue constructs [36].

10.3 Types of Extrusion Mechanisms of EBB

Extrusion mechanisms form the foundation on which the functioning, resolution, and biological outcomes of an EBB process depend. Different extrusion modes influence shear stress, flow rate, cell viability, and having ability to handle different viscosities of bioink. The three primary methods of extrusion commonly used in EBB are pneumatic, piston-driven, and screw-driven systems. Each modality has its advantages as well as other design considerations which depend on the type of targeted tissue, bioink formulation, and intended structural fidelity.

Figure 10.2 shows a schematic representation of EBB systems: (a) pneumatic-driven extrusion bioprinting, where air pressure is applied to push bioink out of a nozzle. The controlled pressure forces the ink downward to form a continuous printed filament, and this system is commonly used for low-to-medium-viscosity bioinks; (b) piston-driven bioprinting, where a mechanical plunger compresses the bioink to extrude it through a nozzle, providing more consistent flow and making it better suited for higher-viscosity bioinks compared to pneumatic systems; and (c) screw-driven bioprinting, where a rotating screw inside the cartridge pushes the bioink downward through the nozzle. The mechanical rotation provides highly controlled and continuous extrusion, making this system suitable for printing high-viscosity, composite bioinks with improved flow stability, with the bioink exiting the nozzle to form a precise printed construct layer by layer.

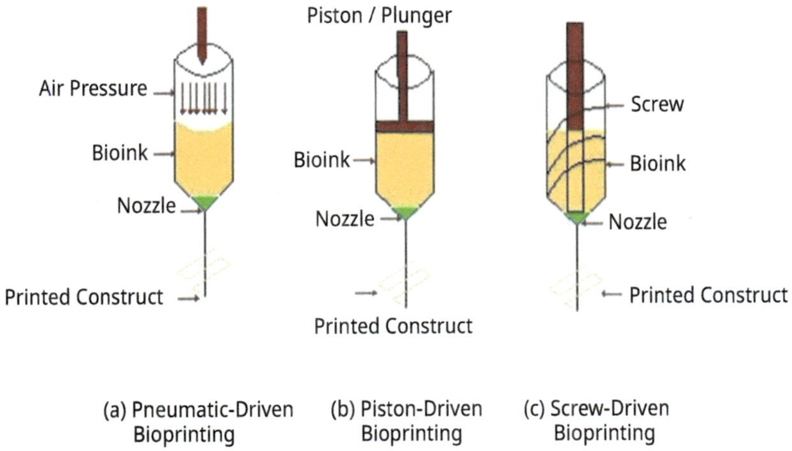

Figure 10.2: Types of extrusion mechanisms of extrusion-based bioprinting.

10.3.1 Pneumatic Extrusion Bioprinting

Pneumatic extrusion bioprinting relies on compressed air generally operating at 20–200 kPa to apply uniform pressure on the reservoir of bioink and lets the bioink pass through the nozzle. This method supports stable laminar flow like in the case of low-to-medium shear-thinning hydrogels like alginate, gelatin, and pluronic F127 [37]. It allows smooth, continuous filament deposition using simple hardware components and low maintenance. However, the high viscosity of these bioinks puts the pneumatic system at a disadvantage when higher pressures are needed. It often results in decrease in precision and the possibility of air bubbles entrapment, which affects accuracy in extrusion and print fidelity. Pressure stabilization delays during the start/stop cycles which can also reduce the accuracy of fine features [38]. It is clear from the recent studies that further optimization of parameters like nozzle diameter, extrusion pressure, and printing speed will be essential for achieving high printability and shape fidelity with pneumatic extrusion. While pneumatic extrusion is still widely used due to its simplicity and effectiveness, other modes of extrusion, such as screw-based or progressive cavity-driven extrusion, have advantages over pneumatic systems in flow control, precision, and reduction in cell damage especially for complex or heterogeneous bioinks [10, 39]. Pneumatic extrusion operates by applying compressed air to the bioink reservoir, generating pressure that drives the bioink through the nozzle as shown in Figure 10.2. Pressure regulators and feedback control systems enable modulation of flow rate. The table 10.1 shows application of pneumatic extrusion system.

10.3.1.1 Advantages of Pneumatic Extrusion Bioprinting

1) Smooth and continuous filament deposition takes place with defined rate due to uniform pressure distribution.
2) Pneumatic extrusion allows gentle and non-contact application of force for the maintenance of cell viability at high levels, especially for sensitive cell types.
3) Lack of direct mechanical force minimizes bioink contamination and material degradation.
4) Pneumatic systems are well suited for temperature-sensitive and biologically active bioinks, including cell-laden hydrogels.
5) Design features make sterilization and cartridge replacement easy, thus increasing the reproducibility while printing.
6) The system also lends itself very well to scalable and automated bioprinting due to its simple pressure control architecture.

10.3.1.2 Limitation of Pneumatic Extrusion Bioprinting

1) The compressibility of air is something that limits precise control over extrusion rate; consequently, delayed responses and pressure fluctuations arise.
2) Pneumatic extrusion is not very reliable for high-viscosity bioinks since, under such conditions, higher pressures are required, which may also affect print fidelity.
3) Inconsistencies in filament diameter and reduced printing accuracy arise due to variations in bioink rheology.
4) Shift-start control is another rather difficult aspect, as it will sometimes cause filament tailing across the print.
5) Shear stress may be induced by high pressures during operation, thus compromising the viability of cells encapsulated within bioinks.
6) The system itself is sensitive to pressure instabilities or air leaks, which will affect reproducibility.

10.3.2 Piston Extrusion Bioprinting

Piston-driven systems use a mechanical actuator typically a linear motor or stepper-motor-driven plunger to directly displace the bioink inside the cartridge. Piston-type bioprinting systems work by using a mechanical piston directly displacing the bioink within a cartridge or syringe, through the nozzle. It allows precise control over flow rate and extrusion pressure which results in the deposition of continuous filaments layer by layer. This helps improve printability and supports better structural accuracy in hydrogel constructs [42]. The table 10.2 shows application of piston extrusion sys-

Table 10.1: Application of pneumatic extrusion system.

S. no.	Case study	Bioink/ material used	Key experimental insight	Outcome/application demonstrated	References
1.	Soft tissue construct fabrication	Alginate and Pluronic F-127	Optimized pressure (~40 kPa), 27 G nozzle, temp. control smooth flow	~77% print accuracy, no filament breakage, ideal for soft shear-thinning inks	[38]
2.	Vascular channel bioprinting using sacrificial ink	Pluronic F127 (sacrificial) and GelMA matrix	Controlled pneumatic flow enabled clean deposition of sacrificial strands	Formation of perfusable microvascular networks after ink removal	[1]
3.	Multilayer skin-tissue constructs	Alginate-collagen hydrogel	Pressure-regulated extrusion smooth stacking, no clogging	>85% cell viability, strong mechanical integrity suitable for skin models	[40]
4.	Cartilage-mimetic scaffolds	Hyaluronic acid-rich hydrogels and chondrocytes	Low-shear pneumatic delivery reduced cell damage	Stable scaffold geometry with high cell survival and cartilage-like properties	[41]

tem. The displacement of the piston is usually controlled by a stepper motor which allows the rate of displacement and volumetric flow of the bioink to be precisely controlled. This is a direct mechanical actuation, so it is consistently stable and responsive. Consistent extrusion can be achieved by applying force acts directly on the bioink, which minimizes delays and fluctuations observed in pneumatic systems. The motion of the piston itself generates the pressure needed to extrude the bioink. Depending on the material's viscosity and yield stress, the amount of pressure can be balanced to ensure printability and cell viability. This method is mostly favorable for printing cell-laden hydrogels and other sensitive bioinks for achieving high-resolution and reproducible constructs with minimum risk of nozzle clogging and better structural fidelity [3, 43].

10.3.2.1 Advantages of Piston Extrusion Bioprinting

1) Extrusion through piston movement lends mechanical force directly, ensuring a steadier and more controllable flow of bioink with respect to pneumatic systems.
2) The system accommodates bioinks from medium-to-high-viscosity states for enhanced fidelity of prints.
3) There is less reliance on gaseous pressure, which minimizes response delays and leads to an optimized start-stop mechanism during printing.

4) Piston extrusion is volumetric and accurate while dispensing which gives a well-defined filament diameter.
5) Without compressed air any fluctuating background pressure is reduced, which emphasizes repeatability.
6) It allows precise delivery of materials such that it can be used in applications that require high geometric accuracy.

10.3.2.2 Limitations of Piston Extrusion Bioprinting

1) High shear stress may be induced by mechanical compression, which might ultimately affect cell viability in cell-laden bioinks.
2) The presence of additional mechanical components means increased maintenance requirements as compared to pneumatic systems.
3) Sudden changes in the rate of extrusion will be limited by the mechanical inertia of the piston.
4) If bioink rheology is not properly controlled, there will be backflow or pressure buildup.
5) The system may not be suitable for bioinks, which are exceedingly high viscous or loaded with particles, due to possible clogging.
6) Due to the direct contact of the piston with the bioink, sterilization and cleaning can be more complex.

10.3.3 Screw-Driven Extrusion Bioprinting

Screw-driven extrusion system is operated by displacing the bioink continuously toward the nozzle by using either a rotating screw or a progressing cavity pump. It helps to achieve a pulsation-free and stable flow of bioink. The rotation speed of the screw is directly controlled by the speed of screw rotation and allows volumetric flow for accurate regulation of extrusion pressure and filament diameter. Screw-driven extrusion provides consistent deposition without compressing like pneumatic systems. It is very responsive, especially for composite hydrogels, highly viscous polymer blends, and particle-laden bioinks. This gradual displacement helps reduce shear stress and improves cell viability during printing. It also enables load-bearing tissues like bone and cartilage to be fabricated with higher mechanical fidelity [4]. The Table 10.3 shows the applications of screw driven extrusion system. Screw-driven extrusion uses a rotating screw inside a chamber to convey bioink toward the nozzle tip. This mechanism has recently gained traction for high-performance bioprinting.

Table 10.2: Applications of piston extrusion system.

S. no.	Step/ stage	Case study example	Bioink/ material used	Key advantage observed	Outcome/ application	References
1.	High-viscosity printing	High-viscosity cartilage bioinks	GelMA + chondrocytes	Precise volumetric flow control allows smooth extrusion	Improved filament uniformity, viable chondrocyte growth, and ECM production	[43]
2.	Reinforced constructs for bone	Bone-mimetic HA scaffolds	Alginate-collagen + hydroxyapatite	Handles high viscosity even with fillers	Increased compressive strength and mineralization for bone regeneration	[5]
3.	Load-bearing tissue printing	Nanofiber-composite hydrogel scaffolds	Cellulose nanofiber + GelMA	Stable, continuous filament at high viscosity	High structural fidelity and osteogenic differentiation support	[18]
4.	Defect-repair and clinical use	Clinical-grade bioinks for cartilage repair	Collagen-rich formulations	Insensitive to compressibility reliable extrusion	Suitable for defect repair constructs in clinical settings	[27]

10.3.3.1 Advantages of Screw-Driven Extrusion Bioprinting

1) The continuous flow of material results in excellent stability during extrusion; thus, screw-driven extrusion has very good process control.
2) The system is, therefore, best suited for high-viscosity and particulate composite bioinks; they can comprise higher densities of particle-laden materials.
3) The screw precisely controls the volume and makes the filament more uniform, which will lead to higher fidelity in prints.
4) There is no flow pulsation in screw extrusion. Thus, layer-by-layer deposition takes place smoothly.
5) Tolerance to sustained extrusion through long printing periods is evident, making the system suitable for large or complex constructs.
6) The improved flow control gives better retention shapes and structural integrity within printed constructs.

10.3.3.2 Limitations of Screw-Driven Extrusion Bioprinting

1) High mechanical shear generated by the shear displacement results in a possible reduction in cell viability of the cell-laden bioinks.
2) The screw-driven systems are having more complicated designs, thereby leading to high costs of fabrication and maintenance.
3) Cleaning and sterilization are challenging due to the intricate internal screw mechanism.
4) Compared to piston-driven systems, the start–stop control is not very rapid.
5) The system may be unsuitable for low-viscosity bioinks because it becomes hard to control precisely.
6) Such mechanical complexity increases the chances of the material heating up or degrading when subjected to prolonged operation.

Table 10.3: Applications of screw-driven extrusion system.

S. no.	Application/case study	Bioink/material used	Key experimental insight/principle	Outcome/ application demonstrated	References (example)
1.	High-viscosity/highly loaded bioinks (viscous, composite, loaded with particles)	Hydrogel + micro-/ nanoparticles (e.g., alginate + α-TCP)	Use of screw-driven or twin-screw extrusion enables handling of viscous/ nanoparticle-laden bioinks that pneumatic extrusion struggles with.	Improved printability, homogeneous mixing of particles/cells, stable filament deposition even for dense inks	[44]
2.	Bone/hard tissue/ bone-scaffold bioprinting	Hydrogel + bioceramics/calcium phosphate particles (e.g., α-TCP, HAp)	Screw extrusion-based systems allow deposition of hydrogel–ceramic composite bioinks suitable for bone regeneration; mechanical integrity and composite mixing can be achieved.	Constructs with improved mechanical strength, mineral content, potential for bone tissue engineering	[45]

Table 10.3 (continued)

S. no.	Application/case study	Bioink/material used	Key experimental insight/principle	Outcome/ application demonstrated	References (example)
3.	Multi-component/multi-material bioinks requiring uniform mixing (e.g., composites, gradients, and cell + particles)	Alginate + α-TCP micro-/ nanoparticles + osteoblast cells (or similar composite hydrogels)	Use of a semi-automated twin-screw extruder head allows real-time mixing of multiple components (polymers, particles, and cells), producing homogeneous bioinks and preventing sedimentation or aggregation.	Uniform particle–cell distribution, reproducible scaffolds with good biological (cell viability) and mechanical properties	[44]
4.	Use of high-viscosity or viscoelastic hydrogels/complex rheological inks (e.g., non-Newtonian, shear thinning)	Various bioinks with shear-thinning/viscoelastic behavior; high polymer content hydrogels	Screw-driven extrusion provides greater volumetric control and pressure to extrude viscous/ non-Newtonian bioinks reliably, improving printability over pneumatic methods.	Successful filament deposition, maintenance of filament continuity and shape fidelity even with challenging rheology	[46]

10.4 Bioink Requirements for EBB

Bioinks suitable for extrusion should be able to balance printability, strength, and biocompatibility to support functional tissue constructs. Rheological properties include shear thinning and viscoelasticity allowing smooth extrusion and stability for 3D printing avoiding shear stress and maintaining cell viability [47]. When it comes to extrusion bioprinting, finding the right viscosity range along with clear shear-thinning behavior is critical for filament continuity, nozzle clogging prevention, and high-resolution pattern formation [31]. It improves printability and biological function through optimization of the viscosity and crosslinking mechanism enhancers such as natural and synthetic hydrogel components using multi-component bioink. Different crosslinking techniques like photopolymerization, ionic, enzymatic, or thermal crosslinking ensures printability and stabilization after printing [49]. These mechanical properties should be tunable to the stiffness of the target tissue. This can include bioinks like GelMA which is improved by adding Laponite to improve rheology and print fidelity while not compromising on the cellular health. Printing is not the end in itself, but the stage where mechanical stability must be put in place since bioinks will also be subjected to handle weight due to subsequent layers and will distribute load without losing the geometry. By controlling the stiffness, yield stress, and elastic modulus, the printed construct can imitate the mechanical behavior of native ECM [50]. Crosslinking dynamics and microgel assembly techniques can improve shape retention, microporosity, and self-healing to support complex tissue architecture and function of cells. Additionally, biocompatibility and cell viability are based on the choice of cytocompatible polymers, minimizing toxic photoinitiators, and allowing nutrient diffusion across the printed matrix. In general, an EBB requires careful balance in flow behavior, structural stability after printing, and a suitable microenvironment for the encapsulated cells survival and differentiation [46].

10.4.1 Viscosity and Shear-Thinning Behavior

Viscosity plays a very important role in the bioink extrusion process used in EBB. The shear-thinning hydrogels are capable of decreasing their viscosity under shear stress and can recover it again after extrusion. This property of hydrogels allows for hassle-free extrusion, which reduces the pressure applied for extrusion, shear stress on loaded cells for better viability, and shape fidelity of the printed filaments [51]. Optimal viscosity requirements for the bioinks range from 30 to 6,000 mPa · s depending on the nozzle size and printing pressure to balance in ease of extrusion against filament stability [47]. Studies on gelatin–alginate composites show that extrusion pressure and print quality are dependent on storage and loss moduli, with an ideal range for the loss tangent of 0.25–0.45 being a good compromise between integrity and uniform extrusion [51]. The presence of rheological modifiers such as layered nanoparticles or nanocellulose may improve viscosity and shear-thinning properties to ensure better printability while maintaining cell viability. Machine learning models have also been developed to predict viscosity of bioink based on composition and shear rate, thus optimizing the formulation to achieve desired extrusion characteristics [52].

Figure 10.3 shows the key parameters that determine the viscosity of a bioink. Factors like molecular weight and concentration directly influence thickness. Temperature affects the flow behavior of thermoresponsive gels. Additives like nanocellulose, collagen, or nanoparticles can increase structural strength, while the degree of crosslinking further controls network density and flow properties.

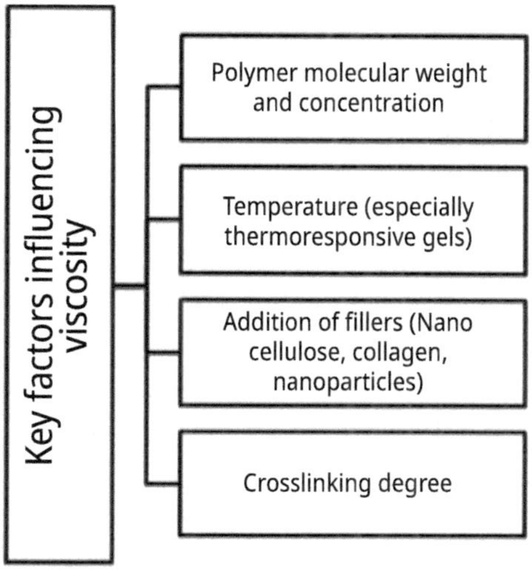

Figure 10.3: Factors affecting viscosity.

10.4.2 Crosslinking Compatibility

Post-extrusion stability of the printed structure depends on crosslinking strategies. These strategies provide mechanical integrity and shape fidelity and preserve the cell viability. There are various crosslinking methods that are commonly used like ionic, covalent, enzymatic, and photo-crosslinking, depending on the bioink's composition and application. Photo-crosslinking is widely used for hydrogels like GelMA because gelation is rapid without significant cytotoxicity. Crosslinking using calcium ions for alginate or iron(III) for carboxymethyl cellulose-based bioinks increases the mechanical stability and has allowed longer integrity with high cell viability [47]. Novel methods like double-crosslinking systems use an internal and external mechanism for improved structural integrity and shape fidelity, as referred in Potere et al. [49]. Enzymatic crosslinking with horseradish peroxidase and hydrogen peroxide leads to fast gelation with good cell viability. One of those is solenoid valve-controlled crosslinking that improves precision and minimizes residual toxic agents. Therefore, successful crosslinking strategies should strike a balance between maintaining mechanical strength and cytocompatibility in bioprinted scaffolds [35].

Figure 10.4 presents the commonly used crosslinking strategies to stabilize bioinks after extrusion. Ionic crosslinking using Ca^{2+} with alginate forms rapid gel networks. Photo-crosslinking uses UV/visible light to polymerize materials like GelMA. Thermo-responsive systems gel with temperature-induced micelle formation, while enzymatic crosslinking relies on enzymes such as thrombin or transglutaminase to form covalent bonds. Together, these methods give structural integrity and biological performance to printed scaffold.

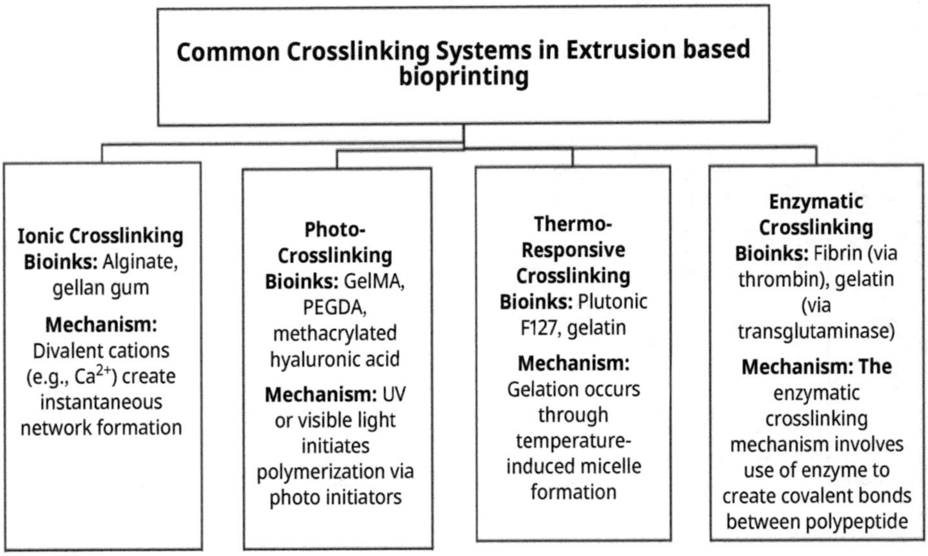

Figure 10.4: Crosslinking methods used for extrusion-based bioprinting.

10.4.3 Biocompatibility and Cell Viability

In EBB, bioinks should provide a compatible microenvironment that is similar to the cells ECM. This is required for cell adhesion, proliferation, and differentiation. It also ensures sufficient nutrient and oxygen diffusion throughout the cell. Such bioinks are collagen, GelMA, hyaluronic acid, and dECM, which provide viability and biological functionality to cells because of their ECM-derived biochemical. There are blends of bioink prepared for scaffold printing such as alginate-GelMA blends, alginate-gelatin blend, and alginate-hydroxyapatite blend. This well-formulated composite of bioinks provides good printability along with biological activity that supports cell growth [53]. For bioprinting, it is necessary to maintain cell viability above 80%, while the bioinks do not cause cytotoxicity. Failing to fulfil any of the above requirements can cause failure of scaffold in body. Ying et al. [53] showed that proper optimization of GelMA has high survival rates of cells and supports cell growth within printed constructs. Advancement in nanocomposite bioinks has incorporated materials like cellulose or conductive polymer which has led to obtaining better biocompatibility and functionality without compromising cell viability [54].

Figure 10.5 represents the factors affecting cell survival during EBB. High shear stress can physically damage cells, while improper temperature conditions can harm thermosensitive bioinks. Crosslinking which includes UV light can affect cellular health. Mechanical stiffness of the printed matrix also plays a role by regulating transduction of cells, which affects the long-term cell function.

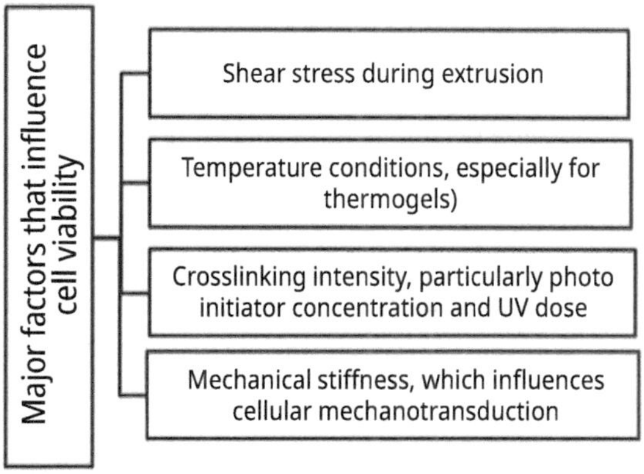

Figure 10.5: Factors affecting cell viability.

10.4.4 Mechanical Stability and Print Fidelity

In order to preserve shape fidelity, bioinks need to have required yield stresses to prevent spreading as well as rapid gelation kinetics immediately after printing. These considerations are very important when it comes to maintaining multilayered 3D-printed structures without collapse. The elastic behavior of bioinks should also be tunable to match the stiffness of the target tissue ensuring mechanical compatibility and biological functions [50]. Advanced bioinks like nano-engineered ionic-covalent entanglement (NICE) become more mechanically stiff and elastic for printing taller, complex structures with high fidelity [55]. dECM bioinks combined with photo-crosslinkers such as vitamin B_2 have the potential to increase mechanical properties similar to native tissue. This enhancement improves printability as well as cell viability [56]. Rheological properties like shear-thinning and Herschel-Bulkley flow characteristics play an important role in cell protection during extrusion while maintaining shape fidelity [55]. Overall, achieving balance of flow properties, crosslinking speed, and architecture of scaffold design is necessary for stable 3D constructs with high integrity.

10.5 Technological Advances in Extrusion-Based Bioprinting

10.5.1 Multi-material Extrusion

Bioprinting the scaffold using multi-material extrusion involves the simultaneous extrusion of two or more bioinks with the combination of biomaterials like polycaprolactone (PCL) with cell-laden hydrogels. This combination has to closely replicate the heterogeneous composition of native tissues. It will create gradients of mechanical and biological properties that are required for designing complex tissues like bone–cartilage and vascularized tissues [37]. Precise spatial control is available for materials through different techniques like side-by-side printing, core-shell extrusion, and advanced multi-reservoir systems which enhance the functional complexity of printed constructs [57]. The challenges include maintenance of high inter-material adhesion to avoid failure and cross-contamination between bioinks during the actual printing continuous multi-material extrusion with very quick switches between bioinks, and OCT monitoring is the latest advancement in printing accuracy and fewer material deposition errors at interfaces [58]. Multi-extrusion systems constructed inexpensively expand accessibility, democratized access, and enabled complex, multimaterial tissue models featuring high cellular viability and remarkably close structural fidelity [59].

10.5.2 Coaxial Nozzle Systems

Extrusion of concentric core-shell structures with outer shells providing mechanical support and inner core carrying cells or growth factors is an application of coaxial nozzle bioprinting. This method is very useful for vascular tissue engineering and drug delivery scaffolds. It enables fabrication of perfusable, cell-laden tubular constructs with different cell types such as endothelial and fibroblast cells. Advantages of coaxial bioprinting includes creating a cocultures by putting different cell populations in core and shell regions which in the end might enhance functionality of the tissue and mimics the similarities in native bones or osteochondral tissues [60]. Thus, optimizing flow rate and nozzle design becomes essential parameter to maintain stable core-shell structures, allow proper gelation, and ensure cell survival during printing. The challenges can be while optimizing extrusion parameters for preventing mixing of different layers and ensuring consistency in the mechanical properties without compromising on cell survival. Recent developments include low-cost DIY coaxial bioprinters and enzymatically crosslinkable bioinks that allow for rapid gelation and high cell viability, thus enabling greater access and use for complex tissue fabrication [18].

10.5.3 Integration with Microfluidics

The integration of bioprinting skills and microfluidic chips allows precise control over nutrient flow and vascularization, giving rise to advanced organ-on-a-chip (OoC) platforms. These OoC platforms resemble in vivo tissue microenvironments in a highly representative manner. The combination allows the construction of continuous perfusion, waste removal, and real-time monitoring while maintaining dynamic culture conditions that support cell survival [61, 62]. The major challenges are developing cheap, reproducible systems that can handle tissue structure and functionality while working with different cell types and biomaterials. With advances of automated bioprinting integrated with robotic handling of microfluidic chips, the output and consistency were improved. The vascularized tissue models which included multicellularity with stable microvascular networks were sustained for longer culture periods [62].

10.5.4 Automation and AI in Bioprinting

Automation and artificial intelligence (AI) are rapidly integrated with bioprinting for optimization of workflows, reproducibility, and rapid-prototyping ability. AI integration has accelerated the capabilities of optimization of bioink compositions and designing printing parameters. It has improved overall printing fidelity and cell viability while reducing trial-and-error experimentation. Robotics facilitates scalability and precision in bioprinting processes supporting personalized implants and complex tissue constructs with consistent quality. They allow prediction of tissue growth and maturation after printing thus facilitating the application of regenerative medicine and organ transplantation which is unable due to donor shortages. Despite promising advances, challenges still remain in integrating AI with diverse biomaterials and complex tissue architectures to fully automated, intelligent bioprinting platforms [63].

10.6 Advantages and Limitations of EBB

EBB is most commonly methods in 3D bioprinting due to its versatility and ability to process a wide range of bioinks. It is used in most of the research work to produce large clinically relevant tissue constructs. However, the technique is associated with limitations in resolution, cell viability, and bioink engineering. Advantages and disadvantages are critical in assisting researchers in determining the different printing strategies combined with bioink formulations they should use for specific tissue applications.

10.6.1 Advantages of EBB

10.6.1.1 Print High-Viscosity Hydrogel Systems

A different advantage of EBB is that it has capability to extrude high-viscosity bioinks approximately from 30 to 6,000 mPa · s. Bioink with such viscosity would be incompatible with inkjet or laser-based printing methods. These viscous hydrogels include alginate, gelatin, GelMA, and collagen blends. They form self-supporting filaments that allow high shape fidelity and enhance mechanical strength of the printed scaffold. This conclusion has been repeatedly emphasized in high-impact reviews like Groll et al. [27] and Murphy and Atala [1].

10.6.1.2 Ability to Incorporate High Cell Densities

EBB supports the use of with high cell density bioinks approximately 10^6–10^8 cells/mL without causing nozzle clogging. Extrusion is based on mechanical or pneumatic force rather than heat or droplet-based mechanisms. This makes it suitable for making the cell-rich tissues, including cartilage, liver, and tumor microenvironments [64].

10.6.1.3 Good Structural Stability in Printed Constructs

Structural strength is very important because of using viscous hydrogels. They retain their shape after deposition and show excellent layer-by-layer integrity and dimensional fidelity. This property is particularly important for load-bearing tissue like bone, cartilage, and vascular scaffolds, where mechanical integrity is paramount [8].

10.6.1.4 Flexibility in Fabrication of Large Tissue Constructs

EBB enables the printing of macroscale constructs with centimeter-scale dimensions, overcoming a limitation in other bioprinting technologies. This capability makes the EBB particularly suitable for creating large tissues and organ segments, including bone grafts, meniscal scaffolds, and muscle constructs [4].

10.6.2 Limitations of EBB

10.6.2.1 High Shear Stress

A key limitation of EBB is reduction in cell viability as cells are subjected to high shear stress. These can cause mechanical damage, apoptosis, or a loss of phenotype in the cells. Shear stress rises with increasing narrowness of the nozzles, higher extrusion speeds, and increased viscosity of the bioink. In various studies, cell viability reductions ranging between 10% and 40% were related to printing parameters, emphasizing the careful optimization of extrusion conditions in more detail [1].

10.6.2.2 Lower Resolution Compared to Inkjet or Laser Bioprinting

Typical EBB resolution ranges between 100 and 500 µm, which is significantly lower than the 10–50 µm resolution achievable with inkjet- or laser-assisted bioprinting. This makes the process unsuitable for several applications requiring finer resolutions, like microtissue patterning, capillary-scale vascular networks, and neuronal architectures [65].

While EBB is well suited for large constructs, complex geometries with many materials, fine internal features, or lattice-like structures can be very time-consuming. Additional multi-material switching and crosslinking steps further reduce throughput, making EBB inefficient for very complex designs [66].

10.6.2.3 Requirement of Rheological Optimization of Bioinks

Printing in EBB relies strongly on the careful tuning of the bioink rheology, including viscosity, yield stress, shear-thinning behavior, and crosslinking kinetics. Poor rheology can easily result in clogging of the nozzle, filament spreading, or low structural fidelity. This was mentioned in several major reviews as one of the most critical bottlenecks to further develop EBB bioinks [31].

10.7 Applications of EBB

10.7.1 Skin Tissue Engineering

Skin is the highly complex organ of the body, and it comes in direct contact with the external environmental. Skin acts as a shield against the UV damage, physical and any external harmful agent [12, 13]. An ideal skin should have the biocompatibility, mechanical properties, as well as the interconnected porosity which can allow the cell for transferring the nutrients [67]. 3D bioprinting is an innovative strategy which helps in overcoming the current limitation for manufacturing the skin tissues, which is caused due to poor vascularization, absence of hair follicles, and sweat gland [12]. EBB is widely used for 3D bioprinting that helps the researchers to print multiple biomaterials, skin cells, and chemical signals layer by layer to mimic ECM. EBB is mostly used for generating skin or soft tissue [68]. Hydrogel is the most common material for generation of the skin graft. dECM is able to mimic the complex functional and structural features of ECM. Khoshnood and Zamanian [69] used porcine skin for developing novel bioink dECM-based bioink consisting of different structural proteins, glycosaminoglycans, and different biochemical signals which support the cell adhesion, proliferation, and differentiation for obtaining the ECM remodeling. 3D-printed skin has better structural fidelity and potential for vascularization which indicates that EBB-based printing helps in treating complex skin defects and chronic wounds.

10.7.2 Bone Tissue Engineering

Bone helps in obtaining the rigid structure of musculoskeletal system. It is highly mineralized tissue. Bone repair is the major challenge worldwide due to limited graft availability, donor site morbidity, and infection risk [70]. EBB is mostly used in bone tissue regeneration because it can easily print composite scaffolds combining natural hydrogels like alginate, gelatin, and collagen with bioceramics such as hydroxyapatite (HAp), β-tricalcium phosphate (β-TCP), and bioactive glass. These composites are suitable for mimicking the mineralized ECM of native bone. It also helps to provide osteoconductive signals that help in differentiation of mesenchymal stem cells (MSCs). EBB constructs help in obtaining mechanically reinforced structure. These structures are capable of sustaining high stresses and maintaining stability under load [1, 71]. EBB supports the layer-by-layer deposition which supports the mineral content and porosity in the gradients to obtain nutrient diffusion and vascular infiltration. Because of these features, EBB is suitable for printing customized bone graft, segmental bone defect repair, orthopedic implant integration, and patient-specific bone graft fabrication. Hydrogel-based scaffold is mostly used in EBB. These hydrogels are combined with thermoplastic polymers or ceramics which integrated with nanoparticles, nanofibers, or carriers for enhancing stiffness and osteoconductivity [72]. Major hurdles for clinical translation of EBB constructs are to obtain mechanical stability, nutrients, and oxygen supply and to print human-sized grafts [42].

10.7.3 Cartilage Tissue Engineering

Cartilage is avascular and a neural connective tissue. It is highly hydrated and consists of chondrocytes which is surrounded by ECM. ECM is made up of water (~70%), proteoglycans (with glycosaminoglycans, GAGs), and type-II collagen fibers. Because of this unique composition, cartilage has load-bearing capacity and resilience to compressive force. Cartilage lacks self-repairing capability because of lacks of vascularization and slow proliferation of chondrocytes. Conventional treatments like autologous chondrocytes implant, cartilage grafts, and microfracture do not fully restore native hyaline cartilage [73].

EBB helps in obtaining cartilage's architecture and microenvironment by layer-by -layer deposition of cells and biomaterials. Different natural and synthetic hydrogels like alginate, gelatin, and nanofibrillated cellulose are the common materials for preparing the bioink for cartilage bioprinting. These materials have water retention, biocompatibility, and ECM mimicking properties [74]. Different studies suggest that hydrogel printed scaffold helps in ECM deposition, chondrocyte viability, and obtaining the cartilage like phenotype. However, obtaining structural complexity and mechanical properties similar to native tissue is still challenging. Hydrogels lack in providing adequate stiffness, structural fidelity, and durability to provide long-term solution. To overcome these limitation polymers like polycaprolactone (PCL), reinforcing particles and composites bioink are combined with hydrogels to print scaffold which has balanced biocompatibility and mechanical properties [75]. EBB is the most promising approach for engineered cartilage replacement for mimicking the structural and functional properties of native ECM.

10.8 Case Studies on EBB

EBB has emerged as a central platform in regenerative medicine due to its capability to process highly viscous biomaterials, incorporate high cell densities, and fabricate clinically relevant, load-bearing constructs. Its ability to precisely deposit multimaterial systems makes it particularly advantageous for tissues requiring hierarchical architecture, structural robustness, and heterogeneous microenvironments. The following sections highlight major application domains where EBB has demonstrated significant impact.

10.8.1 Case Study: Print Accuracy and Filament Stability in Pneumatic Extrusion

A recent study by Hibbert et al. [38] on optimizations of pneumatic extrusion bioprinting parameters for a pluronic F-127 and alginate hybrid hydrogel achieved stable filament formation and around 77% printing accuracy using a 27 G nozzle, with pneumatic pressure of approximately 40 kPa and print-head speed close to 8 mm/s. The study demonstrated the way in which tuning extrusion pressure, nozzle size, and temperature could be used to overcome general problems like filament instability and poor resolution in pneumatic extrusion of shear-thinning hydrogels. Pneumatic extrusion is a practical and feasible technique for printing hydrogels of suitable rheological properties, balancing bioink compatibility, printability, and ease of setup. Such characteristics make it an interesting option for producing soft tissue constructs, microchannel networks, and scaffolds with sacrificial bioinks. The simplicity of the method with the ability to produce the continuous and smooth filament is generally used in tissue engineering and biological model fabrication. However, in case of high-precision or complex bioinks, other extrusion methods like screw-based dispensers may provide better process control and precision [38].

10.8.2 Case Study: Predictive Flow Rate Modeling for Optimizing Pneumatic Extrusion Bioprinting

Another research done by Arjoca et al. [76] focuses on improvement of pneumatic extrusion bioprinting by the determination of hydrogel flow rate and the extrusion speed through a cylindrical nozzle. In this study, the authors used non-Newtonian fluid modeling to predict both extrusion speed and swell ratio, which allows estimating of the printing speeds that were required for getting specific filament diameters under different pressure conditions. To confirm these predictions, they bioprinted three-layer of hydrogel grids using extrusion parameters and printing speeds to identical conditions. This led to enhancement of filament's morphology and scaffold integrity. The authors concluded that the early-stage flow rate measurements can greatly reduce complexity in optimizing printing parameters while ensuring accurate filament deposition and reducing shear stress on cells. This is important for maintaining cell viability and structural fidelity during bioprinting. Overall the methodology provides a step-by-step guide for adjusting pneumatic pressure and printing speed to achieve a consistent filament that is essential in soft tissue engineering and scaffold fabrication where precision in filament's dimensions is essential [76].

10.9 Future Directions

10.9.1 Advanced Rheological Engineering and Bioink Design

In the future, bioink development will focus on the precise engineering of rheological properties that can balance printability and biological functions together. It will also focus on emphasis on shear-thinning behavior for smooth extrusion and immediate recovery of shape fidelity. Alginate-based bioinks reinforced with lysozyme nanofibers exhibit improved shear thinning, with the recovery of ~90%, printability, and cell viability, highlighting the importance of pre-crosslinking and nanofiber content:

1. Composite bioinks combining methacrylated κ-carrageenan and hydroxyapatite possess tunable rheological and mechanical properties that can benefit both printability and cell viability, highlighting the role of chemical modification and filler incorporation.
2. Rheological parameters such as yield stress, shear-thinning, and recovery behavior are critically determined by the factors for extrusion bioprinting performance and cell survival, using mathematical models aiming for optimized printing conditions which can give minimum cell damage.
3. The incorporation of nanomaterials (gold nanoparticles, MXene nanosheets, Laponite) enhances the parameters of conductivity, rheology, printability, and mechanical properties while ensuring that high cell viability. Overall, controlling the

rheology and crosslinking enhances printing fidelity, cell viability, and tissue-specific functionality in extrusion bioprinting [32].

10.9.2 Multi-material and Multimodal Bioprinting

Multi-material bioprinting permits the fabrication of complex heterogeneous tissue constructs that can be used to recreate the natural tissue microenvironments better than any other single-material approaches. Coaxial and triaxial nozzles help in providing the layered structures of vascularity. The hybrid extrusion–inkjet and extrusion–microfluidic systems allow simultaneous deposition of materials with distinct mechanical and biochemical properties. Real-time mixing lays the foundation for dynamic adjustment of bioink composition and allows precise heterogeneity needed for various tissue interfaces, such as osteochondral and tendon bone [77]. These advancements will further facilitate the development of graded, hierarchical, and vascularized tissues with improved structural and functional biomimetics toward tissue engineering applications [78].

10.9.3 In Situ and In Vivo Bioprinting

In situ bioprinting allows the direct deposition of bioinks into the wounds or tissue defects during surgery for personalized and precise repair of tissues. Imaging-guided, robotic, and handheld bioprinters allow the controlled printing on irregular, curved, or moving surfaces which increases the fidelity and flexibility in the clinical environment. Studies have shown that in situ bioprinting promotes wound healing and skin regeneration via cell proliferation, angiogenesis, and ECM synthesis, with applications in burn care, chronic wounds, and full-thickness skin damages [79]. Adding bioactive components like platelet-rich plasma or photosynthetic microalgae in bioinks can enhance the bioprinting for tissue repair by modulating inflammation, fostering vascularization, and relieving hypoxic effects [80]. Commercially available robotic bioprinters have shown efficacy in animal models for enhancing quality of wound healing by not interrupting normal repair processes suggesting stronger clinical translation potential. Handheld bioprinters have the advantage of portability and it is easy to use. Thus, some of the limitations posed by traditional systems can be overcome, thereby broadening the scope of in situ bioprinting in skin, cartilage, bone, and muscle regeneration [81].

10.9.4 Microfluidics and Automation Integration

Integrating microfluidics with EBB enhances control over cell encapsulation, nutrient delivery, and biochemical gradients, enabling fabrication of complex, heterogeneous tissue constructs with improved vascularization potential. Microfluidic printheads rely on rapid mixing and switching of bioinks to enable higher resolution and control over precise spatial positioning of multiple materials and cell types within a single construct [82]. These automated systems, when integrated with AI intelligence for optimization options, would then close the loop for process feedback. This will eliminate the inconsistencies of printing which can arise from the human interpretation of the process and allow some dynamic change during fabrication. Such further techniques are required for scaling up the production of hierarchical, vascularized tissues and organs on a chip with least manual intervention. This is more transferrable to clinical practice and high-throughput tissue engineering. There is still much work to be done to completely validate these approaches for clinical routine and standards for widespread accessibility in clinical practice [83].

10.9.5 Real-Time Monitoring and On-Printer Bioreactors

In bioprinting, real-time monitoring can be applied to imaging tools such as OCT and multiphoton microscopy to evaluate layer fidelity, cell distribution, and structural integrity throughout the fabrication process. Fluorescence imaging, complemented by portable digital microscopes, provides non-invasive and in situ visualization of cell dispersion which allows for immediate detection of anomalies. Embedded sensors in the constructs measure parameters such as pH, oxygen, and temperature to give continuous feedback regarding the microenvironment. On-printer bioreactors, such as FABRICA platform, help in the perfusion and early-stage maturation of 3D-bioprinted tissues which supports viability of cells with real-time monitoring and controlled culture condition. These integrated monitoring and bioreactor systems reduce uncertainty in viability assessments after printing, thus accelerating tissue development, although these technologies still require enrichment for routine clinical implementation [84].

10.9.6 4D Bioprinting and Shape-Morphing Materials

Scaffolds printed with shape-changing materials like smart hydrogels or polymers which are time dependent can remodel or self-assemble at later periods; they respond to different environmental stimuli like temperature, pH, or electromagnetic fields. This system furnishes the fabrication of dynamic structures, such as self-folding vasculature, adaptive grafts, and organoid models that reflect developmental and physiological processes. Many shape-changing mechanisms respond to stimuli, like differential swelling, shape-memory effects, or near-infrared-triggered; an emerging trend is to use computational models to analyze and design the shape changes of bioprinted constructs, thus enabling the function of the constructs. Though advances, challenges still exist to increase the smart bioink options, improve printing strategies, and enable the translation of these systems into clinical tissue engineering applications [67].

10.9.7 Clinical Translation and Regulatory Integration

Due to advancement in bioprinting technology, there will be an increased necessity to develop regulatory frameworks and Good Manufacturing Practice (GMP) compliant protocols. Currently, efforts are focused on defining the quality standards for bioink, scale-up processes as well as clear approval pathways for bioprinted devices. Therefore, collaboration is necessary between researchers, clinicians, and regulatory agencies to facilitate the transition of EBB from laboratory settings into routine clinical practice [85].

10.10 Conclusion

EBB has proven itself as a foundational technology in tissue engineering and regenerative medicine owing to various factors such as versatility and compatibility with highly viscous bioinks and high cell densities. This has made EBB an attractive translational bioprinting technology because of its ability to create structures from bone and cartilage scaffolds to models of complex soft tissue and organs. Even with this advance, many challenges still remain like shear-induced cellular damage, low resolution of printing, and requirement for complex rheological optimization. Developing new online monitoring systems like coaxial multi-material extrusion, rheological adaptive bioinks, and 4D bioprinting strategies is further enhancing this field. As biology, engineering, and computational designing work together, extrusion bioprinting is shifting from experimental lab oratories to routine and clinical application. Continuous development in EBB promises to give rise to patient-specific fabrication of future tissues and organs to push boundaries in regenerative medicine and improve therapeutic success for patients.

References

[1] Murphy, S. V. & Atala, A. (Aug. 2014). 3D bioprinting of tissues and organs. Nature Biotechnology, 32(8), 773–785. doi: 10.1038/nbt.2958.

[2] Imrie, P. & Jin, J. (May 2025). 4D bioprinting: keeping the technology alive. Macromolecular Materials and Engineering, 310(5), doi: 10.1002/mame.202400386.

[3] Rossi, A. et al. (Jun. 2024). Biomaterials for extrusion-based bioprinting and biomedical applications. Frontiers in Bioengineering and Biotechnology, 12, doi: 10.3389/fbioe.2024.1393641.

[4] Ozbolat, I. T. & Hospodiuk, M. (Jan. 2016). Current advances and future perspectives in extrusion-based bioprinting. Biomaterials, 76, 321–343. doi: 10.1016/j.biomaterials.2015.10.076.
[5] Zhang, Y. S. et al. (Nov. 2021)3D extrusion bioprinting. Nature Reviews Methods Primers, 1(1), 75. doi: 10.1038/s43586-021-00073-8.
[6] Bakirci, E., Adib, A. A., Ashraf, S. F. & Feinberg, A. W. (Apr. 2025). Advancing extrusion-based embedded 3D bioprinting via scientific, engineering, and process innovations. Biofabrication, 17(2), 023002. doi: 10.1088/1758-5090/adb7c3.
[7] Placone, J. K. & Engler, A. J. (Apr. 2018). Recent advances in extrusion-based 3D printing for biomedical applications. Advanced Healthcare Materials, 7(8), doi: 10.1002/adhm.201701161.
[8] Cui, X. et al. (Aug. 2020). Advances in extrusion 3D bioprinting: a focus on multicomponent hydrogel-based bioinks. Advanced Healthcare Materials, 9(15), doi: 10.1002/adhm.201901648.
[9] Ramesh, S. et al. (Mar. 2021). Extrusion bioprinting: recent progress, challenges, and future opportunities. Bioprinting, 21, e00116. doi: 10.1016/j.bprint.2020.e00116.
[10] Fisch, P., Holub, M. & Zenobi-Wong, M. (Jan. 2021). Improved accuracy and precision of bioprinting through progressive cavity pump-controlled extrusion. Biofabrication, 13(1), 015012. doi: 10.1088/1758-5090/abc39b.
[11] Mei, X. et al. (2025)Integrating microfluidic and bioprinting technologies: advanced strategies for tissue vascularization. Lab Chip, 25(5), 764–786. doi: 10.1039/D4LC00280F.
[12] Woods, P., Smith, C., Clark, S. & Habib, A. (Aug. 2024). Integrating pneumatic and thermal control in 3D bioprinting for improved bio-ink handling. Designs, 8(4), 83. doi: 10.3390/designs8040083.
[13] Wei, Q., An, Y., Zhao, X., Li, M., Zhang, J. & Cui, N. (Dec. 2025). Optimal design of multi-biomaterials mixed extrusion nozzle for 3D bioprinting considering cell activity. Virtual and Physical Prototyping, 20(1), doi: 10.1080/17452759.2024.2438897.
[14] Lombardi, L., Scalzone, A., Ausilio, C., Gentile, P. & Tammaro, D. (Jun. 2025). Optimizing nozzle design in extrusion-based 3D bioprinting to minimize mechanical stress and enhance cell viability. International Journal of Bioprinting, 025190182. doi: 10.36922/IJB025190182.
[15] McCauley, P. J., Fromen, C. A. & Bayles, A. V. (Oct. 2025). Cell viability in extrusion bioprinting: the impact of process parameters, bioink rheology, and cell mechanics. Rheologica Acta, 64(9–10), 497–515. doi: 10.1007/s00397-025-01504-z.
[16] Reina-Romo, E., Mandal, S., Amorim, P., Bloemen, V., Ferraris, E. & Geris, L. (Aug. 2021). Towards the experimentally-informed in silico nozzle design optimization for extrusion-based bioprinting of shear-thinning hydrogels. Frontiers in Bioengineering and Biotechnology, 9, doi: 10.3389/fbioe.2021.701778.
[17] Jergitsch, M. et al. (Jul. 2025)Fabrication and validation of an affordable DIY coaxial 3D extrusion bioprinter. Scientific Reports, 15(1), 22978. doi: 10.1038/s41598-025-06478-9.
[18] Banigo, A. T., Nauta, L., Zoetebier, B. & Karperien, M. (Mar. 2025). Hydrogel-based bioinks for coaxial and triaxial bioprinting: a review of material properties, printing techniques, and applications. Polymers (Basel), 17(7), 917. doi: 10.3390/polym17070917.
[19] Du Chatinier, D. N., Figler, K. P., Agrawal, P., Liu, W. & Zhang, Y. S. (Jul. 2021). The potential of microfluidics-enhanced extrusion bioprinting. Biomicrofluidics, 15(4), doi: 10.1063/5.0033280.
[20] Garciamendez-Mijares, C. E. et al. (Jul. 2023)Development of an affordable extrusion 3D bioprinter equipped with a temperature-controlled printhead. International Journal of Bioprinting, 9(6), 0244. doi: 10.36922/ijb.0244.
[21] Guo, R. & Tang, W. (Jul. 2024). Optimizing printhead design for enhanced temperature control in extrusion-based bioprinting. Micromachines, 15(8), 943. doi: 10.3390/mi15080943.
[22] Cui, Y., Jin, R., Zhang, Y., Yu, M., Zhou, Y. & Wang, L.-Q. (Aug. 2024). Cellulose nanocrystal-enhanced thermal-sensitive hydrogels of block copolymers for 3D bioprinting. International Journal of Bioprinting, 7(4), 397. doi: 10.18063/ijb.v7i4.397.

[23] Lee, K. Y. & Mooney, D. J. (Jan. 2012). Alginate: properties and biomedical applications. Progress in Polymer Science, 37(1), 106–126. doi: 10.1016/j.progpolymsci.2011.06.003.
[24] Zhu, M., Wang, Y., Ferracci, G., Zheng, J., Cho, N.-J. & Lee, B. H. (May 2019). Gelatin methacryloyl and its hydrogels with an exceptional degree of controllability and batch-to-batch consistency. Scientific Reports, 9(1), 6863. doi: 10.1038/s41598-019-42186-x.
[25] Zhang, Y. et al. (2021)3D composite bioprinting for fabrication of artificial biological tissues. International Journal of Bioprinting, 7(1), 299. doi: 10.18063/IJB.V7I1.299.
[26] Crosby, C. O. (Apr. 2024). Open-source extrusion 3D bioprinters: trends and recommendations. Bioprinting, 38, e00336. doi: 10.1016/j.bprint.2024.e00336.
[27] Groll, J. et al. (Nov. 2018)A definition of bioinks and their distinction from biomaterial inks. Biofabrication, 11(1), 013001. doi: 10.1088/1758-5090/aaec52.
[28] Vaishya, R., Patralekh, M. K., Vaish, A., Agarwal, A. K. & Vijay, V. (Jul. 2018). Publication trends and knowledge mapping in 3D printing in orthopaedics. Journal of Clinical Orthopaedics and Trauma, 9(3), 194–201. doi: 10.1016/j.jcot.2018.07.006.
[29] Paxton, N., Smolan, W., Böck, T., Melchels, F., Groll, J. & Jungst, T. (Nov. 2017). Proposal to assess printability of bioinks for extrusion-based bioprinting and evaluation of rheological properties governing bioprintability. Biofabrication, 9(4), 044107. doi: 10.1088/1758-5090/aa8dd8.
[30] Gillispie, G. J. et al. (Sep. 2023). The correlation between rheological properties and extrusion-based printability in bioink artifact quantification. Materials & Design, 233, 112237. doi: 10.1016/J.MATDES.2023.112237.
[31] Amorim, P. A., D'Ávila, M. A., Anand, R., Moldenaers, P., Van Puyvelde, P. & Bloemen, V. (Jun. 2021). Insights on shear rheology of inks for extrusion-based 3D bioprinting. Bioprinting, 22, e00129. doi: 10.1016/J.BPRINT.2021.E00129.
[32] Ramesh, S. et al. (Mar. 2021). Extrusion bioprinting: recent progress, challenges, and future opportunities. Bioprinting, 21, e00116. doi: 10.1016/J.BPRINT.2020.E00116.
[33] GhavamiNejad, A., Ashammakhi, N., Wu, X. Y. & Khademhosseini, A. (Sep. 2020). Crosslinking strategies for 3D bioprinting of polymeric hydrogels. Small, 16(35), doi: 10.1002/smll.202002931.
[34] Yeleswarapu, S., Dash, A., Chameettachal, S. & Pati, F. (Sep. 2023). 3D bioprinting of tissue constructs employing dual crosslinking of decellularized extracellular matrix hydrogel. Biomaterials Advances, 152, 213494. doi: 10.1016/j.bioadv.2023.213494.
[35] Wu, J. et al. (Aug 2025). A novel 3D bioprinting crosslinking method based on solenoid valve control. Macromolecular Bioscience, 25(8), doi: 10.1002/mabi.202500039.
[36] Soliman, B. G. et al. (Aug. 2020). Stepwise control of crosslinking in a one-pot system for bioprinting of low-density bioinks. Advanced Healthcare Materials, 9(15), doi: 10.1002/adhm.201901544.
[37] Jiang, T., Munguia-Lopez, J. G., Flores-Torres, S., Kort-Mascort, J. & Kinsella, J. M. (Mar. 2019). Extrusion bioprinting of soft materials: an emerging technique for biological model fabrication. Applied Physics Reviews, 6(1), doi: 10.1063/1.5059393.
[38] Hibbert, M., Viljoen, J. M. & Du Plessis, L. H. (Apr 2023). Print parameter optimisation for a Pluronic F-127 and alginate hybrid hydrogel. Bioprinting, 30, e00257. doi: 10.1016/j.bprint.2022.e00257.
[39] Kim, S. H., Park, S. J., Xu, B., Lee, J. H., An, S. J. & Cha, M. (Dec. 2022). Development of polycaprolactone grafts with improved physical properties and body stability using a screw extrusion-type 3D bioprinter. International Journal of Bioprinting, 9(2), 652. doi: 10.18063/ijb.v9i2.652.
[40] Albanna, M. et al. (Feb. 2019)In situ bioprinting of autologous skin cells accelerates wound healing of extensive excisional full-thickness wounds. Scientific Reports, 9(1), 1856. doi: 10.1038/s41598-018-38366-w.
[41] Schwab, A., Levato, R., D'Este, M., Piluso, S., Eglin, D. & Malda, J. (2020). Printability and shape fidelity of bioinks in 3D bioprinting. Chemical Reviews 2020, 120, 11028–11055. doi: 10.1021/acs.chemrev.0c00084.

[42] Xing, F., Xiang, Z., Rommens, P. M. & Ritz, U. (May 2020). 3D bioprinting for vascularized tissue-engineered bone fabrication. Materials (Basel)., 13(10), 2278. doi: 10.3390/ma13102278.

[43] Tarassoli, S. P., Jessop, Z. M., Jovic, T., Hawkins, K. & Whitaker, I. S. (Oct. 2021). Candidate bioinks for extrusion 3D bioprinting – a systematic review of the literature. Frontiers in Bioengineering and Biotechnology, 9, doi: 10.3389/fbioe.2021.616753.

[44] Bhattacharyya, A., Janarthanan, G., Tran, H. N., Ham, H. J., Yoon, J. & Noh, I. (Jul. 2021). Bioink homogeneity control during 3D bioprinting of multicomponent micro/nanocomposite hydrogel for even tissue regeneration using novel twin screw extrusion system. Chemical Engineering Journal, 415, 128971. doi: 10.1016/j.cej.2021.128971.

[45] Tolmacheva, N., Bhattacharyya, A. & Noh, I. (Feb. 2024). Calcium phosphate biomaterials for 3D bioprinting in bone tissue engineering. Biomimetics, 9(2), 95. doi: 10.3390/biomimetics9020095.

[46] Chen, X. B. et al. (Oct. 2023). Biomaterials / bioinks and extrusion bioprinting. Bioactive Materials, 28, 511–536. doi: 10.1016/j.bioactmat.2023.06.006.

[47] Gao, T. et al. (Jun. 2018)Optimization of gelatin–alginate composite bioink printability using rheological parameters: a systematic approach. Biofabrication, 10(3), 034106. doi: 10.1088/1758-5090/aacdc7.

[48] Potere, F. et al. (Dec. 2024). Double-crosslinked dECM bioink to print a self-sustaining 3D multi-layered aortic-like construct. Bioprinting, 44, e00368. doi: 10.1016/j.bprint.2024.e00368.

[49] Shin, Y. J., Shafranek, R. T., Tsui, J. H., Walcott, J., Nelson, A. & Kim, D.-H. (Jan. 2021). 3D bioprinting of mechanically tuned bioinks derived from cardiac decellularized extracellular matrix. Acta Biomater, 119, 75–88. doi: 10.1016/j.actbio.2020.11.006.

[50] Habib, M. A. & Khoda, B. (Apr. 2022). Rheological analysis of bio-ink for 3D bio-printing processes. Journal of Manufacturing Processes, 76, 708–718. doi: 10.1016/j.jmapro.2022.02.048.

[51] Kiyotake, E. A., Douglas, A. W., Thomas, E. E., Nimmo, S. L. & Detamore, M. S. (Sep. 2019). Development and quantitative characterization of the precursor rheology of hyaluronic acid hydrogels for bioprinting. Acta Biomater, 95, 176–187. doi: 10.1016/j.actbio.2019.01.041.

[52] Ying, G., Jiang, N., Yu, C. & Zhang, Y. S. (Dec. 2018). Three-dimensional bioprinting of gelatin methacryloyl (GelMA). Bio-Design and Manufacturing, 1(4), 215–224. doi: 10.1007/s42242-018-0028-8.

[53] Cai, Y., Chang, S. Y., Gan, S. W., Ma, S., Lu, W. F. & Yen, -C.-C. (Oct. 2022). Nanocomposite bioinks for 3D bioprinting. Acta Biomater, 151, 45–69. doi: 10.1016/j.actbio.2022.08.014.

[54] Chimene, D. et al. (Mar. 2018)Nanoengineered ionic–covalent entanglement (NICE) bioinks for 3D bioprinting. ACS Applied Materials and Interfaces, 10(12), 9957–9968. doi: 10.1021/acsami.7b19808.

[55] Jang, J., Kim, T. G., Kim, B. S., Kim, S.-W., Kwon, S.-M. & Cho, D.-W. (Mar. 2016). Tailoring mechanical properties of decellularized extracellular matrix bioink by vitamin B2-induced photo-crosslinking. Acta Biomater, 33, 88–95. doi: 10.1016/j.actbio.2016.01.013.

[56] Richard, C., Neild, A. & Cadarso, V. J. (2020). The emerging role of microfluidics in multi-material 3D bioprinting. Lab Chip, 20(12), 2044–2056. doi: 10.1039/C9LC01184F.

[57] Wang, J., Xu, C., Yang, S., Wang, L. & Xu, M. (Mar. 2023). Continuous and highly accurate multi-material extrusion-based bioprinting with optical coherence tomography imaging. International Journal of Bioprinting, 9(3), 707. doi: 10.18063/ijb.707.

[58] Zgeib, R., Wang, X., Zaeri, A., Zhang, F., Cao, K. & Chang, R. C. (Aug. 2023). Development of a low-cost quad-extrusion 3D bioprinting system for multi-material tissue constructs. International Journal of Bioprinting, 10(1), 0159. doi: 10.36922/ijb.0159.

[59] Hong, S., Kim, J. S., Jung, B., Won, C. & Hwang, C. (2019). Coaxial bioprinting of cell-laden vascular constructs using a gelatin–tyramine bioink. Biomaterials Science, 7(11), 4578–4587. doi: 10.1039/C8BM00618K.

[60] Yu, F. & Choudhury, D. (Jun. 2019). Microfluidic bioprinting for organ-on-a-chip models. Drug Discovery Today, 24(6), 1248–1257. doi: 10.1016/j.drudis.2019.03.025.

[61] Fritschen, A. et al. (Jul. 2024). High-scale 3D-bioprinting platform for the automated production of vascularized organs-on-a-chip. Advanced Healthcare Materials, 13(17), doi: 10.1002/adhm.202304028.
[62] Huang, G. et al. (2024)Applications, advancements, and challenges of 3D bioprinting in organ transplantation. Biomaterials Science, 12(6), 1425–1448. doi: 10.1039/D3BM01934A.
[63] Heinrich, M. A. et al. (Jun. 2019). 3D bioprinting: from benches to translational applications. Small, 15(23), doi: 10.1002/smll.201805510.
[64] Guida, L., Cavallaro, M. & Levi, M. (Dec. 2024). Advancements in high-resolution 3D bioprinting: exploring technological trends, bioinks and achieved resolutions. Bioprinting, 44, e00376. doi: 10.1016/j.bprint.2024.e00376.
[65] Dong, L., Xiao, Y., Li, Y. & Shi, R. (2024). A collision detection algorithm based on sphere and EBB mixed hierarchical bounding boxes. IEEE Access, 12, 62719–62729. doi: 10.1109/ACCESS.2024.3392920.
[66] Kirillova, A., Maxson, R., Stoychev, G., Gomillion, C. T. & Ionov, L. (Dec. 2017). 4D biofabrication using shape-morphing hydrogels. Advanced Materials, 29(46), doi: 10.1002/adma.201703443.
[67] Vijayavenkataraman, S., Lu, W. F. & Fuh, J. Y. H. (Sep. 2016). 3D bioprinting of skin: a state-of-the-art review on modelling, materials, and processes. Biofabrication, 8(3), 032001. doi: 10.1088/1758-5090/8/3/032001.
[68] Khoshnood, N. & Zamanian, A. (Dec. 2020). Decellularized extracellular matrix bioinks and their application in skin tissue engineering. Bioprinting, 20, e00095. doi: 10.1016/j.bprint.2020.e00095.
[69] Wang, M. et al. (Apr. 2025). Mechanical and biological properties of 3D printed bone tissue engineering scaffolds. Frontiers in Bioengineering and Biotechnology, 13, doi: 10.3389/fbioe.2025.1545693.
[70] Bose, S., Vahabzadeh, S. & Bandyopadhyay, A. (2013). Bone tissue engineering using 3D printing. Materials Today, 16(12), 496–504. doi: 10.1016/j.mattod.2013.11.017.
[71] Madhavarapu, S. et al. (Jun. 2025)3D-printed polymer scaffolds for vascularized bone regeneration using mineral and extracellular matrix deposition. Regenerative Engineering and Translational Medicine, 11(2), 512–523. doi: 10.1007/s40883-024-00371-z.
[72] Wu, Y., Kennedy, P., Bonazza, N., Yu, Y., Dhawan, A. & Ozbolat, I. (Jan. 2021). Three-dimensional bioprinting of articular cartilage: a systematic review. Cartilage, 12(1), 76–92. doi: 10.1177/1947603518809410.
[73] Naranda, J., Bračič, M., Vogrin, M. & Maver, U. (Jul. 2021). Recent advancements in 3D printing of polysaccharide hydrogels in cartilage tissue engineering. Materials (Basel), 14(14), 3977. doi: 10.3390/ma14143977.
[74] Debnath, S., Agrawal, A., Jain, N., Chatterjee, K. & Player, D. J. (2025). Collagen as a bio-ink for 3D printing: a critical review. Journal of Materials Chemistry B, 13(6), 1890–1919. doi: 10.1039/D4TB01060D.
[75] Arjoca, S., Bojin, F., Neagu, M., Păunescu, A., Neagu, A. & Păunescu, V. (Jan 2024). Hydrogel extrusion speed measurements for the optimization of bioprinting parameters. Gels, 10(2), 103. doi: 10.3390/gels10020103.
[76] Hassan, S. et al. (Nov 2022). Tunable and compartmentalized multimaterial bioprinting for complex living tissue constructs. ACS Applied Materials and Interfaces, 14(46), 51602–51618. doi: 10.1021/acsami.2c12585.
[77] Ravanbakhsh, H., Karamzadeh, V., Bao, G., Mongeau, L., Juncker, D. & Zhang, Y. S. (Dec. 2021). Emerging technologies in multi-material bioprinting. Advanced Materials, 33(49), doi: 10.1002/adma.202104730.
[78] Douglas, A., Chen, Y., Elloso, M., Levschuk, A. & Jeschke, M. G. (Feb. 2025). Bioprinting-by-design of hydrogel-based biomaterials for in situ skin tissue engineering. Gels, 11(2), 110. doi: 10.3390/gels11020110.

[79] Wang, X., Yang, C., Yu, Y. & Zhao, Y. (Jan. 2022). In situ 3D bioprinting living photosynthetic scaffolds for autotrophic wound healing. Research, 2022, doi: 10.34133/2022/9794745.

[80] Pazhouhnia, Z., Beheshtizadeh, N., Namini, M. S. & Lotfibakhshaiesh, N. (Sep. 2022). Portable hand-held bioprinters promote in situ tissue regeneration. Bioengineering & Translational Medicine, 7(3), doi: 10.1002/btm2.10307.

[81] Chand, R., Kamei, K. & Vijayavenkataraman, S. (Feb. 2025). Advances in microfluidic bioprinting for multi-material multi-cellular tissue constructs. Cell Therapy Engineering Connect, 1(1), 1. doi: 10.69709/CellEngC.2024.111335.

[82 Ma, J., Wang, Y. & Liu, J. (2018). Bioprinting of 3D tissues/organs combined with microfluidics. RSC Advances, 8(39), 21712–21727. doi: 10.1039/C8RA03022G.

[83] Smith, L. J., Li, P., Holland, M. R. & Ekser, B. (May 2018). FABRICA: a bioreactor platform for printing, perfusing, observing, & stimulating 3D tissues. Scientific Reports, 8(1), 7561. doi: 10.1038/s41598-018-25663-7.

[84] Mladenovska, T., Choong, P. F., Wallace, G. G. & O'Connell, C. D. (Aug. 2023). The regulatory challenge of 3D bioprinting. Regenerative Medicine, 18(8), 659–674. doi: 10.2217/rme-2022-0194.

Maneesh Dubey, Ruchin Kacker*, Sanjay Singh, Amit Arora

Chapter 11
Bioprinting in Reformative Medicine

Abstract: Bioprinting has emerged as a groundbreaking technology within reformative medicine, offering unprecedented capabilities for restoring, replacing, and enhancing biological tissues and organs. Reformative medicine goes beyond traditional regenerative approaches by integrating precision, personalization, and predictive methodologies to develop patient-specific therapeutic solutions. Bioprinting, with its ability to spatially control the deposition of cells, biomaterials, and signaling factors, plays a pivotal role in reshaping the future of medical treatments.

This chapter explores the synergistic relationship between bioprinting technologies and the core principles of reformative medicine. It begins with an overview of the conceptual framework of reformative medicine, emphasizing its personalized, dynamic, and ethically driven orientation. The chapter then presents a detailed examination of various bioprinting modalities – such as inkjet, extrusion, laser-based, and stereolithography – and their respective advantages in reformative therapeutic contexts.

Special attention is given to bioink development, stem cell applications, and scaffold-free strategies, all of which enhance tissue compatibility and functional integration. Real-world clinical applications are reviewed, including skin regeneration, orthopedic repair, vascularized tissue fabrication, and organoid-based disease models. Furthermore, the chapter highlights the transformative role of artificial intelligence in optimizing design, predicting biological responses, and enabling real-time process monitoring in bioprinting workflows.

Challenges related to scalability, bioink stability, regulatory approval, and ethical considerations are critically assessed. The chapter concludes by envisioning a future where bioprinting, integrated with smart biomaterials and AI, becomes a cornerstone of reformative medicine, enabling personalized treatments and decentralized healthcare delivery systems.

By bridging engineering, biology, and computational intelligence, bioprinting in reformative medicine represents a paradigm shift toward truly personalized and curative healthcare solutions.

***Corresponding author: Ruchin Kacker,** Department of ME, SISTec, Bhopal, Madhya Pradesh, India, e-mail: ruchinkacker@sistec.ac.in (institutional); ruchinkacker@gmail.com
Maneesh Dubey, Department of ME, IIT Madras, Chennai
Sanjay Singh, Department of ME, SISTec, Bhopal, Madhya Pradesh, India
Amit Arora, Department of DEECE, Galgotias University, Uttar Pradesh, India

 | https://doi.org/10.1515/9783111719993-011

Keywords: Bioprinting, reformative medicine, personalized medicine, regenerative medicine, bioinks, tissue engineering, stem cells, artificial intelligence, organoids, 3D printing in healthcare

11.1 Definition and Scope of Reformative Medicine

Reformative medicine represents a progressive evolution from conventional therapeutic models, focusing not merely on the repair of damaged tissues but on the reconstruction, replacement, and enhancement of biological function using advanced biotechnologies. At its core, reformative medicine encompasses elements of regenerative medicine, precision medicine, tissue engineering, artificial intelligence (AI), and biofabrication, all integrated to create personalized and predictive healthcare solutions.

Unlike traditional regenerative medicine – which aims primarily to restore the structure and function of impaired tissues – reformative medicine seeks to proactively intervene at earlier stages of disease progression and customize therapies to the molecular and cellular profile of individual patients. This is achieved through the incorporation of bioprinting technologies, enabling the fabrication of complex, multicellular structures with controlled spatial distribution of cells, growth factors, and biomaterials tailored to patient-specific needs [1].

Reformative medicine holds promise in several domains, including oncology, neurology, orthopedics, and organ transplantation, where conventional treatments often fall short. With advances in 3D bioprinting, researchers can now engineer tissues such as vascular grafts, cartilage, and even miniaturized organoids that mimic native physiological function [2]. These innovations offer not only restorative solutions but also platforms for disease modeling, drug screening, and predictive diagnostics.

The scope of reformative medicine is thus vast and multidisciplinary. It requires collaborative integration of biology, engineering, data science, and clinical medicine to transition from reactive treatments to preventive and curative modalities. As such, bioprinting technologies serve as a vital enabler of reformative medicine, transforming theoretical possibilities into clinical realities.

11.1.1 Role of Bioprinting in Transforming Medical Paradigms

Bioprinting has emerged as a transformative force in reformative medicine, redefining how we approach the treatment and understanding of human diseases. Traditional medical paradigms often rely on donor tissues, prosthetics, or pharmacological interventions that offer limited personalization, may cause immune rejection, and typically treat symptoms rather than root causes. In contrast, bioprinting enables the fabrication of biologically functional tissues and organs using a patient's own cells and bioactive materials, thereby significantly reducing immunological risks and improving therapeutic efficacy [3].

One of the most profound impacts of bioprinting is its ability to bridge the gap between laboratory innovation and clinical translation. With layer-by-layer deposition technologies, bioprinting can replicate native tissue architecture, enabling the construction of customized implants, vascularized tissue constructs, and disease-specific organoids for both therapeutic and diagnostic purposes [4]. For instance, bioprinted cardiac patches and tracheal grafts are already being explored in preclinical models, offering hope for treatment-resistant cases in cardiovascular and respiratory medicine [5].

Moreover, bioprinting plays a central role in advancing the goals of precision and personalized medicine. Using patient-specific imaging data, such as MRI or CT scans, tissues can be designed to match anatomical dimensions and physiological properties with high accuracy. Additionally, bioprinted disease models allow for drug screening and toxicity testing in patient-derived cellular environments, which greatly enhances predictive capabilities in treatment design [6].

By integrating AI with bioprinting platforms, real-time quality control, process optimization, and predictive modeling have become possible, further propelling the transition from empirical treatments to data-driven, patient-centered care [7].

In essence, bioprinting serves as both a tool and a catalyst for transforming medical paradigms – shifting healthcare from standardized, reactive models to adaptive, proactive, and regenerative systems.

11.1.2 Objectives and Structure of the Chapter

This chapter aims to explore the emerging role of bioprinting in reformative medicine, focusing on how it is reshaping the diagnosis, treatment, and reconstruction of human tissues and organs. The central objective is to elucidate the potential of bioprinting as a tool that extends beyond regenerative healing into proactive, personalized, and curative interventions, aligned with the broader vision of reformative healthcare.

Key objectives of this chapter are to:

- Define the concept and scope of reformative medicine in the context of biomedical innovation.
- Trace the technological evolution of bioprinting, highlighting key breakthroughs and milestones.
- Examine the interdisciplinary integration of AI, biomaterials, and tissue engineering in bioprinting.
- Discuss clinical and translational applications, such as personalized tissue grafts, organoids, and bioengineered implants.

- Identify current challenges, ethical concerns, and regulatory landscapes affecting clinical deployment.
- Envision the future directions of bioprinting in reformative medicine, particularly its potential for personalized therapies and decentralized biofabrication.

To accomplish these goals, the chapter is structured into several key sections:
- **Section 11.1** introduces the foundational concepts of reformative medicine and outlines the trajectory of bioprinting innovation.
- **Section 11.2** details the transition from regenerative to reformative medicine and explores various bioprinting techniques and materials.
- **Section 11.3** presents clinical case studies, therapeutic applications, and AI integration in reformative bioprinting.
- **Section 11.4** addresses ongoing challenges, ethical dimensions, and emerging opportunities.
- **Section 11.5** concludes with a synthesis of insights and a forward-looking perspective on the role of bioprinting in the next generation of medicine.

11.1.3 Historical Development and Key Milestones

The evolution of bioprinting is rooted in the convergence of additive manufacturing, biomaterials science, and cellular biology. The concept of three-dimensional printing was first introduced in the 1980s for industrial prototyping; however, it was not until the early 2000s that this technology was adapted for biological applications [8]. One of the earliest milestones was the inkjet printing of cells by Thomas Boland and colleagues in 2003, which demonstrated the potential of modifying standard desktop printers to deposit living cells without significant loss of viability [9].

This breakthrough initiated a wave of innovation, leading to the development of more refined techniques such as extrusion-based and laser-assisted bioprinting (LAB). By 2008, researchers had successfully printed multilayered skin tissue, marking one of the first functional bioprinted constructs with potential therapeutic application [10].

The 2010s witnessed accelerated progress with the introduction of vascularized tissue constructs, a crucial step toward the fabrication of complex organs. The development of bioinks – formulations that combine living cells with biomaterials – further enabled the printing of tissues with tailored mechanical and biological properties [11]. Around the same time, the incorporation of patient-specific medical imaging into the printing process began to support custom-designed implants and disease models.

A significant milestone was achieved in 2019, when Israeli researchers bioprinted the first miniature heart using a patient's own cells, complete with vascular structures, chambers, and cellular alignment – although not yet functionally contractile, it symbolized a leap toward organ-scale bioprinting [12].

Today, bioprinting is being integrated with AI, robotics, and microfluidics, creating intelligent platforms capable of automated tissue fabrication and real-time quality control. As clinical translation advances, regulatory frameworks are gradually adapting to accommodate bioprinted therapeutics, signaling the dawn of a new medical paradigm [13].

11.2 From Regenerative to Reformative Approaches

The field of regenerative medicine has traditionally focused on the repair or replacement of damaged tissues and organs, primarily through cell therapies, scaffolding, and stem cell-based regeneration. While successful in many domains – such as skin regeneration, bone healing, and corneal repair – regenerative medicine often aims to restore existing biological structures, rather than redesigning or optimizing them for individualized or enhanced functionality [14].

Reformative medicine, by contrast, represents an evolutionary leap that combines regenerative aims with customization, adaptability, and therapeutic intelligence. It does not merely seek to regenerate tissues but aspires to reform them – tailoring biological constructs to specific patient needs, disease phenotypes, and even predictive risks using digital, biofabrication, and AI-integrated methods [15]. This transition is fueled by advances in bioprinting, which enables precise spatial placement of cells, biomaterials, and growth factors to fabricate complex, functional tissues and organ analogs.

Unlike conventional regeneration, reformative approaches facilitate modular, on-demand biofabrication using digital blueprints derived from patient imaging (e.g., CT and MRI), genetic profiles, or disease simulations. For example, rather than regenerating a standard cartilage implant, reformative bioprinting could produce a biomechanically optimized cartilage patch tailored to the patient's gait, anatomy, and degeneration profile [16]. Table 11.1 presents an overview of bioprinting techniques.

Further, reformative medicine embraces adaptive intelligence, where machine learning and real-time feedback systems can predict tissue behavior, optimize bioprinting parameters, and personalize post-implantation outcomes [17]. This integration pushes medicine toward anticipatory and personalized therapeutic models – treating disease not just based on existing pathology, but also on predicted tissue responses and dynamic biological feedback.

In summary, reformative bioprinting bridges the gap between standard regenerative approaches and precision, AI-augmented medicine, making healthcare proactive, personalized, and functionally restorative at an unprecedented scale.

Table 11.1: Overview of bioprinting techniques.

Feature	Extrusion-based	Inkjet	Laser-assisted	Stereolithography
Resolution	Medium-low	High	Ultra-high	High-ultra-high
Speed	Bioink viscosity	Medium	High (wide range)	High
Low	High (layer-wise)	Low	Wide range	Low-medium
Cell viability	High (moderate shear)	High (low stress)	Ultra-high (no shear)	Moderate (light/initiator)
Material versatility	High	Low (ink viscosity)	High	Limited (photo-curable)
Cost	Low-medium	Medium	High	Medium-high
Complexity of constructs	Medium	Medium	High	Very high

11.2.1 Core Technologies in Bioprinting

Bioprinting technologies have rapidly evolved over the past two decades, enabling the fabrication of complex biological constructs with increasing precision, speed, and cell viability. These technologies form the foundation of reformative bioprinting, allowing for the generation of customized and functional tissues. The three primary bioprinting modalities are inkjet, extrusion, and LAB, with newer approaches such as stereolithography gaining prominence for their precision and scalability [18].

11.2.1.1 Inkjet and Extrusion-Based Bioprinting

Inkjet bioprinting, adapted from conventional inkjet printing, uses thermal or piezoelectric actuators to deposit droplets of bioink in a controlled manner. It offers high speed and resolution but is generally limited to low-viscosity bioinks and suffers from challenges related to droplet consistency and cell sedimentation [19].

Extrusion-based bioprinting, one of the most widely used techniques, operates by forcing bioinks through a nozzle using pneumatic, piston, or screw mechanisms. It allows the deposition of highly viscous materials and supports a wider range of bioinks, including those laden with cells and growth factors [20]. Although resolution is lower compared to inkjet systems, extrusion bioprinting enables the printing of large, cell-dense constructs with clinically relevant dimensions, making it a key enabler in reformative medicine [21].

11.2.1.2 Laser-Assisted Bioprinting

LAB employs focused laser pulses to propel bioink droplets from a donor layer onto a substrate. This technique provides exceptional resolution, minimal shear stress, and high cell viability, making it particularly suitable for sensitive or rare cell types [22]. The absence of a nozzle also eliminates the risk of clogging, and the precision of laser targeting is advantageous for applications like neuronal or vascular patterning.

LAB is increasingly being used to print layered skin tissues, vascular networks, and neural scaffolds, aligning closely with the objectives of reformative bioprinting, where precision and spatial control are crucial [23]. Table 11.2 presents a comparison of bioinks.

Table 11.2: Comparison of bioinks.

Property/ category	**Natural bioinks (e.g., collagen, gelatin, alginate, hyaluronic acid, fibrin chitosan)**	**Synthetic bioinks (e.g., PEG, PCL PLGA, PVA, PEEK)**
Source	Derived from biological sources (animals, plants, and microbes)	Chemically synthesized
Biocompatibility	Generally excellent, mimic native extracellular matrix (ECM), contain cell-binding sites	Variable, can be less biocompatible often require functionalization to improve call interaction
Biodegradability	Generally good, often enzymatic degradation; kinetics can be less controllable	Highly tunable, degradation rates can be precisely controlled by polymer design
Mechanical properties	Often poor mechanical strength, low stiffness: highly variable batch-to-batch	Generally superior mechanical strength and stiffness, highly reproducible and tunable
Printability	Good rheological properties (shear-thinning): can be challenging to maintain shape fidelity due to rapid degradation or weak initial strength	Can be tailored for various printing methods; often require photo crosslinking for rapid gelation and shape fidelity
Cell Interactions	Promote cell adhesion, proliferation, and differentiation due to inherent biomimicry and recognition sites	Often inert; require chemical modification (e.g., RGO peptides) to enhance cell adhesion and biological cues
Batch-to-batch variability	High variability due to natural origin, leading to inconsistent properties	Low variability, highly reproducible due to precise chemical synthesis
Tunability	Limited inherent tenability; modifications (e.g., methacrylation) required for photocrosslinking or improved mechanics	High tunability in terms of mechanical properties, degradation rates, and functionalization

Table 11.2 (continued)

Property/ category	Natural bioinks (e.g., collagen, gelatin, alginate, hyaluronic acid, fibrin chitosan)	Synthetic bioinks (e.g., PEG, PCL PLGA, PVA, PEEK)
Immune response	Generally low, but can be immunogenic if not purified properly (e.g., animal-derived proteins)	Can be tailored to be nan immunogenic, but some synthetic components or degradation products may elicit response
Cost	Generally more affordable (e.g., alginate) but some highly purified natural products can be expensive	Can vary widely, some advanced synthetic polymers are expensive

11.2.1.3 Stereolithography and Emerging Techniques

Stereolithographic bioprinting (SLA) utilizes photo-crosslinkable bioinks cured layer by layer using UV or visible light. SLA offers ultra-high resolution, smooth surface finishes, and the ability to create intricate internal architectures [24]. Although the selection of compatible bioinks is currently limited, ongoing innovations in photopolymerizable hydrogels and visible-light curing are expanding its applications in soft tissue and organoid bioprinting [25].

Emerging techniques, such as acoustic, magnetic, and volumetric bioprinting, are also under investigation for their potential to create high-throughput, volumetric, and contact-free biofabrication environments, which may significantly accelerate reformative applications [26].

Together, these core technologies constitute the engine of reformative medicine, enabling the fabrication of personalized, functional, and intelligent biological constructs that go beyond repair – toward proactive and transformative healthcare solutions.

11.3.1 Biomaterials and Bioinks for Reformative Applications

Biomaterials form the foundation of bioprinting systems, serving as the structural and biological support for embedded cells during and after printing. In reformative medicine, the selection and design of bioinks – combinations of biomaterials, cells, and bioactive molecules – are critical not only for biocompatibility and printability, but also for functional integration, responsiveness, and patient-specific adaptation [27]. The evolution from conventional scaffold materials to smart, stimuli-responsive bioinks marks a key step toward intelligent and personalized tissue engineering.

11.3.1.1 Natural and Synthetic Hydrogels

Natural hydrogels, such as alginate, gelatin, collagen, hyaluronic acid, and fibrin, are widely used in bioprinting due to their biocompatibility, cell-adhesion properties, and resemblance to the native extracellular matrix (ECM). Gelatin methacryloyl, in particular, is a tunable natural derivative that supports cell proliferation, differentiation, and matrix remodeling [28].

On the other hand, synthetic hydrogels, such as polyethylene glycol (PEG), pluronic F-127, and polyvinyl alcohol (PVA), offer mechanical strength, degradation control, and consistent chemical properties. However, they typically require surface modification to support cell adhesion and bioactivity [29].

In reformative applications, hybrid systems combining natural and synthetic hydrogels are gaining attention for their synergistic properties – achieving both biological relevance and structural fidelity in complex tissue constructs [30].

11.3.1.2 Stimuli-Responsive and Smart Bioinks

A significant advancement in reformative medicine is the use of smart or stimuli-responsive bioinks, which can alter their properties in response to changes in pH, temperature, light, magnetic fields, or biochemical stimuli. These bioinks enable adaptive behavior – such as shape transformation, drug release, or dynamic remodeling – offering a responsive interface between the printed construct and the biological environment [31].

Photo-crosslinkable hydrogels, for instance, allow precise spatial and temporal control over gelation, enhancing the resolution and mechanical performance of printed tissues [32]. Magnetically responsive hydrogels can be guided to specific locations or activated post-implantation using external magnetic fields, a promising approach for targeted regenerative or reformative interventions [33].

In addition, decellularized ECM (dECM)-based bioinks, derived from native tissues, offer tissue-specific biochemical cues, promoting more effective cell differentiation and functional integration. dECM inks are particularly valuable in applications such as myocardial, hepatic, or neural reformative constructs [34].

In sum, the rational design and selection of bioinks – incorporating biological cues, mechanical tunability, and responsiveness – play a pivotal role in achieving the dynamic, personalized goals of reformative medicine.

11.3 Bioprinting Applications in Reformative Medicine

11.3.1 Personalized Implants and Tissue Grafts

One of the most transformative applications of bioprinting in reformative medicine lies in the development of personalized implants and tissue grafts, tailored to individual anatomical and pathological profiles. Unlike traditional grafts, which are often generic or allogeneic, bioprinted constructs can be patient-specific, structurally and biologically customized to match the target tissue's shape, function, and cellular composition [35].

11.3.1.1 Anatomical Precision and Functional Integration

Bioprinting enables the creation of implants with precise anatomical geometry derived from patient imaging data such as MRI or CT scans. This allows for the development of grafts that fit exactly into the defect site, reducing complications such as inflammation, immune rejection, or mechanical mismatch [36]. For example, bioprinted auricular, cranial, or mandibular implants using cartilage-forming cells embedded in biocompatible hydrogels have demonstrated improved integration and cosmetic outcomes [37].

In reformative medicine, functionality is equally important. Bioinks loaded with progenitor or stem cells, growth factors, and ECM proteins can guide in situ differentiation and vascularization, enabling long-term tissue regeneration rather than passive replacement [38].

11.3.1.2 Soft and Hard Tissue Applications

Bioprinting has been applied to both soft tissues, such as skin, blood vessels, cardiac and neural tissues, and hard tissues, such as bone and cartilage. In bone tissue engineering, for instance, the combination of calcium phosphate-based bioinks with osteogenic cells supports mineralization and osseointegration, offering viable alternatives for maxillofacial and orthopedic repair [39].

In skin regeneration, multilayered skin constructs comprising epidermal and dermal layers have been successfully bioprinted using keratinocytes and fibroblasts, improving wound healing and scar reduction in chronic ulcers and burn patients [40].

11.3.1.3 Clinical Translation and Challenges

Despite promising preclinical and early clinical outcomes, several challenges hinder widespread clinical translation. These include ensuring long-term mechanical stability and biocompatibility; scaling up constructs without compromising cell viability; achieving vascularization and innervation in large grafts; and navigating complex regulatory and ethical frameworks [41].

Nevertheless, ongoing advancements in bioink development, imaging-guided design, and bioreactor maturation technologies are bringing us closer to a future where bioprinted, personalized implants become routine in reconstructive and regenerative medicine.

11.3.3 On-Demand Bioprinting and Emergency Medicine Applications

The concept of on-demand bioprinting – fabricating tissues or organs precisely when and where they are needed – is rapidly gaining traction in reformative medicine. In emergency and battlefield settings, space missions, or disaster zones, the ability to bioprint personalized grafts on-site holds transformative potential. This approach bypasses the delays and limitations associated with centralized manufacturing, enabling real-time, patient-specific interventions in critical care scenarios [50].

11.3.3.1 Portable Bioprinters and Field Deployments

Recent innovations in miniaturized and mobile bioprinting systems have allowed bioprinting technologies to move beyond the laboratory. Handheld bioprinters, such as the Biopen developed in Australia, allow surgeons to directly deposit cell-laden bioinks onto damaged cartilage or skin during surgery, enabling in situ tissue reconstruction [51].

Military medicine has particularly embraced this innovation. The U.S. Armed Forces Institute of Regenerative Medicine (AFIRM) has supported the development of deployable bioprinting platforms capable of printing skin patches and bone scaffolds on-site for wounded soldiers [52].

11.3.3.2 Space and Remote Applications

Bioprinting in extreme or remote environments, such as space stations or submarines, is an emerging field of inquiry. NASA has collaborated with various academic institutions to explore bioprinting under microgravity conditions, which may help overcome some terrestrial challenges such as sedimentation, scaffold collapse, and vascularization issues [53].

In space-based missions, the ability to print bone, skin, or blood vessels from astronauts' own cells could be crucial for long-term survival and autonomy. Such autonomous biofabrication systems could also contribute to future interplanetary healthcare infrastructure [54].

11.3.3.3 Challenges in Point-of-Care Bioprinting

Despite promising results, on-demand bioprinting still faces significant hurdles like sterility and environmental control in non-clinical environments; supply chain logistics for bioink storage and preservation; training of personnel in device operation and post-printing protocols; and quality assurance and real-time validation of constructs prior to implantation [55].

To mitigate these challenges, current research is focused on developing preloaded, shelf-stable bioink cartridges, automated printing protocols, and closed-loop feedback systems guided by AI and imaging data. These advancements are expected to accelerate the deployment of bioprinting in emergency and resource-constrained settings.

11.3.4 Bioprinted Organoids for Drug Screening and Disease Modeling

Bioprinted organoids – miniaturized, three-dimensional tissue constructs that replicate key structural and functional features of human organs – are increasingly used in reformative medicine for drug screening, toxicity testing, and disease modeling. By integrating stem cell technology, tissue engineering, and bioprinting, researchers can now fabricate organoids that provide physiologically relevant in vitro platforms, significantly enhancing the predictability and personalization of therapeutic responses [56].

11.3.4.1 Advancing Preclinical Drug Testing

Traditional 2D cell cultures and animal models often fail to capture the complexity of human physiology, leading to poor drug translation success rates. Bioprinted organoids derived from patient-specific cells and printed with biofunctional hydrogels allow for high-throughput drug screening in a microenvironment that mirrors native tissue architecture [57].

For example, liver and cardiac organoids have been developed to test hepatotoxicity and cardiotoxicity of novel drug compounds, allowing pharmaceutical developers to identify potential side effects earlier in the drug development pipeline [58]. Moreover, tumor organoids bioprinted from patient-derived cancer cells are now enabling personalized oncology trials in vitro, providing predictive data on individual tumor responses to chemotherapy or immunotherapy [59].

11.3.4.2 Disease Modeling and Precision Medicine

In addition to pharmacological testing, bioprinted organoids are being used to model a range of genetic, infectious, and degenerative diseases. Neurological organoids, for instance, are helping researchers understand diseases like Parkinson's, Alzheimer's, and autism spectrum disorders by recreating brain tissue microenvironments for observational and interventional research [60].

Similarly, bioprinted intestinal, renal, and pulmonary organoids have shown promise in modeling diseases such as cystic fibrosis, chronic kidney disease, and COVID-19, respectively. These models are especially important for studying host-pathogen interactions, immune responses, and treatment efficacy [61].

11.3.4.3 Integration with Artificial Intelligence (AI)

The convergence of bioprinting and AI is further revolutionizing disease modeling. AI algorithms are now being used to optimize printing parameters, cellular distributions, and material compositions for enhanced organoid functionality [62]. Moreover, AI-powered image analysis and machine learning tools facilitate real-time assessment of organoid health, morphology, and drug response, enabling adaptive experimental design.

This integration is pivotal for precision medicine, where patient-specific data can be used to bioprint and test organoids that guide clinical decision-making. It also significantly reduces the reliance on animal testing and accelerates regulatory approval processes [63].

11.3.5 Ethical and Regulatory Considerations in Bioprinting Applications

As bioprinting moves from research to clinical application, it brings with it a host of ethical and regulatory challenges that must be critically addressed to ensure safe, equitable, and responsible use in reformative medicine. These challenges pertain to issues such as patient consent, biofabrication of human organs, use of stem cells, and the regulatory pathways that govern their clinical translation [64].

11.3.5.1 Ethical Implications of Creating Human Tissues and Organs

The ability to fabricate living human tissues, and potentially entire organs, raises profound questions about the definition of life, ownership of bioprinted constructs, and moral boundaries in regenerative medicine. For instance, bioprinting brain organoids capable of rudimentary neural activity invites ethical debate around sentience, consciousness, and identity [65].

There is also concern over the commercialization of bioprinted tissues – who owns the product, especially when derived from a patient's own cells? This could lead to ethical dilemmas around intellectual property rights and equitable access. Some argue for the classification of bioprinted organs as "common goods" that should not be commodified [66].

11.3.5.2 Informed Consent and Data Privacy

Bioprinting frequently relies on genetic, imaging, and cellular data from individuals. Ensuring informed consent, data security, and transparency about how personal biological materials and data are used is critical. Special attention must be paid to vulnerable populations, including children, the elderly, and socioeconomically disadvantaged groups [67].

The convergence of AI in bioprinting also raises concerns regarding algorithmic biases, opaque decision-making processes, and the traceability of outcomes – issues that can compromise patient safety and undermine public trust [68].

11.3.5.3 Regulatory Frameworks and Standards

Currently, regulatory agencies such as the US Food and Drug Administration (FDA) and the European Medicines Agency (EMA) lack clear, universally accepted frameworks for evaluating bioprinted tissues and organs. Most constructs fall under the umbrella of either medical devices, biologics, or combination products, creating regulatory ambiguity [69].

Efforts are underway to establish standardized guidelines for bioink characterization, scaffold integrity, sterility, and functional validation. These include initiatives from ASTM International and ISO for bioprinting-related standards [70].

Global harmonization of regulations and collaboration between scientists, clinicians, ethicists, and policymakers will be essential to bridge the gap between laboratory innovation and bedside application.

11.4 Challenges, Ethics, and Future Directions

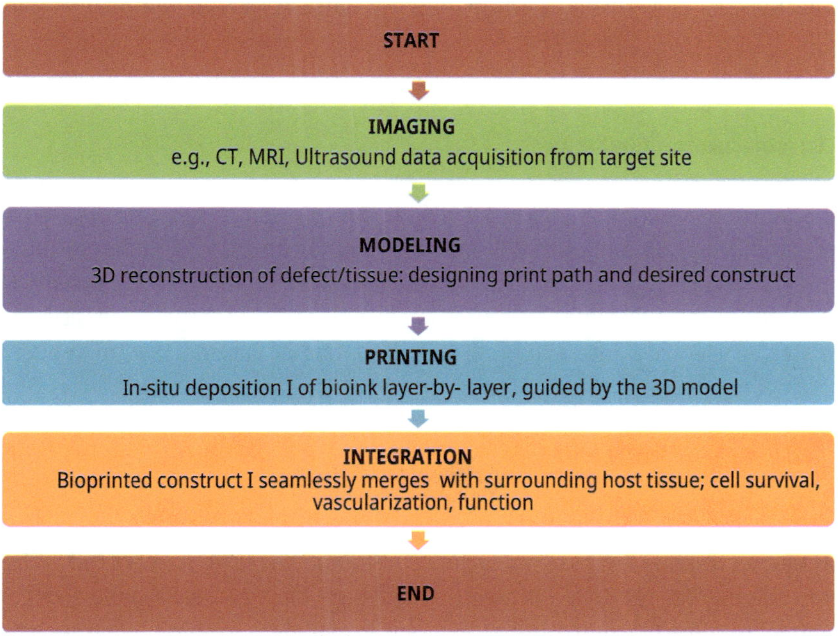

Figure 11.1: Workflow of in situ bioprinting.

11.4.1 Technical and Biological Limitations

Despite its transformative potential, bioprinting in reformative medicine still faces several technical and biological limitations that impede widespread clinical adoption. These challenges relate to the precision of printing processes, viability of printed tissues, scalability, vascularization, and integration of constructs with host tissue [71].

11.4.1.1 Print Resolution and Structural Fidelity

A major technical limitation is achieving high-resolution printing while maintaining cell viability and structural integrity. Many existing bioprinters cannot replicate the microscale features necessary for the complex architecture of native tissues, especially in organs such as the kidney, liver, or lungs, where microvasculature plays a critical role [72]. Figure 11.1 illustrates the workflow involved in in situ bioprinting.

Shear stress during extrusion or laser exposure in LAB may damage delicate cells or biomolecules, compromising the functionality and survival of the printed constructs [73].

11.4.1.2 Vascularization Challenges

One of the most formidable biological hurdles is the creation of functional vascular networks within bioprinted tissues. Without sufficient perfusion, cells in larger tissue constructs experience hypoxia and nutrient deprivation, leading to necrosis [74]. While strategies such as coaxial bioprinting, angiogenic factor incorporation, and sacrificial material use are being explored, true biomimetic vascularization remains elusive.

11.4.1.3 Bioink Constraints

The development of ideal bioinks – materials that mimic the ECM, support cell viability, and are suitable for printing – remains a challenge. Most natural bioinks like collagen or alginate offer biocompatibility but lack mechanical strength, whereas synthetic ones like PEG derivatives provide strength but lack biological cues [75]. Hybrid bioinks are a promising solution, but optimizing their composition remains complex.

11.4.1.4 Cell Source and Maturation

Access to autologous, pluripotent, or stem cell populations that can differentiate and mature appropriately in printed environments is a continuing limitation. Furthermore, post-printing tissue maturation, requiring bioreactors, mechanical stimulation, or biochemical gradients, adds time and complexity to the production pipeline [76].

11.4.1.5 Scalability and Standardization

While laboratory-scale bioprinting has demonstrated remarkable proof-of-concept, scaling up to clinically relevant tissue sizes and ensuring batch-to-batch consistency remain difficult. The lack of universal printing protocols, automated quality controls, and regulatory standardization further complicate commercialization efforts [77].

11.4.2 Ethical Dilemmas in Emerging Bioprinting Technologies

As bioprinting transitions from laboratory innovation to clinical application, it increasingly presents ethical dilemmas that intersect with evolving societal values, technological capabilities, and biomedical goals. While many of these concerns overlap with broader debates in regenerative medicine and biotechnology, bioprinting introduces unique questions regarding human identity, equity, autonomy, and the nature of life itself [78].

11.4.2.1 Creation of Human-Like Tissues and Organoids

The capacity to fabricate functional, patient-specific tissues and organs – including organoids that mimic aspects of brain function – raises challenging questions about moral status and personhood. When bioprinted brain organoids exhibit spontaneous electrical activity or responsiveness, it prompts ethical scrutiny over whether such constructs could possess rudimentary consciousness or experience pain [79].

This is further complicated by the use of embryonic stem cells or induced pluripotent stem cells in printing human tissues, which brings debates around beginning-of-life ethics to the forefront [80].

11.4.2.2 Justice, Access, and Global Inequity

Bioprinting technologies are currently resource-intensive and limited to well-funded institutions. If left unchecked, this could exacerbate global health disparities by offering cutting-edge treatments only to privileged populations. Equitable access to bioprinted organs and therapies – especially in low- and middle-income countries – is an urgent ethical concern [81].

In addition, questions persist about who gets priority when donor cells are limited, and how much personalization is ethical or economically feasible in publicly funded healthcare systems [82].

11.4.2.3 Consent and Donor Rights

Using a patient's cells or genetic material for bioprinting raises issues about informed consent, data ownership, and post-printing usage. For example, should patients have control over how their cells are used after donation? Can they object to commercial applications or future research uses? Transparent consent models must evolve to address these complexities [83].

Furthermore, in AI-assisted bioprinting, ethical tensions emerge around algorithmic bias and opacity in decision-making, especially when machine learning algorithms influence choices about tissue composition, patient suitability, or treatment pathways [84].

11.4.2.4 Dual-Use Risks and Regulation

The same bioprinting technologies designed for healing could be misused – for instance, in bioenhancement, weaponized biology, or unregulated cosmetic tissue fabrication. This "dual-use dilemma" necessitates preemptive regulation, ethical foresight, and international governance structures [85].

Ethical oversight should include multidisciplinary ethics committees, public engagement, and ongoing bioethics education for scientists and clinicians involved in bioprinting research and practice.

11.4.3 Role of AI and Machine Learning in Reformative Bioprinting

Artificial intelligence (AI) and machine learning (ML) are rapidly transforming bioprinting by enhancing precision, automation, and data-driven decision-making across the design–fabrication–validation continuum. In the context of reformative medicine, where personalized and dynamic tissue constructs are critical, AI plays a pivotal role in optimizing biofabrication parameters, predicting construct performance, and accelerating clinical translation [86].

11.4.3.1 Design Optimization and Predictive Modeling

One of the most promising applications of AI in bioprinting is the use of deep learning and generative models for design optimization. AI can analyze vast datasets – from medical imaging to cellular behavior – to generate patient-specific digital blueprints that guide the geometry, cell placement, and material distribution of printed tissues [87]. Figure 11.2 illustrates the function of AI in bioprinting.

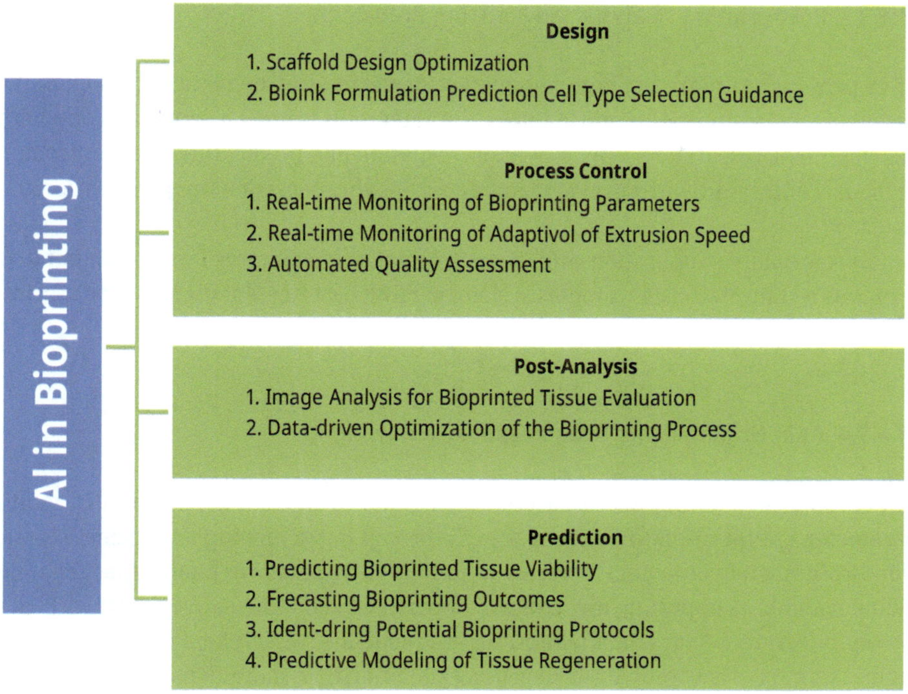

Figure 11.2: Role of AI in bioprinting.

Machine learning algorithms also enable predictive modeling of post-printing outcomes, such as construct maturation, mechanical integrity, and biological function. This allows researchers to pre-screen designs in silico, saving time, reducing cost, and improving safety [88].

11.4.3.2 Process Control and Quality Assurance

AI-integrated bioprinters are increasingly equipped with real-time sensors, computer vision, and feedback loops that monitor temperature, pressure, nozzle speed, and bioink rheology. These systems use ML algorithms to autocorrect deviations, ensuring high-fidelity deposition and reproducibility across batches [89].

For example, convolutional neural networks can detect microscopic anomalies during printing and adjust parameters on the fly to prevent construct failure. Such closed-loop systems are essential for regulatory compliance and clinical scalability [90].

11.4.3.3 Post-printing Analysis and Function Prediction

After printing, AI tools facilitate automated image analysis to evaluate cell viability, vascularization, and tissue morphology. By integrating time-lapse microscopy with ML classifiers, researchers can track tissue evolution and predict functional outcomes, such as contractility in cardiac patches or insulin secretion in pancreatic constructs [91].

In reformative applications, this means AI not only enhances fabrication but also serves as a clinical decision-support system, guiding post-implantation care or reprinting if needed.

11.4.3.4 AI in Organoid and Drug Response Modeling

In organoid bioprinting for disease modeling and drug testing, AI excels in multiparameter optimization. It can assess high-throughput screening data, gene expression profiles, and compound libraries to predict drug response phenotypes for individual patients – supporting the core aim of personalized reformative therapies [92].

By integrating omics data with AI-driven modeling, researchers can also identify biomarkers for tissue growth or degeneration, offering a more dynamic and precise approach to regenerative diagnostics and treatment.

11.4.3.5 Limitations and Ethical Considerations

While AI significantly enhances bioprinting capabilities, it also introduces ethical and practical challenges, such as data privacy, algorithmic transparency, and bias in training data. Furthermore, there is a growing need for regulatory frameworks that address the use of AI in clinical bioprinting, especially when autonomous decision-making is involved [93].

Collaborations between bioengineers, data scientists, ethicists, and clinicians will be key to responsibly harnessing AI for reformative bioprinting.

11.4.4 Vision for the Future: Toward In Situ and On-Demand Printing

The future of bioprinting in reformative medicine is not only about achieving functional tissue constructs in controlled laboratory environments but also about enabling in situ and on-demand bioprinting – printing tissues directly at the point of care, during surgeries, in remote settings, or even in extreme environments like battlefields or outer space. This evolution reflects a shift toward real-time, patient-specific, and context-responsive regenerative solutions [94].

11.4.4.1 From Laboratory Constructs to In-Body Printing

In situ bioprinting aims to print living tissues directly into or onto the body to repair damaged or diseased areas without the need for traditional grafting. Technologies like the Biopen, developed in Australia, allow surgeons to deposit stem cell-laden hydrogels intraoperatively, regenerating cartilage or bone within the surgical site itself [95].

In cardiac or dermal regeneration, robotic-assisted bioprinters are under development to enable precision-guided, layered cell deposition on wounds, potentially reducing recovery time and eliminating donor site morbidity. Future iterations may be combined with imaging tools (e.g., intraoperative MRI/ultrasound) to guide and monitor the printing process in real time [96].

11.4.4.2 On-Demand Bioprinting for Decentralized Medicine

On-demand bioprinting refers to localized, just-in-time fabrication of tissues or organ components based on a patient's immediate clinical need. This concept is particularly promising for military medicine, disaster relief, remote hospitals, and space missions. Organizations like NASA and the U.S. Department of Defense are exploring portable bioprinting units capable of printing skin, bone, or blood vessels on-site [97].

Such systems, integrated with AI-driven imaging and diagnostics, could help clinicians triage, design, and fabricate grafts or patches customized for traumatic injuries within hours. This vision supports the development of mobile biofabrication laboratories, turning hospitals, ambulances, or even spacecraft into regenerative medicine facilities.

11.4.4.3 AI and 4D Printing as Enablers of Real-Time Regeneration

Future advances in AI-guided printing will enable in situ systems to dynamically adapt print parameters during the process, informed by real-time sensor feedback. This is especially important for printing in moving or deforming anatomical regions, such as beating hearts or expanding lungs [98].

Simultaneously, 4D bioprinting – where printed constructs evolve shape or function in response to stimuli (e.g., pH, temperature, and pressure) – offers exciting possibilities for smart, self-assembling implants that can integrate seamlessly once printed inside the body [99].

11.4.4.4 Strategic Roadmap and Milestones

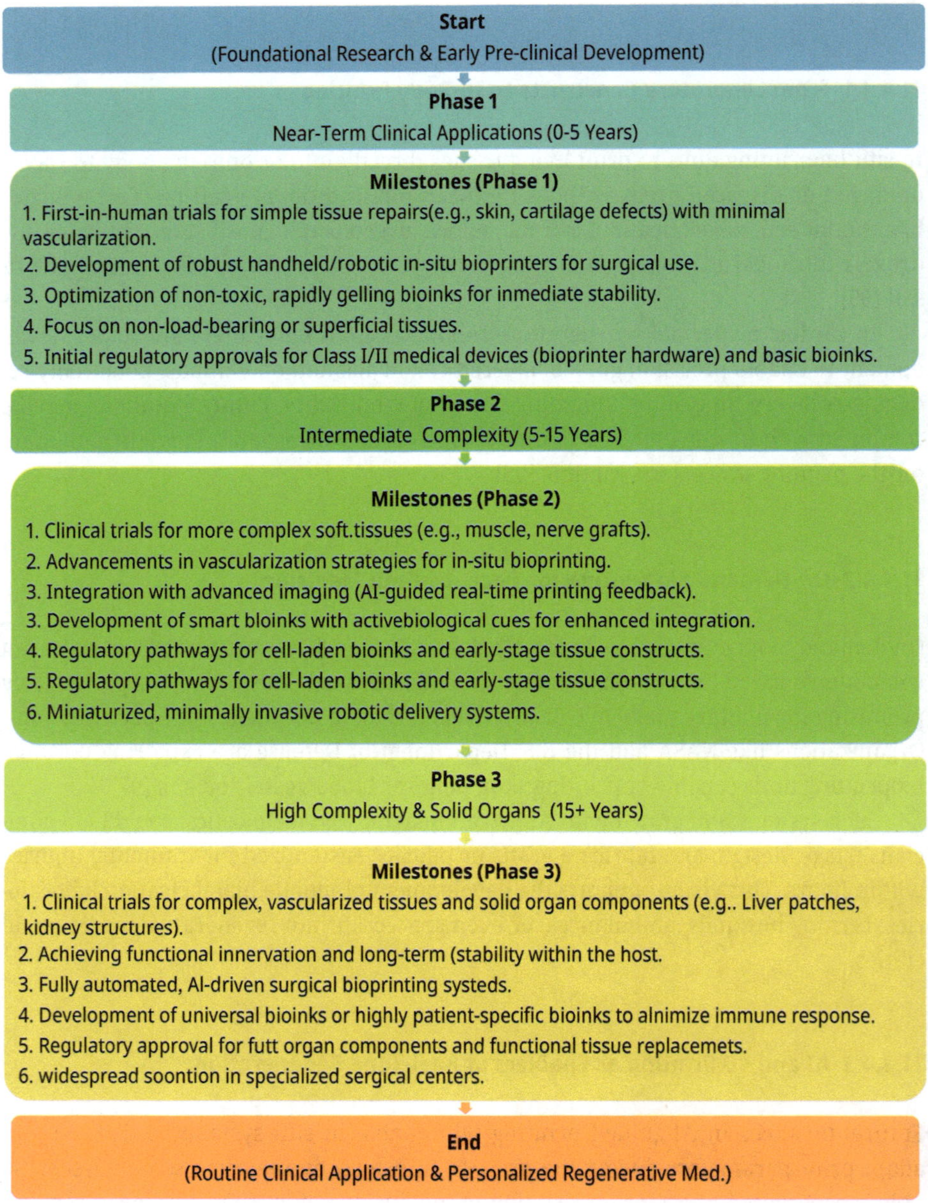

Figure 11.3: Future roadmap for clinical translation.

To realize in situ and on-demand bioprinting, the following milestones are anticipated:
- **2025–2027**: Pilot trials of in situ skin and cartilage printing using handheld or robotic devices; integration with imaging systems.
- **2028–2030**: Portable, AI-integrated biofabrication platforms for trauma and battlefield settings; remote printing in space environments.
- **2030 onward:** Clinical use of complex in situ printed constructs (e.g., vascularized muscle or nerve tissues); incorporation of 4D bioprinting in surgery.

Progress will depend on multi-sectoral collaboration, advances in bioink stability and transport, autonomous robotic systems, and standardized clinical protocols. Figure 11.3 illustrates the future roadmap for clinical translation.

11.5 Conclusion

11.5.1 Summary of Insights

This chapter has explored the foundational principles, technological enablers, clinical applications, and future trajectory of bioprinting in reformative medicine. Beginning with the definition and scope of reformative medicine, we traced its evolution alongside advancements in tissue engineering, biomaterials, and regenerative therapies. The emergence of bioprinting – particularly when enhanced by AI, bioinformatics, and patient-specific modeling – has shifted the paradigm from conventional treatment to dynamic biological restoration.

We examined major bioprinting techniques (inkjet, extrusion, laser-assisted, and stereolithography) and discussed their integration with stem cells, growth factors, and advanced biomaterials to engineer complex tissue constructs. Applications across personalized implants, wound healing, disease modeling, and organoid-based drug screening have demonstrated the real-world potential of bioprinting to address both degenerative and traumatic conditions.

Ethical, regulatory, and biological challenges – such as vascularization, standardization, access, and consent – remain critical hurdles. However, ongoing innovations in AI-driven design, in situ printing, and smart bioinks suggest a clear path toward scalable, safe, and personalized regenerative solutions.

11.5.2 Bioprinting as a Pillar of Future Reformative Medicine

Looking ahead, bioprinting is poised to become a core pillar of reformative medicine, enabling on-demand, patient-specific therapeutic solutions that transcend the limitations of donor-based transplants or synthetic prosthetics. The vision of printing tissues directly onto or within the patient, in operating rooms, battlefields, or remote clinics, is no longer speculative – it is rapidly materializing through multidisciplinary convergence.

By synergizing clinical insights, biofabrication, AI, and real-time diagnostics, bioprinting can support a healthcare model that is restorative rather than palliative, adaptive rather than static, and precise rather than generalized.

To fully realize this potential, future strategies must emphasize:

- Cross-sectoral collaboration among clinicians, engineers, policymakers, and ethicists
- Investment in education, infrastructure, and regulatory frameworks
- Commitment to equity and accessibility

Ultimately, bioprinting reflects the next frontier in medicine – not merely repairing the body but rebuilding it, intelligently and ethically, from the ground up.

Acknowledgments: The author gratefully acknowledges the contributions of researchers, clinicians, and interdisciplinary collaborators whose pioneering work in bioprinting, regenerative medicine, AI, and biomaterials formed the scientific foundation of this chapter.

Special thanks are extended to institutions actively advancing translational bioprinting, including the Wake Forest Institute for Regenerative Medicine (WFIRM), the UCL Centre for 3D Bioprinting, and the Indian Council of Medical Research (ICMR), for their publicly available resources and case studies.

The author also thanks the editorial team of this book for their guidance, support, and encouragement throughout the development of this chapter.

Glossary of Terms

Bioprinting A form of 3D printing that involves layer-by-layer deposition of bioinks containing living cells and biomaterials to create tissue-like structures.

Reformative medicine A progressive field of medical science focused on restoring, regenerating, or replacing damaged or diseased tissues and organs through advanced therapeutic technologies.

Bioink A biomaterial formulation that includes living cells and is suitable for printing via a bioprinter.

In situ bioprinting Bioprinting conducted directly at the site of injury or within the body during surgery, allowing immediate application and tissue integration.

On-demand bioprinting Fabrication of biological constructs in real time based on patient-specific clinical needs, often in decentralized or emergency settings.

Extrusion bioprinting A bioprinting technique where continuous streams of bioink are extruded through a nozzle to form 3D structures.

Laser-assisted bioprinting (LAB) A high-precision method that uses focused laser pulses to transfer bioink droplets onto substrates.

4D bioprinting An extension of 3D bioprinting where printed constructs change over time in response to environmental stimuli.

Organoid A 3D miniature tissue culture that resembles an organ and is used for research or therapeutic purposes.

AI-driven biofabrication The integration of artificial intelligence into the design, optimization, and monitoring of bioprinting processes.

References

[1] Murphy, S. V., & Atala, A. (2014). 3D bioprinting of tissues and organs. Nature. biotechnology, 32(8), 773–785. 10.1038/nbt.2958.

[2] Groll, J., Boland, T., Blunk, T., Burdick, J. A., Cho, D. W., Dalton, P. D., D'Arrigo, E., Gribbon, M. E., Guler, U., Goudswaard, I. J., Jüngst, T., Kim, W. K., Kucukgul, C., Lee, S. J., Li, Y., Mahns, P., Mironov, V. A., Moroni, L., Müller, M., & Wu, D. J. (2016). Biofabrication: Reappraising the definition of an evolving field. Biofabrication, 8(1), 013001. https://doi.org/10.1088/1758-5090/8/1/013001.

[3] Mandrycky, C., Wang, Z., Kim, K., & Kim, D. H. (2016). 3D bioprinting for engineering complex tissues. Biotechnology Advances, 34(4), 422–434. https://doi.org/10.1016/j.biotechadv.2016.01.006.

[4] Ozbolat, I. T. (2015). Bioprinting scale-up tissue and organ constructs for transplantation. Trends in Biotechnology, 33(7), 395–400. https://doi.org/10.1016/j.tibtech.2015.04.005.

[5] Gao, G., Ahn, M., Cho, W. W., Zang, J., & Cho, D. W. (2018). Bioprinting for personalized medicine. Advanced Drug Delivery Reviews, 132, 129–151. https://doi.org/10.1016/j.addr.2018.06.012.

[6] Heinrich, M. A., Bansal, R., Lammers, T., Zhang, Y. S., Schiffelers, R. M., & Prakash, J. (2019). 3D-bioprinted mini-brain: A novel approach to investigate neurodegenerative diseases. Advanced Healthcare Materials, 8(23), e1901407. https://doi.org/10.1002/adhm.201901407.

[7] Gudapati, H., Dey, M., & Ozbolat, I. (2016). A comprehensive review on droplet-based bioprinting: Past, present and future. Biomaterials, 102, 20–42. https://doi.org/10.1016/j.biomaterials.2016.06.012.

[8] Murphy, S. V., & Atala, A. (2016). Organ engineering – Combining stem cells, biomaterials, and bioreactors to produce bioengineered organs for transplantation. Nature Reviews Materials, 1(2), 16015. https://doi.org/10.1038/natrevmats.2016.15.

[9] Boland, T., Xu, T., Damon, B., & Cui, X. (2006). Application of inkjet printing to tissue engineering. Biotechnology Journal, 1(9), 910–917. https://doi.org/10.1002/biot.200600088.

[10] Koch, L., Deiwick, A., Schlie, S., Michael, S., Gruene, M., Coger, V., & Chichkov, B. N. (2012). Skin tissue generation by laser cell printing. Biotechnology & Bioengineering, 109(7), 1855–1863. https://doi.org/10.1002/bit.24479.

[11] Malda, J., Visser, J., Melchels, F. P. W., Jüngst, T., Hennink, W. E., Dhert, W. J. A., Groll, J., & Hutmacher, D. W. (2013). 25th anniversary article: Engineering hydrogels for biofabrication. Advanced Materials, 25(36), 5011–5028. https://doi.org/10.1002/adma.201301824.

[12] Noor, N., Shapira, A., Edri, R., Gal, I., Wertheim, L., & Dvir, T. (2019). 3D printing of personalized thick and perfusable cardiac patches and hearts. Advanced Science, 6(11), 1900344. https://doi.org/10.1002/advs.201900344.

[13] Zhang, Y. S., Yue, K., Aleman, J., Mollazadeh-Moghaddam, K., Bakht, S. M., Yang, J. et al. (2017). 3D bioprinting for tissue and organ fabrication. Annals of Biomedical Engineering, 45(1), 148–163. https://doi.org/10.1007/s10439-016-1681-4.
[14] Mason, C., & Dunnill, P. (2008). A brief definition of regenerative medicine. Regenerative Medicine, 3(1), 1–5. https://doi.org/10.2217/17460751.3.1.1.
[15] Mironov, V., Trusk, T., Forgacs, G., & Markwald, R. R. (2009). Organ printing: Computer-aided jet-based 3D tissue engineering. Trends in Biotechnology, 27(9), 505–512. https://doi.org/10.1016/j.tibtech.2009.06.002.
[16] Tao, Y., You, F., Sun, L., Mokasdar, A., & Zhang, Y. (2013). Bioprinting towards organ fabrication: Challenges and future trends. Biofabrication, 5(1), 014101. https://doi.org/10.1088/1758-5082/5/1/014101.
[17] Srivastava, S., Norfleet, J., Shah, P., & Ghosh, S. (2021). Artificial intelligence-assisted bioprinting: Toward next-generation tissue engineering. Frontiers in Bioengineering and Biotechnology, 9, 652611. https://doi.org/10.3389/fbioe.2021.652611.
[18] Hospodiuk, M., Dey, M., Sosnoski, D., & Ozbolat, I. T. (2017). The bioink: A comprehensive review on bioprintable materials. Biotechnology Advances, 35(2), 217–239. https://doi.org/10.1016/j.biotechadv.2016.12.006.
[19] Xu, T., Zhao, W., Zhu, J. M., Albanna, M. Z., Yoo, J. J., & Atala, A. (2013). Complex heterogeneous tissue constructs containing multiple cell types prepared by inkjet printing technology. Biomaterials, 34(1), 130–139. https://doi.org/10.1016/j.biomaterials.2012.09.055.
[20] Ozbolat, I. T., & Hospodiuk, M. (2016). Current advances and future perspectives in extrusion-based bioprinting. Biomaterials, 76, 321–343. https://doi.org/10.1016/j.biomaterials.2015.10.076.
[21] Cui, H., Nowicki, M., Fisher, J. P., & Zhang, L. G. (2017). 3D bioprinting for organ regeneration. Advanced Healthcare Materials, 6(1), 1601118. https://doi.org/10.1002/adhm.201601118.
[22] Guillemot, F., Souquet, A., Catros, S., Guillotin, B., Lopez, J., Faucon, M., J., H., & R, J. (2010). High-throughput laser printing of cells and biomaterials for tissue engineering. Acta Biomaterialia, 6(7), 2494–2500. https://doi.org/10.1016/j.actbio.2010.02.008.
[23] Koch, L., Deiwick, A., Franke, A., Schwanke, K., Haverich, A., Zweigerdt, R., & Chichkov, B. N. (2018). Laser bioprinting of human induced pluripotent stem cells – The effect of printing and biomaterials on cell survival, pluripotency, and differentiation. Biofabrication, 10(3), 035005. https://doi.org/10.1088/1758-5090/aacb36.
[24] Zhu, W., Holmes, B., Glazer, R. I., & Zhang, L. G. (2016). 3D printed nanocomposite matrix for the study of breast cancer bone metastasis. Nanomedicine, 12(1), 69–79. https://doi.org/10.1016/j.nano.2015.09.006.
[25] Lim, K. S., Schon, B. S., Mekhileri, N. V., Brown, G. C., Chia, C. M., & Prabakar, S. (2016). New visible-light photoinitiating system for improved print fidelity in gelatin-based bioinks. ACS Biomaterials Science and Engineering, 2(10), 1752–1762. https://doi.org/10.1021/acsbiomaterials.6b00170.
[26] Lee, A., Hudson, A. R., Shiwarski, D. J., Tashman, J. W., Hinton, T. J., Yerneni, S., & Feinberg, A. W. (2019). 3D bioprinting of collagen to rebuild components of the human heart. Science, 365(6452), 482–487. https://doi.org/10.1126/science.aav9051.
[27] Chimene, D., Lennox, K. K., Kaunas, R. R., & Gaharwar, A. K. (2016). Advanced bioinks for 3D printing: A materials science perspective. Annals of Biomedical Engineering, 44(6), 2090–2102. https://doi.org/10.1007/s10439-016-1610-6.
[28] Yue, K., Trujillo-de Santiago, G., Alvarez, M. M., Tamayol, A., Annabi, N., & Khademhosseini, A. (2015). Synthesis, properties, and biomedical applications of gelatin methacryloyl (GelMA) hydrogels. Biomaterials, 73, 254–271. https://doi.org/10.1016/j.biomaterials.2015.08.045.

[29] Highley, C. B., Rodell, C. B., & Burdick, J. A. (2015). Direct 3D printing of shear-thinning hydrogels into self-healing hydrogels. Advanced Materials, 27(34), 5075–5079. https://doi.org/10.1002/adma.201501103.
[30] Jang, J., Park, H. J., Kim, S. W., Kim, H., Park, J. Y., Na, S. J., Kim, H. J., Kang, H. W., & Han, D. W. (2017). 3D printed complex tissue construct using stem cell-laden decellularized extracellular matrix bioinks for cardiac repair. Biomaterials, 112, 264–274. https://doi.org/10.1016/j.biomaterials.2016.10.021.
[31] Koons, G. L., Diba, M., & Mikos, A. G. (2020). Materials design for bone-tissue engineering. Nature Reviews Materials, 5(8), 584–603. https://doi.org/10.1038/s41578-020-0205-2.
[32] Lin, H., Zhang, D., Alexander, P. G., Yang, G., Tan, J., Cheng, A. W., J., W., J., W., W., W., W., B., W., Z., & W, F. (2013). Application of visible light-based projection stereolithography for live cell-scaffold fabrication with designed architecture. Biomaterials, 34(2), 331–339. https://doi.org/10.1016/j.biomaterials.2012.09.043.
[33] Basara, G., & Zorlutuna, P.. (2020). Magnetically controllable 3D-printed cardiac tissue constructs for in vitro modeling. Advanced Materials Technologies, 5(4), 1900715. https://doi.org/10.1002/admt.201900715.
[34] Pati, F., Jang, J., Ha, D. H., Kim, S. W., Rhie, J. W., Shim, J. H., Kim, M. J., Cho, D. W., & Bae, H.. (2014). Printing three-dimensional tissue analogues with decellularized extracellular matrix bioink. Nature Communications, 5, 3935. https://doi.org/10.1038/ncomms4935.
[35] Murphy, S. V., & Atala, A.. (2014). 3D bioprinting of tissues and organs. Nature Biotechnology, 32(8), 773–785. https://doi.org/10.1038/nbt.2958.
[36] Kang, H. W., Lee, S. J., Ko, I. K., Kengla, C., Yoo, J. J., & Atala, A.. (2016). A 3D bioprinting system to produce human-scale tissue constructs with structural integrity. Nature Biotechnology, 34(3), 312–319. https://doi.org/10.1038/nbt.3413.
[37] Zhang, Q., Shi, Y., Zhou, M., Zhang, L., Yu, X., Jin, L., Tang, W., & Zhang, Y.. (2019). In vivo cartilage regeneration using scaffolds with gradient pore sizes fabricated by a 3D bioprinting system. ACS Applied Materials and Interfaces, 11(45), 41658–41668. https://doi.org/10.1021/acsami.9b14275.
[38] Ma, X., Yu, C., Wang, P., Yang, J., Valerius, M. T., Sundin, B. M., J., M., & F, A.. (2018). Rapid 3D bioprinting of decellularized extracellular matrix with regionally varied mechanical properties and biomimetic microarchitecture. Biomaterials, 185, 310–321. https://doi.org/10.1016/j.biomaterials.2018.09.020.
[39] Wang, L., Wu, Y., Hu, T., Guo, B., & Ma, P. X.. (2020). 3D printed bioactive citrate-based scaffold for bone regeneration. Bioactive Materials, 5(1), 82–91. https://doi.org/10.1016/j.bioactmat.2020.01.001.
[40] Baltazar, T., Merola, J., Catarino, C., Mitchell, R., & Ferreira, F. C.. (2020). Skin tissue engineering: An update on 3D bioprinting and biomedical applications. Biomedical Materials, 15(5), 052003. https://doi.org/10.1088/1748-605X/ab86a4.
[41] Zhang, B., Gao, L., Ma, L., Luo, Y., Yang, J., & Liu, J.. (2022). Bioprinting of patient-specific renal constructs for clinical translation. Advanced Healthcare Materials, 11(9), 2102253. https://doi.org/10.1002/adhm.202102253.
[42] Ozbolat, I. T.. (2015). Bioprinting scale-up tissue and organ constructs for transplantation. Trends in Biotechnology, 33(7), 395–400. https://doi.org/10.1016/j.tibtech.2015.04.005.
[43] Ma, X., Qu, X., Zhu, W., Li, Y. S., Yuan, S., Zhang, H., Liu, J., & Atala, A.. (2016). Deterministically patterned biomimetic human iPSC-derived hepatic model via rapid 3D bioprinting. Proceedings of the National Academy of Sciences of the United States of America, 113(8), 2206–2211. https://doi.org/10.1073/pnas.1524335113.
[44] Homan, K. A., Kolesky, D. B., Skylar-Scott, M. A., Herrmann, J., Obuobi, H., Moisan, A., & Lewis, J. A.. (2016). Bioprinting of 3D convoluted renal proximal tubules on perfusable chips. Scientific Reports, 6, 34845. https://doi.org/10.1038/srep34845.

[45] Noor, N., Shapira, A., Edri, R., Gal, I., Wertheim, L., & Dvir, T.. (2019). 3D printing of personalized thick and perfusable cardiac patches and hearts. Advanced Science, 6(11), 1900344. https://doi.org/10.1002/advs.201900344.

[46] Gaetani, R., Doevendans, P. A., Metz, C. H., Alblas, J., Messina, E., Giacomello, A., & A, S.. (2012). Cardiac tissue engineering using tissue printing technology and human cardiac progenitor cells. Biomaterials, 33(6), 1782–1790. https://doi.org/10.1016/j.biomaterials.2011.11.026.

[47] Joung, D., Truong, V., Neitzke, C. C., Guo, S. Z., Walsh, P. J., Monat, J. R., Lee, S. J., Li, B., & Zhang, L. G.. (2018). 3D printed stem-cell derived neural progenitors generate spinal cord scaffolds. Advanced Functional Materials, 28(39), 1801850. https://doi.org/10.1002/adfm.201801850.

[48] Hakobyan, D., Kerobyan, N., Mandrycky, C., Dey, M., Macdonald, D., & Ozbolat, I. T.. (2021). Bioprinting of pancreatic pseudo-islets with functional vascular networks. Biofabrication, 13(3), 035020. https://doi.org/10.1088/1758-5090/abf08d.

[49] Bishop, E. S., Mostafa, S., Pakvasa, M., Luu, H. H., Lee, M. J., Wolf, J. M., & H, L.. (2017). 3-D bioprinting technologies in tissue engineering and regenerative medicine: Current and future trends. Genes and Diseases, 4(4), 185–195. https://doi.org/10.1016/j.gendis.2017.10.005.

[50] Gudapati, H., Dey, M., & Ozbolat, I. T.. (2016). A comprehensive review on droplet-based bioprinting: Past, present and future. Biomaterials, 102, 20–42. https://doi.org/10.1016/j.biomaterials.2016.06.012.

[51] Di Bella, C., Duchi, S., O'Connell, C. D., Blanchard, R., Augustine, C., Yue, Z., & G, G.. (2018). In situ handheld three-dimensional bioprinting for cartilage regeneration. Journal of Tissue Engineering and Regenerative Medicine, 12(3), 611–621. https://doi.org/10.1002/term.2520.

[52] Atala, A., & Frampton, J. P.. (2020). The biofabrication frontier: A perspective. Science, 368(6491), 990–991. https://doi.org/10.1126/science.aba4181.

[53] Kang, H.-W., Kengla, C., & Atala, A.. (2019). 3D bioprinting in space: A frontier in regenerative medicine. Regenerative Medicine, 14(7), 659–662. https://doi.org/10.2217/rme-2019-0027.

[54] Blaber, E. A., Dvorochkin, N., Lee, C., Alwood, J. S., Yousuf, R., Pianetta, P., L., M., L., R., & L, A.. (2015). Microgravity influences on stem cell-derived tissues: Implications for tissue engineering and regenerative medicine in space. Stem Cells and Development, 24(21), 2605–2621. https://doi.org/10.1089/scd.2015.0191.

[55] Zhu, W., Qu, X., Zhu, J., Ma, X., Patel, S., Liu, J., & J, P.. (2017). Direct 3D bioprinting of prevascularized tissue constructs with complex microarchitecture. Biomaterials, 124, 106–115. https://doi.org/10.1016/j.biomaterials.2017.02.001.

[56] Takebe, T., & Wells, J. M.. (2019). Organoids by design. Science, 364(6444), 956–959. https://doi.org/10.1126/science.aaw7906.

[57] Zhang, Y. S., Arneri, A., Bersini, S., Shin, S. R., Zhu, K., Goli-Malekabadi, Z., & W, D.. (2016). Bioprinting 3D microfibrous scaffolds for engineering endothelialized myocardium and heart-on-a-chip platforms. Biomaterials, 110, 45–59. https://doi.org/10.1016/j.biomaterials.2016.09.020.

[58] Lee, J., Sutcliffe, M., Li, B., Matz, J., Wong, C., Linderman, J. R., & H, S.. (2021). 3D bioprinted human liver tissue for personalized drug screening. Lab on a Chip, 21(1), 189–200. https://doi.org/10.1039/D0LC00889A.

[59] Kim, J., Koo, B. K., & Knoblich, J. A.. (2020). Human organoids: Model systems for human biology and medicine. Nature Reviews Molecular Cell Biology, 21(10), 571–584. https://doi.org/10.1038/s41580-020-0259-3.

[60] Lancaster, M. A., Renner, M., Martin, C. A., Wenzel, D., Bicknell, L. S., Hurles, M. E., & A, J.. (2013). Cerebral organoids model human brain development and microcephaly. Nature, 501(7467), 373–379. https://doi.org/10.1038/nature12516.

[61] Zhao, Y., Yao, R., Ouyang, L., Ding, H., Zhang, T., Zhang, K., & Chen, J.. (2014). Three-dimensional printing of HUVECs with ECM and its application in a microfluidic chip for drug screening. Biofabrication, 6(4), 045009. https://doi.org/10.1088/1758-5082/6/4/045009.
[62] Tamay, D. G., Usal, T. D., Alagoz, A. S., Yucel, D., Hasirci, N., & Hasirci, V.. (2019). 3D and 4D bioprinting of polymers for tissue engineering applications. Frontiers in Bioengineering and Biotechnology, 7, 164. https://doi.org/10.3389/fbioe.2019.00164.
[63] Mittal, R., Woo, F. W., Castro, C. S., Cohen, M. A., Karanxha, J., Mittal, J., & Khademhosseini, A.. (2019). Organ-on-chip models: Implications in drug discovery and clinical applications. Journal of Cellular Physiology, 234(6), 8352–8380. https://doi.org/10.1002/jcp.27788.
[64] Murphy, S. V., De Coppi, P., & Atala, A.. (2020). Opportunities and challenges of translational 3D bioprinting. Nature Biomedical Engineering, 4(4), 370–380. https://doi.org/10.1038/s41551-020-0535-1.
[65] Lavazza, A., & Massimini, M.. (2018). Cerebral organoids: Ethical issues and consciousness assessment. Journal of Medical Ethics, 44(9), 606–610. https://doi.org/10.1136/medethics-2018-104845.
[66] Hyun, I.. (2017). Engineering ethics and self-regulation in stem cell science. Cell Stem Cell, 21(3), 275–279. https://doi.org/10.1016/j.stem.2017.08.006.
[67] Schaefer, G. O., Emanuel, E. J., & Wertheimer, A.. (2009). The obligation to participate in biomedical research. JAMA, 302(1), 67–72. https://doi.org/10.1001/jama.2009.957.
[68] Gerke, S., Minssen, T., & Cohen, G.. (2020). Ethical and legal challenges of artificial intelligence-driven healthcare. Artificial Intelligence in Healthcare, 2, 295–336. https://doi.org/10.1016/b978-0-12-818277-2.00018-6.
[69] Christensen, K., Rybicki, F. J., & Mitsouras, D.. (2015). Three-dimensional printing with patient-specific data: Review of medical applications. Journal of the American College of Radiology, 12(10), 1151–1159. https://doi.org/10.1016/j.jacr.2015.06.014.
[70] Mironov, V., Kasyanov, V., Drake, C., & Markwald, R.. (2008). Organ printing: Promises and challenges. Regenerative Medicine, 3(1), 93–103. https://doi.org/10.2217/17460751.3.1.93.
[71] Ozbolat, I. T., & Hospodiuk, M.. (2016). Current advances and future perspectives in extrusion-based bioprinting. Biomaterials, 76, 321–343. https://doi.org/10.1016/j.biomaterials.2015.10.076.
[72] Mandrycky, C., Wang, Z., Kim, K., & Kim, D. H.. (2016). 3D bioprinting for engineering complex tissues. Biotechnology Advances, 34(4), 422–434. https://doi.org/10.1016/j.biotechadv.2016.01.006.
[73] Zhang, Y. S., Yue, K., Aleman, J., Mollazadeh-Moghaddam, K., Bakht, S. M., Yang, J., & Khademhosseini, A.. (2017). 3D bioprinting for tissue and organ fabrication. Annals of Biomedical Engineering, 45(1), 148–163. https://doi.org/10.1007/s10439-016-1681-4.
[74] Kolesky, D. B., Truby, R. L., Gladman, A. S., Busbee, T. A., Homan, K. A., & Lewis, J. A.. (2014). 3D bioprinting of vascularized, heterogeneous cell-laden tissue constructs. Advanced Materials, 26(19), 3124–3130. https://doi.org/10.1002/adma.201305506.
[75] Chimene, D., Lennox, K. K., Kaunas, R. R., & Gaharwar, A. K.. (2016). Advanced bioinks for 3D printing: A materials science perspective. Annals of Biomedical Engineering, 44(6), 2090–2102. https://doi.org/10.1007/s10439-016-1610-6.
[76] Heinrich, M. A., Bansal, R., Lammers, T., Zhang, Y. S., Schiffelers, R. M., & Prakash, J.. (2019). 3D-bioprinted mini-brain: A novel tool for preclinical drug screening. Advanced Drug Delivery Reviews, 140, 101–103. https://doi.org/10.1016/j.addr.2019.01.006.
[77] Murphy, S. V., & Atala, A.. (2014). 3D bioprinting of tissues and organs. Nature Biotechnology, 32(8), 773–785. https://doi.org/10.1038/nbt.2958.
[78] Jorfi, M., D'Avanzo, C., Kim, D. Y., & Irimia, D.. (2018). Three-dimensional models of the human brain development and disease. Advanced Healthcare Materials, 7(17), e1700726. https://doi.org/10.1002/adhm.201700726.

[79] Lavazza, A.. (2021). Human cerebral organoids and consciousness: A double-edged sword. Journal of Medical Ethics, 47(3), 161–168. https://doi.org/10.1136/medethics-2020-106548.
[80] Lo, B., & Parham, L.. (2009). Ethical issues in stem cell research. Endocrine Reviews, 30(3), 204–213. https://doi.org/10.1210/er.2008-0046.
[81] Solomon, M. Z., Gusmano, M. K., & Maschke, K. J.. (2016). The ethical imperative and moral challenges of engaging patients and the public with evidence. Health Affairs, 35(4), 583–589. https://doi.org/10.1377/hlthaff.2015.1190.
[82] Isasi, R., Kleiderman, E., & Knoppers, B. M.. (2016). Editing policy to fit the genome? Science, 351(6271), 337–339. https://doi.org/10.1126/science.aad9424.
[83] Chadwick, R., & Berg, K.. (2001). Solidarity and equity: New ethical frameworks for genetic databases. Nature Reviews Genetics, 2(4), 318–321. https://doi.org/10.1038/35066099.
[84] Morley, J., & Floridi, L.. (2020). The limits of empowerment: How to reframe the role of mHealth tools in the healthcare ecosystem. Science and Engineering Ethics, 26(3), 1159–1183. https://doi.org/10.1007/s11948-019-00125-9.
[85] Moreno, J. D.. (2013). Dual-use and the ethical responsibility of scientists. The American Journal of Bioethics, 13(6), 28–34. https://doi.org/10.1080/15265161.2013.784551.
[86] Ghosh, S., Yao, J., & Tan, W.. (2021). Artificial intelligence in 3D bioprinting for tissue engineering and regenerative medicine. Advanced Healthcare Materials, 10(19), 2100598. https://doi.org/10.1002/adhm.202100598.
[87] Srivastava, M., Dash, D., Srivastava, R., & Sinha, A.. (2022). AI-based design and optimization in tissue engineering: Current trends and future perspectives. Biotechnology & Bioengineering, 119(2), 361–373. https://doi.org/10.1002/bit.27961.
[88] Paulsen, S. J., & Miller, J. S.. (2015). Tissue vascularization through 3D printing: AI-driven modeling of angiogenesis and perfusion. Biomedical Engineering and Computational Biology, 7, 1–7. https://doi.org/10.4137/bmecb.s13253.
[89] Noor, N., Shapira, A., & Dvir, T.. (2020). AI-assisted quality control in biofabrication: A paradigm shift in smart biomanufacturing. Trends in Biotechnology, 38(4), 378–387. https://doi.org/10.1016/j.tibtech.2019.12.001.
[90] Hospodiuk, M., Dey, M., Sosnoski, D., & Ozbolat, I. T.. (2017). The bioink properties of 3D bioprinting. Biomaterials, 140, 203–215. https://doi.org/10.1016/j.biomaterials.2017.06.036.
[91] Kolesky, D. B., Homan, K. A., Skylar-Scott, M. A., & Lewis, J. A.. (2016). Three-dimensional bioprinting of thick vascularized tissues. Proceedings of the National Academy of Sciences of the United States of America, 113(12), 3179–3184. https://doi.org/10.1073/pnas.1521344113.
[92] Barata, D., Hutmacher, D. W., Hennessy, R. J., & Loessner, D.. (2023). Machine learning in organoid bioprinting: Predictive models for regenerative and translational outcomes. Trends in Biotechnology, 41(3), 214–226. https://doi.org/10.1016/j.tibtech.2022.07.009.
[93] Morley, J., & Floridi, L.. (2020). The limits of empowerment: How to reframe the role of AI in the healthcare ecosystem. Science and Engineering Ethics, 26(3), 1159–1183. https://doi.org/10.1007/s11948-019-00125-9.
[94] Murphy, S. V., De Coppi, P., & Atala, A.. (2020). Opportunities and challenges of translational 3D bioprinting. Nature Biomedical Engineering, 4(4), 370–380. https://doi.org/10.1038/s41551-020-0535-1.
[95] Di Bella, C., Duchi, S., O'Connell, C. D., Blanchard, R., Augustine, C., Yue, Z., & G, G.. (2018). In situ handheld three-dimensional bioprinting for cartilage regeneration. Journal of Tissue Engineering and Regenerative Medicine, 12(3), 611–621. https://doi.org/10.1002/term.2520.
[96] Zhang, B., Luo, Y., Ma, J., Luo, Z., Lu, Q., Huang, Y., & Liu, J.. (2021). Robotic-assisted in situ 3D bioprinting for minimally invasive cartilage repair. Biofabrication, 13(2), 025034. https://doi.org/10.1088/1758-5090/abde86.

[97] Kang, H.-W., Kengla, C., & Atala, A.. (2019). 3D bioprinting in space: A frontier in regenerative medicine. Regenerative Medicine, 14(7), 659–662. https://doi.org/10.2217/rme-2019-0027.
[98] Noor, N., Shapira, A., Edri, R., Gal, I., Wertheim, L., & Dvir, T.. (2019). 3D printing of personalized thick and perfusable cardiac patches and hearts. Advanced Science, 6(11), 1900344. https://doi.org/10.1002/advs.201900344.
[99] Miao, S., Cui, H., Nowicki, M., Xia, L., Zhou, X., Lee, S. J., & L, R.. (2017). 4D bioprinting: Advancing biomedical applications. Trends in Biotechnology, 35(9), 910–922. https://doi.org/10.1016/j.tibtech.2017.06.012.

Koyel Ghosal, Nikita Saini, Durba Pal, and Bodhisatwa Das*

Chapter 12
Bioprinting of Structures Using Viable Cells, Biomaterials, and Living Molecules

Abstract: Bioprinting is a technology that combines additive manufacturing and tissue engineering, with enormous potential. 3D organ equivalents are developed through the fabrication of scaffolds utilizing a bioink that can be used for various applications, like skin, liver, heart, vasculature, etc. The primary rationale behind the development of 3D bioprinting is either the manufacturing of artificial organs for implantation in a patient post-organ failure, where a donor is not available, or the fabrication of 3D microtissues for screening and performance evaluation of therapeutics and vaccines. 3D bioprinted scaffolds should have optimum mechanical, rheological, and biological properties that support their stability and can be used for further applications. The scaffold can be printed using various methods, such as extrusion-based, inkjet-based, and laser-assisted printing, depending on the application. The choice of bioinks, cells, and bioactive molecules depends upon the requisite tissue characteristics, mechanical integrity, and biological functionality. Optimization of factors such as bioink viscosity, nozzle diameter, and extrusion pressure plays a crucial role in minimizing shear stress and maintaining high cell viability in 3D bioprinting. Composite bioinks and cell-laden hydrogels have shown significant advances and potential applications in regenerative medicine. In this chapter, we will focus on various types of cell-laden bioinks, selection and optimization of bioprinting methods, biomaterials, and bioactive molecules in bioprinting, with their impact on tissue engineering and regenerative medicine applications.

Keywords: Bioprinting, bioinks, hydrogels, tissue engineering, regenerative medicine

12.1 Introduction

In 1991, Vacanti and Langer first introduced the idea of tissue engineering in a study that became an emerging area of research. The goal was to design personalized treatments that could help the body heal by regenerating, remodeling, and growing damaged tissues [1]. This technology has led to the development of biomaterials that can

***Corresponding author: Bodhisatwa Das,** Department of Biomedical Engineering, IIT Ropar, Rupnagar 140001, Punjab, India, e-mail: bodhisatwa.das@iitrpr.ac.in
Koyel Ghosal, Nikita Saini, Durba Pal, Department of Biomedical Engineering, IIT Ropar, Rupnagar 140001, Punjab

 | https://doi.org/10.1515/9783111719993-012

be used for drug testing and to create bioactive scaffolds that imitate real tissue, both for laboratory experiments and for actual use in the body through transplantation [2].

Creating these scaffolds is a detailed process that involves combining specific types of cells, bioactive substances like growth factors, and a scaffold material that aids in cell survival, growth, and mimics the natural environment of the tissue being targeted. A diverse range of materials can be used to make these scaffolds, which include both natural and synthetic polymers, hydrogels, ceramics, metals, and polymer-based composites, mainly because they are biocompatible. These materials can be shaped into 2D or 3D structures that support cell growth and interaction. Traditional 2D cell cultures, like those grown in dishes or flat scaffolds, encourage cells to multiply quickly, but they eventually stop growing once the cells are confluent. Scientists have designed 3D cell cultures that offer a more realistic and desirable environment for the cells to grow and function, thereby overcoming limitations and enhancing nutrient availability [3].

Bioprinting, a technique that utilizes additive manufacturing to generate scaffolds by depositing layers of bioink materials containing living cells, is based on 3D designs made using software called computer-aided design. Using this software, complex 3D tissues and organs can be designed that are functional and biologically relevant by selecting the right combination of biomaterials, cells, and signaling molecules like growth and differentiation factors [4]. These printed constructs have few applications, such as drug testing, delivery of genes or biomolecules, disease modeling, tissue regeneration, and biohybrid robotics. The advantage of bioprinting is that it offers reasonable control over the design and development of these structures. Researchers have shown that several types of tissues, as well as various organs, such as cartilage, bones, heart muscle tissue, heart valves, blood vessels, and trachea, have been successfully bioprinted [5].

Although both 3D printers and bioprinters build scaffold layers, layer by layer using a specific material, they are designed for very different purposes. Conventional 3D printers, which have been in use for a longer duration, usually print with materials like metals, rubber, resins, and plastics. These are particularly useful in making implants, tools, and other medical devices.

On the other hand, bioprinters are explicitly made to print biological materials, called bioinks. These bioinks often contain living cells from humans or animals. Bioprinters use special methods, like scaffolding and crosslinking, to help printed structures grow and resemble real tissues in both shape and function. Most 3D printers melt and extrude plastic that hardens into a solid form. Bioprinters, however, print using soft materials like gels and liquids, and can even print in droplets without touching the surface. They can print materials such as Matrigel, sugary syrups, and thick pastes, making them useful not only in healthcare but also in areas like food technology. The main goal of bioprinting is to offer a better option than using tissue implants from the same person (autologous) or from donors (allogeneic), and to reduce or even eliminate the need for animal testing when studying diseases and developing new treatments [5].

Bioprinting can be distinguished into three stages: pre-bioprinting, bioprinting, and post-bioprinting. Each stage influences the subsequent steps and affects the performance of the fabricated constructs. For organ fabrication to get an adequate number of cells, tissue biopsy, and cell expansion techniques are essential in pre-bioprinting. To achieve accuracy, medical imaging is necessary for generating high-resolution designs in bioprinting. It is crucial to select biomaterials that solidify at the optimum rate to ensure that the printed structures support high cell viability and fidelity. However, there is a need to advance bioprinters that possess a high degree of mobility, operate for a longer duration, and can be compact as well as cost-effective. Finally, the maturation of bioprinted cells depends on the conditions maintained during the post-printing phase [6].

Several types of technologies are used in 3D bioprinting, with the four major ones being extrusion, inkjet, laser-assisted, and stereolithography bioprinting [5]. In extrusion bioprinting, a specific amount of bioink is pushed using mechanical force or air pressure through the nozzle, allowing the creation of 3D shapes. Inkjet-based bioprinting works by using either heat or sound waves to release droplets of bioink, which may include cells. Not only bioinks but also other types of biomaterials can be printed using this printing technology. In laser-assisted bioprinting, an intense laser beam is used to generate pressure, which allows the biomaterial to deposit onto a surface for printing. Stereolithography, on the other hand, uses a photochemical process to create 3D models layer by layer by selectively curing a photopolymer resin with a UV laser [4].

Bioprinting involves many challenges. The key components – cells, bioinks, and bioprinters – each present unique biological, technical, and ethical issues. Additionally, there are concerns about the potential effectiveness and affordability of this technology in clinical settings. Due to these factors, it may be challenging to implement 3D bioprinting widely in everyday medical practice [7]. Another major challenge in bioprinting is successfully integrating printed structures into the human body, particularly developing proper functional vascular and neural networks in 3D-printed tissues. Unlike mechanical implants like stents or pacemakers, bioprinted implants contain living cells, which makes their behavior inside the body more unpredictable. Factors like cell movement, changes in cell type after printing, potential to cause cancer, and abnormal cell development can all be affected by the patient's unique genetic makeup [8].

One of the biggest challenges in bioprinting is the ethical side concern. A significant issue is the reluctance to carry out clinical trials. Since it would not be ethical to test bioprinted organ transplants on healthy people, designing these trials becomes complicated. The use of autologous cells from patients further complicates the distinction between treatment and natural body response, making it difficult to interpret. Even after proper clinical trials, it becomes difficult because once an organ is implanted, the intervention is irreversible. Getting consent from patients can be challenging when associated risks are involved. Without trials and clinical evidence, approval by regulatory agencies such as the FDA is difficult, and the rapid pace of research and new developments in the field of bioprinting makes regulators even more cautious [7].

12.2 Bioprinting Methods

3D bioprinting can be generally categorized into four major types: -

12.2.1 Extrusion-Based Bioprinting (Pressure-Assisted Bioprinting)

Extrusion-based bioprinting (EBB) utilizes extrusion to form 3D shapes and structures. In this method, materials like solutions, pastes, or dispersions are pushed out in a steady stream through a tiny nozzle or microneedle [9]. It uses a computer-guided system to continuously print bioinks, which are usually thick, gel-like materials. This process works by layering the bioink through a nozzle that moves in all directions (x, y, and z) while the printing platform can be adjusted to help shape the final 3D structure. There are two major types of extrusion-based methods: pneumatic-based, which utilizes controlled air pressure to dispense the bio ink, and piston or screw-based, which mechanically pushes the material through the nozzle. Viscosity of bioinks can range from 30 to 6×10^7 mPas. EBB works well with different materials with varying viscosities. Thick, high-viscosity materials help build strong scaffolds, while thinner ones are better for supporting cell activities. It's crucial to achieve an optimum balance between mechanical strength and biological function [10]. One benefit of using extrusion-based bioprinting to create tissue scaffolds is that they can handle a broad range of cell densities in the bioink, even reaching levels like those found in real tissues (around 10^8–10^9 cells per mL). This helps in saving the time needed for cells to grow and develop before the scaffold can be implanted [11]. The fact is that it is generally cost-effective and easy to use. However, one of the main downsides is that it has lower printing resolution, which makes it hard to accurately control how cells are arranged in the final structure [12].

Applications: EBB has been used in several studies to design different tissue models. For example, HepG2 liver cells were printed inside alginate to build a liver model [13]. In another study, researchers used collagen bioink to recreate intestinal villi mixed with Caco-2 cells [14]. Johnson and colleagues used this technique to build a nervous system structure using cervical ganglia and hippocampal neurons [15]. A similar approach was used to print thick, vascularized heart patches using a hydrogel mixed with a patient's cells [16]. Also, a bioink was developed using alginate and nanocellulose, encapsulating chondrocytes and stem cells to produce a cartilage-type structure [17].

12.2.2 Inkjet-Based Bioprinting (Droplet-Based Bioprinting)

Similar to conventional 2D inkjet printers, it is also a form of noncontact printing. It is further divided into three types: thermal, electrostatic, and piezoelectric inkjet bioprinting [18, 19]. In piezoelectric inkjet printing, an actuator creates sound waves inside the chamber to help in the formation of droplets [20]. For the electrostatic type, droplets are produced by generating a voltage pulse between an electrode and a pressure plate. Heat is supplied inside the bioink chamber, which creates pressure that pushes the bioink out to form droplets in thermal inkjet bioprinting. It can produce droplets as small as 40 µm, leading to better resolution. This method avoids mechanical damage to cells, leading to potentially high cell viability [18].

Applications: DBB has been used to develop skin tissue by printing keratinocytes that represent the epidermis and fibroblasts for dermal layers, with collagen used as the dermal matrix [21]. This method has also been used to print bone tissue using a mixture of acrylated peptides, acrylated polyethylene glycol, and human mesenchymal stem cells (hMSCs) from bone marrow [22]. In another study, Graham et al. (2017) utilized an approach to create kidney-like tissue using human embryonic kidney cells along with MSCs [23]. It is used in cosmetology to print skin tissue by exuding tiny droplets of biological material, like a mixed solution of stem cells, melanocytes, keratinocytes, and fibroblast cells [24].

12.2.3 Laser-Assisted Bioprinting (LAB)

This bioprinting method was first developed for printing metals, but has shown great potential to print biological materials like DNA and even organs [25]. LAB uses a laser to deposit biomaterials onto a surface. This machine has three major parts, which include a pulsed laser, a ribbon coated with liquid biological materials placed on a thin metal layer, and a receiving surface. When the laser hits the ribbon, it causes the biological material to evaporate and form droplets that land on the receiving surface [26]. To facilitate adherence and proliferation of the transferred cells, the surface is coated with a biopolymer or cell culture medium. To print hydrogels, cells, proteins, and even ceramic materials, LAB commonly utilizes the nanosecond lasers with UV or near-UV wavelengths [27, 28]. The print resolution can range from very tiny (pico-scale) to micro-scale, and it's influenced by several factors such as the thickness and flow behavior of the bio-materials, laser energy, how well the surface holds liquid (wettability), and how fast and accurately the structure is printed [29, 30]. It minimizes mechanical stress to the cells due to its noncontact nature. This technology can be automated, enabling large-scale tissue bioprinting.

Application: Scientists have shown that laser-based bioprinting can print different types of cells, including human dermal fibroblasts, mouse muscle cells (C2C12), human fibroblasts, breast cancer cells (MCF-7), and rat neural stem cells [30–32]. A breakthrough happened in 2013 when Michael and his team successfully used LAB to create Graftskin, a type of skin substitute, marking an important milestone in this field [33].

12.2.4 Stereolithography (SLA)-Based Bioprinting

SLA, a nozzle-free, solid freeform technology, which was developed in the 1980s [34]. It works by using light to harden a liquid, light-sensitive polymer into a solid shape. SLA utilizes digital micromirror devices to adjust the intensity of light and cure light-sensitive polymers. This bioprinting method is mainly used to build structures from materials like acrylics and epoxies that can be hardened by light. As more photo-crosslinkable polymers are being developed, it's now possible to use multiple types of resin in a single print [9]. It works through a top-down printing process that is managed by digital light projection. In comparison to other solid freeform methods, SLA offers the highest level of printing accuracy and supports a growing variety of materials. The thickness of the final construct primarily controls the total duration of the printing process [35].

Application: Stereolithographic methods have been successfully combined with medical imaging to help improve disease diagnosis, plan surgeries more effectively, and enhance the design and fit of prosthetics and implants. This technology also contributes significantly to improving the outcomes of complex surgical procedures. Looking ahead, stereolithography is expected to become a key tool in the field of regenerative medicine [36]. A visible light-based SLA 3D bioprinting technique was used to design a dome-shaped structure that closely resembles the shape of the human corneal stroma [37].

The different 3D bioprinting techniques are illustrated in Figures 12.1(a), 12.1(b), 12.1(c), 12.1(d) and detailed comparison of the four bioprinting techniques, including their bioink characteristics, advantages and disadvantages is provided in table 12.1.

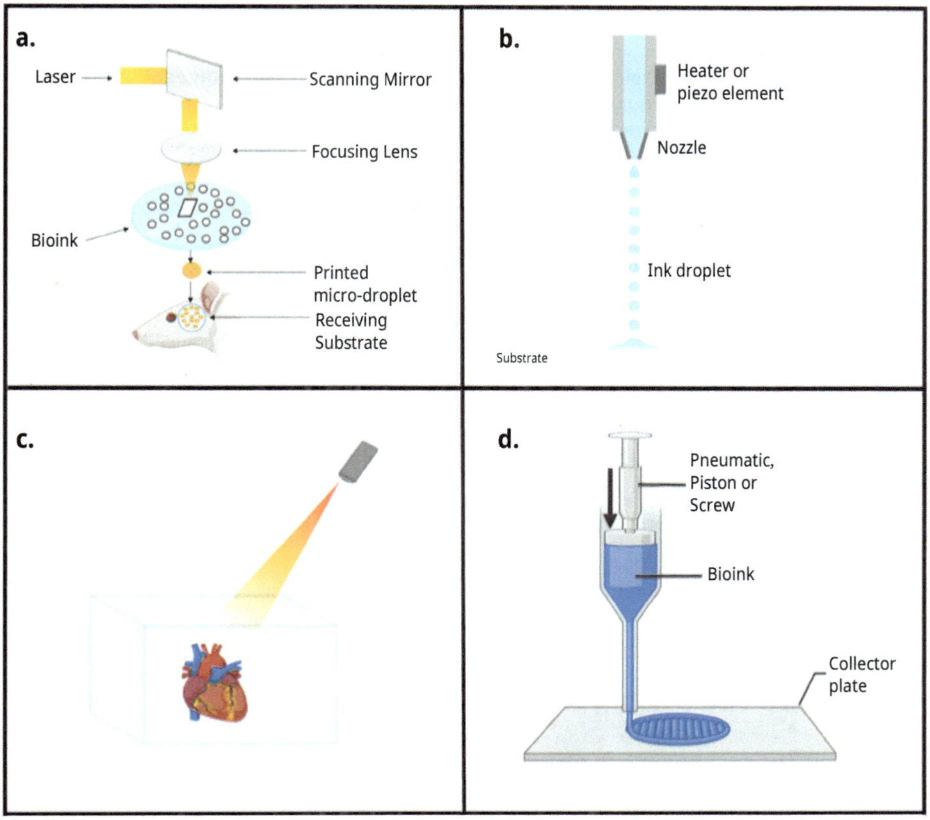

Figure 12.1: Illustration of 3D bioprinting techniques. (a) Laser-assisted bioprinting, (b) inkjet bioprinting, (c) stereolithography bioprinting, and (d) extrusion-based bioprinting.

Table 12.1: A comparison between the four different bioprinting methods based on composition, feasibility, advantages, and disadvantages is given below.

Methods	Cell viability	Bioink characteristics	Advantages	Disadvantages	References
Extrusion-based bioprinting	40–97%	Low adhesion and surface tension, shear thinning, and fast gelation	It can print biomaterials with varying viscosities and different cell concentrations, utilizing direct incorporation and homogeneous cell distribution.	Cell viability is moderate, low printing speed, and medium resolution.	[38–41]

Table 12.1 (continued)

Methods	Cell viability	Bioink characteristics	Advantages	Disadvantages	References
Inkjet-assisted bioprinting	80%	It offers low viscosity, rapid gelation, and a nonfibrous nature	Low cost, it can print different cell types with high resolution	Potential mechanical and thermal stress to cells, not suitable for printing material with high viscosity & high cell density	[26, 41–45]
Laser-assisted bioprinting	90%	It offers rapid gelation and low surface tension	No mechanical stress to cells, high cell viability, Versatile and adaptable, Ability to print complex structures with high resolution	Coating the bioinks on the laser-absorbing materials layer by layer is cumbersome and time-consuming.	[30, 31, 41]
Stereolithography	85%	It provides high mechanical strength and stability	Printing speed is high with high fabrication accuracy, and it can print photocurable hydrogel layers layer by layer.	Specifically applicable to photopolymers, the possibility of causing harm to human skin and DNA on exposure to UV light	[46, 41]

12.3 Bioinks

Bioinks are specialized inks made from biomaterials incorporating cells. They can be used to develop complex biological 3D scaffolds using 3D bioprinting technologies. Mimicking organs using 3D printing technology aims to attain mechanical and physiological characteristics similar to those of real organs. Consequently, bioinks play a pivotal role in mitigating these qualities, and they must ensure cellular protection during bioprinting procedures, such as extrusion and unsuitable environments [47]. An optimal bioink should possess high mechanical integrity, printability, a similar rate of biodegradation comparable to tissue regeneration, the ability to promote cell adhesion, be non-immunogenic, and nontoxic [48]. These bioinks must meet several mechanical, biological, and overlapping requirements, such as sufficient hydration to enable nutrient diffusion, rapid gelation to maintain shape fidelity, extrusion through fine needles supported by shear thinning properties, protection of cells from shear stresses ensured by viscoelasticity, and uniform encapsulation of cells achieved through optimum viscosity [49]. Different types of tissue constructs or models have been developed using a variety of biomaterials as bioink. For instance, collagen and gelatin, like natural polymers, have been employed extensively as they contain arginine-glycine-aspartate (RGD) motifs, which play a key role in the adhesion and migration of cells [50]. However, because these materials tend to have poor mechanical properties, different combinations of biomaterials have been developed with additives to develop multi-material bioinks that exhibit superior properties compared to traditional single-material-based bioinks. The physicochemical properties of the resulting multicomponent bioinks should enable printing [51].

12.3.1 Types of Bioinks

Bioinks can be categorized into two types: scaffold-based and scaffold-free bioinks.

12.3.1.1 Scaffold-Based Bioink

Scaffold-based bioprinting is the predominant technology for tissue building. Scaffolds are essential for tissue regeneration, as they provide a substrate for adhesion of cells and deliver biological signals that promote cell differentiation [52, 53]. Scaffolds with high porosity typically provide a substantial surface area that facilitates cell adhesion and angiogenesis.

Hydrogel-Based Bioinks

Hydrogels are ideal for application as tissue scaffolds owing to numerous advantageous properties. They are typically biocompatible and biodegradable, ensuring safety in interaction with biological tissues. Numerous hydrogels incorporate natural cell-binding sites that facilitate critical biological processes, including attachment, spreading, proliferation, and differentiation. Moreover, some hydrogels can undergo chemical modification to facilitate crosslinking via light, hence improving their structural integrity and functionality in biological applications [54].

Natural Polymer-Based Hydrogels

Hydrogels derived from natural polymers, such as proteins and polysaccharides, represent the most appealing biofabrication inks because of their swelling networks, which facilitate oxygen permeability and provide an adequately hydrated environment for cell growth, nutrient absorption, and the diffusion of water-soluble metabolites [55].

Collagen

Collagen, a highly appealing polymer, is widely explored in the tissue engineering domain. It is a key element of ECM in most tissues, along with a significant component of musculoskeletal tissue. Collagen scaffolds are naturally occurring triple-helical proteins that are biocompatible and typically elicit negligible immune reactions [56]. Collagen also promotes attachment, adhesion, and cell proliferation [48]. However, collagen type I has been utilized in bioprinting, but several drawbacks exist. It takes almost 30–40 min at 37 °C for complete gelation. Generally, at low temperatures, it remains liquid, and as the temperature rises, it develops a fibrous structure. This slow gelation process hampers 3D bioprinting. Diamantides et al. [57] showed how riboflavin photo-crosslinking and pH affected the rheological characteristics and printability of collagen. Their results showed that while the gelation kinetics itself had no discernible effect on printability, the shape fidelity of the construct throughout the collagen gelation process was substantially reliant on pH. In addition, because gravity pulls the cells down before gelation occurs, the deposited cells in collagen are not uniformly distributed. Collagen requires supportive hydrogels due to its low mechanical qualities, instability, and the problems mentioned above.

Alginate

Alginate is one of the most widely used naturally occurring polysaccharides. Having unique qualities such as low cost, biocompatibility, and flexibility with different printing methods makes it an ideal polymer for bioprinting [58]. It can gel up quickly, making it a valuable material for tissue engineering, therapeutics, cell encapsulation, and delivery of cells [59]. However, it exhibits poor cell adhesion when compared to other natural polymers. Some researchers combined alginate with other natural polymers, such as fibrinogen and gelatin, to address this issue [60]. Li et al. (2017) utilized gelatin-alginate as a bioprinted scaffold for skin wound healing. Before printing the scaffold, mesenchymal stem cells (MSCs) were introduced into the bone marrow of mice [61]. In another research performed by Do et al. (2017), alginate and polylactic-co-glycolic acid were employed to develop a drug delivery device using 3D printing technology [62].

Gelatin

Gelatin is primarily obtained from collagen and is produced by hydrolyzing natural collagen with an acid, alkali, or hot water [63]. The majority of proteolytic enzymes can hydrolyze gelatin into amino acids and peptides because the conversion of collagen into gelatin yields molecules with different molecular weights [64]. Many functional groups will leak out as collagen hydrolyzes to create gelatin. According to Lukin et al. (2022), these functional groups give gelatin distinct qualities via binding to cross-linkers or specific ligands. Gelatin is therefore both biocompatible and biodegradable [65]. Gelatin has low immunogenicity, contains the arginine-glycine-aspartate (RGD) sequence, is water soluble, and noncytotoxic. It also encourages cell adhesion. Due to these characteristics, gelatin hydrogel, namely gelatin methacryloyl, is typically utilized for direct ink writing printing [66, 67]. Due to its intrinsically low mechanical strength, gelatin in its original form is rarely utilized for bioprinting. Gelatin is often crosslinked using chemical agents like glutaraldehyde to overcome this limitation [68]. Through a nucleophilic addition and subsequent dehydration, along the gelatin polymer chain, the free amino group combines with the two glutaraldehyde groups to produce imine linkages known as Schiff bases. The pH of the surrounding environment frequently affects how much gelation occurs in gelatin-based systems. Proton-accepting or proton-donating molecules are extremely sensitive to pH changes, which can change how they behave. Hepatocytes were bioprinted utilizing extrusion-based bioprinting and encapsulated in gelatin in a noteworthy application. The hepatocytes not only sustained viability but also preserved their biological capabilities for more than two months [48].

Chitosan

Deacetylation of chitin yields chitosan, a linear polysaccharide molecule with numerous uses in tissue engineering, including the development of scaffolds, cartilage regeneration, hemostatic and antimicrobial devices, and wound dressings [69]. It is easily soluble in dilute acidic environments below its pK_a (pH = 6.5), whereas chitin remains insoluble in solvents [70]. Chitosan has been utilized in extrusion-based bioprinting (EBB) to fabricate perfusable vessel-like microfluidic channels, with crosslinking facilitated by sodium hydroxide (NaOH) as an ionic crosslinker. The chitosan polymer and crosslinker solution were simultaneously extruded using a coaxial nozzle apparatus, allowing the crosslinker solution in the inner core to diffuse outward into the polymer, thereby creating hollow tubular structures [71]. In a study chitosan along with polyethylene glycol diacrylate utilized as a bioink for scaffold fabrication using the stereolithography approach [72].

Hyaluronic Acid

Hyaluronic acid (HA) is a linear non-sulfated glycosaminoglycan that is extensively present across connective, epithelial, and neural tissues. It is a major ECM component of cartilage, and it has therapeutic promise for osteoarthritis, just like collagen type I. HA is made up of repeated D-glucuronic acid and *N*-acetyl-D-glucosamine disaccharides connected by β-1,4 and β-1,3 glycosidic linkages. Three functional groups, the glucuronic carboxyl, secondary hydroxyl, and *N*-acetyl groups, are principally responsible for its chemical action [48]. It is essential in tissue engineering due to its superior bio-resorbability, biodegradability, and biocompatibility, as well as its nonthrombogenic, nonadhesive, and nonimmunogenic properties, and its capacity to make flexible hydrogels. Kreimendahl et al. [73] employed HA and fibrin as a bioink to develop a material using FRESH bioprinting. The combination allowed better vascularization for a low-viscosity solution, achieving excellent spatial resolution [73]. Horder et al. fabricated gel spheroids with 1% hyaluronic acid to ensure a homogeneous distribution of hyaluronic acid and optimal viability of seed cells for the breast cancer adipose tissue model [74].

Fibrin

Fibrin is a naturally occurring biopolymer that aids in the healing process. Fibrin prevents excessive bleeding and encourages the release of soluble components by utilizing a fibrous three-dimensional network of randomly aligned fibers. It is formed from soluble fibrinogen, primarily activated by thrombin, leading to the formation of a matrix [75]. The fibrin polymer's γ chains can covalently crosslink with coagulation factor XII, resulting in a durable fibrin network that withstands protease degradation [76]. Due to the fibrinogen solution's low viscosity, the development of scaffolds via extrusion bioprinting is challenging. To solve this, a solution was prepared by mixing thrombin and fibrinogen and utilized in the fabrication of scaffolds to enhance the printed solution viscosity [77]. Hence, adding other biomaterials to the fibrinogen during the preparation of the solution and incorporating a crosslinker can improve the printability of the fibrin [78]. Thrombin and fibrinogen can be bioprinted from distinct cartridges, then mixed to create a hydrogel. In a study, neural cells encapsulated in fibrin gel were bioprinted in an alternating fashion, resulting in viable neural constructs with potential applications in neural engineering [79].

Synthetic Polymer-Based Hydrogels

Synthetic polymers can undergo chemical modification with both crosslinkable functional groups and domains that enhance the mechanical strength and structural properties of bioprinted structures. This allows for the meticulous engineering of the polymer backbone architecture to include either domains that respond to the external stimuli or cell-adhesive domains that feature the RGD sequence [48].

Polyethylene Glycol (PEG)

A linear polymer, PEG, extensively utilized in pharmaceutical applications, is available in a variety of chemical forms (linear or multi-arm) and molecular weights [80]. Although hydrophilic PEG is inadequate for 3D bioprinting alone, it is frequently combined with polyglycol diacrylate (PGDA) or polyethylene glycol methacrylate (PEGMA) to formulate bioinks [81, 82]. Despite its hydrophobic properties, PEG-based polymers, such as PEGMA, facilitate cell encapsulation and viability, including that of osteoblasts [83]. Combining PEG with other polymers, such as PEGDA and alginate, markedly improves mechanical strength, elevating the elastic modulus from around 5 to 75 kPa [84]. Furthermore, PEG functions as a proficient linker for polymer conjugation in bioink compositions. A study combined bioactive glass nanoparticles with PEGMA and hydroxyapatite, utilizing the mixture for bioprinting hMSCs) [85]. Notably, cell viability was recorded alongside an elevated compressive modulus of approximately 358 kPa.

Pluronic® F-127

Pluronics, or Poloxamers, are FDA-approved, triblock copolymers composed of polyethylene oxide/polypropylene oxide that exhibit a solution-to-gel transition in aqueous solutions when the temperature exceeds a lower critical gelation temperature (LCGT) [86]. It also facilitates the development of thermosensitive hydrogels with flexible characteristics such as gelation concentration and respective time under physiological conditions [87–91]. F127 is extensively utilized as a drug and cell carrier due to its lower toxicity, reverse thermal gelation properties, substantial drug loading capacity, and ability to gel at low concentrations in physiological environments. It is also suitable for cell printing due to its biological inertness, gelation at temperatures between 10 and 40 °C (depending on concentration), extensive viscosity range, and minimum stress on cells [86, 92]. Furthermore, F127 can be readily removed post-printing by reducing the temperature below its LCGT. The study conducted by Vashi et al. [93] demonstrated that bone marrow stromal cells could interact inside a 3D Pluronic® matrix, with adipogenesis commencing after 4 days of culture [93]. UV light can polymerize Pluronic® for its application in bioink; however, the intensity and type of the radiation may have an impact on the viability of cells [94]. Also, the photo-initiator concentration may affect the metabolic activity of cells.

Polyvinyl Alcohol (PVA)

PVA, a synthetic polymer formed by the polymerization of the repeating units of $(C_2H_4O)_n$ that dissolves readily in water, and can be synthesized through the decomposition of polyvinyl acetate. The structure comprises several hydroxyl groups along its backbone, making it highly hydrophilic. This enables the formation of hydrogen bonds. Due to these properties, PVA is widely recognized for its effectiveness in producing thin films. The presence of -OH radicals facilitates the combination of PVA with different types of polymers, hence enhancing its flow and mechanical characteristics, two essentials that are vital for applications in 3D printing and bioinks [95]. The viscoelastic properties and tunable viscosity of PVA render it especially advantageous for bioprinting via extrusion techniques, as these qualities are influenced by the degree of polymerization, concentration, and temperature [96–99]. Masri et al. [100] discovered that incorporating synthetic polymers such as PVA and crosslinkers like genipin into gelatin mixtures significantly increases the hydrogel's strength and stability [100].

Decellularized Matrix-Derived Bioinks

The ECM of tissues derived from their native cells is known as decellularized matrix (dECM), which has been recognized as a possible natural biomaterial for tissue engineering, intended to sustain, replace, or regenerate damaged tissues. The dECM can easily be extracted from various animal tissues or organs, such as small intestines, skin, and urinary bladder, using suitable decellularization methods, thereby simulating the structure and composition of the natural ECM and facilitating a hostile environment for cells [101, 102]. Diverse dECMs exert distinct effects on various cell types, with innovations involving the use of synthetic polymers to tailor dECMs for specific requirements [103]. dECM bioinks are employed in the fabrication of tissues and organs, such as liver, heart, skin, cartilage, and adipose tissue. When stem cells are used, the presence of macromolecules such as growth factors encourages cell division and proliferation. Growth factors influence cellular differentiation, adhesion, migration, and proliferation, and are crucial for intercellular communication [104]. Artificial tissue constructs design has significantly advanced science in domains, including drug screening, regenerative medicine, and disease modeling. The integration of human lung fibroblast-derived extracellular matrix (fd-ECM) into a collagen hydrogel established an angiogenic microenvironment for human umbilical vein endothelial cell (HUVECs), showing a synergistic interaction between fd-ECM and angiogenic growth factors within the 3D structure [105]. When an ECM was made from mechanically stretched cardiac fibroblasts, the metabolic activity of ventricular cells increased [106]. The study indicated that a glycosaminoglycan linked to a proteoglycan was accountable for the observed effect [106]. dECM serves as a superior allogenic or xenogeneic biomaterial utilized in tissue engineering, resulting in several commercial products, including SurgiSIS®, Alloderm®, and Synergraft® [107].

Microcarrier

Biomaterials that integrate a microcarrier compound system represent an additional type of bioink formulated for 3D bioprinting. It serves as a reinforcement block in the construction of frameworks with an extensive surface area for cell transfer. Microcarriers can typically be composed of natural materials like gelatin, cellulose, collagen, or synthetic materials like glass, dextran, or plastic. A significant benefit of using it is the increased cell density, coupled with good cell survival in bioinks [108]. They also enhance the compressive modulus of constructs, facilitate stem cell differentiation into specific lineages, and preserve phenotype even at high cell densities. These microcarriers can be used in EBB. The utilization of high cell density while maintaining viability makes this method attractive. Levato et al. [109] found that MSCs pre-seeded on polylactic acid (PLA) microcarriers within hydrogels had enhanced interaction, aggregation, and osteogenic differentiation compared to the cells that were suspended in hydrogels [109].

12.3.1.2 Scaffold-Free Bioink

Scaffold-free cell suspensions have garnered significant interest for developing tissues or organs using cell aggregates, which can exist as mono or multicellular formations, including cell sheets, pellets, spheroids, and, more recently, tissue strands as fundamental components. This method involves collecting, harvesting, and extracting target cells without disturbing them or using any chemical or enzymatic treatments. The time needed for tissue building in these bioinks is reduced due to a higher cell seeding density from the start, along with faster cell proliferation and migration compared to scaffold-based bioinks. This strategy encompasses the self-assembly of cells and the formation of structures resulting from cell-cell interactions [110].

Tissue Spheroids

Tissue spheroids, which are densely packed clusters of living cells, are proposed as fundamental units for 3D bioprinting. The development of these spheroids involves three essential stages. Initially, cellular spheroids with high cell density are produced within a designated timeframe, depending on the cell type and fabrication method, during which the cells aggregate and fuse. In the second stage, the spheroids undergo significant proliferation. Ultimately, multicellular aggregates are formed and subsequently used as bioink for 3D bioprinting of complex tissue architectures. A variety of traditional methods are utilized to create cell spheroids, such as the hanging drop method, hydrogel microwells, spinner flasks, microfluidic systems, and magnetic levitation. Kuo et al. (2017) successfully generated high-throughput multicellular spheroids using a polydimethylsiloxane (PDMS)-based hanging drop technique within 24 h. The hydrophobic nature of PDMS, combined with its contact angle of 99°, allows for effective droplet retention during spheroid formation.

Cell Pellet

The cell pellet method utilizes centrifugation or gravitational force to aggregate cells at the base of a conical tube. Once the pellets are formed, they may be transferred to a micropipette or mold, where cohesiveness is increased, facilitated by intercellular contacts. This method is a simple technique for developing cell aggregates without the need for special equipment. Nonetheless, it possesses constraints, such as restricted diffusion of oxygen, which substantially reduces cell viability after 24 h [111]. Cell pellet-derived bioink has been utilized in extrusion-based bioprinting (EBB), wherein the pellet was extruded into a confined space formed by a 3D-printed agarose support mold. The agarose mold supported cell aggregation, which led to the development of tubular heterocellular nerve grafts [112].

Tissue Strand

To create tissue strands, the high-density targeted cells are compacted and injected into hollow alginate tubes with controlled permeability and mechanistic properties. The tubes are subsequently eliminated via ionic decoupling, resulting in cellular aggregates that develop into cylindrical threads. The obtained tissue strands serve as bioink, which is fed into a custom-designed bioprinter head and extruded [113]. To bioprint native-like tissue structures, Yu et al. (2016) developed scaffold-free tissue strands as bioink, eliminating the requirement for any scaffold or mold support during the procedure [114].

12.3.1.3 Bioactive Molecules

Various bioink constituents and strategies have been investigated to optimize the biocompatibility and effectiveness of 3D bioprinted structures. Various mitogenic factors such as IGF-II, BMP-2, and FGF-2 have been included in bioinks to promote cellular proliferation and tissue growth. For example, constructs using BMP-2 increased ALP expression in myogenic cells, whereas FGF-2 exhibited minimal osteogenic activity, illustrating the selective influence of specific growth factors [115–117]. Spatial regulation of tissue development has been achieved via the localized deposition of biomolecules, including TGF-β1, BMP-2, Noggin, and GDF-5, onto acellular dermis substrates, resulting in selective bone formation in BMP-2-printed regions [118]. Bioinks developed from blood plasma and alginate exhibit potential in skin tissue engineering by facilitating stem cell proliferation, differentiation, and suitable tissue layer formation post-printing, utilizing the inherent ECM-like characteristics of plasma proteins such as fibrinogen and albumin [119–121]. To enhance cell preservation during low-temperature processing, cryo-bioinks including PEG, ectoine, and trehalose were synthesized. These inks safeguarded red blood cells during freezing and thawing, preserving their morphology and viability after droplet-based extrusion printing [122]. In addition, ultrashort peptides with self-assembly properties were used to create rigid hydrogels characterized by high water content and exceptional shape fidelity. These hydrogels facilitated fast alignment and elongation of encapsulated MSCs, demonstrating excellent biocompatibility and durability in vivo, thus rendering them appropriate for regenerative medicine and drug screening [123]. M13 phages, modified with integrin- and calcium-binding motifs, were combined with alginate to create bioinks that improved osteogenic differentiation and cell survival after printing. These phage-based inks provide adjustable molecular characteristics and self-assembly properties, representing an innovative approach to developing bioinks with specific bioactivity [124]. The figure 12.2 shows the various bioink systems.

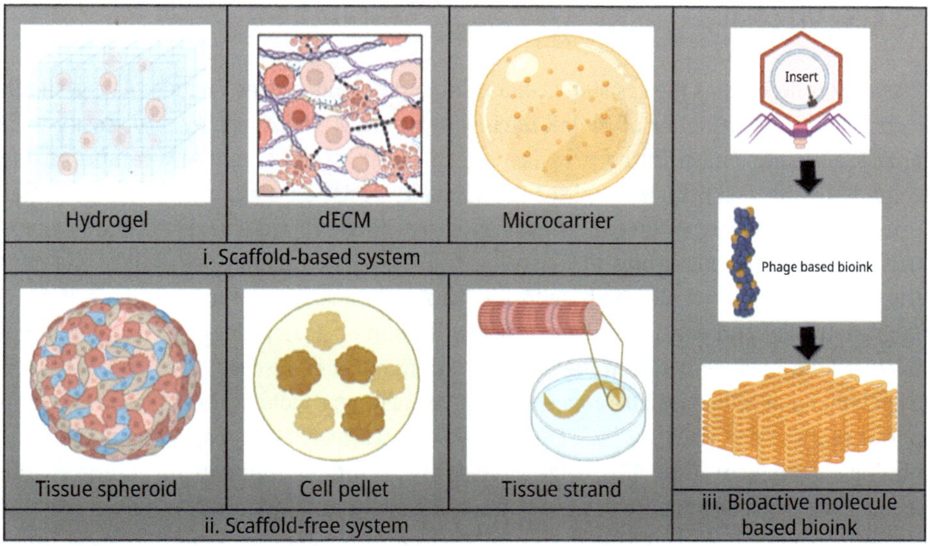

Figure 12.2: Bioinks can be classified into (i) scaffold-based systems, which utilize biomaterials (e.g., hydrogels or dECM-like scaffolds) to offer mechanical support and facilitate cell encapsulation, enabling growth of cells within a predefined architecture. Examples include hydrogels (left), decellularized extracellular matrix scaffolds (middle), and microcarrier supportive gel matrices (right); (ii) scaffold-free systems, which depend on the self-assembly of cell spheroids, cell pellet, or tissue strands to build constructs that mimic native tissue organization without supplementary scaffold materials; and (iii) bioactive molecule-based bioinks, which integrate biofunctional cues such as peptides, proteins, or phage-displayed molecules. These deliver biological signals to direct cellular behavior, differentiation, or tissue development, and are frequently incorporated into printed constructions to improve biofunctionality.

12.4 Optimization/Parameters of Bioinks

Printability characterization is divided into pre-printing and post-printing stages. In nozzle-based systems, the material is extruded through a narrowing passage, and after deposition, it must quickly solidify to retain its shape and form a 3D structure. The printing rate is essential for success, emphasizing the differences between injectable and printable hydrogels [125]. The rheological parameters during printing influence the shape fidelity, printability, and cell viability, whereas post-crosslinking affects bioink stability, mechanical integrity, and cellular functioning [126]. The properties of the final construct are dependent upon cell density, proliferation, migration, and integration. Printing requires balancing between mechanical demands and cell viability.

12.4.1 Viscosity

Viscosity is defined as the resistance of a fluid to flow under stress, which plays a significant role in the behavior of bioink during 3D printing. The interplay of viscosity with nozzle diameter and printing pressure affects shear stress, potentially compromising cellular health [127]. Bioinks with high viscosity resist spreading and collapse after printing, thereby preserving structural integrity; however, they necessitate higher extrusion pressures, increasing shear stress, and risking cell damage as well as filament fracture [128]. Additionally, high viscosity can result in reduced porosity, hindering cell migration [129] and causing uneven cell distribution or nozzle clogging [125]. Ideal bioinks strike a balance between low concentration and high viscosity [129]. Factors such as polymer molecular weight, concentration, branching, rheological modifiers, and temperature influence viscosity [126, 130, 131]. Viscosity affects cell encapsulation and morphological integrity [130, 132]. Higher viscosity facilitates filament formation, while lower viscosity leads to spreading [126, 131]. Shear-thinning materials are preferred for high-viscosity DBB and EBB bioinks [133]. Viscosity is typically assessed alongside printability and rheological properties through oscillatory sweeps for modulus (G', G'') and shear sweeps for viscosity (η) [126].

12.4.2 Crosslinking Methods

When constructing a 3D bioprinting system, it is essential to select a suitable crosslinking method for the intended applications [134]. Crosslinking strategies are critical for establishing the structural integrity, printability, and cytocompatibility of hydrogel-based bioinks. Physically crosslinked hydrogels are established via non-covalent interactions, including hydrogen bonding, ionic forces, or hydrophobic interactions [135]. These are generally reversible and exhibit shear-thinning and self-healing properties; however, they frequently possess inadequate mechanical strength and are sensitive to environmental conditions, rendering them inappropriate for load-bearing or long-term applications [136]. Conversely, chemical crosslinking, which entails the formation of covalent bonds between polymer chains, markedly improves mechanical stability and durability, particularly for in vivo applications [137, 138]. However, potent chemical crosslinkers such as glutaraldehyde may present cytotoxic hazards to encapsulated cells [137]. Cytocompatible crosslinking techniques, including enzymatic or photo-crosslinking with biocompatible photoinitiators, are frequently favored. The nature and degree of crosslinking significantly affect the rheological characteristics of the bioink, such as viscosity and gelation kinetics, which directly influence print fidelity, resolution, and the mechanical strength of the final construct [139, 140]. Attaining balance among swift gelation (to preserve shape integrity), mechanical reinforcement, and a biocompatible milieu is essential for the efficacy of bioprinted tissues [140]. Ultimately, selecting the suitable crosslinking strategy is contingent upon the material and application, and constitutes a critical design parameter in the domain of biofabrication [136, 140].

12.4.3 Shear-Thinning Properties

Shear-thinning behavior, where viscosity decreases as shear rate increases, is an essential attribute for bioinks, facilitating smooth extrusion during printing without the need for excessive force [141, 142]. Upon deposition, the ink swiftly reverts to its original viscosity, aiding in the maintenance of the printed structure's morphology and fidelity [143, 144]. This attribute reduces shear stress on the encapsulated cells, boosting cell viability after printing [145]. Rheological models, including the Power-law and Herschel–Bulkley equations, are frequently employed to characterize shear-thinning behavior and enhance ink formulations for printability [54]. However, excessive shear-thinning bioinks may exhibit inadequate mechanical integrity, necessitating post-printing stabilization [146]. Consequently, shear-thinning inks are frequently utilized alongside secondary crosslinking methods, such as UV, ionic, or enzymatic crosslinking, to enhance mechanical strength and the long-term stability of constructs. Polymers such as alginate, gelatin, hyaluronic acid, and xanthan gum are commonly employed to optimize the shear-thinning characteristics, hence improving both extrusion efficacy and structural integrity [54]. Hybrid bioinks, including gellan gum and sodium alginate, demonstrated shear-thinning characteristics advantageous for extrusion, whereas ionic crosslinking with calcium ions (Ca^{2+}) enhanced their mechanical strength and stability [148]. Furthermore, enzymatic crosslinking methods have been utilized to enhance the mechanical strength of shear-thinning bioinks. Shi et al. (2022) employed tyrosinase to enzymatically crosslink gelatin methacrylamide and collagen-based bioinks, resulting in improved mechanical properties while preserving cytocompatibility in the final structures [148]. These results affirm that the incorporation of shear-thinning properties with suitable secondary crosslinking methods is essential for effective biofabrication.

12.4.4 Shape fidelity

Structural precision, commonly known as shape fidelity, denotes the degree to which a bioprinted object mimics its original model [149]. Attaining excellent shape fidelity is crucial for preserving the structure of extruded filaments and supporting complex characteristics such as pores and internal passages [129]. For cell-laden bioinks, it is vital to maintain the spatial structure of the construct during and after the printing process, maintaining consistent resolution, geometry, and overall shape during subsequent cell culture [130, 150]. This fidelity primarily relies on a balance of bioink characteristics – specifically shear-thinning behavior, shape recovery, and yield stress. The swelling behavior, governed by the material's charge density and crosslinking degree, is crucial; an increased crosslinking density results in a reduced swelling ratio, which improves shape fidelity but may impede nutrient and oxygen passage [126]. A strategic combination of two hydrogel varieties – one to sustain cell viability and the other to provide mechanical strength – can further improve fidelity [126]. The faster recovery of the structure post-extrusion reduces deformation, such as drooping, and gives adequate time to efficient post-printing crosslinking [151]. Other techniques, like printing within a supporting bath, have demonstrated efficacy in preserving structural precision [152]. However, print precision typically decreases when the size of the construct is reduced. To counter this, printing resolution and fidelity can be enhanced by modifying the path width and height, using fine nozzles, and low extrusion rates, as shown in Figure 12.3 [150].

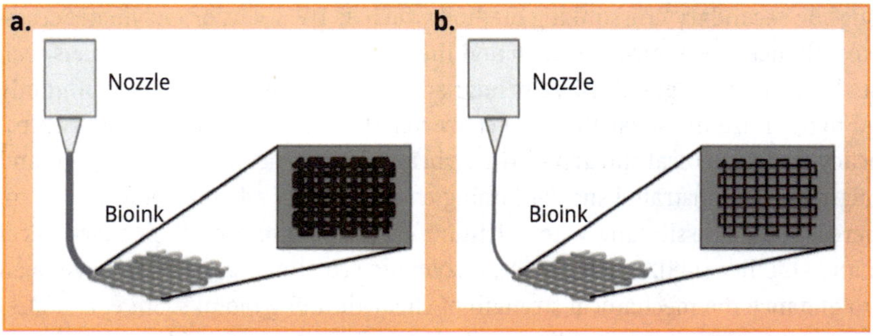

Figure 12.3: Effect of nozzle diameter on the bioink: (a) A wider nozzle produces a thicker and less defined filament with decreased resolution, whereas (b) a narrower nozzle results in a narrower flow with improved structural fidelity and resolution.

12.5 Applications in Regenerative Medicine and Organ Engineering

12.5.1 Drug Screening

Designing drug screening systems using 3D bioprinting is a promising new technique. For testing and screening the interactions between the tested drugs and the cells, bioprinting could evenly distribute the cells over the surfaces of a microdevice, which is much more desirable than traditional manual screening methods [153, 154]. Chang et al. (2010) created an EBB, pneumatically-driven bioprinter to develop a drug testing platform for the liver using immortalized hepatocytes encapsulated in alginate. To screen for the efficacy and toxicity of the drug, this system can distinguish between the drug metabolism capacities of various mammalian tissues and replicate their in vivo microenvironments [155].

12.5.2 Bone 3D Bioprinting

Patient-customized implants that fit the shape and mechanical properties of the respective fractured bone region can be made via 3D bioprinting [156], by being able to develop multilayered structures that can increase the stability of the implant via simulating the complex structure of natural bone tissue [157]. This can lower the rejection rates, hasten the healing process, and lead to increased chances of assimilation of the transplant by surrounding tissue. Tortelli et al. (2009) implanted the mouse osteoclasts and osteoblast precursors on porous ceramic scaffolds to establish a 3D bone *model* in vitro [158]. Zhu et al. (2020) used 3D-printed nano-ink, composed of hydroxyapatite nanoparticles, which are suspended in hydrogel, to mimic a bone-specific environment to study breast cancer bone invasion [159].

12.5.3 Liver Tissue Bioprinting

The liver has a strong regeneration ability compared to other organs. A person with liver injury or liver-associated disease can receive a transplant from a healthy donor [160]. However, due to the scarcity of healthy donors and the lengthy process of self-liver tissue regeneration, bioprinting liver tissue through tissue engineering is particularly important. Many researchers have studied liver bioprinting [161]. In comparison to conventional printing methods, 3D printing provides precise liver size and shape for patients undergoing liver resection [162]. A new method has been used to sustain cell functionality and activity for an extended period [163]. The method develops structures known as "canaliculi" that resemble the liver's hepatic cords by utilizing bioprinting technology. Collagen matrix is used to culture both primary hepatocytes and "canaliculus" structures. The primary hepatocytes' activity and functionality on different ECM-based hydrogels [164] are assessed via a biomimetic ECM system. After that, cells can be sustained for up to 1 month. In addition to this, a further increase in cellular activity would facilitate more applications of bioprinted liver tissue. Arai et al. (2017) used an artificial scaffold to develop a 3D culture system using an ink-jet bioprinter to study hepatocytes by facilitating the interactions between asialoglycoprotein receptors and galactosylated alginate gels [165]. Moya et al. (2018) developed a liver-on-a-chip-based microfluidic channel to monitor oxygen concentration using inkjet-based bioprinting [166]. The figure 12.4 shows usuages of 3D bioprinting in various biomedical applications.

12.5.4 Skin

The largest organ, which protects the body from attack by foreign agents, thereby maintaining the overall integrity of the body. Bioprinting helps in the development of skin substitutes to repair or replace damaged skin tissue. Laser-assisted bioprinting technology has been in use to print bio-skin. Using LAB technology, Michael et al. (2013) successfully made and transplanted skin substitutes to nude mice. After 11 days, the graft adhered to the wound and then proliferated and differentiated.

12.5.5 Cardiac Tissue

Cardiac tissue engineering develops functionally engineered tissue and organs or in vitro models to study disease mechanisms and drug discovery, or as an in vivo transplant to address the shortage of organs for transplantation [167–169]. In one study, Xu et al. [60] fabricated bioengineered cardiac pseudo tissue with the primary focus on contractile cardiac hybrids and a "half-heart" structure with beating cell responses using the inkjet bioprinting method [170]. In another study, the bioprinting of a cardiac tissue model with spontaneous synchronized contractions in vitro using cardiomyocyte-laden hydrogels [171].

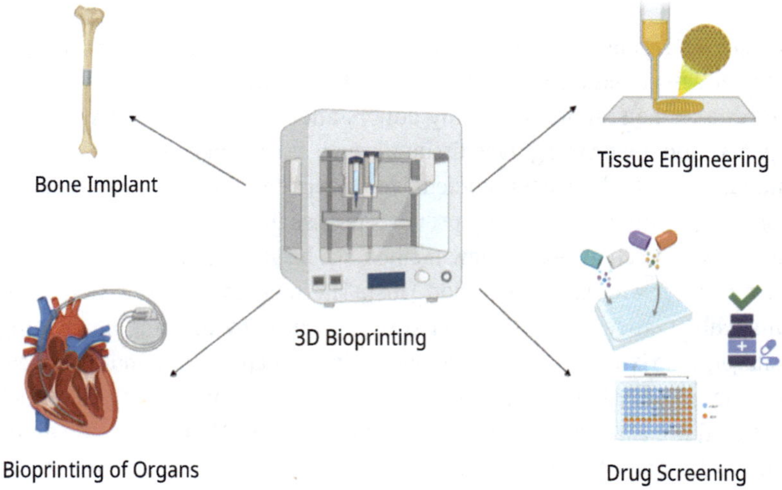

Figure 12.4: Depicts the uses of 3D bioprinting. It displays a 3D bioprinter employed in tissue engineering for creating scaffold-based tissues, in producing bone implants, in drug testing to evaluate the effectiveness of medications on printed tissue models, and in organ bioprinting for generating functional organs.

12.6 Conclusion

3D bioprinting signifies a revolutionary approach to tissue engineering and regenerative medicine, providing the capability to construct complex, functional tissues and organs. This chapter explored the four primary bioprinting techniques: extrusion-based, inkjet-based, laser-assisted, and stereolithography, along with their respective advantages and drawbacks. The selection and optimization of bioinks, particularly hydrogels and polymers like collagen, alginate, gelatin, and Pluronic acid, are essential in influencing the mechanical strength, cell viability, and print fidelity of the bioinks. Both scaffold-based and scaffold-free approaches have various benefits, depending on the specific application. Despite the significant advancements, challenges persist, especially regarding vascularization, neural integration, and ethical issues related to therapeutic translation. However, through ongoing research and innovation, bioprinting is progressively transitioning from experimental laboratories to real-life clinical applications. It demonstrates significant potential for personalized medicine, drug testing, organ transplantation, and more applications, suggesting a promising future for regenerative therapies.

Abbreviations

FRESH	freeform reversible embedding of suspended hydrogels
SLA	Stereolithography
EBB	Extrusion-based bioprinting
DBB	Droplet-based bioprinting
dECM	Decellularized extracellular matrix
IGF-II	Insulin-like growth factor II
BMP-2	Bone morphogenetic protein-2
FGF-2	Fibroblast growth factor-2
GDF-5	Growth and differentiation factor-5
TGF-β1	Transforming growth factor beta 1
ECM	Extracellular matrix
HA	Hyaluronic acid
PEG	Polyethylene glycol
MSC	Mesenchymal stem cell
ALP	Alkaline phosphatase
LAB	Laser-assisted bioprinting
MSCs	Mesenchymal stem cells
LCGT	Lower critical gelation temperature
hMSCs	Human mesenchymal stem cells

References

[1] Stapenhorst, F., Dos Santos, M. G., Prestes, J. P., Alcantara, B. J., Borges, M. F. & Pranke, P. (Jun. 2021). Bioprinting: A promising approach for tissue regeneration. Bioprinting, 22, e00130. doi: 10.1016/j.bprint.2021.e00130.

[2] Zhu, W., Ma, X., Gou, M., Mei, D., Zhang, K. & Chen, S. (Aug. 2016). 3D printing of functional biomaterials for tissue engineering. Current Opinion in Biotechnology, 40, 103–112. doi: 10.1016/j.copbio.2016.03.014.

[3] Kačarević, Ž. P. et al. (Nov. 2018). An Introduction to 3D Bioprinting: Possibilities, Challenges and Future Aspects. Materials (Basel), 11(11), 2199. doi: 10.3390/ma11112199.

[4] Hong, N., Yang, G., Lee, J. & Kim, G. (Jan. 2018). 3D bioprinting and its *in vivo* applications. Journal of Biomedical Materials Research, 106(1), 444–459. doi: 10.1002/jbm.b.33826.

[5] Zhang, X. & Zhang, Y. (Jul. 2015). Tissue Engineering Applications of Three-Dimensional Bioprinting. Cell Biochemistry and Biophysics, 72(3), 777–782. doi: 10.1007/s12013-015-0531-x.

[6] Datta, P., Barui, A., Wu, Y., Ozbolat, V., Moncal, K. K. & Ozbolat, I. T. (Sep. 2018). Essential steps in bioprinting: From pre- to post-bioprinting. Biotechnology Advances, 36(5), 1481–1504. doi: 10.1016/j.biotechadv.2018.06.003.

[7] Jovic, T. H., Combellack, E. J., Jessop, Z. M. & Whitaker, I. S. (Nov. 2020). 3D Bioprinting and the Future of Surgery. Frontiers in Surgery, 7, 609836. doi: 10.3389/fsurg.2020.609836.

[8] Matai, I., Kaur, G., Seyedsalehi, A., McClinton, A. & Laurencin, C. T. (Jan. 2020). Progress in 3D bioprinting technology for tissue/organ regenerative engineering. Biomaterials, 226, 119536. doi: 10.1016/j.biomaterials.2019.119536.

[9] Chia, H. N. & Wu, B. M. (Dec. 2015). Recent advances in 3D printing of biomaterials. Journal of Biological Engineering, 9(1), 4. doi: 10.1186/s13036-015-0001-4.

[10] Little, C. J., Bawolin, N. K. & Chen, X. (Aug. 2011). Mechanical properties of natural cartilage and tissue-engineered constructs. Tissue Engineering Part B: Reviews, 17(4), 213–227. doi: 10.1089/ten.TEB.2010.0572.

[11] Ning, L. & Chen, X. (2017). A brief review of extrusion-based tissue scaffold bio-printing. Biotechnology Journal, 12(8), 1600671. doi: 10.1002/biot.201600671.

[12] Agarwal, T. et al. (May 2021). Recent advances in bioprinting technologies for engineering cardiac tissue. Materials Science and Engineering: C, 124, 112057. doi: 10.1016/j.msec.2021.112057.

[13] Chang, R., Emami, K., Wu, H. & Sun, W. (Dec. 2010). Biofabrication of a three-dimensional liver micro-organ as an in vitro drug metabolism model. Biofabrication, 2(4), 045004. doi: 10.1088/1758-5082/2/4/045004.

[14] Kim, W. & Kim, G. H. (Feb. 2018). An innovative cell-printed microscale collagen model for mimicking intestinal villus epithelium. Chemical Engineering Journal, 334, 2308–2318. doi: 10.1016/j.cej.2017.12.001.

[15] Johnson, B. N. et al. (Apr. 2016). 3D printed nervous system on a chip. Lab on a Chip, 16(8), 1393–1400. doi: 10.1039/C5LC01270H.

[16] "3D Printing of Personalized Thick and Perfusable Cardiac Patches and Hearts – Noor – 2019 – Advanced Science – Wiley Online Library". Available: https://advanced.onlinelibrary.wiley.com/doi/10.1002/advs.201900344

[17] Markstedt, K., Mantas, A., Tournier, I., Martínez Ávila, H., Hägg, D. & Gatenholm, P. (May 2015). 3D Bioprinting Human Chondrocytes with Nanocellulose–Alginate Bioink for Cartilage Tissue Engineering Applications. Biomacromolecules, 16(5), 1489–1496. doi: 10.1021/acs.biomac.5b00188.

[18] Gudapati, H., Dey, M. & Ozbolat, I. (Sep. 2016). A comprehensive review on droplet-based bioprinting: Past, present and future. Biomaterials, 102, 20–42. doi: 10.1016/j.biomaterials.2016.06.012.

[19] Kim, J. D., Choi, J. S., Kim, B. S., Chan Choi, Y. & Cho, Y. W. (May 2010). Piezoelectric inkjet printing of polymers: Stem cell patterning on polymer substrates. Polymer, 51(10), 2147–2154. doi: 10.1016/j.polymer.2010.03.038.
[20] Wijshoff, H. (Jun. 2010). The dynamics of the piezo inkjet printhead operation. Physics Reports, 491(4), 77–177. doi: 10.1016/j.physrep.2010.03.003.
[21] Lee, V. et al. (Jun. 2014). Design and Fabrication of Human Skin by Three-Dimensional Bioprinting. Tissue Eng Part C Methods, 20(6), 473–484. doi: 10.1089/ten.tec.2013.0335.
[22] "Inkjet-bioprinted acrylated peptides and PEG hydrogel with human mesenchymal stem cells promote robust bone and cartilage formation with minimal printhead clogging – Gao – 2015 – Biotechnology Journal – Wiley Online Library." Available: https://analyticalsciencejournals.onlinelibrary.wiley.com/doi/10.1002/biot.201400635
[23] Graham, A. D., Olof, S. N., Burke, M. J., Armstrong, J. P. K., Mikhailova, E. A., Nicholson, J. G., Box, S. J., Szele, F. G., Perriman, A. W., & Bayley, H. (2017). High-Resolution Patterned Cellular Constructs by Droplet-Based 3D Printing. Scientific reports, 7(1), 7004. https://doi.org/10.1038/s41598-017-06358-x.
[24] Velasquillo, C., Galue, E. A., Rodriquez, L., Ibarra, C. & Ibarra-Ibarra, L. G. (Jan. 2013). Skin 3D Bioprinting. Applications in Cosmetology. Journal of Cosmetics, Dermatological Sciences and Applications, 3(1, Art. no. 1), doi: 10.4236/jcdsa.2013.31A012.
[25] Dinca, V. et al. (Feb. 2008). Directed Three-Dimensional Patterning of Self-Assembled Peptide Fibrils. Nano Lett, 8(2), 538–543. doi: 10.1021/nl072798r.
[26] Jana, S. & Lerman, A. (Dec. 2015). Bioprinting a cardiac valve. Biotechnology Advances, 33(8), 1503–1521. doi: 10.1016/j.biotechadv.2015.07.006.
[27] Catros, S. et al. (Jun. 2011). Laser-assisted bioprinting for creating on-demand patterns of human osteoprogenitor cells and nano-hydroxyapatite. Biofabrication, 3(2), 025001. doi: 10.1088/1758-5082/3/2/025001.
[28] Trombetta, R., Inzana, J. A., Schwarz, E. M., Kates, S. L. & Awad, H. A. (Jan. 2017). 3D Printing of Calcium Phosphate Ceramics for Bone Tissue Engineering and Drug Delivery. Annals of Biomedical Engineering, 45(1), 23–44. doi: 10.1007/s10439-016-1678-3.
[29] Guillemot, F., Souquet, A., Catros, S. & Guillotin, B. (Apr. 2010). Laser-assisted cell printing: Principle, physical parameters versus cell fate and perspectives in tissue engineering. Nanomedicine (London), 5(3), 507–515. doi: 10.2217/nnm.10.14.
[30] Guillemot, F. et al. (Jul. 2010). High-throughput laser printing of cells and biomaterials for tissue engineering. Acta Biomater, 6(7), 2494–2500. doi: 10.1016/j.actbio.2009.09.029.
[31] Barron, J. A., Wu, P., Ladouceur, H. D. & Ringeisen, B. R. (Jun. 2004). Biological laser printing: A novel technique for creating heterogeneous 3-dimensional cell patterns. Biomedical Microdevices, 6(2), 139–147. doi: 10.1023/b:bmmd.0000031751.67267.9f.
[32] Ringeisen, B. R. et al. (2004). Laser printing of pluripotent embryonal carcinoma cells. Tissue Engineering, 10(3–4), 483–491. doi: 10.1089/107632704323061843.
[33] Michael, S. et al. (Mar. 2013). Tissue Engineered Skin Substitutes Created by Laser-Assisted Bioprinting Form Skin-Like Structures in the Dorsal Skin Fold Chamber in Mice. PLOS ONE, 8(3), e57741. doi: 10.1371/journal.pone.0057741.
[34] Melchels, F. P. W., Feijen, J. & Grijpma, D. W. (Aug. 2010). A review on stereolithography and its applications in biomedical engineering. Biomaterials, 31(24), 6121–6130. doi: 10.1016/j.biomaterials.2010.04.050.
[35] Wang, Z., Abdulla, R., Parker, B., Samanipour, R., Ghosh, S. & Kim, K. (Dec. 2015). A simple and high-resolution stereolithography-based 3D bioprinting system using visible light crosslinkable bioinks. Biofabrication, 7(4), 045009. doi: 10.1088/1758-5090/7/4/045009.
[36] "Stereolithographic 3D Bioprinting for Biomedical Applications", ResearchGate. Available: https://www.researchgate.net/publication/282743555_Stereolithographic_3D_Bioprinting_for_Biomedical_Applications

[37] Mahdavi, S. S., Abdekhodaie, M. J., Kumar, H., Mashayekhan, S., Baradaran-Rafii, A. & Kim, K. (Jul. 2020). Stereolithography 3D Bioprinting Method for Fabrication of Human Corneal Stroma Equivalent. Annals of Biomedical Engineering, 48(7), 1955–1970. doi: 10.1007/s10439-020-02537-6.
[38] Chien, K. B., Makridakis, E. & Shah, R. N. (Jun. 2013). Three-dimensional printing of soy protein scaffolds for tissue regeneration. Tissue Engineering Part C: Methods, 19(6), 417–426. doi: 10.1089/ten.TEC.2012.0383.
[39] Chien, K. B., Aguado, B. A., Bryce, P. J. & Shah, R. N. (Nov. 2013). In vivo acute and humoral response to three-dimensional porous soy protein scaffolds. Acta Biomater, 9(11), 8983–8990. doi: 10.1016/j.actbio.2013.07.005.
[40] Lim, T. C., Chian, K. S. & Leong, K. F. (Sep. 2010). Cryogenic prototyping of chitosan scaffolds with controlled micro and macro architecture and their effect on in vivo neo-vascularization and cellular infiltration. Journal of Biomedical Materials Research, 94(4), 1303–1311. doi: 10.1002/jbm.a.32747.
[41] Jamieson, C. et al. (Feb. 2021). A Review of Recent Advances in 3D Bioprinting With an Eye on Future Regenerative Therapies in Veterinary Medicine. Frontiers in Veterinary Science, 7, 584193. doi: 10.3389/fvets.2020.584193.
[42] Okamoto, T., Suzuki, T. & Yamamoto, N. (Apr. 2000). Microarray fabrication with covalent attachment of DNA using bubble jet technology. Nature Biotechnology, 18(4), 438–441. doi: 10.1038/74507.
[43] Xu, T., Jin, J., Gregory, C., Hickman, J. J. J. J. & Boland, T. (Jan. 2005). Inkjet printing of viable mammalian cells. Biomaterials, 26(1), 93–99. doi: 10.1016/j.biomaterials.2004.04.011.
[44] Duan, B., Hockaday, L. A., Kang, K. H. & Butcher, J. T. (May 2013). 3D bioprinting of heterogeneous aortic valve conduits with alginate/gelatin hydrogels. Journal of Biomedical Materials Research, 101(5), 1255–1264. doi: 10.1002/jbm.a.34420.
[45] Hockaday, L. A. et al. (Sep. 2012). Rapid 3D printing of anatomically accurate and mechanically heterogeneous aortic valve hydrogel scaffolds. Biofabrication, 4(3), 035005. doi: 10.1088/1758-5082/4/3/035005.
[46] Ali, M., Pages, E., Ducom, A., Fontaine, A. & Guillemot, F. (Sep. 2014). Controlling laser-induced jet formation for bioprinting mesenchymal stem cells with high viability and high resolution. Biofabrication, 6(4), 045001. doi: 10.1088/1758-5082/6/4/045001.
[47] Rutz, A. L., Lewis, P. L. & Shah, R. N. (Aug. 2017). Toward next-generation bioinks: Tuning material properties pre- and post-printing to optimize cell viability. MRS Bulletin, 42(8), 563–570. doi: 10.1557/mrs.2017.162.
[48] Hospodiuk, M., Dey, M., Sosnoski, D. & Ozbolat, I. T. (Mar. 2017). The bioink: A comprehensive review on bioprintable materials. Biotechnology Advances, 35(2), 217–239. doi: 10.1016/j.biotechadv.2016.12.006.
[49] Cooke, M. E. & Rosenzweig, D. H. (Feb. 2021). The rheology of direct and suspended extrusion bioprinting. APL Bioengineering, 5(1), 011502. doi: 10.1063/5.0031475.
[50] Davidenko, N. et al. (Aug. 2016). Evaluation of cell binding to collagen and gelatin: A study of the effect of 2D and 3D architecture and surface chemistry. Journal of Materials Science: Materials in Medicine, 27(10), 148. doi: 10.1007/s10856-016-5763-9.
[51] Colosi, C. et al. (2016). Microfluidic Bioprinting of Heterogeneous 3D Tissue Constructs Using Low-Viscosity Bioink. Advanced Materials, 28(4), 677–684. doi: 10.1002/adma.201503310.
[52] Badhe, R. V. et al. (Feb. 2017). A composite chitosan-gelatin bi-layered, biomimetic macroporous scaffold for blood vessel tissue engineering. Carbohydrate Polymers, 157, 1215–1225. doi: 10.1016/j.carbpol.2016.09.095.
[53] McBeth, C., Lauer, J., Ottersbach, M., Campbell, J., Sharon, A. & Sauer-Budge, A. F. (Jan. 2017). 3D bioprinting of GelMA scaffolds triggers mineral deposition by primary human osteoblasts. Biofabrication, 9(1), 015009. doi: 10.1088/1758-5090/aa53bd.

[54] Gungor-Ozkerim, P. S., Inci, I., Zhang, Y. S., Khademhosseini, A. & Dokmeci, M. R. (May 2018). Bioinks for 3D bioprinting: An overview. Biomaterials Science, 6(5), 915–946. doi: 10.1039/C7BM00765E.

[55] Tajik, S., Garcia, C. N., Gillooley, S. & Tayebi, L. (Mar. 2023). 3D Printing of Hybrid-Hydrogel Materials for Tissue Engineering: A Critical Review. Regenerative Engineering and Translational Medicine, 9(1), 29–41. doi: 10.1007/s40883-022-00267-w.

[56] Guvendiren, M., Molde, J., Soares, R. M. D. & Kohn, J. (Oct. 2016). Designing Biomaterials for 3D Printing. ACS Biomaterials Science & Engineering, 2(10), 1679–1693. doi: 10.1021/acsbiomaterials.6b00121.

[57] Diamantides, N. et al. (Jul. 2017). Correlating rheological properties and printability of collagen bioinks: The effects of riboflavin photocrosslinking and pH. Biofabrication, 9(3), 034102. doi: 10.1088/1758-5090/aa780f.

[58] Gudapati, H., Dey, M. & Ozbolat, I. (Sep. 2016). A comprehensive review on droplet-based bioprinting: Past, present and future. Biomaterials, 102, 20–42. doi: 10.1016/j.biomaterials.2016.06.012.

[59] Pawar, S. N. & Edgar, K. J. (Apr. 2012). Alginate derivatization: A review of chemistry, properties and applications. Biomaterials, 33(11), 3279–3305. doi: 10.1016/j.biomaterials.2012.01.007.

[60] Xu, T., Baicu, C., Aho, M., Zile, M. & Boland, T. (Sep. 2009). Fabrication and characterization of bio-engineered cardiac pseudo tissues. Biofabrication, 1(3), 035001. doi: 10.1088/1758-5082/1/3/035001.

[61] Liu, C., Qin, W., Wang, Y., Ma, J., Liu, J., Wu, S., & Zhao, H. (2021). 3D Printed Gelatin/Sodium Alginate Hydrogel Scaffolds Doped with Nano-Attapulgite for Bone Tissue Repair. *International Journal of Nanomedicine, 16*, 8417–8432. https://doi.org/10.2147/IJN.S339500.

[62] Do, A. V., Akkouch, A., Green, B., Ozbolat, I., Debabneh, A., Geary, S., & Salem, A. K. (2017). Controlled and Sequential Delivery of Fluorophores from 3D Printed Alginate-PLGA Tubes. *Annals of biomedical engineering, 45*(1), 297–305. https://doi.org/10.1007/s10439-016-1648-9.

[63] Tan, H., Tu, Z., Jia, H., Gou, X. & Ngai, T. (Apr. 2018). Hierarchical Porous Protein Scaffold Templated from High Internal Phase Emulsion Costabilized by Gelatin and Gelatin Nanoparticles. Langmuir, 34(16), 4820–4829. doi: 10.1021/acs.langmuir.7b04047.

[64] Mikhailov, O. V. (Jan. 2023). Gelatin as It Is: History and Modernity. International Journal of Molecular Sciences, 24(4, Art. no. 4), doi: 10.3390/ijms24043583.

[65] Lukin, I. et al. (Jun. 2022). Progress in Gelatin as Biomaterial for Tissue Engineering. Pharmaceutics, 14(6, Art. no. 6), doi: 10.3390/pharmaceutics14061177.

[66] Sakai, S., Hirose, K., Taguchi, K., Ogushi, Y. & Kawakami, K. (Jul. 2009). An injectable, *in situ* enzymatically gellable, gelatin derivative for drug delivery and tissue engineering. Biomaterials, 30(20), 3371–3377. doi: 10.1016/j.biomaterials.2009.03.030.

[67] Bertassoni, L. E. et al. (Apr. 2014). Direct-write bioprinting of cell-laden methacrylated gelatin hydrogels. Biofabrication, 6(2), 024105. doi: 10.1088/1758-5082/6/2/024105.

[68] "Physically and Chemically Crosslinked Gelatin Gels – Hellio – 2006 – Macromolecular Symposia – Wiley Online Library". Accessed: May 27, 2025. Available: https://onlinelibrary.wiley.com/doi/10.1002/masy.200650904

[69] "Chitosan-based biomaterials for tissue engineering – ScienceDirect." [Online]. Available: https://www.sciencedirect.com/science/article/pii/S0014305712004181

[70] Xu, Z. (2017). Solubility of Polysaccharides. BoD – Books on Demand.

[71] Zhang, Y., Yu, Y. & Ozbolat, I. T. (Jul. 2013). Direct Bioprinting of Vessel-Like Tubular Microfluidic Channels. Journal of Nanotechnology in Engineering and Medicine, 4(020902), doi: 10.1115/1.4024398.

[72] Mosesson, M. W. (2005). Fibrinogen and fibrin structure and functions. *Journal of Thrombosis and Haemostasis, 3*(8), 1894–1904. https://doi.org/10.1111/j.1538-7836.2005.01365.x.

[73] Kreimendahl, F., Kniebs, C., Tavares Sobreiro, A. M., Schmitz-Rode, T., Jockenhoevel, S. & Thiebes, A. L. (Jan. 2021). FRESH bioprinting technology for tissue engineering – The influence of printing process and bioink composition on cell behavior and vascularization. Journal of Applied Biomaterials & Functional Materials, 19, 22808000211028808. doi: 10.1177/22808000211028808.
[74] Horder, H. et al. (Apr. 2021). Bioprinting and Differentiation of Adipose-Derived Stromal Cell Spheroids for a 3D Breast Cancer-Adipose Tissue Model. Cells, 10(4, Art. no. 4), doi: 10.3390/cells10040803.
[75] Laurens, N., Koolwijk, P. & De Maat, M. P. M. (May 2006). Fibrin structure and wound healing. Journal of Thrombosis and Haemostasis, 4(5), 932–939. doi: 10.1111/j.1538-7836.2006.01861.x.
[76] England, S., Rajaram, A., Schreyer, D. J. & Chen, X. (Mar. 2017). Bioprinted fibrin-factor XIII-hyaluronate hydrogel scaffolds with encapsulated Schwann cells and their *in vitro* characterization for use in nerve regeneration. Bioprinting, 5, 1–9. doi: 10.1016/j.bprint.2016.12.001.
[77] Laki, K. (Jul. 1951). The polymerization of proteins: The action of thrombin on fibrinogen. Archives of Biochemistry and Biophysics, 32(2), 317–324. doi: 10.1016/0003-9861(51)90277-9.
[78] Pitacco, P., Sadowska, J. M., O'Brien, F. J. & Kelly, D. J. (Jan. 2023). 3D bioprinting of cartilaginous templates for large bone defect healing. Acta Biomater, 156, 61–74. doi: 10.1016/j.actbio.2022.07.037.
[79] Xu, T. et al. (Jul. 2006). Viability and electrophysiology of neural cell structures generated by the inkjet printing method. Biomaterials, 27(19), 3580–3588. doi: 10.1016/j.biomaterials.2006.01.048.
[80] Gref, R. et al. (Oct. 2000). 'Stealth' corona-core nanoparticles surface modified by polyethylene glycol (PEG): Influences of the corona (PEG chain length and surface density) and of the core composition on phagocytic uptake and plasma protein adsorption. Colloids and Surfaces B: Biointerfaces, 18(3), 301–313. doi: 10.1016/S0927-7765(99)00156-3.
[81] 2025. Mechanical Properties, Cytocompatibility and Manufacturability of Chitosan:PEGDA Hybrid-Gel Scaffolds by Stereolithography | Annals of Biomedical Engineering. Accessed: May, 30, [Online]. Available https://link.springer.com/article/10.1007/s10439-016-1643-1.
[82] Kim, J. S., Hong, S. & Hwang, C. (2016). Bio-ink Materials for 3D Bio-printing. Journal of International Society for Simulation Surgery, 3(2), 49–59. doi: 10.18204/JISSiS.2016.3.2.049.
[83] Benoit, D. S. W., Durney, A. R. & Anseth, K. S. (Jun. 2006). Manipulations in Hydrogel Degradation Behavior Enhance Osteoblast Function and Mineralized Tissue Formation. Tissue Engineering, 12(6), 1663–1673. doi: 10.1089/ten.2006.12.1663.
[84] Hockaday, L. A. et al. (Aug. 2012). Rapid 3D printing of anatomically accurate and mechanically heterogeneous aortic valve hydrogel scaffolds. Biofabrication, 4(3), 035005. doi: 10.1088/1758-5082/4/3/035005.
[85] Gao, G., Schilling, A. F., Yonezawa, T., Wang, J., Dai, G. & Cui, X. (2014). Bioactive nanoparticles stimulate bone tissue formation in bioprinted three-dimensional scaffold and human mesenchymal stem cells. Biotechnology Journal, 9(10), 1304–1311. doi: 10.1002/biot.201400305.
[86] Gioffredi, E. et al. (Jan. 2016). Pluronic F127 Hydrogel Characterization and Biofabrication in Cellularized Constructs for Tissue Engineering Applications. Procedia CIRP, 49, 125–132. doi: 10.1016/j.procir.2015.11.001.
[87] Gilbert, J. C., Hadgraft, J., Bye, A. & Brookes, L. G. (Oct. 1986). Drug release from Pluronic F-127 gels. International Journal of Pharmaceutics, 32(2), 223–228. doi: 10.1016/0378-5173(86)90182-1.
[88] Yang, Y., Wang, J., Zhang, X., Lu, W. & Zhang, Q. (Apr. 2009). A novel mixed micelle gel with thermo-sensitive property for the local delivery of docetaxel. Journal of Controlled Release, 135(2), 175–182. doi: 10.1016/j.jconrel.2009.01.007.
[89] Guzmán, M., García, F. F., Molpeceres, J. & Aberturas, M. R. (Feb. 1992). Polyoxyethylene-polyoxypropylene block copolymer gels as sustained release vehicles for subcutaneous drug administration. International Journal of Pharmaceutics, 80(1), 119–127. doi: 10.1016/0378-5173(92)90269-8.

[90] Brunet-Maheu, J.-M., Fernandes, J. C., De Lacerda, C. A., Shi, Q., Benderdour, M. & Lavigne, P. (Sep. 2009). Pluronic F-127 as a Cell Carrier for Bone Tissue Engineering. Journal of Biomaterials Applications, 24(3), 275–287. doi: 10.1177/0885328208096534.

[91] Khattak, S. F., Bhatia, S. R. & Roberts, S. C. (May 2005). Pluronic F127 as a Cell Encapsulation Material: Utilization of Membrane-Stabilizing Agents. Tissue Engineering, 11(5–6), 974–983. doi: 10.1089/ten.2005.11.974.

[92] "Three-dimensional tissue constructs built by bioprinting – Karoly Jakab, Brook Damon, Adrian Neagu, Anatolij Kachurin, Gabor Forgacs, 2006." Available: https://journals.sagepub.com/doi/10.1177/0006355X2006043003004033

[93] Vashi, A. V. et al. (Feb. 2008). Adipose differentiation of bone marrow-derived mesenchymal stem cells using Pluronic F-127 hydrogel *in vitro*. Biomaterials, 29(5), 573–579. doi: 10.1016/j.biomaterials.2007.10.017.

[94] Johnson, M. (Jan. 2011). Public sector e-procurement: A study of benefits from e-markets in the local government sector. International Journal of Services Technology and Management, 16(1), 1–27. doi: 10.1504/IJSTM.2011.041975.

[95] Johari, N., Adabavazeh, Z. & Baino, F. (Sep. 2025). PVA-based bioinks for 3D bioprinting: A comprehensive review of their applications in tissue engineering. Bioprinting, 49, e00419. doi: 10.1016/j.bprint.2025.e00419.

[96] Bazhenov, V. E. et al. (Feb. 2025). The Utilization of Polyvinyl Alcohol (PVA) Filaments for the Three-Dimensional Printing of Water-Soluble Patterns for Investment Casting. Journal of Manufacturing and Materials Processing, 9(2, Art. no. 2), doi: 10.3390/jmmp9020048.

[97] A Multi-State Comparative Coarse-Grained Modeling of Semi-Crystalline Poly(vinyl alcohol) | Macromolecules. Available https://pubs.acs.org/doi/10.1021/acs.macromol.4c03146.

[98] Upadhyay, P., Gupta, M. K. & Upadhyay, S. (2025). Bioink technology in 3D bioprinting and their improvement. In Handbook of 3D Printing in Biomedical Applications. CRC Press.

[99] Setayeshmehr, M., Hafeez, S., Van Blitterswijk, C., Moroni, L., Mota, C. & Baker, M. B. (Jan. 2021). Bioprinting Via a Dual-Gel Bioink Based on Poly(Vinyl Alcohol) and Solubilized Extracellular Matrix towards Cartilage Engineering. International Journal of Molecular Sciences, 22(8, Art. no. 8), doi: 10.3390/ijms22083901.

[100] Masri, S., Maarof, M., Aziz, I. A., Idrus, R. & Fauzi, M. B. (Feb. 2023). Performance of hybrid gelatin-PVA bioinks integrated with genipin through extrusion-based 3D bioprinting: An in vitro evaluation using human dermal fibroblasts. International Journal of Bioprinting, 9(3), 677. doi: 10.18063/ijb.677.

[101] Crapo, P. M., Gilbert, T. W. & Badylak, S. F. (Apr. 2011). An overview of tissue and whole organ decellularization processes. Biomaterials, 32(12), 3233–3243. doi: 10.1016/j.biomaterials.2011.01.057.

[102] Yao, Q., Zheng, Y.-W., Lan, Q.-H., Kou, L., Xu, H.-L. & Zhao, Y.-Z. (Nov. 2019). Recent development and biomedical applications of decellularized extracellular matrix biomaterials. Materials Science and Engineering: C, 104, 109942. doi: 10.1016/j.msec.2019.109942.

[103] Tissue Engineered Bio-Blood-Vessels Constructed Using a Tissue-Specific Bioink and 3D Coaxial Cell Printing Technique: A Novel Therapy for Ischemic Disease – Gao – 2017 – Advanced Functional Materials – Wiley Online Library. Available https://advanced.onlinelibrary.wiley.com/doi/10.1002/adfm.201700798.

[104] Dzobo, K., Motaung, K. S. C. M. & Adesida, A. (Sep. 2019). Recent Trends in Decellularized Extracellular Matrix Bioinks for 3D Printing: An Updated Review. International Journal of Molecular Sciences, 20(18), 4628. doi: 10.3390/ijms20184628.

[105] Du, P., Suhaeri, M., Ha, S. S., Oh, S. J., Kim, S.-H. & Park, K. (May 2017). Human lung fibroblast-derived matrix facilitates vascular morphogenesis in 3D environment and enhances skin wound healing. Acta Biomater, 54, 333–344. doi: 10.1016/j.actbio.2017.03.035.

[106] Guo, Y. et al. (Nov. 2013). Extracellular Matrix of Mechanically Stretched Cardiac Fibroblasts Improves Viability and Metabolic Activity of Ventricular Cells. International Journal of Medical Sciences, 10(13), 1837–1845. doi: 10.7150/ijms.6786.

[107] Gilbert, T. W., Sellaro, T. L. & Badylak, S. F. (Jul. 2006). Decellularization of tissues and organs. Biomaterials, 27(19), 3675–3683. doi: 10.1016/j.biomaterials.2006.02.014.

[108] Zhang, Z., Wang, B., Hui, D., Qiu, J. & Wang, S. (Aug. 2017). 3D bioprinting of soft materials-based regenerative vascular structures and tissues. Composites Part B: Engineering, 123, 279–291. doi: 10.1016/j.compositesb.2017.05.011.

[109] Levato, R., Visser, J., Planell, J. A., Engel, E., Malda, J. & Mateos-Timoneda, M. A. (Jul. 2014). Biofabrication of tissue constructs by 3D bioprinting of cell-laden microcarriers. Biofabrication, 6(3), 035020. doi: 10.1088/1758-5082/6/3/035020.

[110] Ovsianikov, A., Khademhosseini, A. & Mironov, V. (Apr. 2018). The Synergy of Scaffold-Based and Scaffold-Free Tissue Engineering Strategies. Trends in Biotechnology, 36(4), 348–357. doi: 10.1016/j.tibtech.2018.01.005.

[111] Khalil, M. et al. (Jan. 2001). Human hepatocyte cell lines proliferating as cohesive spheroid colonies in alginate markedly upregulate both synthetic and detoxificatory liver function. Journal of Hepatology, 34(1), 68–77. doi: 10.1016/S0168-8278(00)00080-5.

[112] Owens, C. M., Marga, F., Forgacs, G. & Heesch, C. M. (Nov. 2013). Biofabrication and testing of a fully cellular nerve graft. Biofabrication, 5(4), 045007. doi: 10.1088/1758-5082/5/4/045007.

[113] Sun, H., Jia, Y., Dong, H., Dong, D. & Zheng, J. (Jun. 2020). Combining additive manufacturing with microfluidics: An emerging method for developing novel organs-on-chips. Current Opinion in Chemical Engineering, 28, 1–9. doi: 10.1016/j.coche.2019.10.006.

[114] Yu, Y., Moncal, K. K., Li, J., Peng, W., Rivero, I., Martin, J. A., & Ozbolat, I. T. (2016). Three-dimensional bioprinting using self-assembling scalable scaffold-free "tissue strands" as a new bioink. *Scientific reports*, 6, 28714. https://doi.org/10.1038/srep28714.

[115] Goldman, R. (Feb. 2004). Growth Factors and Chronic Wound Healing: Past, Present, and Future. Advances in Skin & Wound Care, 17(1), 24.

[116] Grazul-Bilska, A. T. et al. (2003). Wound healing: The role of growth factors. Drugs of Today, 39(10), 787. doi: 10.1358/dot.2003.39.10.799472.

[117] Miller, E. D., Phillippi, J. A., Fisher, G. W., Campbell, P. G., Walker, L. M. & Weiss, L. E. Inkjet Printing of Growth Factor Concentration Gradients and Combinatorial Arrays Immobilized on Biologically-Relevant Substrates. Combinatorial Chemistry & High Throughput Screening, 12(6), 604–618. doi: 10.2174/138620709788681907.

[118] Cooper, G. M. et al. (May 2010). Inkjet-Based Biopatterning of Bone Morphogenetic Protein-2 to Spatially Control Calvarial Bone Formation. Tissue Engineering Part A, 16(5), 1749–1759. doi: 10.1089/ten.tea.2009.0650.

[119] Elowsson, L., Kirsebom, H., Carmignac, V., Mattiasson, B. & Durbeej, M. (Mar. 2013). Evaluation of macroporous blood and plasma scaffolds for skeletal muscle tissue engineering. Biomaterials Science, 1(4), 402–410. doi: 10.1039/C2BM00054G.

[120] Gruene, M. et al. (Mar. 2011). Adipogenic differentiation of laser-printed 3D tissue grafts consisting of human adipose-derived stem cells. Biofabrication, 3(1), 015005. doi: 10.1088/1758-5082/3/1/015005.

[121] Koch, L. et al. (2012). Skin tissue generation by laser cell printing. Biotechnology and Bioengineering, 109(7), 1855–1863. doi: 10.1002/bit.24455.

[122] Assal, R. E. et al. (2014). Bio-Inspired Cryo-Ink Preserves Red Blood Cell Phenotype and Function During Nanoliter Vitrification. Advanced Materials, 26(33), 5815–5822. doi: 10.1002/adma.201400941.

[123] Loo, Y., Lakshmanan, A., Ni, M., Toh, L. L., Wang, S. & Hauser, C. A. E. (Oct. 2015). Peptide Bioink: Self-Assembling Nanofibrous Scaffolds for Three-Dimensional Organotypic Cultures. Nano Lett, 15(10), 6919–6925. doi: 10.1021/acs.nanolett.5b02859.

[124] Lee, D.-Y., Lee, H., Kim, Y., Yoo, S. Y., Chung, W.-J. & Kim, G. (Jan. 2016). Phage as versatile nanoink for printing 3-D cell-laden scaffolds. Acta Biomater, 29, 112–124. doi: 10.1016/j.actbio.2015.10.004.
[125] Jungst, T., Smolan, W., Schacht, K., Scheibel, T. & Groll, J. (Feb. 2016). Strategies and Molecular Design Criteria for 3D Printable Hydrogels. Chemical Reviews, 116(3), 1496–1539. doi: 10.1021/acs.chemrev.5b00303.
[126] Deo, K. A., Singh, K. A., Peak, C. W., Alge, D. L. & Gaharwar, A. K. (Mar. 2020). Bioprinting 101: Design, Fabrication, and Evaluation of Cell-Laden 3D Bioprinted Scaffolds. Tissue Engineering Part A, 26(5–6), 318–338. doi: 10.1089/ten.tea.2019.0298.
[127] Kyle, S., Jessop, Z. M., Al-Sabah, A. & Whitaker, I. S. (2017). 'Printability' of Candidate Biomaterials for Extrusion Based 3D Printing: State-of-the-Art. Advanced Healthcare MMaterials, 6(16), doi: 10.1002/adhm.201700264.
[128] Karvinen, J. & Kellomäki, M. (Jul. 2023). Design aspects and characterization of hydrogel-based bioinks for extrusion-based bioprinting. Bioprinting, 32, e00274. doi: 10.1016/j.bprint.2023.e00274.
[129] Li, H., Tan, C. & Li, L. (Dec. 2018). Review of 3D printable hydrogels and constructs. Materials & Design, 159, 20–38. doi: 10.1016/j.matdes.2018.08.023.
[130] Li, J., Wu, C., Chu, P. K. & Gelinsky, M. (Apr. 2020). 3D printing of hydrogels: Rational design strategies and emerging biomedical applications. Materials Science and Engineering: R: Reports, 140, 100543. doi: 10.1016/j.mser.2020.100543.
[131] Hölzl, K., Lin, S., Tytgat, L., Van Vlierberghe, S., Gu, L. & Ovsianikov, A. (2016). Bioink properties before, during and after 3D bioprinting. Biofabrication, 8(3), doi: 10.1088/1758-5090/8/3/032002.
[132] Kačarević, Ž. P. et al. (2018). An introduction to 3D bioprinting: Possibilities, challenges and future aspects. Materials, 11(11), doi: 10.3390/ma11112199.
[133] Gopinathan, J. & Noh, I. (2018). Recent trends in bioinks for 3D printing. Biomaterials Research, 22(1), doi: 10.1186/s40824-018-0122-1.
[134] GhavamiNejad, A., Ashammakhi, N., Wu, X. Y. & Khademhosseini, A. (Sep. 2020). Crosslinking Strategies for Three-Dimensional Bioprinting of Polymeric Hydrogels. Small, 16(35), e2002931. doi: 10.1002/smll.202002931.
[135] Bertlein, S. et al. (2017). Thiol–Ene Clickable Gelatin: A Platform Bioink for Multiple 3D Biofabrication Technologies. Advanced Materials, 29(44), 1703404. doi: 10.1002/adma.201703404.
[136] Xu, C., Lee, W., Dai, G. & Hong, Y. (Mar. 2018). Highly Elastic Biodegradable Single-Network Hydrogel for Cell Printing. ACS Applied Materials & Interfaces, 10(12), 9969–9979. doi: 10.1021/acsami.8b01294.
[137] Effective Light Directed Assembly of Building Blocks with Microscale Control – Dinh – 2017 – Small – Wiley Online Library. Available https://onlinelibrary.wiley.com/doi/10.1002/smll.201700684.
[138] GhavamiNejad, A., Hashmi, S., Vatankhah-Varnoosfaderani, M. & Stadler, F. J. (Feb. 2016). Effect of H2O and reduced graphene oxide on the structure and rheology of self-healing, stimuli responsive catecholic gels. Rheologica Acta, 55(2), 163–176. doi: 10.1007/s00397-015-0906-3.
[139] Mandrycky, C., Wang, Z., Kim, K. & Kim, D.-H. (2016). 3D Bioprinting for Engineering Complex Tissues. Biotechnology Advances, 34(4), 422–434. doi: 10.1016/j.biotechadv.2015.12.011.
[140] Lim, K. S., Galarraga, J. H., Cui, X., Lindberg, G. C. J., Burdick, J. A. & Woodfield, T. B. F. (Oct. 2020). Fundamentals and Applications of Photo-Cross-Linking in Bioprinting. Chemical Reviews, 120(19), 10662–10694. doi: 10.1021/acs.chemrev.9b00812.
[141] Ouyang, L., Yao, R., Zhao, Y. & Sun, W. (Sep. 2016). Effect of bioink properties on printability and cell viability for 3D bioplotting of embryonic stem cells. Biofabrication, 8(3), 035020. doi: 10.1088/1758-5090/8/3/035020.
[142] Chimene, D., Lennox, K. K., Kaunas, R. R. & Gaharwar, A. K. (Jun. 2016). Advanced Bioinks for 3D Printing: A Materials Science Perspective. Annals of Biomedical Engineering, 44(6), 2090–2102. doi: 10.1007/s10439-016-1638-y.

[143] Three-dimensional printing of complex biological structures by freeform reversible embedding of suspended hydrogels. Available https://www.science.org/doi/10.1126/sciadv.1500758.
[144] Hong, S. et al. (2015). 3D Printing of Highly Stretchable and Tough Hydrogels into Complex, Cellularized Structures. Advanced Materials, 27(27), 4035–4040. doi: 10.1002/adma.201501099.
[145] Schwab, A., Levato, R., D'Este, M., Piluso, S., Eglin, D. & Malda, J. (Oct. 2020). Printability and Shape Fidelity of Bioinks in 3D Bioprinting. Chemical Reviews, 120(19), 11028–11055. doi: 10.1021/acs.chemrev.0c00084.
[146] Highley, C. B., Rodell, C. B. & Burdick, J. A. (Sep. 2015). Direct 3D Printing of Shear-Thinning Hydrogels into Self-Healing Hydrogels. Advanced Materials, 27(34), 5075–5079. doi: 10.1002/adma.201501234.
[147] Shi, Y. et al. (Mar. 2018). Tyrosinase-doped bioink for 3D bioprinting of living skin constructs. Biomedical Materials, 13(3), 035008. doi: 10.1088/1748-605X/aaa5b6.
[148] Chen, Y. et al. (Jul. 2020). 3D Bioprinting of shear-thinning hybrid bioinks with excellent bioactivity derived from gellan/alginate and thixotropic magnesium phosphate-based gels. Journal of Materials Chemistry B, 8(25), 5500–5514. doi: 10.1039/d0tb00060d.
[149] Townsend, J. M., Beck, E. C., Gehrke, S. H., Berkland, C. J. & Detamore, M. S. (Apr. 2019). Flow behavior prior to crosslinking: The need for precursor rheology for placement of hydrogels in medical applications and for 3D bioprinting. Progress in Polymer Science, 91, 126–140. doi: 10.1016/j.progpolymsci.2019.01.003.
[150] 'Printability' of Candidate Biomaterials for Extrusion Based 3D Printing: State-of-the-Art – Kyle – 2017 – Advanced Healthcare Materials – Wiley Online Library. Available https://advanced.onlinelibrary.wiley.com/doi/full/10.1002/adhm.201700264.
[151] Dorishetty, P., Dutta, N. K. & Choudhury, N. R. (Jul. 2020). Bioprintable tough hydrogels for tissue engineering applications. Advances in Colloid and Interface Science, 281, 102163. doi: 10.1016/j.cis.2020.102163.
[152] Li, H. et al. (Aug. 2018). Automatic quantification of crypt architecture in ex vivo gastrointestinal epithelium for high-resolution microendoscopic. In *Tenth International Conference on Digital Image Processing (ICDIP 2018)*, SPIE. 1454–1461. doi: 10.1117/12.2502831.
[153] Huh, D. D. & Kim, D.-H. (Apr. 2015). JALA Special Issue: Microengineered Cell- and Tissue-Based Assays for Drug Screening and Toxicology Applications. Journal of Laboratory Automation, 20(2), 79–81. doi: 10.1177/2211068215574458.
[154] "Biomimetic 3D Tissue Models for Advanced High-Throughput Drug Screening – Ki-Hwan Nam, Alec S. T. Smith, Saifullah Lone, Sunghoon Kwon, Deok-Ho Kim, 2015". https://journals.sagepub.com/doi/full/10.1177/2211068214557813
[155] Chang, R., Emami, K., Wu, H., & Sun, W. (2010). Biofabrication of a three-dimensional liver micro-organ as an in vitro drug metabolism model. Biofabrication, 2(4), 045004. https://doi.org/10.1088/1758-5082/2/4/045004
[156] Ashammakhi, N. et al. (Apr. 2019). Advancing Frontiers in Bone Bioprinting. Advanced Healthcare Materials, 8(7), e1801048. doi: 10.1002/adhm.201801048.
[157] Bracaglia, L. G., Smith, B. T., Watson, E., Arumugasaamy, N., Mikos, A. G. & Fisher, J. P. (Jul. 2017). 3D printing for the design and fabrication of polymer-based gradient scaffolds. Acta Biomater, 56, 3–13. doi: 10.1016/j.actbio.2017.03.030.
[158] Tortelli, F., Pujic, N., Liu, Y., Laroche, N., Vico, L., & Cancedda, R. (2009). Osteoblast and osteoclast differentiation in an in vitro three-dimensional model of bone. *Tissue engineering. Part A, 15*(9), 2373–2383. https://doi.org/10.1089/ten.tea.2008.0501
[159] Zhu, W., Holmes, B., Glazer, R. I., & Zhang, L. G. (2016). 3D printed nanocomposite matrix for the study of breast cancer bone metastasis. Nanomedicine : nanotechnology, biology, and medicine, 12 (1), 69–79. https://doi.org/10.1016/j.nano.2015.09.010.

[160] Zein, N. N. et al. (Dec. 2013). Three-dimensional print of a liver for preoperative planning in living donor liver transplantation. Liver Transplantation, 19(12), 1304–1310. doi: 10.1002/lt.23729.
[161] Bale, S. S. et al. (Sep. 2014). In vitro platforms for evaluating liver toxicity. Experimental Biology and Medicine (Maywood), 239(9), 1180–1191. doi: 10.1177/1535370214531872.
[162] "Transplantation: 3D printing of the liver in living donor liver transplantation – PubMed." Available: https://pubmed.ncbi.nlm.nih.gov/24126562/
[163] Nakao, Y., Kimura, H., Sakai, Y. & Fujii, T. (Jun. 2011). Bile canaliculi formation by aligning rat primary hepatocytes in a microfluidic device. Biomicrofluidics, 5(2), 22212. doi: 10.1063/1.3580753.
[164] "Tissue specific synthetic ECM hydrogels for 3-D in vitro maintenance of hepatocyte function – PubMed." Available: https://pubmed.ncbi.nlm.nih.gov/22475531/
[165] "Fabrication of 3D-culture platform with sandwich architecture for preserving liver-specific functions of hepatocytes using 3D bioprinter – Arai – 2017 – Journal of Biomedical Materials Research Part A – Wiley Online Library." https://onlinelibrary.wiley.com/doi/full/10.1002/jbm.a.35905
[166] Moya, A. et al. (Jul. 2018). Online Oxygen Monitoring Using Integrated Inkjet-printed Sensors in a Liver-on-a-chip System. doi: 10.1039/C8LC00456K.
[167] Furman, E. (Oct. 2013). The dynamic state of patents in regenerative medicine. Tissue Engineering and Regenerative Medicine, 10(5), 230–233. doi: 10.1007/s13770-013-1082-0.
[168] "Advent and maturation of regenerative medicine – PubMed." Available: https://pubmed.ncbi.nlm.nih.gov/23176292/
[169] Badylak, S. F. & Nerem, R. M. (Feb. 2010). Progress in tissue engineering and regenerative medicine. Proceedings of the National Academy of Sciences of the United States of America, 107(8), 3285–3286. doi: 10.1073/pnas.1000256107.
[170] Xu, T., Baicu, C., Aho, M., Zile, M. & Boland, T. (Sep. 2009). Fabrication and characterization of bio-engineered cardiac pseudo tissues. Biofabrication, 1(3), 035001. doi: 10.1088/1758-5082/1/3/035001.
[171] Wang, Z., Lee, S. J., Cheng, H.-J., Yoo, J. J. & Atala, A. (Apr. 2018). 3D bioprinted functional and contractile cardiac tissue constructs. Acta Biomater, 70, 48–56. doi: 10.1016/j.actbio.2018.02.007.

N. Vishnudevi*, K. Aravinth*, B. Krishna Kumar*

Chapter 13 Computational Intelligence Usages in Bioprinting

Abstract: Computational intelligence (CI) is revolutionizing bioprinting by enhancing precision, efficiency, and customization in tissue engineering and regenerative medicine. By incorporating artificial intelligence (AI), machine learning (ML), and deep learning (DL), CI optimizes processes, improves material selection, and enables real-time quality assessment, ultimately increasing the accuracy of printed biological structures. One key application of CI in bioprinting is predictive modeling, which allows for accurate simulations of printing processes and material behaviors. These models help minimize errors, optimize printing parameters, reduce material waste, and improve reproducibility. Additionally, advanced image processing techniques analyze and refine bio-printed constructs to ensure their structural integrity and functionality. AI-driven robotics also play a crucial role in automating bioprinting systems. Features such as autonomous calibration, adaptive control mechanisms, and self-correcting algorithms enhance precision while reducing the need for human intervention. Moreover, DL frameworks facilitate cell pattern recognition, enabling the creation of complex, multi-cellular structures that closely mimic natural tissue architecture. Despite its many advantages, CI in bioprinting still faces challenges, including computational complexity, limited data availability, and ethical concerns related to AI-driven decision-making. Future developments will likely focus on enhancing algorithms, integrating multi-modal data sources, and improving real-time monitoring to further refine bioprinting technologies. This chapter explores the expanding role of CI in bioprinting, highlighting recent advancements, potential applications, and ongoing challenges. By bridging AI and biomedical engineering, CI is paving the way for more efficient and precise fabrication techniques, ultimately driving progress in personalized medicine and tissue engineering.

Keywords: Computational intelligence, machine learning, bioprinting, tissue fabrication, artificial intelligence

---

***Corresponding author: N. Vishnudevi,** Department of Electronics Engineering (VLSI), Velammal College of Engineering and Technology, Viraganoor, Madurai 625 009, Tamil Nadu, India, e-mail: Vichu0408@gmail.com
***Corresponding author: K. Aravinth,** Velammal College of Engineering and Technology, Madurai, Tamil Nadu, India, e-mail: aravinthkarthik2006@gmail.com
***Corresponding author: B. Krishna Kumar,** Velammal College of Engineering and Technology, Madurai, Tamil Nadu, India, e-mail: krishnakumarb2005@gmail.com

 | https://doi.org/10.1515/9783111719993-013

13.1 Introduction to Bioprinting and Computational Intelligence

13.1.1 Overview of Bioprinting

Bioprinting is a disruptive technology that sprawls in the nexus of biotechnology, materials science, and engineering. It is a process that layers bioinks, living cells, biomaterials and growth factors in a sequential deposition in order to construct complex biological compositions and synthetic tissues that resemble native tissue designs. Bioprinting, being a subset of additive manufacturing, has advanced since the initial two-dimensional (2D) distribution of cells to the current three-dimensional (3D) printing of tissues and organs. It could be used in fields as regenerative medicine, drug testing, cancer modeling, and personalized therapeutics.

Bioprinting presents the basic aim of synthesizing a viable biological construction that is structurally and biologically complementary to human tissues. In order to do this, the printing itself should produce a printing that is highly precise in terms of materials, cell density, cell orientation, and their microenvironment. Even with such impressive progress, bioprinting remains fraught with several dire issues, especially when it comes to recapitulating vascularization, life span, and mechanical integrity of printed tissue.

13.1.2 Emergence of Computational Intelligence in Biomedicine

Computational intelligence (CI) can be taken as the use of artificial intelligence (AI), machine learning (ML), and deep learning (DL) methods to address complex, nonlinear, and data-intensive problems. Within the sphere of biomedicine, CI facilitates predictive analytics, automatic decision-making, and brilliant data interpretation, which are needed to cope with the complexity of biological systems.

Within recent years, CI became more and more integrated in biomedical technologies, such as diagnostics, imaging, genomics, and robotic surgery. It perfectly suits addressing the fluctuation and randomness of biological processes since it knows how to learn and adjust to new data. With massive biomedical data, CI systems can identify patterns, streamline processes, and offer live insights.

The collision of CI and biomedicine signifies an enormous shift toward precision healthcare, through which information-based methods may tailor solutions, anticipate patient outcomes, and optimize clinical processes. In the framework of this larger model, bioprinting has become an excellent candidate in terms of CI integration since the task requires multi-variable optimization, process management, and interpretation of the biological data stream.

13.1.3 Intersection of Bioprinting and CI

The incorporation of CI into bioprinting will not result in an enhancement of the current programs; it will be the change that marks the new period in the way the biological structures are thought about, manufactured, and tested. Traditional bioprinting processes are trial and error, hands-on calibrations, and fixed protocols; this is a leading cause of inefficiency, variability, and cost highs. The limitations of automation, real-time learning, and predictive analytics complicate this, but CI delivers real-time data-driven flexibility on a dynamic basis to the process.

To give an example, the process of accepting massive data sets that involve printing parameters and subsequent post-print tissue testing can be carried out with the use of a machine learning (ML) algorithm. Such models are capable of suggesting favorable combinations of parameters, including nozzle speed, pressure, and bioink rheology, as well as regular quality production due to the identification of complex, nonlinear correlations between them. Further, they can use reinforcement learning models to dynamically adjust print settings during the print process based on sensor response and adapt to any variation in material or environmental conditions.

In analyzing data in an imaging system during and after printing, DL DL (especially convolutional neural networks (CNNs)) can be vital. These systems allow detecting defects automatically, evaluating the quality of layers layer-by-layer, and monitoring cell viability without destruction. Therefore, CI-enabled imaging modalities minimize waste and increase reproducibility, which is essential to translational and clinical contexts.

The second field with possibilities is simulation and virtual prototyping. Structural integrity and biological response of a printed construct may be simulated through predictive modeling with the use of AI, even before the physical printing process is undertaken. This not only enhances the speed of the cycle development but also lessens the use of expensive biological materials and reliance on the use of animals.

Moreover, CI helps in closed-loop control systems integration. Having sensors and actuators integrated into it, a bioprinter is able to gather real-time information about flow dynamics, temperature, or pressure and have intelligent algorithms process it to make adjustments in real-time. This feedback loop is critical to preserving geometric fidelity, and as well as permitting and responding to variability in bioink composition/environment.

Musical cooperation of CI and bioprinting continues in the field of personal medicine. With patient-specific anatomical data, i.e., data provided by MRI or CT data, CI systems may model custom anatomies that perfectly fit a patient's anatomy and pathology. This would allow customized implants and grafts to come very real, not just in form but also in cellular makeup and action.

At that, CI transforms bioprinting, currently based on a set of rules and semi-automated, to an intelligent and adaptive system with the ability to improve itself and make real-time decisions. The integration of CI will be an essential part of realizing the precision, scalability, and personalization that next-generation biomedical applications demand as tissue engineering increasingly becomes a clinical reality.

Table 13.1: Comparison of Traditional Bioprinting vs. CI-Integrated Bioprinting.

Feature	Traditional Computing	CI-Integrated Bioprinting
Process Control	Manual/Static	Adaptive and Dynamic
Optimization Approach	Trial-and-error	Data-Driven Modeling
Real-Time Monitoring	Limited	Automated and Continuous
Error Correction	Post-process	In-process via AI Feedback
Design Flexibility	Fixed Structures	Intelligent Multi-cell Arrangements
Output Consistency	Variable	High Accuracy and Repeatability

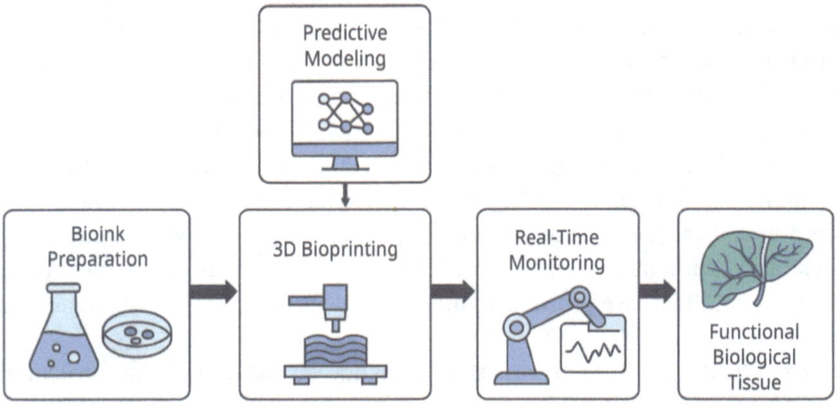

Figure 13.1: CI- Enhanced Bioprinting.

13.1.4 Objectives and Scope of the Chapter

In this chapter, reader examines the increasing engagement of CI into the process of the bioprinting development, paying particular attention to the arising issues and bioethics, as well as perspectives on the way to the next stage of development of this field in regard to the envisioned interconnection of CI and bioprinting development. It aims to provide a comprehensive overview of how CI technologies, such as ML, DL, and intelligent robotics, are being applied to various aspects of the bioprinting process.

The scope includes:

- Analyzing core CI applications in predictive modeling, material optimization, image-based validation, and robotic automation
- Identifying technical challenges like data scarcity, model accuracy, and reproducibility

- Addressing ethical considerations, including autonomy, consent, data ownership, and societal impact
- Exploring emerging innovations and future directions in intelligent, patient-specific bioprinting

The chapter helps to develop a better insight into the role of computational tools in the future of personalized medicine, regenerative therapies, biofabrication, and human-machine symbiosis in healthcare by connecting the fields of biofabrication and AI.

13.2 Bioprinting Processes and Material Challenges

13.2.1 Fundamentals of Bioprinting Technologies

Bioprinting is a type of additive manufacturing where bioinks, which are composed of living cells and biomaterials, are used to create tissue-like structures in layers. This method is also used to simulate the intricate microarchitecture of the native tissues by incubating cells in a well-defined spatial location. There are three major bioprinting modalities, namely, inkjet bioprinting, extrusion bioprinting, and laser-aided bioprinting. All the methods include their own peculiarities, both in their benefits and limitations related to resolution, throughput, and biological compatibility.

Inkjet bioprinting is based on the controlled expulsion of small bioink droplets by the controlled thermal or piezoelectric actuator. It is noncontact so there is little chance of contamination and due to the speed of its dispensing, it is very efficient at producing patterns over large surfaces. Nevertheless, it is not usually applicable to high-viscosity bioinks and could have issues with high repeatability in creating the right type of droplets when growing cells or when cell balling or clogging has to be done. The method is most appropriate when relatively thin layers need to be deposited in a short time, usually when the application is printing of skin or some simple epithelial tissue.

However, **extrusion bioprinting** entails the constant deposition of bioink under pneumatic or mechanical action, or solenoid-driven claws. This makes it quite popular because it is able to support a broad variation in bioink viscosity, such as those containing high cell densities or hydrogel combinations. Whereas such an approach allows producing more elaborate and bulkier structures, it can independently impose shear stress on cells, which may compromise cell viability and functionality. Temperature control systems can also be configured to be able to provide stabilization to the bioink during the process with the help of extrusion systems.

In **laser-assisted bioprinting**, a line of pressure or microbubbles is created with the help of a focused laser beam, propelling the droplets of bioink to the substrate. It does away with the problem of nozzle clogging and enables high-resolution printing with accurate cell positioning. Its centimeter precision is suitable for microscale manipulations of applications, e.g., tissue engineering in vascular or nanoscale neural tissue. But spectral resolution and the associated laser systems can be very expensive and demand special substrates, which can restrict their wide use, particularly in low-resource research.

However, there exist new hybrid methods that are bringing together the various methods into one platform by exploiting the drawbacks and advantages of each other. An example is the so-called multimode systems that blend inkjet and extrusion, which can toggle between fine resolution body and bulk deposition, leading to better structural stability without loss of resolution. On the same note, 4D bioprinting, in which the constructs are programmed to evolve over time under the influence of signals, is further stretching the limits of bioprinting to what has currently been done.

All in all, the choice of bioprinting method utilized will be dictated by the purpose of that method, the required resolution, the composition of bioink utilized, and the preferred cell viability. With the advance of the field, hardware, software, and material innovation will further hone the ability of these building blocks of the bioprinting technologies.

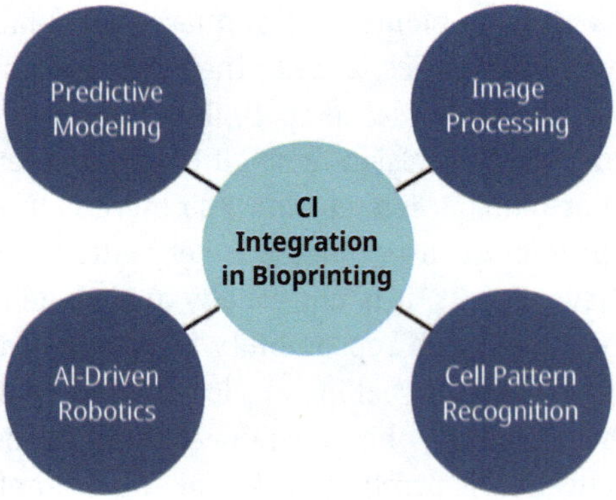

Figure 13.2: CI integration in bioprinting.

13.2.2 Bioink Composition and Limitations

Bioinks are a critical component of the bioprinting process. They must be biocompatible, printable, and supportive of cell proliferation. Common bioink components include **natural polymers** (e.g., alginate, collagen, gelatin) and **synthetic polymers** (e.g., PEG and PLA).

However, there are major challenges:

- **Printability** versus **cell viability**: High-viscosity materials offer better print resolution but can harm embedded cells.
- **Mechanical strength** versus **degradation rate**: Balancing structural support with timely biodegradation is crucial.
- **Cell encapsulation** and **spatial organization** remain complex due to a lack of control over differentiation and cell signaling post-printing.

Table 13.2: Comparison of bioink materials based on biocompatibility, printability, mechanical strength, and degradation rate.

Bioink type	Material example	Biocompatibility	Printability	Mechanical strength	Degradation rate
Natural polymer	Alginate	High	Moderate	Low	Moderate
Natural polymer	Collagen	Very high	Low	Very low	Fast
Synthetic polymer	PEG	Moderate	High	High	Slow
Composite	Gelatin + alginate	High	Good	Medium	Moderate

13.2.3 Challenges in Structural Integrity and Vascularization

Achieving the necessary mechanical integrity and vascular complexity remains difficult. Most tissues require multi-layered, vascularized networks for nutrient transport, and cell survival. Traditional printing strategies often fail to replicate such intricate geometries.

CI-based approaches (explored in Section 13.3) aim to resolve these limitations by predicting structure viability, optimizing layer thickness, and designing microvascular layouts algorithmically. However, current experimental limitations prevent the full realization of vascularized constructs at scale.

To bridge this gap, researchers are increasingly leveraging generative design algorithms and bioinspired modeling techniques that mimic the hierarchical structure of natural vasculature. These computational tools use biological principles to guide the placement and branching of microchannels, ensuring both structural efficiency and physiological relevance. In silico simulations further enable the evaluation of fluid dynamics within these networks, optimizing for oxygen delivery, shear stress distribution, and waste removal.

In spite of these advancements, other problems like cell compatibility in terms of cell types, printability of channels, and degradation of materials over time still exist. A large proportion of bioinks do not even have enough mechanical strength or resolution to sustain delicate vascular structures, devoid of collapsing or deforming throughout the manufacturing process. Incorporation of sacrificial inks, photopolymerizable hydrogels, and cell-laden materials is promising insofar as hybrid printing, but requires better control structures and better coordination between hardware and computational modeling.

Concurrently, bioprinting with multiple materials and coaxial extrusion is being developed to build perfusable vascular tube architecture with functional tissue. They have to combine these methods with real-time monitoring and feedback to guarantee accuracy and reproducibility, ideally at least in the case of printing constructs destined for clinical translation.

Additionally, a post-printing maturation of tissues, in bioreactor conditioning or dynamic perfusion culture, is increasingly seen as a necessary step toward increasing stability and biological functionality of printed vasculature. In this case as well, CI may be instrumental in tracking the environment in which growth occurs, cell behavior forecasting, and environmental alteration to foster the growth of the vascular network development.

In summary, albeit the recreation of the complete complexity of vascularized tissues is still a daunting task, CI-based design and modeling tools are slowly emerging to put the field to the test further. Further advancements will be facilitated through the improvement of experimental tools, the proliferation of the biofabrication toolboxes, and close cross-disciplinary cooperation between engineers, biologists, and data scientists.

13.2.4 Integration Challenges and Print Fidelity

Bioprinting of hybrid structures (that comprise soft and hard tissues) in high resolution is still at its inception. Differences in printing parameters, the environment, and biogink characteristics cause variations in print fidelity and print repeatability.

It is highly possible to have faulty tissue construction due to minor errors in nozzle pressure, ambient temperature, or layer alignment, without direct feedback. Moreover, unexpected deformation after printing leads to poor functionality because of inter-layer bonding and cell migration.

The discrepancy in the rheological behavior of the varying bioinks is one of the fatal impediments to fidelity maintenance. The success of printing composites that contain soft hydrogels and rigidity in one does make uniform deposition difficult. Such variations may cause delamination, irregular surface topology or the insufficient support of overhanging structures. To tackle such disparities, it is essential to achieve a fine coordination of extrusion, temperature control, and curing.

The tissues, e.g., cartilage, bonding of bones, or neural scaffolds, may require much greater details of microscale resolution than usually achievable with conventional printing systems. Mechanical weak spots, as well as defective cell adhesion and poor integration with host tissue after implantation, can be induced by inconsistencies at the micro-level. Developments in bioprinting are underway, including the use of multi-axis robots and microfluidic systems in order to achieve better spatial resolution and interlayer bonding.

To reduce these obstacles, scholars are using CI tools that can dynamically monitor and control the printing process. Real-time sensing platforms combined with an ML algorithm can find abnormalities and automatically change user-set parameters, such as flow rate, temperature, or layer alignment. Labeling accuracy, as well as making the printing less prone to error, this closed-loop feedback enhances the reproducibility over many print runs.

Besides, predictive modeling will be able to evaluate the thermal and mechanical response of printed structures at different environmental conditions. Such observations can be used to make corrections or compensations in advance to account for the anticipated distortions or material shrinkage, maintaining geometric and functional integrity.

Additional validation methods to ensure the quality of complex bioprinted constructs include high-resolution imaging, mechanical stress tests, and viability assays that post-printed grade. By utilizing DL to analyze image, layer uniformity, pore distribution, and cell dispersion can be analyzed quickly, and provide quantitative measures of print fidelity.

Overall, it is possible to state that high-fidelity fabrication in hybrid bioprinting is a complex issue that depends on a variety of variables, both biological and mechanical. Nonetheless, with the incorporation of intelligent monitoring, realistic materials engineering, and real-time CI regulation, the treasure trail of guaranteeing and functional tissue fabrication is becoming more plausible than before.

13.3 Computational Intelligence in Bioprinting

13.3.1 Role of AI in Design and Process Optimization

AI algorithms allow the automatic regulation of the work of bioprinting sites through large volumes of data and find the best printing conditions. AI can track pattern recognition and review historical data to adjust nozzle pressure, control temperature, and determine printing speed in real-time.

Print test: Trial and error is minimized when using AI-based optimization. As an example, reinforcement learning algorithms allow for continuous optimization of printing results through learning from previous trials. They are able to determine such trade-offs as resolution-cell viability or speed-accuracy.

Design customization: data mapping patient-specific anatomy to 3D structures is also supported using AI, enhancing graft compatibility in regenerative medicine.

Moreover, the use of AI-driven generative design algorithms enables them to generate complex geometries themselves, which could not be developed manually. These designs are not only efficient in terms of shape, but also in structural strength, diffusion of nutrients, and biomechanics. The AI design phase involves simulating biological conditions, making the end product have a higher likelihood of mimicking native tissue behavior once implanted.

The other sector where AI can be helpful is the application of multi-objective optimization. Bioprinting has such a complexity of results due to a balance of many variables, including ink viscosity, layer height, cell density, and crosslinking rate. Genetic programming, evolutionary algorithms, and Bayesian optimization are also finding use in finding these desired sets of parameters to meet multiple performance objectives.

AI also plays a significant part in predicting failures and developing in advance to eliminate them before they occur. With the ability to identify hard-to-detect faults in print dynamics, including a change in the extrusion rate or a thermal drift, the AI models will trigger a warning of a possible defect before it physically occurs, slightly cutting down on material waste and print yield.

In addition, the incorporation of AI in the manufacturing process, specifically in CAD (computer-aided design) and CAM (computer-aided manufacturing) workflow, makes the entire fabrication pipeline much more streamlined. AI minimizes manual portions of image segmentation of MRI or CT scans, mesh generation, and print path planning, thereby decreasing the time-to-print.

Finally, the combination of AI and bioprinting changes the entire discipline into an educated process based on data analysis. This transition not only further increases the level of reproducibility and customization but also opens the door to entirely autonomous biomanufacturing systems that could provide fully automated production with low supervision from human workers.

13.3.2 Machine Learning for Predictive Modeling and Error Detection

ML allows predicting how bioink behaves and how tissues develop with time. The models of supervised learning are trained against the material-property datasets to predict:

- Gelation timing
- Structural collapse risks
- Long-term cellular viability

These both assist in lessening paper wastage of materials and printing fiascos since numerous kinds of print are tested in the model before the actual production. Unsupervised ML, such as clustering algorithms, will assist in classifying the various types of tissues according to the behavior of cell growth. Moreover, the anomaly detection algorithms help to track sensor signals and identify preliminary printing faults, false security, space filling curves, information security, and ensure that these errors will be eliminated as quickly as possible.

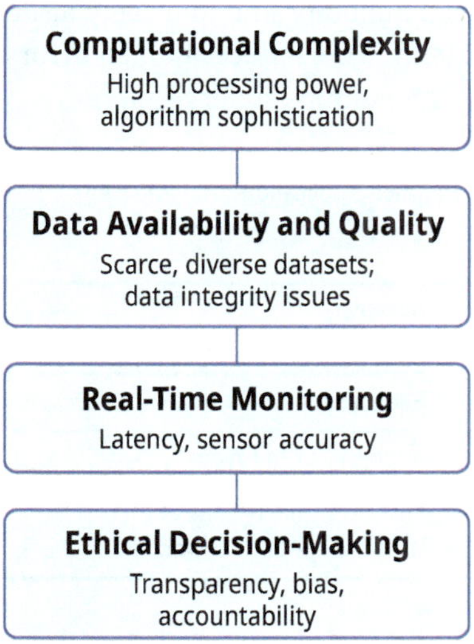

Figure 13.3: Challenges in CI-based bioprinting.

13.3.3 Deep Learning for Image Analysis and Tissue Mapping

CNNs as well as DL contribute significantly to designing 3-D printed design analysis, segmentation of medical images, and quality control automation. DL models and microscopy imaging can find flaws, cell population discrepancies, or pore size or shape irregularities. This enables:
- Real-time visual inspection
- Automated feedback loops
- Enhanced reproducibility

Besides, DL assists in tissue mapping by learning intricate patterns in cell patterns and reproducing the same in the successive layers. This is necessary in the case of printing of vascular structures or pathways of neurons, where the spatial adherence is pivotal.

13.3.4 CI-Based Automation and Robotic Integration

CI extends beyond data modeling into robotics and system automation. In modern setups:
- Robotic arms use CI algorithms to position substrates and bioinks with micron-scale precision.
- **Autonomous calibration systems** adjust hardware components without human input.
- **Self-correcting control loops** use feedback from embedded sensors to dynamically adjust the print environment.

For example, an intelligent robotic system can detect a humidity shift and compensate by altering print speed or ink viscosity, ensuring fidelity. This reduces human errors, boosts scalability, and enables continuous printing with minimal supervision.

Table 13.3: Overview of computational intelligence techniques and their applications and impact in bioprinting.

CI technique	Application	Impact
AI	Print parameter optimization	Reduces trial/error and improves speed
ML	Predictive modeling of bioink behavior	Increases print reliability
DL	Image-based tissue defect detection	Enhances quality control
Robotics + CI	Autonomous positioning and adaptive calibration	Reduces human intervention

13.4 Ethical Issues in CI-Driven Bioprinting

13.4.1 Ethical Implications of Human Tissue and Organ Creation

Bioprinting capable of producing human-like tissues and even organ prototypes raises deep ethical questions:
- Should we create organs-on-demand?
- Can printed tissues be used for human transplantation?
- Who owns or regulates these synthetic biological constructs?

These questions challenge our current understanding of life, identity, and the sanctity of the human body. Creating tissues using **patient-derived stem cells** blurs boundaries between natural and artificial, complicating bioethics, and consent laws.

There's also the risk of **"organ black markets"** or unauthorized use of bioengineered organs, prompting the need for strong governance.

13.4.2 Algorithmic Bias and Data Ethics

The use of AI and ML in bioprinting is inherently data-driven, making the quality and inclusivity of training datasets a critical determinant of system performance. In cases where the datasets are nondiverse, especially based on ethnicity, age, gender, or genetic backgrounds, there is a possibility that the resulting algorithms do not generalize the outputs to other populations. Such misrepresentation may accidentally result in poor tissue modeling, wrong predictions, and poor clinical outcomes.

As an example, an AI model that was trained primarily on patient data specific to the Western population could fail to consider atypical biological and anatomical peculiarities specific to South Asian, African, or Indigenous populations. It may influence such critical parameters of bioprinting as cell distribution density, geometry of the scaffold, or vascularization method. This inequality has the potential of perpetuating the current health inequality instead of lowering it.

Moreover, biased data might lead the AI systems to overfit on the prevailing patterns and consider biological characteristics that are statistically overrepresented, ignoring rare, or minor ones. This may jeopardize the equity and performance of patient-specific bioprinting use. Subsequently, the creation of AI models in this area should be followed by strict procedures of dataset auditing and validation in order to make it inclusive and not affected by errors.

Informed consent as to the use of the information is another urgent issue. Patients tend to deposit anatomical, cellular, or even genomic information without knowing how that information will be processed, stored, or recycled, especially when it will be meshed with complex AI systems. Patients do not have ready access to the strength of data usage, areas of possible risks, or output applications, as there is the opaqueness of the ML pipelines.

In order to tackle these difficulties, transparency, accountability, and explainability in developing AI models ought to be highlighted as ethical frameworks. Patients must become perfectly aware of the ways of collecting the data and their intended use, along with the possible access to the information by third parties. Additionally, data governance should be carried out by interdisciplinary ethics committees that make sure the protocols of consent are well-built and that patient rights are not violated.

Long-term efforts to reduce equity and human-centered design issues in AI tools will need to include the construction of culturally and biologically diverse sets of data, as well as the propagation of fair and equal access to data resources. Such measures result not only in enhancing the durability of bioprinting systems but also in keeping up the ethical standards that are required to enable safe and inclusive biomedical innovations.

13.4.3 Intellectual Property and Ownership Issues

Who owns the design of a printed organ?
- The hospital?
- The AI that created it?
- The patient whose data was used?

Bioprinting powered by CI often results in **autonomously generated designs**, raising ambiguity about ownership rights. This poses challenges in applying **traditional IP laws** to:

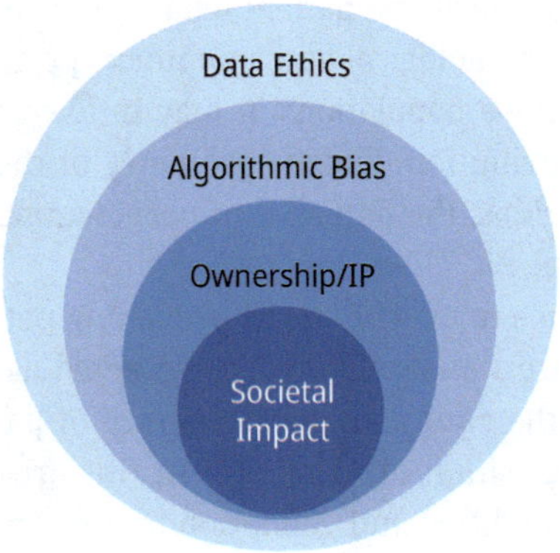

Figure 13.4: Ethical considerations in computational bioprinting.

- AI-generated 3D models
- Adaptive printing workflows
- Customized grafts based on proprietary algorithms

Further complications occur when algorithms trained on **open-source data** are commercialized.

13.4.4 Regulatory and Legal Frameworks

Laws and ethical regulations have not yet caught up with the rapid evolution of computational bioprinting. Key challenges include:
- Lack of **universal legal definitions** for bio-fabricated tissues
- Uncertainty in **clinical trial requirements** for AI-designed tissues
- Absence of standards for **automated decision-making** in surgical implants

Current ethical frameworks (e.g., Belmont Report and CIOMS guidelines) offer limited guidance for **AI-based decision-making** in regenerative medicine.

To navigate this, ethical committees must evolve from static review bodies to **adaptive AI ethics panels**, capable of reviewing algorithmic outcomes and feedback loops in real-time.

13.5 Future Perspectives and Conclusion

13.5.1 Evolving Trends in CI-Bioprinting Integration

Over the past decade, CI has shifted from basic automation to sophisticated, autonomous systems capable of:

- Predictive analytics in tissue morphology
- Real-time defect detection
- Autonomous printing decisions

Recent progress includes:
- Generative AI for organ design
- Federated learning to handle diverse bio-data without compromising privacy
- Use of **digital twins** to simulate biological responses pre-printing

These trends mark a transition from reactive to proactive bioprinting.

13.5.2 Interdisciplinary Collaborations and Research

The fusion of CI and bioprinting demands cross-disciplinary partnerships:
- **Biomedical engineers** must work with **computer scientists** to tailor algorithms for tissue behavior.
- **Ethicists** and **legal experts** are vital in crafting frameworks for algorithmic accountability.
- **Pharmaceutical companies** are exploring CI-printed tissue as testing platforms for drugs, reducing animal trials.

Future research must bridge domains such as:
- Neuroscience × CI for brain tissue bioprinting
- Bioinformatics × DL for genomic-guided printing
- Blockchain × AI for secure, traceable bioprinting pipelines

Table 13.4: Interdisciplinary domains contributing to computational intelligence–driven bioprinting and their respective purposes/impacts.

Domain 1	Domain 2	Purpose/impact
Biomedical engineering	Machine learning	Tissue-specific AI algorithms for accuracy
Bioinformatics	Deep learning	Genome-informed printing models
Ethics	Computer science	Fair, explainable, and transparent AI systems
Neuroscience	Bioprinting	Complex neural tissue fabrication
Regulatory bodies	AI developers	Guidelines for certification and AI audits
Blockchain experts	Medical informatics	Secure biodata tracking across printing stages

13.5.3 Regulatory Innovations and Global Policy Alignment

For CI-enabled bioprinting to move from lab to clinic:
- Standardization of **AI audit trails** is needed for regulatory approval

- Frameworks must assess **algorithmic explainability** and **cybersecurity risks**
- Cross-border cooperation (e.g., WHO, ISO, FDA, CDSCO) can streamline global trials and certifications

Ethical AI must be embedded **by design** – not as an afterthought.

13.5.4 The Vision Ahead

CI-driven bioprinting could, in the next 10–15 years:
- Enable **on-site organ fabrication** in hospitals
- Print **tumor models** for personalized oncology
- Integrate **biosensors** during fabrication for post-implant feedback
- Respond dynamically to patient-specific conditions in real time

The convergence of **cloud-based bioprinting platforms**, **wearable bio-monitors**, and **neural networks** will reshape not only medicine but the very definition of biological repair.

13.6 Future Roadmap of CI-Driven Bioprinting (2025–2040)

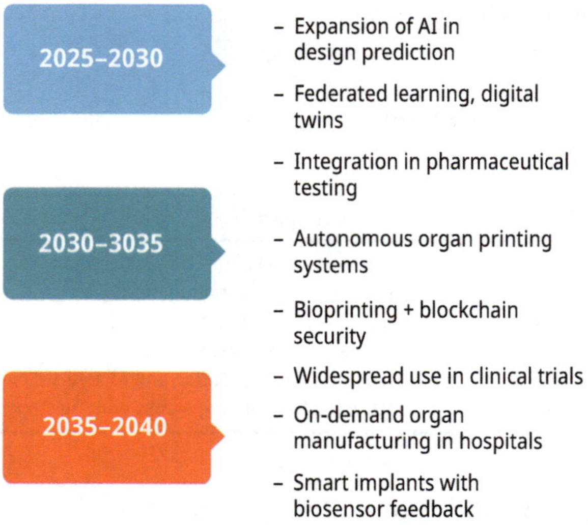

Figure 13.5: Future roadmap of CI-driven bioprinting.

13.6.1 Recapitulation of Key Insights

The integration of CI into bioprinting represents a transformative advancement in biomedical engineering. Throughout this chapter, we have explored the multifaceted ways in which CI – encompassing ML, DL, and autonomous robotic systems – can enhance the design, fabrication, and functional fidelity of bioprinted tissues.

Key contributions of CI include:

Enhanced Precision and Customization: By leveraging data-driven algorithms, CI can fine-tune spatial resolution, control bioink flow rates, and personalize scaffold designs to match individual patient anatomies. This personalization holds great promise for regenerative therapies, especially in addressing patient-specific needs in tissue repair and transplantation.

Improved Predictive Modeling and Process Optimization: Computational simulations informed by historical and real-time data allow for accurate predictions of material behavior, structural stability, and cell viability. Such predictive power reduces trial-and-error iterations and expedites the prototyping process, thereby saving time and resources.

Automation of Bioprinting Workflows: Intelligent robotic systems, integrated with adaptive algorithms, facilitate real-time adjustments to printing parameters, ensuring operational consistency and reducing human intervention. These systems not only boost throughput but also minimize variability between prints.

Real-Time Monitoring and Structural Validation: Through the use of AI-powered imaging and sensor-based feedback loops, it becomes possible to detect deviations, correct defects mid-process, and ensure compliance with structural and biological specifications. This leads to more robust and functional tissue constructs.

Despite these significant strides, several barriers remain. The lack of diverse, high-quality training data limits the generalizability of models across populations. High computational demands, particularly in multi-modal or high-resolution bioprinting, create bottlenecks for real-time implementation. Furthermore, the interpretability of complex AI models poses ethical and operational challenges, especially when human health outcomes are involved.

Looking ahead, bridging these gaps will require a concerted effort from interdisciplinary teams. Future research should focus on the development of standardized datasets, scalable algorithms, and explainable AI (XAI) models tailored to biological systems. As the synergy between CI and bioprinting continues to mature, it will undoubtedly redefine the landscape of personalized medicine and tissue engineering.

13.6.2 Key Ethical and Societal Reflections

We highlighted several ethical concerns:

- **Data privacy** in handling patient-derived biological inputs
- **Equity and access**: Will CI-bioprinted organs only be available to the wealthy?
- **Autonomy**: Can machines decide tissue configuration without human oversight?

Ensuring that **AI systems remain transparent, explainable, and fair** is critical to maintain trust and safety in clinical settings.

13.6.3 Strategic Recommendations

For Researchers:

- Focus on generating high-quality, labeled biomedical data to train robust models.
- Collaborate across disciplines – AI engineers, ethicists, clinicians, and biologists.

For Clinicians:

- Understand the working of AI/ML tools to safely interpret bioprinted outputs.
- Advocate for standardized validation metrics.

For Policymakers & Industry:

- Develop regulatory frameworks addressing **AI explainability**, **algorithmic bias**, and **validation protocols**.
- Incentivize **open-access repositories** and **transparent audit mechanisms**.

For Developers:

- Design AI systems that have lower ethical limitations built-in (e.g. equitability, safety).
- Make sure that it would not go against international health and safety codes.

13.6.4 Final Reflection

Bioforming: The merging of CI with bioprinting is not a technological advancement, but a paradigm shift. It enables individualized, effective, and reproducible tissue engineering, and it forces us to think of new ethical, legal, and social limits.

It is a collaboration of diverse fields and ethical thinking that can make sure that this new science uses itself and benefits all humankind, not harmfully nor greedily, but wisely.

13.7 Challenges in CI-Based Bioprinting

13.7.1 Data Availability and Training Bias

Lack of publicly available high-quality and domain-specific datasets is one of the leading issues in the application of CI in the bioprinting area. Bioprinting involves multimodal data, with effects of cell behavior, material characteristics, and protection healthy systems. Such data tends to be sparse, incomplete, or siloed, so it becomes difficult to apply ML and DL algorithms to these data. Moreover, the data sets in question can be associated with certain bias caused by the unequal samples or too scarce demographic representation, or methodological inconsistencies. Such biases may lead to biased predictive results that are ultimately reflected in the reliability and fairness of CI-made choices in tissue production.

One more urgent issue is the absence of standardized data forms and reporting criteria among laboratories and institutions. That is why this lack of harmonization presents obstacles when it comes to the integration of data and the development of collaborative models. Where data sharing is present, inconsistency in the reporting of experimental parameters, e.g., cell line conditions, printer settings, scaffold chemistries, etc., may add noise into model training and generalization.

Moreover, most models of ML/DL need large amounts of annotated data to discover effective patterns. In the bioprinting field, however, obtaining such annotations not only takes up a lot of time and resources, but they are also validated by experts. This results in the utilization of minimized, selected databases that cannot reflect the entire range of realistic settings of bioprinting.

Training dataset biases can also take the form of overrepresentation of some tissue types, species, or printing methods. Consequently, the models trained on such narrow datasets can show good performance in a specific and constrained condition and be unable to transfer to new materials and other biological contexts or patient-specific adaptations. This again poses a risk to reproducibility, particularly in cases when CI tools are applied in clinical decision-making or regulatory decisions.

In response to these issues, there has been an increasing demand for bioprinting open-access data repositories built in cooperation with academic, industrial, and medical organizations. Such repositories ought to be diverse, transparent, and have an ethical source of biodata. Other methods (data augmentation, transfer learning, and particular generative models) can alleviate the lack of data and the use of sensitive biological material.

To sum up, the effective emancipation of the data sources and the reduction of training bias play a definitive role in using CI in bioprinting in a responsible and efficient manner. Tight data governance systems, interdisciplinary work, and the consistent analysis of the model performance in various conditions will play a significant role in the development of trustworthy and fair AI-powered bioprinting systems.

13.7.2 Model Complexity and Computational Resources

The neural architecture of the CI models of bioprinting tasks, including structural integrity prediction, cell patterning, and real-time monitoring, is usually significantly complex. Such architectures are very computationally costly during training and inference. It needs high-performance computing (HPC) platforms or GPU-accelerated systems that are not available to all research teams. Also, the training of large-scale models requires a lot of energy, which is problematic in terms of sustainability. Finding a trade-off between model performance and resource efficiency presents a major technical and moral dilemma.

Besides, the rising complexity of biological systems that are being modeled demands the need to develop more complex, more profound algorithms. Although DL has proved to have a very strong predictive ability, it is usually at the risk of interpretability and scalability. Due to the growing size and complexity of datasets, as they will now include multi-omics data, imaging inputs, and patient-specific anatomical models, the requirements of memory, processing power, and storage infrastructure grow significantly.

In response to these issues, scientists are starting to investigate lightweight network architectures, model sparse training methods, and federated learning. These alternatives propose to crunch around the computational load at the expense of the predictive accuracy. Such an approach as federated learning specifically enables it to train models on decentralized nodes, providing strong data privacy, as well as reducing the need to outsource such resource-intensive training centers.

Finally, making CI-powered bioprinting technologies more democratically accessible will entail not just the fundamental innovation of algorithms but invest in various kinds of infrastructure, as well. Organizations and governments might feel the need to subsidize open-source systems, cloud AI, and community computing resources to the end that more individuals can become involved in this field that is so quickly evolving.

13.7.3 Reproducibility and Standardization Issues

One of the key shortcomings of the CI-assisted bioprinting research is the absence of standardized protocols and metrics of reproducibility. The discrepancy in the data preprocessing, the model architecture, the hyperparameter tuning, and the validation processes presents an impediment to the comparison of results between different studies. The lack of standardized metrics of bioprinting activities creates another level of difficulty. This heterogeneity not only impedes communal development but also slows down clinical translation. The development of standard evaluation criteria and the open-access repositories of models is the key to the evolution of the field.

Besides methodological variations, some experimental variations, including the nature of the bioinks, cell line, and printing environment conditions, also result in discrepancies in outcomes. There is also a significant variation compared to their performance, even with similar AI algorithms, when differences are varied based on the quality and composition of the training data. This contradiction reduces the applicability and transferability of CI models between laboratories and clinical environments.

Also, data is not documented or shared openly, so that it can be reproducible. Most researchers fail to provide complete details concerning model structures, training examples, or code execution; thus, a researcher has a hard time proving or expanding the work. The most effective methods of increasing transparency should include the publication of reproducible pipelines, standardized datasets, and open-source frameworks that can allow broader use of the technologies.

To provide reliable and stable research and study results, the current requirement is global working groups or standardization committees focusing on CI-driven bioprinting. These organizations may be able to coordinate the best practices, minimal reporting, and benchmarks of performance that every research team may abide by. Such cooperations would smooth the process of innovation and speed up the process of transferring bioprinted constructs safely to the clinic.

13.7.4 Biological Safety and Uncertainty in Predictions

The critical issue with respect to biomedical applications is safety, where predictive uncertainty of CI models is a possible safety risk. In the inexperienced or noisy data conditions, ML algorithms can make significantly confident yet false forecasts. The existence and/ or safety of printed tissues or organs may be compromised by such errors. It is complicated further by the fact that the inner logic of many DL models is hidden, similar to the black box of the systems, and clinicians/researchers might fail to explain or interpret the results of the model. To support the biological safety, it is essential to integrate the uncertainty quantification, XAI, with rigorous validation methods.

Moreover, this is complicated by the fact that biological environments are dynamic. Current models may be unable to predict how cellular behavior would or may change depending on a field of in vivo stimuli. Such a discrepancy of simulated and real-life biological responses can result in non-functionalities or integration failures at the implantation site. Consequently, there must be incorporation of biological feedback loops capable of refining predictions in real-time using live biological indicators.

In addition, regulatory agencies like the FDA and EMA are now also starting to consider how AI-based forecasts can become more reliable in terms of clinical implementation. Having unified measures to measure risks, evaluate performance, and quantify ethical standards will be central to transforming CI-assisted bioprinting systems to life-saving applications. Transparency with pronounced emphasis with decision traceability and the validation process, especially post the print stage, will address the uncertainty that will end up following the algorithmic prediction of regenerative medicine.

13.8 Ethical Issues in Bioprinting

13.8.1 AI and Autonomy in Biomedical Decision-Making

The use of AI in bioprinting systems may make human experts lose their decision-making authority. Even though automation is more precise and efficient, it also evokes ethical issues related to responsibility and visibility. There are also doubts as to who should take responsibility in case of inaccuracy in the fabrication of tissues using AI, whether it is engineers, clinicians, or the AI developers. Human control over essential actions and the creation of AI models that could be applied and understood is crucial to avoid breaches in ethics.

Besides, since AI systems are involved more and more in complex clinical activities, such as type selection of cells or maximization of the pattern of vascularization, there is an increasing need to specify the areas of machine autonomy. The trust taken exclusively in algorithmic results without a certain comprehension might lead to a clinically unsupported result. Consequently, it becomes an ethical mandate to build the concept of explainability and traceability even in AI algorithms, particularly when AI may be applied to ensure the safety of patients.

As a solution to that, a layered form of autonomy should be considered, one in which AI could only make recommendations, but the decision-making should still lie within the hands of qualified humans. It is possible to integrate the rapidity and proficiency of AI and the practical reflection of skilled clinicians in this hybrid model. In addition, the establishment of regulatory standards and audit frameworks that check the decision paths of AI models would be critical in the promotion of trust and ethical adherence of the biomedical AI applications.

13.8.2 Consent, Data Privacy, and Ownership of Biological Designs

Besides privacy and consent, the problem of secondary data application is becoming tense. As soon as a patient agrees to use his/her data to support therapeutic procedures, the issue arises whether or not it can be used in other tasks, such as research work, commercial development, or training AI models. It is imperative to make sure that the patients maintain control over their data repurposing in order to maintain the element of autonomy and ethical transparency.

In addition, the fact that computer models, parameters of simulations, and design files used in applications of AI produce digital versions of biological constructs introduces an entirely new dimension of arguments in the intellectual property discourse. Such digital assets could be easily replicated and changed, and there are some issues of inappropriate use or abuse. Some of the solutions that may be used to protect the ownership rights are licensing agreements, digital rights management (DRM), and blockchain-based traceability.

Also, cross-border bioprinting employment increases regulatory concerns, with various nations prescribing diverse data security principles, medical apparatus categorization, and patient agreement. Aligning such regulatory frameworks will be required to accommodate international research collaboration alongside with ethical standards that are locally considered.

Finally, governance of bioprinted data and constructs should use a patient-centric approach, that is, focus on informed consent, transparency, and equal distribution of benefits. Good faith engagement of the patient in conversations regarding data use and ownership might include the ability to build trust and encourage the safe progression of bioprinting technologies.

13.8.3 Commercialization Versus Humanitarian Use

The ethical dilemma based on equitable access arises from the rapid commercialization of bioprinting technologies. Complex CI-enabled models of bioprinting, as well as bioprinting materials, are also expensive, which may restrict access to more financially equipped facilities or affluent areas. This could intensify unequal access to healthcare in the world. Open innovation, subsidized access in low-resource areas, and public-private partnerships geared toward humanitarian uses of bio-printing should be encouraged by ethical governance.

Furthermore, the patenting and the commercialized approach to research and development of human biological constructs are trivial issues regarding making money. And when proprietary platforms occupy the industry, the innovation and knowledge that are collective might be limited retarding more sciences. The balance between society's benefit and intellectual property rights is an urgent necessity that requires a policy to be developed, more so in the case of life-saving applications.

Secondly, the regulation systems must promote equitable pricing mechanisms and also reward the companies that practice social responsibilities. As an example, such tiered licensing arrangements or international health consortiums might guarantee that life-transforming bioprinting technologies will not belong to affluent countries exclusively. This is because it will be important to address these commercial-humanitarian tensions early and create an innovative yet inclusive bioprinting ecosystem.

13.8.4 Frameworks for Ethical Governance in Bioprinting

The urgent issues of the somewhat comprehensive ethical governance structures that are unique in CI-integrated bioprinting need. Some of the issues that such frameworks should solve are the algorithmic bias, safety certification, auditability, and clinical accountability. An interdisciplinary group consisting of ethicists, technologists, biomedical professionals, and policymakers should be charged with the responsibility of developing dynamic ethical standards. In addition, constant stakeholder interaction and public discourse are the key to earning trust and legitimacy.

Besides technical governance, there is also a consideration of fair access, intellectual property rights, and international regulatory compliance, which should be done. As tissues and organs produced through bioprinting can vary significantly in use, such as cosmetic reconstructions or life-saving transplants, the set of ethical considerations should be relevant and open to changes according to both clinical and research purposes.

Transparency of an algorithmic decision-making is another crucial element in which the AI systems will have the capacity to be auditable, explicable, and accountable in case they have an impact on medical design or therapeutic choice. This can be aided with Ethics-by-Design being a part of the software and hardware development plan, when ethical safeguards would be implemented right at the beginning instead of being tacked on afterward.

Moreover, foreign bodies need to cooperate to avoid such inequalities as security requirements and approval rates of different regions. Establishing international registries of bioprinting experiments alongside AI-powered models would follow the same pattern as drug trials and spark transparency and the ability to compare benchmarks.

Finally, innovation should not be inhibited through governance but, instead, it should be routed responsibly so that this intersection between bioprinting and computing intelligence does not undermine the human principles and values, clinical ethics, and wellbeing of humanity.

13.9 Future Perspectives and Innovations

13.9.1 Integrating Multi-modal Data Sources

An optimistic vision of the future of computational intelligence (CI) in bioprinting is that in the near future the multi-modal data sets that can and should be used in bioprinting applications will be smoothly integrated, varying as they do all the way along the continuum between genomic and proteomic profiling on the one hand, and imaging and biomechanical measurement on the other. With such integration, more detailed models of biological systems can be achieved as well as tissues being made personalized. Highly sophisticated models (such as transformers and graph neural networks (GNNs)) are quite adapted to working with heterogeneous data, which opens the vista of tissue engineering.

Using multi-modal data, the bioprinting platforms will be able to make a more reasonable choice in bioink types, scaffold design, and vasculature approach. As an example, a scan of a patient taken in MRI can be used to complement the cellular metabolism profile in the cellular parts to provide insights into the geometry of the printed tissue as well as cellular composition most adaptable in terms of functionality and regeneration.

Besides, integration enables adaptive learning structures where the performance of printed tissues (e.g., viability after implantation or resistance to applied mechanical stress) can feed back into a future design. With multi-modal fusion, this loop becomes iterative, and hence, bioprinters can move to dynamic learning-based fabrication systems beyond static, one-time structures.

The uniformity of data formats and building systems that are interoperable will play a decisive role in the process of integrating effectively. Further improvements can also involve cloud-based repositories and federated learning models that enable the safe sharing and access to patient data without affecting privacy, and thus further facilitate the collaboration of research and the translation of the results.

Across the board, the issues of genomics, imaging, and real-time sensor information made possible in AI-powered applications can change bioprinting, as an otherwise technical process, into a highly individualized data-guided therapy system.

13.9.2 Advancements in Real-Time AI Monitoring

13.9.2.1 Advancements in Real-Time AI Monitoring

The emerging trends also indicate the creation of AI systems that can deliver real-time monitoring and stream customer feedback in the process of bioprinting. These systems have the ability to identify abnormalities, modify parameters in real-time operations, and provide stable quality. With the help of reinforcement learning and edge AI, it is possible to decrease the latency and improve the responsiveness to a level where printing activities may be comparatively more autonomous but safe.

The present-day monitoring systems built on AI increasingly incorporate the information of multiple sensors, such as visual, thermal, acoustic, and mechanical signals, to form the complete picture of the printing environment. Intelligent systems using real-time analysis of these streams of data can then identify deviations like nozzle clogging, layer overlap, or change in temperature, which in turn would undermine the integrity of the final construct. When detected, corrective measures can be applied on the spot, and waste of materials can be reduced and general reliability can be enhanced.

Moreover, computer vision and DL-based CNNs are in use to conduct live evaluations of printed layers, against digital blueprints, at the micrometer level of accuracy. This layer-by-layer validation flags any anomaly introduced so that it can be removed prior to spreading to the rest of the print, thus improving structural integrity and biological utility.

The emergence of edge AI, in which the data is processed locally on the printing devices, can be seen as a great step in speed and efficiency. Edge-AI eliminates the reliance on network latency, unlike in cloud-based systems, whose services are provided by remote servers. This is crucial more than ever in a bioprinting situations, where time-sensitive and vulnerable biological samples are to be processed.

In addition, the possibility of using reinforcement learning models has been considered, where printing outcomes are used to learn and optimize the control strategies constantly with time. These models will not only respond to the present states, but also make predictions of what would happen in the future by deriving from the cumulative experiences and this will make the bioprinting processes smarter and more adaptable. Safety thresholds and limiting conditions can also be put in such intelligent systems to ensure safety and avoid the occurrence of errors that will possibly harm delicate cell structures or print stability.

A combination of these technologies is leading to semi-autonomous and fully autonomous bioprinters, which will be involved in the performance of multi-step, intricate processes with relatively little human input. Consequently, besides achieving enhanced efficiency of operations, real-time AI monitoring is also opening up an entirely new set of bioprinting opportunities, such as on-site tissue reparation and custom regenerative treatment.

To conclude, in real-time AI monitoring can be considered a pillar of next-generation bioprinting, which has to be fast, precise, and versatile. Increased sensor fusion, low-latency calculation, and intelligent control will continue to drive the move toward data-based, predictive tissue engineering as opposed to trial-based approaches.

13.9.3 Personalized Bioprinting and Patient-Specific Solutions

The personalized bio-printing practice will be a standard practice as the CI models become more accurate and robust, corresponding to the patient-specific dataset used in the design and construction of the tissue. Skin grafting, organ patches, and the usage of AI can optimize cell localization, vesselization, and scaffold development based on individual biological profiles. This transition not only optimizes treatment results but also reduces the possibility of immune rejection.

As medical imaging data, including MRI and CT image files, are becoming more and more integrated into computational processing profiles, a high-fidelity three-dimensional anatomy model of patients can be created. Such digital doubles can be used as templates to design tissue constructs of a more custom-fit nature to reflect both the contour and microstructural characteristics of the desired destination. By so, the bioprinted tissues are able to have enhanced fit and infiltration into the body once placed.

In addition, the ML algorithms can assess the information concerning the genomic, proteomic, and immunologic data of a patient in order to advise on the most promising bioinks and cellular compositions. As an example, AI can be used to predict the immune reaction of a patient toward specific biomaterials or cell types, and based on such a prediction, the clinician could alter the bioprinting plan upfront to avoid inflammation and rejection.

More sophisticated scaffold design is also getting the benefit of CI-driven modeling. Silicon-based generation design can test thousands of geometries of the scaffold in silico, to identify the best scaffold configurations to support cell attachment, nutrient diffusion, and subsequent tissue regeneration. Such designs are not only anatomically tailored but also made efficient with the view of healing faster and integrating with native tissue.

In medical practice, personalized bioprinting has the potential to transform therapeutic processes to those with congenital deformations, trauma healing, or degenerative disorders. It is possible to fabricate autologous tissue constructs by using the cells of a patient via biopsies that are minimally invasive, hence there is hardly any necessity to use donor tissues or use lifelong immunosuppressive medications.

Moreover, incorporating patient-specific bioprinting into biomanufacturing facilities in hospitals is a positive indication toward point-of-care technologies. Assisted by the automation of design processes based on AI algorithms and cloud storage of information resources, the production of custom therapeutic constructs has become accessible and possible within a clinical time frame, shortening the wait time and positively affecting the scalability of personalized medicine.

To summarize, the combination of CI and bioprinting technologies will change the regenerative healthcare landscape. Besides having enhanced precision and efficacy of delivery, personalized bioprinting is a step closer to realizing a long-term goal of individualized, assisted by intelligent machines, treatment using tissues engineered specifically for targets.

13.9.4 Interdisciplinary Collaboration in CI and Bioprinting

Bioprinting is too complex to be undertaken in only one field because it requires the cooperation of such fields as biomedical engineering, AI, material science, ethics, and clinical medicine. Research on cross-institutional bodies and collective forums will stimulate discoveries in the future. To boost development in this frontier area, funding agencies and academic institutions are supposed to motivate cross-disciplinary trainings, cross-disciplinary project collaborations, and knowledge-sharing ecosystems.

The key to avoiding this issue of interdisciplinary discontinuity is that there should be a common ground in the form of language and a format of communication to use so as to bridge the gap. As an illustration, AI specialists should have basic knowledge about the biological processes, and biomedical researchers have to become fluent in the terms of data science. This common literacy may, in turn, be nurtured through cross-training programs, dual-degree programs, and interdisciplinary workshops, and will allow more unified and fruitful collaborations.

Wet laboratories, computation facilities, and clinical test settings shared through one roof in a collaborative research center are becoming the innovation model. Such hubs enable high-velocity prototyping, iterated feedback among computational models and experimental data, and facilitate bench-to-bedside translation. Besides, these arrangements promote the early inclusion of clinicians, which enables technologies to be developed keeping in mind the real-life applicability and patient outcomes.

It is also essential to include ethical scholars and policymakers in collaborative networks. Bioprinting technologies, such as bioprinting, are an up-and-coming tool on the road to clinical and commercial application, and the problems of data privacy, patient consent, equitable access, and the influence that bioprinting will have on society in the long term are gaining paramount importance. These challenges can be intricate to handle, but multidisciplinary advisory boards will assist in changing this situation and help decide on whether the technological advancement will be in line with ethical principles.

Moreover, the global collaboration in cloud-based platforms and open-source repositories can be implemented through methods that allow researchers to communicate in real-time data, tools, and models. The digital infrastructures help reduce barriers to entry for emerging researchers and enhance an inclusive and collaborative culture at the geographical and institutional level.

University-industry and public-private partnerships are also a key graph point in the scaling of bioprinting technologies in the form of international consortia. These alliances allow a collective pooling of resources, pooling of risk, and aligning the R&D objective with healthcare needs. Moreover, collaborative funding processes will facilitate long-term impacts and high-impact research projects that might prove to be too ambitious or expensive to be undertaken by a single institution.

To sum up, computing intelligence and bioprinting fusion is not merely a technological activity but a highly interdisciplinary activity. The further development will rest on the establishment of collaborative ecosystems, where different expertise intersects, ideas flow freely, and solutions are created together in the interest of science and society.

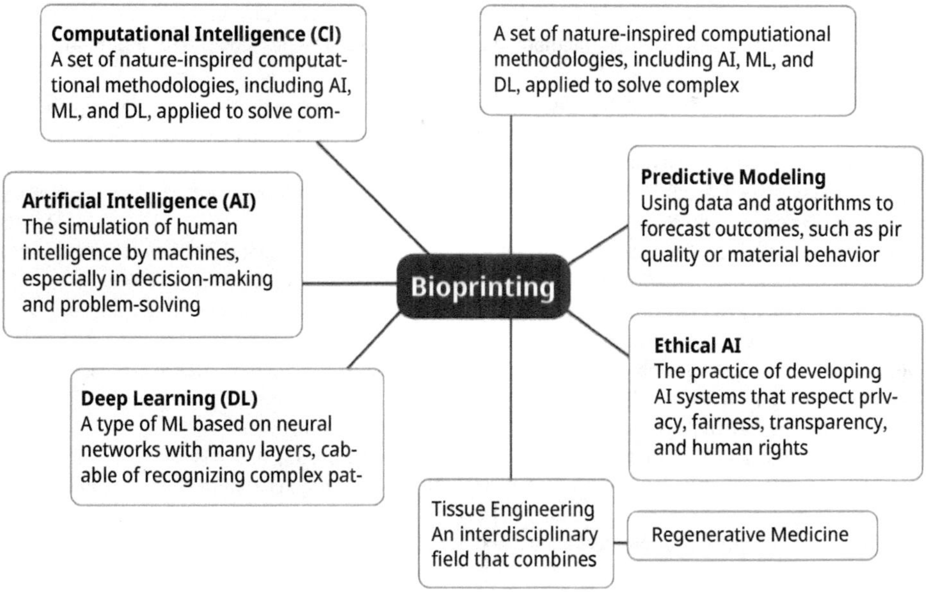

Figure 13.6: Role of computational intelligence in bioprinting and regenerative medicine.

References

[1] World Health Organization. (2021). Ethics and Governance of Artificial Intelligence for Health. WHO Press.

[2] Yang, Y., Wang, H., & Li, H. (2021). Artificial intelligence-enabled biofabrication: From intelligent design to smart manufacturing. Bio-Design and Manufacturing, 4, 313–328.

[3] Sun, W., Starly, B., Daly, A. C., & Burdick, J. A. (2020). 3D printing of tissue engineering scaffolds: A focus on emerging strategies. Advanced Healthcare Materials, 9(1), 1900973.

[4] Liu, Y., Zheng, Y., & Wu, S. (2020). Machine learning for bioprinting: From bioink design to printed constructs. Acta Biomaterialia, 101, 15–35.

[5] Varkey, M., Atala, A., & Yoo, J. J. (2019). Ethical issues in 3D bioprinting. Journal of Tissue Engineering and Regenerative Medicine, 13(1), 1–14.

[6] Wang, X. (2019). Advanced polymers for organ 3D bioprinting. Microsystems & Nanoengineering, 5, 17.

[7] Noor, N., Shapira, A., Edri, R., Gal, I., Wertheim, L., & Dvir, T. (2019). 3D printing of personalized thick and perfusable cardiac patches and hearts. Advanced Science, 6(11), 1900344.

[8] Topol, E. J. (2019). High-performance medicine: The convergence of human and artificial intelligence. Nature Medicine, 25, 44–56.

[9] Floridi, L., Cowls, J., Beltrametti, M., Chatila, R., Chazerand, P., Dignum, V. . . . Vayena, E. (2018). AI4People – An ethical framework for a good AI society. Minds and Machines, 28, 689–707.

[10] Groll, J., Burdick, J. A., Cho, D. W., Derby, B., Gelinsky, M., Heilshorn, S. C. . . . Woodfield, T. B. F. (2018). A definition of bioinks and their distinction from biomaterial inks. Biofabrication, 11(1), 013001.

[11] Ngo, T. D., Kashani, A., Imbalzano, G., Nguyen, K. T. Q., & Hui, D. (2018). Additive manufacturing (3D printing): A review of materials, methods, applications and challenges. Composites Part B, 143, 172–196.

[12] Litjens, G., Kooi, T., Bejnordi, B. E., Setio, A. A. A., Ciompi, F., Ghafoorian, M. . . . Sánchez, C. I. (2017). A survey on deep learning in medical image analysis. Medical Image Analysis, 42, 60–88.

[13] Zhang, Y. S., Yue, K., Aleman, J., Mollazadeh-Moghaddam, K., Bakht, S. M., Yang, J. . . . Khademhosseini, A. (2017). 3D bioprinting for tissue and organ fabrication. Annals of Biomedical Engineering, 45, 148–163.

[14] Choi, Y. J., Yi, H. G., Kim, S. W., & Cho, D. W. 3D cell printing of functional skeletal muscle constructs using skeletal muscle-derived bioink. Advanced Healthcare Materials, 2017(6(6), 1600848.

[15] Mandrycky, C., Wang, Z., Kim, K., & Kim, D. H. (2016). 3D bioprinting for engineering complex tissues. Biotechnology Advances, 34(4), 422–434.

[16] Ozbolat, I. T., & Hospodiuk, M. (2016). Current advances and future perspectives in extrusion-based bioprinting. Biomaterials, 76, 321–343.

[17] Goodfellow, I., Bengio, Y., & Courville, A. (2016). Deep Learning. MIT Press.

[18] LeCun, Y., Bengio, Y., & Hinton, G. (2015). Deep learning. Nature, 521, 436–444.

[19] Murphy, S. V., & Atala, A. (2014). 3D bioprinting of tissues and organs. Nature Biotechnology, 32(8), 773–785.

[20] Bishop, C. M. (2006). Pattern Recognition and Machine Learning. Springer.

Nisha Shankhwar*, Satyendra Singh, Arbind Prasad*

Chapter 14 Integrating Artificial Intelligence with Bioprinting: Smart Design and Optimization of Tissue Constructs

Abstract: The integration of artificial intelligence (AI) with 3D bioprinting is transforming biofabrication from an empirical, operator-dependent practice into a predictive, autonomous, and highly reproducible manufacturing paradigm. Bioprinting involves complex interactions among bioink properties, deposition mechanics, and cellular behavior, which often limit reproducibility and functional outcomes. In this study, we explore how computational approaches can support more predictable formulation design, printing stability, and tissue maturation. By relating hydrogel composition and processing parameters to viscosity, crosslinking behavior, and printability, predictive models help reduce extensive trial-and-error and improve the consistency of extrusion. Image-based analysis provides real-time assessment of filament formation, enabling early detection of thinning, spreading, or irregular flow and guiding timely adjustments to maintain structural fidelity. Adaptive control strategies adjust pressure, speed, or temperature in response to changes during printing, improving uniformity across layers. Computational simulations further extend into the maturation phase by predicting nutrient transport, metabolic activity, and structural development in perfusion bioreactors.

The consolidated framework presented here can support experimental planning, improve the interpretation of variability, and assist in developing more robust protocols suited for tissue-specific applications. While challenges such as data limitations, biological variability, and regulatory requirements remain, the approaches outlined

Acknowledgments: Dr Nisha Shankhwar gratefully acknowledges the financial support provided by the Department of Biotechnology, Ministry of Science and Technology, Government of India, through Project File No. DBT-RA/2022/July/N/2240. The authors thank Prof. Aynur Unal and Dr Mohit Kumar for their consistent guidance and support throughout this work. Dr Shankhwar also extends heartfelt gratitude to her daughter, Vanshika, for her encouragement and understanding.

***Corresponding author: Nisha Shankhwar,** Special Centre for Nanoscience, Jawaharlal Nehru University, New Delhi 110067, India, e-mail: shankhwarnisha3july@gmail.com
***Corresponding author: Arbind Prasad,** Mechanical Engineering Department, Katihar Engineering College (Under the Department of Science, Technology and Technical Education, Government of Bihar), Katihar 854109, Bihar, India, e-mail: arbind.iitg@gmail.com
Satyendra Singh, Special Centre for Nanoscience, Jawaharlal Nehru University, New Delhi 110067, India

 | https://doi.org/10.1515/9783111719993-014

in this chapter offer practical strategies for achieving more reliable and scalable bioprinting.

Keywords: AI-enabled bioprinting, hydrogel optimization, real-time defect detection, adaptive process control, digital twins, tissue maturation, regenerative medicine

14.1 A New Era of Biofabrication: Why AI Matters Now

The integration of artificial intelligence (AI) with bioprinting marks a profound transition from an empirical, skill-dependent craft to a reproducible, predictive, and intelligent biofabrication ecosystem [1, 2]. Traditional 3D bioprinting relies heavily on manual parameter tuning, iterative prototyping, and operator intuition, all of which introduce variability and limit scalability[3]. Challenges such as unpredictable hydrogel rheology, complex crosslinking behavior, nozzle-induced shear stresses, filament sagging, interlayer fusion failures, and inconsistent cell viability underscore the limits of human-guided optimization [4, 5]. These issues become even more pronounced when producing large, heterogeneous, or vascularized tissues. AI provides a transformative toolkit to address these long-standing limitations. Machine-learning (ML) models can predict printability and rheology, computer-vision tools enable real-time defect detection, and reinforcement learning (RL) or model predictive control (MPC) can autonomously adjust printing parameters [6, 7]. The application of AI in biofabrication is shown in Figure 14.1. Digital twins further extend AI's impact by simulating long-term maturation behaviors such as oxygen diffusion, ECM deposition, and metabolic evolution. Taken together, AI functions as a "second brain" for bioprinting systems; augmenting, guiding, and stabilizing every stage of the fabrication workflow [8, 9].

By embedding intelligence directly into biofabrication hardware and software, researchers move closer to an era where tissue constructs can be designed, printed, monitored, and matured with unprecedented fidelity and reproducibility [10, 11]. This chapter provides a technically enriched synthesis of existing knowledge, integrating the mechanistic perspectives and studies from cutting-edge AI-bioprinting research.

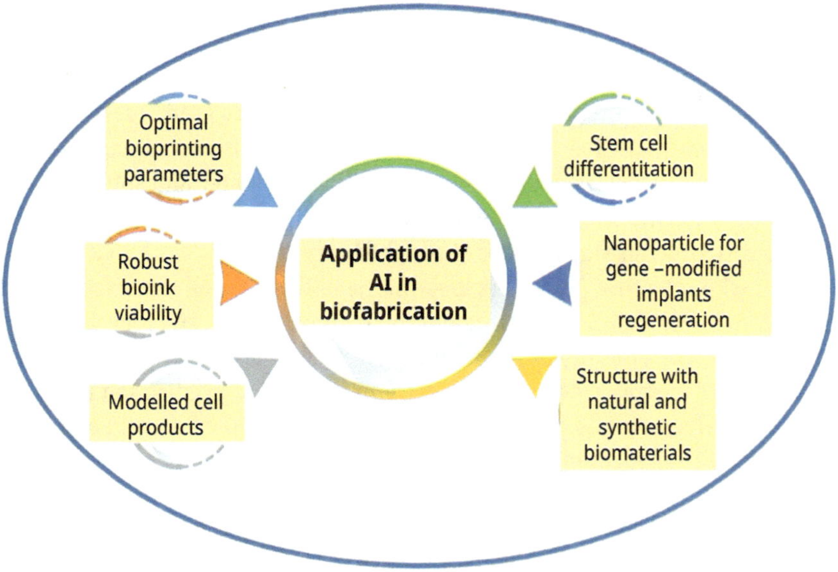

Figure 14.1: Application of AI in Biofabrications.

14.2 The Bioprinting Battlefield: Where Challenges Emerge

14.2.1 Material Complexity and Bioink Behavior

Hydrogel-based bioinks underpin most extrusion and hybrid bioprinting systems due to their cytocompatibility and similarity to native ECM. However, their behavior is inherently complex [12]. Bioinks often exhibit non-Newtonian, shear-thinning behavior; viscoelasticity; yield stress; and time-dependent thixotropy [13]. These rheological properties determine extrusion pressure requirements, filament uniformity, and geometrical fidelity. Small deviations in polymer concentration, molecular weight distribution, or temperature can drastically alter viscosity and gelation kinetics. Shear stresses within the nozzle can reach 1–10 kPa, which may damage sensitive cell types unless viscosity and flow rates are carefully tuned. Thermal and photo-crosslinking kinetics evolve dynamically during deposition, requiring predictive strategies to maintain filament shape [14]. Multimaterial printing introduces interfacial tensions and diffusion-driven instabilities, which modern AI models are now beginning to predict [15]. These complexities form a multidimensional parameter space that surpasses what human-guided trial-and-error can efficiently explore.

14.2.2 Mechanical and Deposition Challenges

During extrusion, pressure fluctuations propagate to the nozzle tip, altering filament thickness and inducing waviness or discontinuities. Temperature gradients across the nozzle influence viscosity in real time [16]. Multimaterial deposition often results in local mechanical inconsistencies, especially in regions where stiffer and softer materials meet. Filament sagging and layer collapse tend to escalate quickly because they depend on yield stress and storage modulus, which are tricky to tune by trial and error [17]. Even when the first few layers look fine, small deviations can stack up and eventually lead to major defects [18]. On top of that, dehydration can creep in during long prints and shift the viscosity of the bioink in ways that aren't always obvious at the start. All of these moving pieces make the process harder to predict and highlight why real-time, AI-driven monitoring and adaptive control are so valuable. Figure 14.2 shows the emerging challenges in bioprinting.

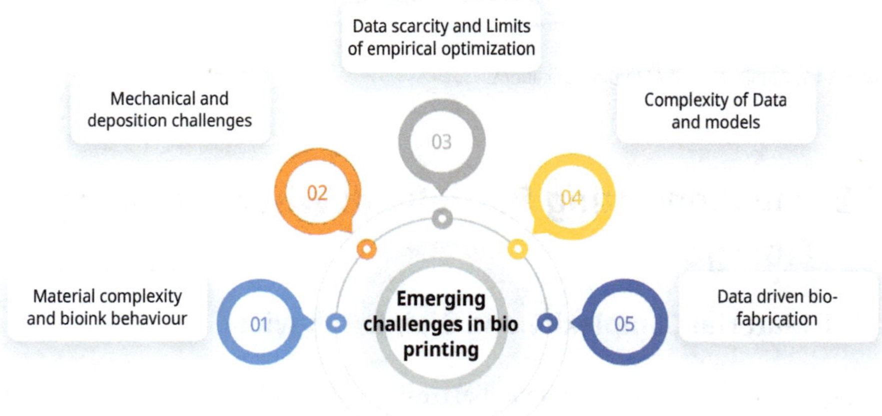

Figure 14.2: Emerging challenges in bioprinting.

14.2.3 Biological Constraints: Cell Viability and Microenvironments

Cells are profoundly sensitive to microenvironmental cues. High extrusion pressures or narrow nozzle diameters increase shear forces that deform or lyse cells. Crosslinking chemistry affects mitochondrial function, DNA integrity, and differentiation trajectories. Post-printing nutrient diffusion is constrained by pore geometry, crosslinking density, and construct thickness [19]. Shear stresses above 5 kPa can reduce viability in MSCs and hepatocytes by 20–40%. Improper gelation timing leads to heterogenous stiffness, affecting cell spreading, proliferation, and lineage commitment [20]. Diffusion limits restrict oxygen penetration to ~200–300 μm, making vascularization and perfusion strategies essential.

14.2.4 Data Scarcity and the Limits of Empirical Optimization

Bioprinting generates heterogeneous data types; imaging, rheology, force sensors, gene expression, perfusion metrics, but datasets are typically small and lack standardized metadata. Human-driven optimization struggles to predict interactions between rheology, printing parameters, cell mechanics, and maturation dynamics.

AI becomes important here because it can capture nonlinear behavior and subtle relationships that are hard to see by hand. It can pull meaningful patterns out of limited or noisy data by weaving physics into the learning process [21, 22]. With enough examples, it can also learn to work across different bioinks, printer formats, and experimental setups, which makes it far more flexible than traditional modeling approaches [6]. These limitations of traditional workflows explain why the field is moving toward data-driven and automated systems.

14.3 Enter AI: Data, Models, and a New Way of Thinking

The growing complexity of bioprinting has pushed the field toward tools that can interpret vast amounts of information and guide decisions with a level of precision that manual expertise cannot consistently achieve. AI has become the bridge between this complexity and actionable insight [23]. Instead of relying solely on trial-and-error tuning or intuition-based parameter choices, modern biofabrication increasingly operates as a data-driven discipline, where predictive modeling, automated interpretation, and multisensor integration shape each step of the process [24]. AI offers a new way of thinking about living material manufacturing, one where data streams converge, emergent patterns are quantified, and every layer of a construct is informed by computational intelligence.

14.13.1 The Rise of Data-Driven Biofabrication

Bioprinting has traditionally involved a vast parameter space that is difficult to navigate: extrusion pressure, nozzle diameter, temperature, print speed, crosslinking intensity, bioink rheology, cell density, and environmental conditions all interact in nonlinear ways. AI introduces a structured method to explore this complexity. Statistical regressors can capture relationships between polymer concentration and shear-thinning behavior [20]. Neural networks trained on printing videos can classify filament stability, layer deformation, and failure modes. Hybrid architectures fuse imaging data with numerical process parameters, allowing models to predict printability or mechanical outcomes with far greater accuracy than isolated approaches [22]. Data-driven biofabrication transforms the field from a craft into a partially automated science, where parameters are optimized by models that learn from thousands of examples rather than by subjective judgment.

14.3.2 Multimodal Data Streams: Sensors, Vision, and Biology

This computational shift is made possible by the diverse sensors integrated into modern bioprinting systems. High-speed cameras track how filaments emerge, adhere, and fuse. Thermal sensors capture real-time cooling and gelation dynamics. Pressure and flow transducers reveal subtle fluctuations in the extrusion path, while load cells monitor mechanical resistance and contact events [25]. In-line spectroscopic tools detect specific chemical signatures during crosslinking or bioink polymerization [26]. As constructs move into perfused bioreactors, oxygen, pH, CO_2, and metabolite sensors provide continuous data on the microenvironment that supports cell survival. Each modality alone offers only a partial view, but together they create rich, multilayered datasets. AI systems use these datasets to uncover hidden correlations, subtle shifts in flow rate that predict nozzle clogging, temperature fluctuations that precede filament thinning, or microenvironment cues that foreshadow hypoxia [27]. This multimodal integration gives bioprinting a new analytical depth and enables real-time interpretation of biological and mechanical processes.

14.3.3 From Raw Signals to Actionable Intelligence

The value of these data streams lies not in their collection, but in their transformation into meaningful predictions. Convolutional neural networks (CNNs) process optical data to quantify filament geometry, identify discontinuities, and flag early-stage defects. Tree-based models like random forests (RFs) and XGBoost provide fast, interpretable predictions of viscosity, yield stress, and bioink stability based on formulation parameters and sensor readings [28]. Physics-informed neural networks go a step further by embedding mechanical laws, flow equations, and biological constraints directly into the learning process, producing models that align with physical reality rather than relying on correlations alone. Digital twins extend this capability across timescales, simulating nutrient transport, oxygen gradients, mechanical stress distributions, and cell proliferation patterns from the moment of printing through days or weeks of maturation [29]. Together, these tools convert raw numerical and visual signals into a dynamic, predictive understanding of both the printing process and the evolving tissue.

14.3.4 AI as the "Second Brain" of Bioprinting Systems

When these computational tools are embedded directly into printers and bioreactors, AI becomes more than an analytical module. AI acts as a second brain for the entire fabrication pipeline. Models can detect anomalies in extrusion and adjust pressure or speed before defects propagate. They can identify the onset of gelation and alter nozzle temperature or crosslinking intensity to preserve filament integrity. During maturation, predictive algorithms estimate nutrient diffusion limits or early signs of hypoxia, prompting adjustments in perfusion flow or biochemical supplementation [30]. In advanced systems, the printer and bioreactor exchange data continuously, allowing the construct's design, printing parameters, and maturation conditions to update in response to one another. The result is a coordinated system in which AI maintains situational awareness, makes decisions in real time, and ensures that every stage of biofabrication remains aligned with the biological and structural objectives of the tissue [31, 32]. In this emerging framework, AI is more of an autonomous collaborator, shaping the engineering of living materials that would be impossible through manual methods alone.

14.4 Designing Better Bioinks: AI as the Materials Scientist

14.4.1 Predicting Rheology, Gelation, and Printability

Hydrogel-based bioinks undergo dynamic rheological transitions from pre-print viscosities to post-print crosslinked structures. Their flow behavior, including shear-thinning, yield stress, viscoelasticity, and thixotropy is determined by molecular interactions among polymers, ions, and crosslinkers [33]. Traditionally, researchers explore only a small portion of this massive formulation space. AI has emerged as a powerful tool to predict rheological profiles from compositional variables. ML models such as RF, Gaussian process regression, and deep neural networks can accurately forecast viscosity curves, storage modulus (G'), loss modulus (G''), gelation time, and printability scores. Studies show that ML models can reach R^2 values of 0.95–0.99, outperforming empirical or rule-based predictions [34]. These tools reduce the number of experiments required, accelerate screening, and identify promising formulations that may be overlooked through intuition alone. By learning the nonlinear interactions between polymer concentration, temperature, degree of functionalization, and crosslinker stoichiometry, AI helps shift bioink development from empirical “tuning” to data-driven formulation engineering [35].

14.4.2 Learning the Viscosity-Viability Trade-off

Bioprinting must balance structural fidelity with biological safety. High-viscosity hydrogels resist deformation and maintain shape fidelity but generate high shear stresses (~1–10 kPa) during extrusion that can compromise cell viability. Low-viscosity hydrogels protect cells but collapse post-printing [36].

AI models help map out how rheology shapes cell survival across different printing conditions, pulling together factors like speed, nozzle size, pressure, and temperature into a single picture. They can estimate how viability changes by predicting the shear stresses cells experience during extrusion, and they can use imaging data from printed filaments to link geometric irregularities to excessive shear or unstable flow [37]. These tools also include fast surrogate models that search through large numbers of possible bioink formulations, making it easier to find combinations that balance print fidelity with healthy cell outcomes.

14.4.3 Inverse Design of Bioink Formulations

Inverse design flips the problem: instead of testing bioinks and measuring properties, researchers specify target performance metrics (*e.g.*, $G' = 1–5$ kPa; viscosity = 30 Pa · s; gelation time = 10 s), and AI proposes the required formulation. Generative models, including variational autoencoders (VAEs), Bayesian optimization, and evolutionary algorithms, can explore theoretical formulation spaces orders of magnitude larger than what is experimentally feasible [38]. AI can suggest compositions involving multiple polymers, nanoparticles, bioactive components, or crosslinking systems, producing candidate bioinks tailored for specific tissues (e.g., cartilage-like stiffness, liver-like porosity, brain-like softness). Inverse design systems are becoming central to next-generation bioink discovery pipelines [39].

14.4.4 Examples of AI-Enabled Bioink Optimization

Studies have shown that AI can streamline bioink design by linking formulation choices to both flow behavior and biological performance. Models have been used to predict alginate viscosity directly from concentration and crosslinking conditions, helping narrow down workable ranges before any lab testing [40]. CNNs have also been trained to classify printability in GelMA systems by examining filament shape and stability. Beyond single-component inks, ML has guided the optimization of composite formulations that incorporate materials like cellulose nanofibrils, PCL blends, and hyaluronic acid hydrogels [41]. In several studies, AI-driven rheology prediction has supported print settings that keep shear exposure low, raising cell viability in MSC and hepatocyte constructs to well above ninety percent. Work in this area consistently shows that AI-assisted tuning reduces printing defects, avoids unstable flow regions, and improves filament continuity [42]. Together, these advances highlight how AI can improve both the fabrication process and the biological outcomes of engineered tissues.

14.5 Watching Every Drop: AI for Real-Time Print Monitoring

Real-time monitoring has moved from a conceptual aim to a deployable technology. Modern systems combine high-resolution optics and lightweight neural networks that analyze each deposited strand as it forms. Convolutional models detect extrusion defects, filament thinning or bulging, discontinuities, nozzle-clogging signatures, and layer misalignment with accuracies exceeding 95% for several defect classes. Recent work demonstrates that this can be done using highly compact hardware: a 2025 MIT-Polimi (Polytechnic University of Milan) platform mounts a miniature digital microscope directly beside the nozzle and uses AI to compare each printed segment to its intended geometry [43]. This modular setup is inexpensive, printer-agnostic, and able to flag anomalies in embedded bioprinting in real time, pushing quality assurance closer to plug-and-play reliability. Complementing this, resource-efficient networks such as BioLite U-Net achieve high Dice scores on real-time video segmentation while running on minimal hardware like Raspberry Pi boards, suggesting that robust defect detection will soon be feasible even on low-cost and mobile bioprinting systems [44]. Beyond binary detection, vision models quantify the evolving geometry of each filament. They measure strand width, height, sagging between supports, fusion between adjacent lines, and deviations from CAD-specified dimensions. These geometric parameters feed temporal models like convolutional neural network-long short-term memory hybrids that track flow oscillations, back-pressure increases, thermal drift, and mechanical perturbations in the printing stage [45]. By connecting geometric trends with physical process cues, these systems generate early warnings before failures propagate through multiple layers. The most advanced platforms integrate this monitoring with automated feedback correction, adjusting pressure, temperature, feed rate, or even recalculating the deposition path on the fly. Prototype printers using these closed-loop strategies show markedly improved reproducibility for complex, millimeter-scale, and organ-shaped constructs.

14.5.1 Hydrogel Formulation Optimization Aided by AI

Bioinks based on hydrogels form the structural and biological microenvironment for cell-laden constructs, so their rheology, crosslinking kinetics, cell-material interactions, and printability must all be calibrated carefully. Traditional trial-and-error formulation is labor-intensive and slow. Recent work uses ML-driven approaches to accelerate hydrogel design. Li et al. [46] review the broader domain of "AI-energized hydrogel design" and show that supervised ML models (RF and neural networks) can predict hydrogel properties (gelation time, modulus, swelling behavior) given component concentrations, crosslinker type, and processing conditions. In the bioprinting context specifically, one study demonstrated an ML-driven predictive model for bioink viscosity based on alginate-gelatin-nano-cellulose compositions (extrusion-based printing) achieving $R^2 \approx 0.99$ and MAE ≈ 0.09 for viscosity predictions [47]. Another investigation compiled a database of roughly 1,200 bioprinting tests across multiple parameter combinations (nozzle size, pressure, temperature) and used neural-network models to classify printability with ~85–90 % sensitivity/specificity [48]. Such advances show how AI can shift hydrogel formulation from heuristics to data-driven design. In practice, high-fidelity hydrogel formulations have translated into improved print outcomes. Chen et al. demonstrated a gelatin-alginate carboxymethyl-chitosan/aldehyde-hyaluronic-acid (GEL-ALG/CMC/AHA) hydrogel, which maintained high cell viability (~91% on day 29) and long-term fidelity of printed constructs in aqueous culture [49]. Although not explicitly AI-optimized, this experimental result illustrates the kind of multivariate outcome one might optimize with ML (viscosity, crosslink kinetics, biocompatibility, and print fidelity). Together, these findings illustrate that AI-driven hydrogel optimization is becoming a viable strategy for improving print fidelity and viability of bioprinted constructs.

14.5.2 Real-Time Defect Detection Using Convolutional Neural Networks

Beyond formulation, the actual printing process introduces defects, filament breakage, porosity, over-/under-extrusion, and misalignment that degrade construct structure, cell distribution, and ultimately function. In other additive-manufacturing domains, the use of convolutional neural networks for defect detection is established. Deep learning (DL) models were applied to SEM images of laser-powder-bed-fusion metal parts to detect cracks and pores, achieving >90% identification accuracy [50]. While these studies are not bioprinting-specific, they establish the feasibility of real-time visual/optical inspection via CNNs. In bioprinting, a "deep learning quality control loop" was recently demonstrated for extrusion-based bioprinting: a closed-loop system uses online imaging, DL segmentation of printed layers, and adaptive parameter feedback to maintain print fidelity. The study reported successful automatic optimization of printing parameters and online monitoring of layer quality [51]. The increasing complexity of bioprinted constructs, particularly those involving intricate cellular architectures like cardiac patches, necessitates robust quality control mechanisms that extend beyond conventional manual inspection [52]. Traditional quality assurance methods are often insufficient to capture the subtle, critical defects that can arise during the bioprinting process, such as filament inconsistencies, cell dispersion anomalies, or void formations, which directly impact the structural integrity and biological function of the printed tissue [53].

14.5.3 Adaptive Extrusion Control: Reinforcement Learning and Model Predictive Control

The printing process itself is a dynamic system: extrusion pressure, nozzle speed, bioink rheology, temperature, and crosslinking kinetics all interact in time and space. To date, most bioprinting systems operate open loop, i.e., fixed parameters. However, control-engineering methods such as MPC or RL could adapt parameters online in response to sensed deviations (filament diameter change, flow rate drift, temperature variations). While directly published studies in bioprinting remain rare, the concept is well-founded in process control literature: frameworks combining RL and MPC have been applied to chemical reactor control [54]. In the bioprinting realm, one can envision an extrusion printer that, during deposition, senses filament diameter via optical or laser sensors, compares to target geometry, and dynamically adjusts pressure, chute speed or temperature *via* an RL agent or MPC loop.

14.5.3.1 Digital Twin Frameworks for Tissue Maturation in Perfusion Bioreactors

A significant hurdle in bioprinting is the post-print maturation phase. Tissue constructs, especially larger ones, require perfusion, nutrient/oxygen transport, mechanical stimulation, and dynamic culture to reach functional-level maturity [55]. To manage this, digital twin frameworks, virtual replicas of a bioreactor system that simulate flow, cell metabolism, and tissue maturation, are emerging. A recent review on "Digital Twins for Tissue Culture Techniques" outlines how mechanistic and data-driven models can integrate sensors and IoT data from perfusion bioreactors to optimize culture conditions, personalize protocols, and provide predictive quality control [56]. One case-study described digital twin integration in 3D bioplotting (scaffold fabrication), where the virtual model tracked scaffold geometry, process parameters and predicted deviations before fabrication [57]. Figure 14.3 shows AI in parameter setting for the fabrication of biomaterials.

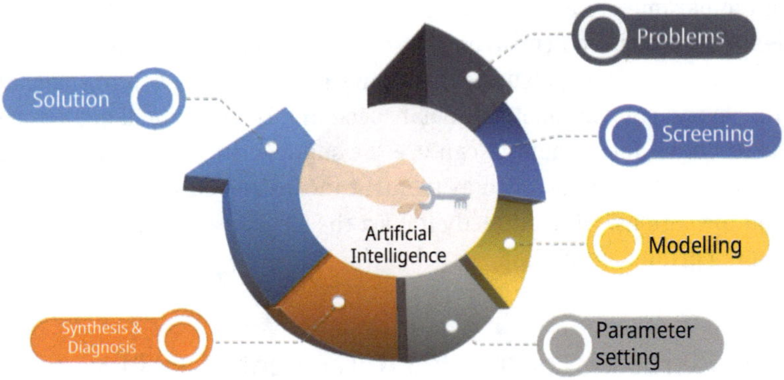

Figure 14.3: Artificial intelligence in parameter setting, modeling, synthesis and diagnosis in biomaterials fabrications.

14.5.3.2 Translational Case-Studies: From Liver on chip to Osteochondral Grafts

Several translational efforts highlight how bioprinting and AI tools might impact engineered tissues [58]. These case-studies illustrate the diversity of tissue targets (cardiac and osteogenic) and the need for integrated control of bioink, printing process, cell viability, and maturation:

i. A bioprinted cardiac patch composed of decellularized cardiac ECM and human cardiac progenitor cells (hCPCs) in a GelMA matrix achieved >75 % hCPC viability post-print and demonstrated angiogenic potential *in vivo* (vascularization in a rat model over 14 days) [59].
ii. A reinforced cardiac tissue patch (RCPatch) combining a stiffness-tuned cardiomyocyte-infiltrated metamaterial and a hydrogel-infiltrated mesh was produced *via* volumetric 3D printing with melt-electrowriting and tested in a large-animal acute myocardial defect, demonstrating hemodynamic destabilization [60].
iii. In bone tissue engineering, a composite hydrogel bioink with human bone-allograft particles achieved ~90 % hMSC viability up to 28 days in a printed scaffold and enhanced osteogenic differentiation [61].
iv. The polymer-biomaterial composite system offers bioactivity and structural support that could be adapted into printable hybrid inks for bone-related constructs. The work shows how moisture-retentive, drug-friendly polymers can create a more responsive healing environment. Shankhwar et al. outline how tailored polymer blends and bioactive additives can be engineered for bioprinted scaffolds that guide tissue growth and integrate with the body more effectively [62, 63].

14.6 Beyond Monitoring: AI That Controls the Printer

Adaptive control is becoming a cornerstone of next-generation bioprinters. RL treats the printer as an evolving environment, learning how pressure, nozzle height, motion parameters, and thermal settings influence print fidelity and cell viability. By repeatedly observing sensor and vision data, RL agents learn to compensate for viscosity drift, batch variation in bioinks, thermal fluctuations, and environmental changes such as humidity. These capabilities are especially powerful for bioinks with shear-thinning or temperature-sensitive behavior, where static parameter sets cannot maintain consistent quality. MPC adds another essential layer by forecasting future states of the print. MPC uses dynamic models to predict shear stress, pressure profiles, temperature distributions, and structural stability, enforcing safe boundaries that protect embedded cells from mechanical or thermal damage. Hybrid RL–MPC systems combine adaptability and safety: MPC defines a physiological and mechanical safe zone, while RL searches for optimal behavior within that space [11, 23]. As real-time monitoring and adaptive control merge, printers become increasingly autonomous. They self-assess layer quality, correct deviations immediately, adapt to new bioink formulations, and scale up prints with reduced operator involvement. Research on robotic-arm–based bioprinting amplifies this trend, enabling multimaterial deposition, improved precision, and in situ bioprinting directly onto tissues or surgical sites [15, 41]. Together, these developments signal a shift toward intelligent, operator-assisting, and eventually operator-independent bioprinting platforms.

14.7 Designing the Architecture of Living Tissues with Generative AI

Generative AI is now central to scaffold and tissue architecture design. Variational autoencoders and generative adversarial models learn from large libraries of scaffold geometries and propose novel designs with optimized porosity, spatial stiffness gradients, nutrient diffusion pathways, and biomimetic structural patterns such as trabecular bone or neural micro-networks [64]. Importantly, these models are no longer constrained to simple geometries. Recent work on model-guided vascular generation can produce full organ-scale synthetic vasculature from inlet to capillary-like branching, in minutes. These vascular trees are computationally optimized for fluid dynamics, shear stress distribution, and manufacturability, and yield watertight meshes ready for slicing [65].

Mechanical and biological performance predictions are increasingly embedded directly into the design loop. Finite-element simulations, computational fluid dynamics, and nutrient-transport solvers evaluate generative designs before printing, optimizing structural durability, perfusion, diffusion, and mechanical stimulation profiles. Once finalized, AI-enhanced slicers convert the architecture into deposition paths that reduce collapse, smooth multimaterial transitions, enforce shear-minimizing trajectories for cell protection, and identify portions that can be printed support-free. These design-simulation-slicing pipelines are enabling scaffolds that push beyond what manual CAD or intuition-driven engineering can achieve.

14.8 When Printing Ends: AI for Growth, Perfusion, and Maturation

Maturation is often the true determinant of tissue functionality, and AI is transforming this "hidden half" of biofabrication. Modern perfusion bioreactors track oxygenation, nutrient concentration, pH, metabolite profiles, and mechanical cues like compression or shear. ML models interpret this data to maintain optimal conditions for cell growth and ECM formation. Digital twins go further by simulating oxygen gradients, nutrient transport, metabolic shifts, ECM deposition patterns, and local stiffness changes over days or weeks. These simulations identify emerging hypoxic zones, predict necrosis onset, and forecast spatial differences in tissue mechanics [66]. Researchers are now testing adaptive perfusion systems that modify flow rates, oxygenation, compression cycles, and biochemical supplementation in real time, guided by digital-twin predictions. Although fully autonomous bioreactors remain in early stages, the foundational elements, predictive modeling, sensor-rich culture chambers, and AI-assisted decision-making are already in place. As these systems become standardized and integrated with printers, maturation will shift from a manual, trial-and-error phase to a controlled, optimized, and reproducible step in tissue manufacturing.

14.8.1 Evidence and Case Studies: What AI-Integrated Bioprinting Achieves

AI-driven printing and maturation are producing measurable improvements across several tissue types. In cardiac patches, real-time defect detection combined with uniform-filament deposition improves electrical continuity and reduces structural discontinuities by up to 40%. Cardiomyocyte viability routinely exceeds 90% in GelMA-based formulations printed with closed-loop control, supporting organized sarcomere formation and synchronized contractions. In hepatic constructs, digital twin–guided perfusion prevents hypoxic zones that typically cause hepatocyte dedifferentiation. ML models predicting albumin secretion and CYP450 activity allow dynamic tuning of culture conditions, significantly extending functional lifespan [67]. Bone and osteochondral constructs benefit especially from generative design and simulation-guided refinement. Trabecular-like architectures with graded stiffness match the mechanical demands of bone while providing diffusion-friendly porosity. AI-optimized slicing strategies maintain the integrity of the cartilage-bone interface and enhance osteogenic and chondrogenic differentiation. Similar successes are reported in neural, adipose, and vascular tissues, where consistent themes emerge: sharper reproducibility, higher cell viability, better structural fidelity, and shorter maturation timelines.

14.8.2 Limits, Risks, and the Reality Check

Despite progress, major constraints remain. Data sparsity, small datasets, inconsistent imaging setups, variable bioink batches, and heterogeneous printer architectures limit model generalization. Researchers increasingly call for standardized metadata, including rheology, extrusion parameters, optics, and environmental conditions, to enable cross-lab comparability. Biological variability introduces another layer of uncertainty: donor differences, passage number, and differentiation state can destabilize ML models trained on narrow datasets [3, 68]. Physics-informed networks and uncertainty-aware architectures help, but are not complete solutions. AI-driven quality assurance must be transparent, auditable, and version-controlled. Automated decision systems used in advanced therapy manufacturing need human oversight, clear risk management, and robust validation. Moreover, many in silico advantages, such as generative vascular networks or digital twin predictions, still lack large-scale in vivo validation. AI accelerates discovery, but it cannot yet reliably model multiscale immune response, long-term tissue remodeling, or host-integration outcomes.

14.8.3 Toward Autonomous Biofabrication Ecosystems

The emerging vision is a closed-loop ecosystem where printers learn from every print, bioreactors adapt to every tissue, and digital twins update with every dataset. Printers will build internal models of bioink behavior, adapt to new materials without manual retuning, and share optimized parameters across networked systems [58]. Bioreactors will pair dense sensor data with predictive simulations to modulate perfusion, mechanical cues, and biochemical signaling in real time. Robotics will automate bioink preparation, cartridge loading, construct retrieval, and bioreactor transfer, enabling clinically scalable manufacturing workflows.

When generative design, adaptive printing, autonomous maturation, and robotic handling are integrated, the result is a continuously improving, self-calibrating biofabrication pipeline. Patient-specific digital twins will feed both scaffold design and maturation targets, supporting personalized, on-demand tissue manufacturing.

14.9 Future Pathways

Near-term progress depends heavily on data: standardized, multimodal datasets; high-resolution monitoring; and multisensor fusion (vision, pressure, spectroscopy, flow). Mid-term goals include validated digital twins, hybrid RL-MPC controllers, automated QA/QC, and ML-guided bioink formulation [69]. Long-term aspirations center on personalized tissues with functional vascularization, multicell organization, and GMP-ready automated workflows [70]. As the technology advances, ethical frameworks, transparent AI systems, and equitable access will be essential to ensure safe and responsible clinical adoption.

14.10 Conclusion: AI as a Co-engineer of Living Tissues

The trajectory of bioprinting is shifting from handcrafted experimentation to intelligent, data-guided manufacturing. Across the entire workflow, AI is reshaping how engineered tissues are designed, fabricated, monitored, and matured. Real-time vision systems and lightweight neural networks have moved quality control from post-print inspection to continuous, in-process oversight. Adaptive controllers built on RL and predictive models stabilize extrusion, protect embedded cells, and maintain fidelity even when materials or environmental conditions drift. Generative models now produce scaffold architectures and vascular networks that surpass what manual design can reasonably achieve, while advanced slicing and simulation tools translate these architectures into manufacturable paths with improved structural performance and biological relevance. Beyond printing itself, AI has become an essential partner in the maturation phase. Digital twins that simulate nutrient transport, oxygen gradients, mechanical cues, and matrix deposition provide early warnings of failure and help tune perfusion and culture conditions to support long-term functionality. These predictive tools reduce the variability that has long hindered tissue engineering and move the field toward reproducible, clinically meaningful outcomes. Taken together, these advances point to an ecosystem in which printers, bioreactors, and design tools exchange information continuously. Such systems learn from every print, adjust culture conditions dynamically, and refine structural designs through iterative feedback. Robotics and integrated sensing will push this evolution further, enabling automated workflows that reduce operator dependency and support regulated, GMP-compatible production. AI's role is no longer limited to isolated tasks. It is emerging as a coordinating intelligence that links design, fabrication, monitoring, and maturation into a cohesive, adaptive pipeline. As datasets grow, standards mature, and regulatory frameworks evolve, the field will move closer to producing complex, personalized tissues at scale. The next decade is likely to bring an era of autonomous biofabrication platforms that operate not as tools directed by researchers, but as collaborative systems that help engineer living structures with a level of precision and predictability that has not been possible before.

In this study, we brought these developments together into a single framework that maps how AI influences every stage of bioprinting. We outlined the current capabilities, highlighted the technologies pushing the field forward, and identified the practical and scientific gaps that still need attention. By synthesizing progress in sensing, modeling, control, design, and maturation, our work offers a coherent view of where AI-integrated bioprinting stands today and where it is headed. This perspective can guide researchers, engineers, and clinicians as they develop the next generation of intelligent biofabrication systems.

References

[1] Javaid, F., Hassan, M. H. U., Butt, E. N., Shafique, F., Khan, A. H., & Pervaiz, R. (Jun 2025). Recent Advances in 3D Bioprinting and Biofabrication. Futuristic Biotechnology, 10–15. doi: 10.54393/fbt.v5i2.170.

[2] Pathak, K. et al. (Dec 2023). 3D printing in biomedicine: Advancing personalized care through additive manufacturing. Exploration of Medicine, 4(6), 1135–1167. doi: 10.37349/emed.2023.00200.

[3] Shankhwar, N., & Prasad, A. (2025). Bioimplants with 3D and 4D Additive Manufacturing Processes. pp. 217–241. doi: 10.1007/978-981-96-9306-1_9.

[4] Ahmad, S., Alam, H., & Thareja, P. (2025). 3D printing of hydrogels: A synergistic approach of rheology and computational fluid dynamics (CFD) modeling. RSC Advances. 15(47). 39369–39390. doi: 10.1039/D5RA04380H.

[5] Yu, K. et al. (Dec 2025). Defects, monitoring, and AI-enabled control in soft material additive manufacturing: A review. Virtual and Physical Prototyping, 20(1). doi: 10.1080/17452759.2025.2588456.

[6] Ye, L. et al. (Oct 2025). Artificial intelligence in rheumatology: A transformative perspective. Journal of Translational Internal Medicine, 13(5), 390–393. doi: 10.1515/jtim-2025-0046.

[7] Song, Y., & Zhang, A. (Sep 2025). From black box to physically interpretable: Trustworthy computing for AI-driven decision-making and control. Journal of Automation and Intelligence. doi: 10.1016/j.jai.2025.09.003.

[8] Sun, Y., & Pan, W. (Nov 2025). Brain organoids: A new paradigm for studying human neuropsychiatric disorders. Frontiers in Neuroscience, 19. doi: 10.3389/fnins.2025.1699814.

[9] Kakni, P., Truckenmüller, R., Habibović, P., & Giselbrecht, S. (Aug 2022). Challenges to, and prospects for, reverse engineering the gastrointestinal tract using organoids. Trends in Biotechnology, 40(8), 932–944. doi: 10.1016/j.tibtech.2022.01.006.

[10] Yücer, S., Sarac, B., & Ciftci, F. (Nov, 2025). Bioprinting revolution: Innovative design of 3D bioactive scaffolds for living organs and transdermal tissues. Bioengineering and Translational Medicine, 10(6), doi: 10.1002/btm2.70080.

[11] Mirshafiei, M., Rashedi, H., Yazdian, F., Rahdar, A., & Baino, F. (Apr 2024). Advancements in tissue and organ 3D bioprinting: Current techniques, applications, and future perspectives. Materials and Design, 240. pp. 112853. doi: 10.1016/j.matdes.2024.112853.

[12] Gogoi, D., Kumar, M., & Singh, J. (Aug 2024). A comprehensive review on hydrogel-based bio-ink development for tissue engineering scaffolds using 3D printing. Annals of 3D Printed Medicine, 15. pp. 100159. doi: 10.1016/j.stlm.2024.100159.

[13] Iyer, K. S. et al. (Jun 2025). Microgel-based bioink for extrusion-based 3D bioprinting and its applications in tissue engineering. Bioactive Materials, 48, 273–293. doi: 10.1016/j.bioactmat.2025.02.003.

[14] Schwab, A., Levato, R., D'Este, M., Piluso, S., Eglin, D., & Malda, J. (Oct 2020). Printability and shape fidelity of bioinks in 3D bioprinting. Chemical Reviews, 120(19), 11028–11055. doi: 10.1021/acs.chemrev.0c00084.

[15] Lai, J. et al. (Jul 2024). 4D bioprinting of programmed dynamic tissues. Bioactive Materials, 37, 348–377. doi: 10.1016/j.bioactmat.2024.03.033.

[16] Vaes, D., & Van Puyvelde, P. (Jul 2021). Semi-crystalline feedstock for filament-based 3D printing of polymers. Progress in Polymer Science, 118. pp. 101411. doi: 10.1016/j.progpolymsci.2021.101411.

[17] Shankhwar, N., Unal, A., & Singh, S. (2025). Nanomedicine in patient-specific clinical trend: Shape memory polymers for emerging biomedical applications and their future prospects. In: Nanomedicine in Translational Research, Elsevier. pp. 309–338. doi: 10.1016/B978-0-443-22257-3.00014-3.

[18] Huo, T., Zhou, L., Bian, X., & Wen, Y. (Jun 2025). Advancing microneedle technology for multiple distinct target organs drug delivery through 3D printing: A comprehensive review. Advanced Composites and Hybrid Materials, 8(3), 266. doi: 10.1007/s42114-025-01336-8.

[19] Rojek, K. O., Ćwiklińska, M., Kuczak, J., & Guzowski, J. (Nov 2022). Microfluidic formulation of topological hydrogels for microtissue engineering. Chemical Reviews., 122(22), 16839–16909. doi: 10.1021/acs.chemrev.1c00798.

[20] Ji, Q., Wang, Y. L., Xia, L. M., Yang, Y., Wang, C. S., & Mei, Y. Q. (Dec 2019). High shear stress suppresses proliferation and migration but promotes apoptosis of endothelial cells co-cultured with vascular smooth muscle cells via down-regulating MAPK pathway. Journal of Cardiothoracic Surgery, 14(1), 216. doi: 10.1186/s13019-019-1025-5.

[21] Wang, Y., Wang, K., & Zhang, C. (Oct 2024). Applications of artificial intelligence/machine learning to high-performance composites. Composites Part B: Engineering, 285. pp. 111740. doi: 10.1016/j.compositesb.2024.111740.

[22] Butler, K. T., Davies, D. W., Cartwright, H., Isayev, O., & Walsh, A. (Jul 2018). Machine learning for molecular and materials science. Nature, 559(7715), 547–555. doi: 10.1038/s41586-018-0337-2.

[23] Robazzi, J. V. S. et al. (Oct 2025). The synergy of artificial intelligence and 3d bioprinting: unlocking new frontiers in precision and tissue fabrication. Advanced Functional Materials. doi: 10.1002/adfm.202509530.

[24] Yaneva, A. et al. (Aug 2023). The progress in bioprinting and its potential impact on health-related quality of life. Bioengineering, 10(8), 910. doi: 10.3390/bioengineering10080910.

[25] Murthy, H., Thakur, N., & Shankhwar, N. (2022). Nickel-based inks for flexible electronics – a review on recent trends. Journal of Advanced Manufacturing Systems. 21(3). 591–624. doi: 10.1142/S0219686722500214.

[26] Hinton, T. J., Lee, A., & Feinberg, A. W. (Mar 2017). 3D bioprinting from the micrometer to millimeter length scales: Size does matter. Current Opinion in Biomedical Engineering, 1. pp. 31–37. doi: 10.1016/j.cobme.2017.02.004.

[27] Matavosian, A. A., & Bonassar, L. J. (Oct 2025). Reimagining bioprinters: Real-time monitoring for quality control of bioprinted constructs and future vision. Biofabrication, 17(4), 042008. doi: 10.1088/1758-5090/ae11d4.

[28] Chen, J., Deng, Y., Bai, G., & Su, G. (Jan 2015). Face image quality assessment based on learning to rank. IEEE Signal Processing Letters, 22(1), 90–94. doi: 10.1109/LSP.2014.2347419.

[29] Iliuţă, M.-E., Moisescu, M.-A., Pop, E., Ionita, A.-D., Caramihai, S.-I., & Mitulescu, T.-C. (Jun 2024). Digital twin – a review of the evolution from concept to technology and its analytical perspectives on applications in various fields. Applied Sciences, 14(13), 5454. doi: 10.3390/app14135454.

[30] Yu, J., Yao, D., Wang, L., & Xu, M. (Jul 2025). Machine learning in predicting and optimizing polymer printability for 3D bioprinting. Polymers (Basel), 17(13), 1873. doi: 10.3390/polym17131873.

[31] Górriz, J. M. et al. (Oct 2020). Artificial intelligence within the interplay between natural and artificial computation: Advances in data science, trends and applications. Neurocomputing, 410, 237–270. doi: 10.1016/j.neucom.2020.05.078.

[32] Gokcekuyu, Y., Ekinci, F., Guzel, M. S., Acici, K., Aydin, S., & Asuroglu, T. (Jul 2024). Artificial intelligence in biomaterials: A comprehensive review. Applied Sciences, 14(15), 6590. doi: 10.3390/app14156590.

[33] Karvinen, J., & Kellomäki, M. (Jul 2023). Design aspects and characterization of hydrogel-based bioinks for extrusion-based bioprinting. Bioprinting, 32, e00274. doi: 10.1016/j.bprint.2023.e00274.

[34] Calafel, M. I., Criado-Gonzalez, M., Aguirresarobe, R., Fernández, M., & Mijangos, C. (2025). From rheological concepts to additive manufacturing assessment of hydrogel-based materials for advanced bioprinting applications. Materials Advances. 6(14). 4566–4597. doi: 10.1039/D5MA00019J.

[35] Elango, J., & Zamora-Ledezma, C. (Aug 2025). Rheological, structural, and biological trade-offs in bioink design for 3D bioprinting. Gels, 11(8), 659. doi: 10.3390/gels11080659.

[36] Oh, D., Shirzad, M., Chang Kim, M., Chung, E.-J., & Nam, S. Y. (Aug 2023). Rheology-informed hierarchical machine learning model for the prediction of printing resolution in extrusion-based bioprinting. International Journal of Bioprinting, 9(6), 1280. doi: 10.36922/ijb.1280.

[37] Malekpour, A., & Chen, X. (Apr 2022). Printability and cell viability in extrusion-based bioprinting from experimental, computational, and machine learning views. Journal of Functional Biomaterials, 13(2), 40. doi: 10.3390/jfb13020040.

[38] Griffin, M. R., Bertram, S. E., Robison, N. P., Panoskaltsis-Mortari, A., Janardan, R., & McAlpine, M. C. (Aug 2025). 3D vector field-guided toolpathing for 3D bioprinting. Communications Engineering, 4(1), 154. doi: 10.1038/s44172-025-00489-0.

[39] Aubin, H. et al. (Sep 2010). Directed 3D cell alignment and elongation in microengineered hydrogels. Biomaterials, 31(27), 6941–6951. doi: 10.1016/j.biomaterials.2010.05.056.

[40] Byrne, R., Carrico, A., Lettieri, M., Rajan, A. K., Forster, R. J., & Cumba, L. R. (Oct. 2024). Bioinks and biofabrication techniques for biosensors development: A review. Materials Today Bio, 28. pp. 101185. doi: 10.1016/j.mtbio.2024.101185.

[41] Sun, J., Yao, K., An, J., Jing, L., Huang, K., & Huang, D. (Aug 2024). Machine learning and 3D bioprinting. International Journal of Bioprinting, 9(4), 717. doi: 10.18063/ijb.717.

[42] Cidonio, G., Glinka, M., Dawson, J. I., & Oreffo, R. O. C. (Jul 2019). The cell in the ink: Improving biofabrication by printing stem cells for skeletal regenerative medicine. Biomaterials, 209. pp. 10–24. doi: 10.1016/j.biomaterials.2019.04.009.

[43] Duran, P. Researchers from MIT and the Polytechnic University of Milan Create Modular, Printer-Agnostic Monitoring Tool for 3D Bioprinting Available: https://3dprintingindustry.com/news/researchers-from-mit-and-the-polytechnic-university-of-milan-create-modular-printer-agnostic-monitoring-tool-for-3d-bioprinting244574/#:~:text=51am00-,0Shares,atlarge%2C"saysColosimo.

[44] Haider, U., Szemet, L., Kelly, D., Sergis, V., Daly, A. C., & Mason, K. (Sep. 2025). BioLite U-Net: Edge-Deployable Semantic Segmentation for In Situ Bioprinting Monitoring. Available: http://arxiv.org/abs/2509.06690.

[45] Kim, H. et al. (Aug 2025). Advances and perspectives in fiber-based electronic devices for next-generation soft systems. Npj Flexible Electronics, 9(1), 84. doi: 10.1038/s41528-025-00465-w.

[46] Li, Z. et al. (Apr 2024). AI energized hydrogel design, optimization and application in biomedicine. Materials Today Bio, 25, 101014. doi: 10.1016/j.mtbio.2024.101014.

[47] Habib, A., Sarah, R., Tuladhar, S., Khoda, B., & Limon, S. M. (2024). Modulating rheological characteristics of bio-ink with component weight and shear rate for enhanced bioprinted scaffold fidelity. Bioprinting. 38. e00332. doi: 10.1016/j.bprint.2024.e00332.
[48] Mace, M. A. M., Reginatto, C. L., Soares, R. M. D., & Fuentefria, A. M. (Apr 2024). Three-dimensional printing of medical devices and biomaterials with antimicrobial activity: A systematic review. Bioprinting, 38. pp. e00334. doi: 10.1016/j.bprint.2024.e00334.
[49] Chen, H. et al. (Apr 2021). A facile, versatile hydrogel bioink for 3D bioprinting benefits long-term subaqueous fidelity, cell viability and proliferation. Regenerative Biomaterials, 8(3). doi: 10.1093/rb/rbab026.
[50] Wen, H., Huang, C., & Guo, S. (May 2021). The application of convolutional neural networks (CNNs) to recognize defects in 3D-printed parts. Materials, 14(10), 2575. doi: 10.3390/ma14102575.
[51] Bonatti, A. F., Vozzi, G., Chua, C. K., & De Maria, C. (Oct 2022). A deep learning quality control loop of the extrusion-based bioprinting process. International Journal of Bioprinting, 8(4), 620. doi: 10.18063/ijb.v8i4.620.
[52] Zhao, X., Chen, Y., Jiang, Y., Radenbaugh, A., Moskwa, J., & Jensen, D., "Machine Learning Approaches for Defect Detection in a Microwell-based Medical Device," Sep. 2024, [Online]. Available: http://arxiv.org/abs/2409.07551
[53] Barjuei, E. S., Shin, J., Kim, K., & Lee, J. (Aug 2024). Precision improvement of robotic bioprinting via vision-based tool path compensation. Scientific Reports, 14(1), 17764. doi: 10.1038/s41598-024-68597-z.
[54] Alhazmi, K., Albalawi, F., & Sarathy, S. M. (May 2021). A Reinforcement Learning-based Economic Model Predictive Control Framework for Autonomous Operation of Chemical Reactors. arXiv:2105.02656.
[55] Shankhwar, N., Saha, P., Zurek-Mortka, M., Thomas, S., & Unal, A. (2022). Tissue engineered products-Translational avenues. Tissue Engineering: Current Status and Challenges. 575–625 doi: 10.1016/B978-0-12-824064-9.00007-1.
[56] Möller, J., & Pörtner, R. (Mar 2021). Digital twins for tissue culture techniques – concepts, expectations, and state of the art. Processes, 9(3), 447. doi: 10.3390/pr9030447.
[57] Ahmed, N., Narayanan, L. K., & Shirwaiker, R. (Oct 2024). A framework for digital twin integration in biofabrication and a scaffold 3D bioplotting case study. Manufacturing Letters, 41. pp. 1182–1191. doi: 10.1016/j.mfglet.2024.09.144.
[58] Shankhwar, N. et al. (February 2025). Integrating advanced synthesis techniques and AI-driven approaches with nanofiber technology: A state-of-the-art approach to wound care management. Next Nanotechnology, 8, pp. 100147. doi: 10.1016/j.nxnano.2025.100147.
[59] Bejleri, D. et al. (Dec 2018). A bioprinted cardiac patch composed of cardiac-specific extracellular matrix and progenitor cells for heart repair. Advanced Healthcare Materials, 7(23). doi: 10.1002/adhm.201800672.
[60] Jones, L. S. et al. (Nov 2025). Volumetric 3D printing and melt-electrowriting to fabricate implantable reinforced cardiac tissue patches. Advanced Materials, 37(45). doi: 10.1002/adma.202504765.
[61] Gharacheh, H., & Guvendiren, M. (Sep 2022). Cell-laden composite hydrogel bioinks with human bone allograft particles to enhance stem cell osteogenesis. Polymers (Basel), 14(18), 3788. doi: 10.3390/polym14183788.
[62] Shankhwar, N. et al. (2016). Electrospun polyvinyl alcohol-polyvinyl pyrrolidone nanofibrous membranes for interactive wound dressing application. Journal of Biomaterials Science, Polymer Edition, 27(3), 247–262. doi: 10.1080/09205063.2015.1120474.
[63] Shankhwar, N. et al. (2016). Novel polyvinyl alcohol-bioglass 45S5 based composite nanofibrous membranes as bone scaffolds. Materials Science and Engineering C, 69, 1167–1174. doi: 10.1016/j.msec.2016.08.018.

[64] Zhang, Z., Zhou, X., Fang, Y., Xiong, Z., & Zhang, T. (Mar 2025). AI-driven 3D bioprinting for regenerative medicine: From bench to bedside. Bioactive Materials, 45. pp. 201–230. doi: 10.1016/j.bioactmat.2024.11.021.
[65] Yiannoudes, S. (Oct 2025). Shaping architecture with generative artificial intelligence: Deep learning models in architectural design workflow. Architecture, 5(4), 94. doi: 10.3390/architecture5040094.
[66] Tokeshi, M. (ed.). (2024). Applications of microfluidic systems in biology and medicine. In: Bioanalysis Vol. 13 Springer Nature Singapore. doi: 10.1007/978-981-97-6540-9.
[67] Zhang, B., Luo, Y., Zhou, X., Gao, L., Yin, X., & Yang, H. (Jun, 2024). GelMA micropattern enhances cardiomyocyte organization, maturation, and contraction via contact guidance. APL Bioengineering, 8(2), doi: 10.1063/5.0182585.
[68] Shankhwar, N. et al. (2025). Background, History, and Introduction to Resorbable Composites for Implants and Fixation Devices. pp. 1–29. doi: 10.1007/978-981-96-9306-1_1.
[69] Shankhwar, N. et al. (2025). Advancing mental healthcare: AI-driven tools, clinical integration, challenges, and future directions. In: Artificial Intelligence and Brain Computer Interfaces in Healthcare. ACADEMIC Press, Elsevier.
[70] Iliadis, I. et al. (Oct 2025). Applications of modern cell therapies: The latest data in ophthalmology. Life, 15(10), 1610. doi: 10.3390/life15101610.

N. Vishnudevi*, T. Thenmozhi*, S. Vijayasharmila*

Chapter 15
Challenges, Ethical Issues, and Perspectives in Bioprinting

Abstract: One new area of biotechnology is three-dimensional bioprinting technology. The primary driver for the development of this technology is the global organ donation scarcity and the necessity for organ transplantation. Three-dimensional (3D) bioethics and its legal implications have not yet received much attention from bioethicists worldwide, especially in Russia. 3D bioprinting poses a number of interdisciplinary challenges related to contemporary science, technology, bioethics, and philosophy in addition to the problems associated with the sophisticated methods of printing human tissues and organs. The practicality of creating these technologies and their morality are among the first concerns surrounding the use of bioprinting to create organs and tissues. This is also crucial to keep an eye on how quickly these technologies are evolving in order to spot and research ethical issues before a therapeutic 3D bioprinting is prepared for general patient use. Stem cells are frequently employed as "building blocks" in the bio-fabrication of human tissue and organs. The "source" of stem cells is the primary ethical concern. Human embryonic stem cell (HESC) use has been widely criticized and has significant ethical and legal restrictions. While assessing the ethics of bioprinting, it is also important to keep in mind that the technology is based on a digital model. According to several authors, the advancement of 3D bioprinting technology causes the "digitalization" of tangible objects, blurs the lines between the real and virtual worlds, and begins to digitize the individual.

Keywords: 3D bioprinting, HESC, three-dimensional (3D) bioprinting, computational modeling, stem cells

***Corresponding author: N. Vishnudevi**, Department of Electronics Engineering (VLSI), Velammal College of Engineering and Technology, Viraganoor, Madurai 625 009, Tamil Nadu, India, e-mail: Vichu0408@gmail.com
***Corresponding author: T. Thenmozhi**, Department of Electronics and Communication Engineering, Velammal College of Engineering and Technology, Viraganoor, Madurai 625 009, Tamil Nadu, India, e-mail: thenvishnu2015@gmail.com
***Corresponding author: S. Vijayasharmila**, Department of Information and Technology, K.L.N. College of Engineering, Madurai, Tamil Nadu, India, e-mail: vijayasharmila.s@gmail.com

 | https://doi.org/10.1515/9783111719993-015

15.1 Introduction

Bioprinting, a revolutionary convergence of biology, engineering, and material science, offers transformative potential for regenerative medicine and organ transplantation. However, alongside its promising applications, bioprinting introduces complex ethical, legal, and social concerns. This chapter explores the multidimensional challenges and ethical issues posed by bioprinting while offering future perspectives.

15.2 Background of Bioprinting

15.2.1 Definition and Concept

Three-dimensional (3D) bioprinting is a specialized form of additive manufacturing that involves the precise layering of biological materials, cells, and biomolecules to fabricate tissue-like structures that imitate natural human tissues and organs [8, 48]. The concept is rooted in traditional 3D printing technology but tailored for biomedical applications. Unlike conventional printing materials such as plastic or metal, bioprinting utilizes bioinks – mixtures of living cells and supportive biomaterials – that are deposited layer by layer to construct complex biological forms [1]. This technology enables the creation of personalized and functional biological constructs that could eventually be used for regenerative medicine, drug testing, and organ transplantation.

The definition of 3D bioprinting encompasses more than just the printing process itself. It also includes the pre-printing phase, which involves imaging, modeling, and computer-aided design (CAD) to develop a digital blueprint of the desired tissue [13]. During printing, various bioprinters use extrusion-based, inkjet, or laser-assisted techniques to deposit bioinks in spatially controlled patterns [10]. Post-printing steps involve maturation and conditioning of the printed structure in bioreactors to promote tissue development and vascularization [7]. This integrative process positions 3D bioprinting at the intersection of engineering, biology, and medicine, with the potential to revolutionize therapeutic strategies and clinical practice [48].

15.2.2 Historical Evolution

The evolution of 3D bioprinting is the result of decades of advancements in both biotechnology and additive manufacturing [8]. The roots of bioprinting can be traced back to the early 1980s with the advent of 3D printing technology. In 1986, Charles Hull's invention of stereolithography laid the groundwork for additive fabrication.

However, it wasn't until the late 1990s and early 2000s that researchers began experimenting with printing living cells [48].

One of the earliest milestones in bioprinting was achieved in 2003 when Dr Thomas Boland of Clemson University adapted a modified inkjet printer to deposit living cells [13]. In subsequent years, bioprinting progressed rapidly with the development of specialized bioinks and advanced printing modalities. By 2010, researchers had successfully printed simple tissues like skin, cartilage, and blood vessels [3].

A notable breakthrough occurred in 2014 when scientists printed functional thyroid glands in mice, demonstrating viability in living organisms Kang et al., 2016a. In 2019, researchers from Tel Aviv University printed a miniature heart using patient-derived cells, symbolizing a major step toward fully functional organs [5]. These milestones reflect both technical progress and growing interdisciplinary collaboration.

15.2.3 Scientific Foundations of Bioprinting

The scientific underpinnings of 3D bioprinting draw from cell biology, materials science, mechanical engineering, and computational modeling [8, 13]. At the core is additive manufacturing, where complex biological structures are constructed layer-by-layer. These layers consist of cells and biomaterials that mimic the native tissue microenvironment, promoting cell-cell and cell-matrix interactions [48].

Bioinks – combinations of living cells and hydrogels – must be optimized for structural support, cell viability, and degradability [1]. Understanding cellular behavior (e.g., proliferation, migration, and differentiation) is key to achieving biologically functional outcomes [6]. Computational modeling and imaging (e.g., MRI and CT) assist in designing patient-specific constructs, while bioreactors provide dynamic conditions post-printing to aid tissue maturation [7].

15.2.4 Techniques and Materials Used in Bioprinting

Bioprinting techniques are broadly classified into inkjet-based, extrusion-based, and laser-assisted methods [10]. Inkjet-based bioprinting uses piezoelectric or thermal mechanisms to deposit bioink droplets. While fast and cell-friendly, it is limited to low-viscosity inks [8].

Extrusion-based printing, which extrudes continuous strands of bioinks, accommodates a wider viscosity range and enables robust structure formation – though it may impose higher stress on cells [13]. Laser-assisted bioprinting offers high precision and avoids nozzle clogging, suitable for delicate cells but expensive and complex [48].

Hydrogel-based bioinks – alginate, gelatin, collagen, and PEG – are favored for biocompatibility [1]. Advanced inks may include growth factors, nanoparticles, or vascularization agents to improve outcomes [2].

15.2.5 Applications in Organ and Tissue Engineering

Bioprinting's most transformative potential lies in tissue and organ engineering [48]. It offers customized implants using autologous cells, reducing rejection risk and transplant wait times [8].

Bioprinted tissues include skin, bone, cartilage, and vasculature. For example, skin constructs can be printed with pigmentation and vasculature for burn treatment, while bone and cartilage models are reinforced with scaffolds for orthopedic use [13]. A major milestone is the development of perfusable vascular networks using sacrificial inks and multi-material techniques [12].

Bioprinted tissues also serve as drug testing and disease modeling platforms, mimicking physiological environments better than 2D cultures [5]. Organoids – miniaturized organs – support research, toxicity screening, and early therapeutic use [2].

15.2.6 Global Organ Shortage and Demand

The global organ shortage is a public health crisis, with demand far exceeding supply [48]. Cultural, ethical, and logistic challenges hinder donation, and many donated organs are unfit for transplantation [6].

Alternatives like mechanical devices and stem cell therapies exist, but are limited. Bioprinting offers personalized, on-demand solutions using patient-derived cells, eliminating dependency on donors and reducing immunosuppression needs (Cui et al., 2017a).

Economically, this can reduce the costs of chronic treatments like dialysis and improve the quality of life [13].

15.2.7 Technical and Engineering Challenges

Several technical barriers hinder widespread clinical use. Vascularization remains one of the largest obstacles – cells inside thick tissues die without blood vessels [12]. While co-printing endothelial cells or using sacrificial channels helps, full vascular maturity is still elusive [48].

Printing resolution is another issue – fine detail reduces scalability, while large-scale printing lacks precision [10]. Multi-cell and multi-material coordination is prone to error, and bioinks often struggle to balance printability, mechanical strength, and biocompatibility [1].

Standardized cell sourcing is also difficult. Autologous cells may be limited in elderly patients, while allogenic or iPSC sources raise ethical or immunological concerns [9]. Additionally, post-printing maturation in bioreactors is still being optimized [7].

15.2.8 Stem Cells in Bioprinting

Stem cells are central to 3D bioprinting, offering regenerative potential and differentiation capacity [6]. Embryonic stem cells (ESCs) are pluripotent but face ethical concerns. Adult stem cells like mesenchymal stem cells (MSCs) are multipotent and immunomodulatory [9].

Induced pluripotent stem cells (iPSCs) provide a patient-specific, ethically sound option for differentiation into various lineages [5]. Bioinks must be carefully formulated to protect stem cells and deliver biochemical cues for tissue development [1].

Organoid bioprinting using stem cells has enabled modeling of liver, kidney, and brain tissue for drug testing and early-stage therapeutic applications [2]. However, challenges remain in controlling differentiation and avoiding teratoma formation [13].

15.3 Scientific and Technical Challenges

15.3.1 Bioink Composition and Standardization

The development of suitable bioinks is one of the most critical scientific and technical challenges in 3D bioprinting, as it directly influences print fidelity, structural integrity, and biological performance of the printed construct. A bioink typically consists of a combination of living cells, biocompatible hydrogels, and sometimes biomolecules such as growth factors or signaling peptides. The ideal bioink must meet a delicate balance of physical, chemical, and biological requirements: it must be printable, nontoxic, support cell viability and proliferation, and mimic the native extracellular matrix (ECM) of the target tissue.

From a materials standpoint, hydrogels such as alginate, gelatin methacryloyl (GelMA), collagen, fibrin, hyaluronic acid, and chitosan are commonly used due to their biocompatibility and ability to form hydrated 3D networks [17]. However, these materials often suffer from poor mechanical strength, necessitating blending with synthetic polymers like polyethylene glycol (PEG) or Pluronic to enhance rheological properties. The viscosity and cross-linking behavior of the bioink must be carefully tuned to allow extrusion or droplet formation during printing, while still maintaining structure post-printing.

A major technical hurdle lies in standardization. Currently, there is no universal protocol for bioink preparation, and variations in cell type, hydrogel concentration, and cross-linking chemistry can lead to inconsistent outcomes across labs and printers [48]. The lack of standardized testing for mechanical strength, degradation rates, and biological response further complicates reproducibility and regulatory approval. Additionally, different tissue types require highly specialized bioinks tailored to their unique mechanical, biological, and biochemical environments – making the development of "one-size-fits-all" bioinks impractical.

Efforts are underway to create modular or tunable bioink platforms, allowing for the customization of properties depending on the intended application. Moreover, the integration of smart bioinks – those that respond to external stimuli such as temperature, pH, or light – is an emerging trend aimed at enhancing functionality and in situ adaptability [18]. Despite these advances, achieving reliable scalability and commercial viability of bioinks remains challenging, particularly for clinical applications.

In conclusion, optimizing bioink composition and establishing standardization protocols are essential for advancing the safety, effectiveness, and reproducibility of bioprinted tissues and organs. This area demands ongoing collaboration between materials scientists, cell biologists, and regulatory experts to create frameworks that balance innovation with practical application.

15.3.2 Printing Resolution and Structural Fidelity

One of the fundamental technical limitations in 3D bioprinting is achieving high printing resolution and structural fidelity, particularly when reproducing complex tissue architectures at the microscale level. Resolution determines how accurately a bioprinter can replicate the geometric details of a digital model, which is critical for replicating hierarchical features such as vascular channels, cell compartments, and organ-specific geometries [13].

Inkjet-based bioprinting systems can offer resolutions below 100 μm, but they are limited to low-viscosity bioinks and often struggle with cell density and viability. Extrusion-based bioprinters, which are more versatile and compatible with a wider range of bioinks, typically achieve resolutions between 100 and 500 μm, but may compromise cell viability due to pressure-induced shear stress [16]. Laser-assisted bioprinting and stereolithography (SLA)-based approaches can achieve superior resolution (<50 μm) and cell placement accuracy, but face limitations in scalability and operational cost [14].

Structural fidelity also depends on the rheological behavior of the bioink during and after deposition, the curing method used (thermal, photo, or chemical crosslinking), and environmental conditions such as humidity and temperature during printing. Misalignment, swelling, or collapse of layers can distort the final construct, particularly for large or multilayered tissues.

Advanced imaging and computational modeling are increasingly integrated into printing workflows to improve accuracy and quality control. Real-time feedback systems using optical coherence tomography or machine learning (ML)-based error detection are under development to monitor and correct print deviations on the fly (Groll et al., 2016).

Continued research in printer technology, bioink rheology, and computational optimization is vital to achieving consistent resolution and fidelity that are essential for mimicking the functional complexity of native tissues and organs.

15.3.3 Vascularization and Nutrient Transport

One of the greatest scientific obstacles in 3D bioprinting is the successful fabrication of vascularized tissues capable of sustaining cellular metabolism, growth, and function over extended periods [20]. In native tissues, a dense vascular network enables the delivery of oxygen and nutrients while removing waste products. Replicating this complex capillary architecture within bioprinted constructs remains a formidable challenge.

Without vascularization, the viability of cells in the interior of thick tissue constructs is compromised due to diffusion limitations, typically restricting effective oxygen diffusion to only 100–200 µm from the nearest blood vessel [12]. Strategies to overcome this include co-printing endothelial cells, using angiogenic growth factors (e.g., VEGF), and incorporating sacrificial materials (e.g., Pluronic F127) that can be removed post-printing to create perfusable channels [20].

Microfluidic bioprinting and hybrid techniques that integrate 3D printing with soft lithography or electrowriting are emerging approaches to generate vascular-like networks with controlled geometry and flow dynamics [19]. However, ensuring long-term perfusion, anastomosis with host vasculature, and functionality under physiological pressure and flow remain critical hurdles for clinical translation.

Additionally, computational modeling of mass transport and hemodynamics is increasingly being used to optimize the design and placement of vascular features in complex constructs, allowing for predictive simulations of nutrient and oxygen distribution [21].

15.3.4 Cell Viability and Functionality

Maintaining high cell viability and functionality throughout the bioprinting process is essential for the success of engineered tissues and organs. Various steps in the process – ranging from bioink preparation, mixing, and extrusion to post-printing culture – can introduce mechanical, thermal, or chemical stresses that impair cell survival and behavior Cui et al., 2017a.

Extrusion-based printing, for example, can subject cells to shear stress depending on nozzle diameter, pressure, and viscosity of the ink. Inkjet systems may cause thermal stress due to rapid heating, while laser-assisted systems pose risks of photothermal damage. Prolonged exposure to UV light in photo-cross-linking can induce DNA damage if not carefully controlled [16].

Beyond mere survival, the ability of printed cells to differentiate, form functional tissue-specific structures, and communicate with their microenvironment is crucial. This is especially important when printing stem cells or iPSCs, where differentiation cues and niche factors must be carefully preserved.

Post-printing, bioreactors, and dynamic culture systems are used to enhance cell maturation and functionality by mimicking physiological conditions such as mechanical loading, fluid shear, and electrical stimulation. Organoids and spheroids are also being explored as building blocks that inherently possess microarchitecture and cell-cell interactions, enhancing functional outcomes [11].

Improving cell viability and performance across different printing modalities remains a core area of research, with innovations in nozzle design, printing protocols, and cell-protective additives showing promising results.

15.3.5 Integration of Multiple Cell Types

Tissues and organs are composed of heterogeneous populations of cells that must interact harmoniously for physiological function. One of the major scientific challenges in bioprinting is the spatial organization and integration of multiple cell types within a single construct. This includes positioning parenchymal cells, supporting stromal cells, endothelial cells, and immune cells in anatomically and functionally appropriate locations Mo-roni et al., 2018a.

Inadequate coordination of these different cell types can result in poor tissue maturation, dysfunction, or even immune rejection. Strategies to address this challenge include multi-head bioprinters that allow the simultaneous deposition of different cell-laden bioinks, layer-by-layer printing of cell-specific architectures, and coaxial extrusion techniques for tubular or layered constructs Kang et al., 2016a.

Recent developments in spheroid and organoid bioprinting also allow the use of pre-organized cell aggregates that self-assemble into tissue-like structures, potentially simplifying the challenge of spatial cell organization. However, issues remain with cell sorting, adhesion, and mechanical integration post-printing.

15.3.6 Scaffold-Free Bioprinting Techniques

Scaffold-free bioprinting seeks to eliminate the use of biomaterial scaffolds and rely solely on the cells' ability to self-assemble and organize into functional tissues. This method aims to replicate developmental biology processes and avoid complications associated with scaffold degradation, immune response, or mismatch in mechanical properties [15].

Techniques such as cell sheet engineering, tissue spheroids, and self-assembling droplets have demonstrated promise in generating scaffold-free tissues. However, these approaches often suffer from long maturation times, limited structural integrity during handling, and difficulty in maintaining predefined geometry.

Scaffold-free methods also require high cell densities, which pose challenges in cell expansion, harvesting, and viability. Therefore, while biologically attractive, scaffold-free bioprinting is not yet widely used in clinical-grade constructs and is largely confined to research and development.

15.3.7 Scalability and Manufacturing Constraints

Transitioning from laboratory-scale prototypes to clinically relevant tissues or organs introduces significant challenges in scalability and manufacturing. Scaling up requires not only printing larger and more complex structures but also ensuring uniformity, sterility, reproducibility, and cost-effectiveness in production [20].

Large-scale bioprinting systems must maintain precise control over parameters such as temperature, humidity, and oxygenation, and allow integration of multiple cell types and materials across large volumes. Batch-to-batch variability and lengthy printing times further complicate scalability.

Moreover, regulatory hurdles increase significantly with scale. Quality control becomes more demanding, and robust validation protocols must be established to meet GMP (good manufacturing practice) requirements for clinical application [48].

Automation, closed-loop bioprinting systems, and artificial intelligence (AI)-based process control are being developed to address these constraints and improve throughput, but widespread adoption is still limited by technological and economic barriers.

15.4 Ethical Challenges in Bioprinting

15.4.1 Moral Status of Bioprinted Tissues and Organs

As 3D bioprinting advances from producing simple tissues to functional organs, it raises fundamental ethical questions about the moral status of these constructs. At the heart of this issue is whether bioprinted tissues – especially those mimicking sentient or functional human organs – should be granted any degree of moral consideration, particularly as their complexity and autonomy increase. While current constructs lack full physiological integration or consciousness, emerging technologies such as bioprinted neural tissues, brain organoids, and functional cardiac systems have blurred traditional distinctions between the artificial and the biological [27].

The moral status of a bioprinted construct depends largely on its level of functionality, origin of the cells, and intended use. Simple tissues like skin patches or cartilage typically do not raise ethical concerns, as they are devoid of sensory, cognitive, or reproductive capacity. However, the creation of bioprinted brain tissues or cerebral organoids, which exhibit neural activity and synaptic behavior, has led ethicists to question at what point such entities might attain moral standing or rights [24]. Some scholars argue that if a bioprinted brain organoid were capable of consciousness or pain perception, even minimally, it would merit ethical protections similar to animals used in research [22]. Additionally, the use of human ESCs or fetal-derived cells in bioprinting raises moral concerns among certain cultural and religious groups, who believe these cells possess intrinsic moral value from conception [25]. The figure 15.1 shows ethical continuum of bioprinted constructs. The table 15.1 shows Ethical frameworks for assessing moral status of bioprinted tissues. The controversy deepens when constructs are developed using human–animal chimeras or genetically modified cells, which challenge notions of species integrity and human identity [27].

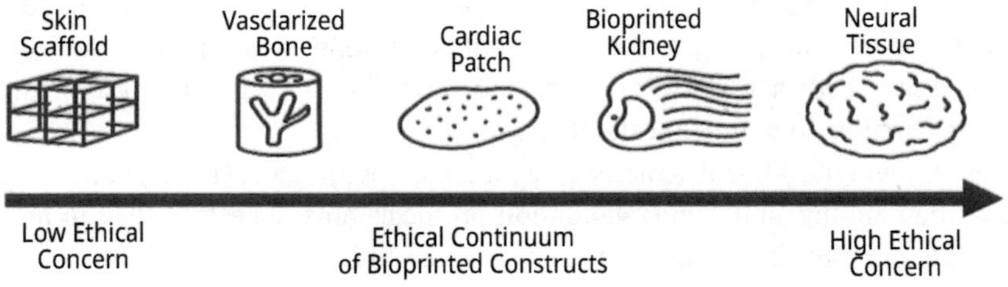

Figure 15.1: Ethical continuum of bioprinted constructs based on complexity and moral consideration.

Table 15.1: Ethical frameworks for assessing moral status of bioprinted tissues.

Framework	Key criteria	Implications
Biological functionality	Degree of physiological activity	Highly functional tissues may warrant protection
Sentience-based framework	Capacity to feel pain or awareness	Neural constructs may gain moral consideration
Source-based ethics	Origin of cells (e.g., ESCs and iPSCs)	Affects acceptability across cultural/religious lines
Human-likeness threshold	Similarity to human tissue/ organs	Higher resemblance = higher ethical concern
Utilitarian consideration	Overall benefit versus harm	Balances scientific value with moral costs

Adapted from [24, 25, 27].

15.4.2 Informed Consent and Donor Cell Ethics

Bioprinting often requires harvesting human cells for tissue engineering. Ethical issues arise when obtaining these cells, especially regarding informed consent and privacy. Donors must be made fully aware of the future uses of their biological materials, particularly if their cells are used to create tissues or organs that could be implanted in others or commercialized [23]. The principle of autonomy mandates that individuals retain control over how their biological materials are used – even after donation. Issues also arise when biobanks or companies fail to disclose the full range of future applications, including bioprinting for reproductive or enhancement purposes.

Furthermore, ethical dilemmas are magnified in low-resource settings where economic disparity may lead to the exploitation of vulnerable populations as sources of stem cells or tissue samples [30]. A robust and transparent consent process that explains risks, future applications, and commercial potential is critical to avoid exploitation and maintain public trust in bioprinting.

15.4.3 Equity and Access to Bioprinted Therapies

As with many advanced medical technologies, 3D bioprinting risks deepening existing healthcare inequities. While bioprinted organs may eventually offer life-saving treatments, they will likely be expensive and accessible only to privileged populations initially. This raises distributive justice concerns – how can these technologies be made equitably available, especially in low- and middle-income countries (LMICs) [29]?

Some propose a tiered-access system or global subsidy programs for LMICs, but practical implementation remains complex. Furthermore, unequal access could lead to a two-tiered healthcare system where wealthier individuals receive bioprinted organs, while others rely on traditional, less effective treatments. Ethical policymaking must consider mechanisms to reduce costs and increase access to prevent exacerbating global health disparities.

15.4.4 Identity, Personhood, and Psychological Impacts

Implanting bioprinted organs, especially neural tissues or facial structures, may affect a patient's perception of self. Philosophical and psychological concerns arise over whether having lab-made organs influences a person's identity or personhood [26]. Would a person with a bioprinted brain or reproductive organ be perceived or treated differently? How does this affect dignity, authenticity, or social integration?

Moreover, recipients may struggle with psychological adaptation to artificial replacements, particularly in the absence of long-term cultural or social acceptance.

This is especially sensitive in the case of facial bioprinting or neurobioprinting, where the constructs influence core features of individuality and cognition.

15.4.5 Use of Bioprinted Tissues in Research and Testing

Bioprinted tissues present new opportunities to reduce animal testing, as they can simulate human physiology more closely than animal models. However, ethical questions arise regarding the degree to which bioprinted constructs can or should be subjected to invasive experimentation. If a brain organoid exhibits electrical activity analogous to sentience, does it deserve similar ethical considerations as sentient lab animals [27]?

Research ethics committees and Institutional Review Boards (IRBs) must adapt protocols to evaluate studies involving bioprinted constructs with potentially emergent or conscious properties. Additionally, there is the question of commercial use of these constructs in drug testing – where corporations benefit economically from materials derived from human donors.

15.4.6 Future-Proofing Ethical Governance

Due to the pace of technological advancement, many ethical frameworks and regulations lag behind innovation. A proactive, anticipatory ethics approach is needed, incorporating interdisciplinary oversight, public deliberation, and scenario forecasting [28]. Regulatory bodies must update definitions of "organ," "person," or "sentience" to accommodate future innovations such as fully autonomous bioengineered constructs or AI-integrated organoids.

Furthermore, ethics education for researchers, clinicians, and engineers involved in bioprinting should be expanded to include topics such as dual-use concerns, biosecurity, and long-term societal impacts. Cross-border ethical harmonization will also become essential to prevent regulatory arbitrage or ethical dumping.

15.5 Legal and Regulatory Considerations

Bioprinting has emerged as a groundbreaking technology that promises to revolutionize regenerative medicine, drug testing, and organ transplantation. However, its rapid growth has far outpaced the development of appropriate legal and regulatory frameworks. This chapter explores the multifaceted legal landscape surrounding bioprinting, focusing on current regulations, existing gaps, international guidelines, and legal liabilities.

15.5.1 Current Legal Frameworks

Bioprinting combines tissue engineering, computer-aided design (CAD), and additive manufacturing to create three-dimensional biological structures. Yet, legal classification of bioprinted products – whether as medical devices, biological products, or drugs – varies widely across jurisdictions.

In the United States, the Food and Drug Administration (FDA) regulates medical devices and biologics under the Federal Food, Drug, and Cosmetic Act (FD&C Act). However, the legal framework lacks specificity for bioprinted tissues and organs [32]. Classification of bioprinted products across jurisdictions are shown in table 15.2. Similarly, in the European Union, the European Medicines Agency (EMA) oversees Advanced Therapy Medicinal Products (ATMPs), under Regulation (EC) No. 1394/2007, which could apply to certain bioprinted tissues [31].

Table 15.2: Classification of bioprinted products across jurisdictions.

Jurisdiction	Regulating body	Classification	Governing regulation
United States	FDA	Device/biologic/drug	FD&C Act, PHSA
European Union	EMA	ATMP	Regulation (EC) No. 1394/2007
Japan	PMDA	Regenerative medicine	Pharmaceuticals and Medical Device Act [35]
India	CDSCO and ICMR	Undefined/in progress	Draft Biomedical Regulations [33]

15.5.2 Gaps in Regulatory Oversight

There are several critical gaps in regulatory oversight:

1. **Ambiguity in Classification**: Bioprinted tissues do not always neatly fall into existing categories of medical products.
2. **Lack of Long-Term Evaluation Standards**: Regulatory agencies lack clear protocols for assessing the long-term viability and functionality of bioprinted tissues [32].
3. **Ethical Concerns Unaddressed**: Issues related to donor cell sources, consent, and potential human enhancement are underregulated.
4. **Custom vs. Mass Production**: Personalized bioprinting challenges mass-market regulatory models.

The Figure 15.2 illustrates regulatory gaps.

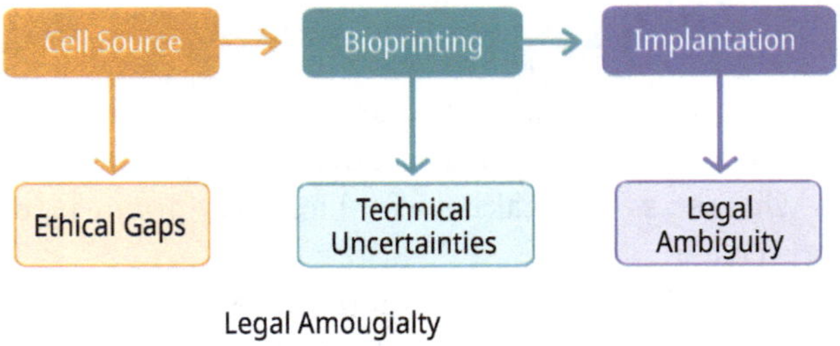

Figure 15.2: Regulatory gaps in the bioprinting life cycle.

15.5.3 FDA and EMA Guidelines

15.5.3.1 FDA Guidelines

The FDA has adopted a case-by-case approach, evaluating bioprinted products under existing pathways. In 2017, it released a discussion paper: *Technical Considerations for Additive Manufactured Devices*, which includes some bioprinting elements. However, no dedicated framework yet exists for complex living tissues [32].

15.5.3.2 EMA Guidelines

The EMA classifies bioprinted products under ATMPs, particularly tissue-engineered products (TEPs). FDA versus EMA approach to bioprinting are shown in table 15.3. However, ambiguity remains around composite products [31].

Table 15.3: FDA versus EMA approach to bioprinting.

Criteria	FDA (USA)	EMA (EU)
Framework	FD&C Act + Guidance	Regulation 1394/2007 (ATMPs)
Cell-scaffold products	Combination Product Pathway	TEP within ATMP category
Custom implants	510(k) or PMA pathway (if device)	Hospital Exemption may apply
Regulatory clarity	Limited	Moderate

15.5.4 Bioprinting and Patent Law

Intellectual property (IP) issues in bioprinting are complex. Key challenges include:

1. **Patentability of Living Constructs**: The U.S. Supreme Court ruling in *Association for Molecular Pathology v. Myriad Genetics* (2013) held that naturally occurring

DNA cannot be patented. This raises questions about the patentability of bioprinted tissues [36].

2. **Overlap Between Software, Hardware, and Biological IP**: Bioprinting platforms involve proprietary CAD software, bioinks, and printers – each subject to different IP laws.
3. **Inventorship and Ownership**: When AI tools design constructs or when donor cells are involved, assigning inventorship becomes contentious.

15.5.4.1 Case Study

Organovo Inc. holds numerous patents for its bioprinting technology. However, ongoing litigation illustrates the difficulty of protecting IP in this evolving space [34].

15.5.5 International Regulations and Harmonization

The global nature of biomedical research necessitates regulatory harmonization. However, major discrepancies exist between the U.S., EU, China, and other regions in how bioprinted products are regulated.

15.5.5.1 Challenges in Harmonization

- Varying definitions of "tissue-engineered products"
- Inconsistent consent and bioethics laws
- Different levels of stringency in product validation [31, 32]

International collaborations such as the International Council for Harmonisation (ICH) have not yet directly addressed bioprinting. The Figure 15.3 shows global regulatory disparity.

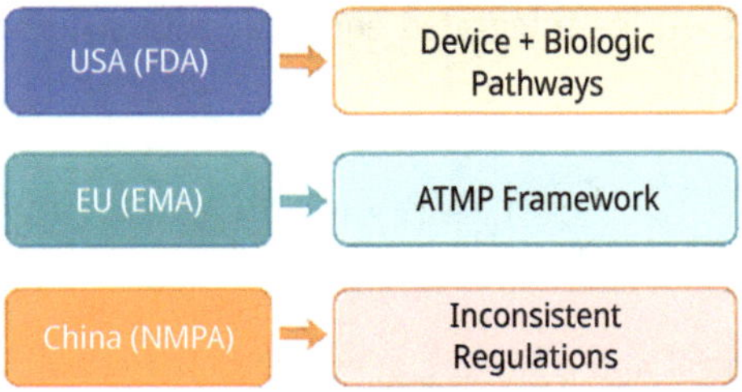

Figure 15.3: Regulatory disparities across nations.

15.5.6 Liability and Malpractice in Bioprinted Organs

The question of legal liability in bioprinting is particularly complex. If a bioprinted organ fails, who is responsible – the software designer, the printer manufacturer, the surgeon, or the biologist who cultured the cells?

15.5.6.1 Key Legal Dilemmas

- **Product Versus Service Liability**: Should a bioprinted organ be treated as a product (like a pacemaker) or a service (like tissue therapy)?
- **Medical Malpractice**: Can physicians be held accountable for implanting organs whose long-term outcomes are uncertain?
- **Insurance Coverage**: Most malpractice and liability insurers do not cover risks associated with experimental bioprinted products. Stakeholder liability matrix in bioprinted organ failure are shown in table 15.4

Table 15.4: Stakeholder liability matrix in bioprinted organ failure.

Stakeholder	Potential liability	Legal defense
Bio-ink supplier	Contaminated input materials	Due diligence records
Bioprinter manufacturer	Device malfunction	Compliance with ISO standards
Software developer	Design flaw in printing model	Licensing agreements
Surgeon	Surgical error/misuse	Informed consent; standard of care
Research lab	Defective biological process	Preclinical evidence; regulatory approval

15.6 Social and Cultural Perspectives

The integration of bioprinting into healthcare and biomedical research is not merely a technical or legal challenge – it also raises significant social and cultural issues. Public perception, media portrayal, cultural beliefs, and religious doctrines all influence how bioprinting is received and whether it will be integrated equitably into society. This section explores these dimensions in detail.

15.6.1 Public Perception and Acceptance

The success of bioprinting technology in clinical and commercial settings is heavily dependent on public trust and acceptance. Research indicates that although many people support regenerative medicine in principle, they harbor concerns about unnatural body modification, unknown long-term effects, and the fear of “playing God” [38].

15.6.1.1 Key Influencing Factors

- **Risk Versus Benefit Understanding:** Public willingness to accept bioprinted tissues increases when the life-saving potential is made clear.
- **Transparency in Communication:** Clear communication from researchers and policymakers can build trust.
- **Educational Outreach:** Public education initiatives positively influence perceptions of bioprinting. The Figure 15.4 shows perception factors.

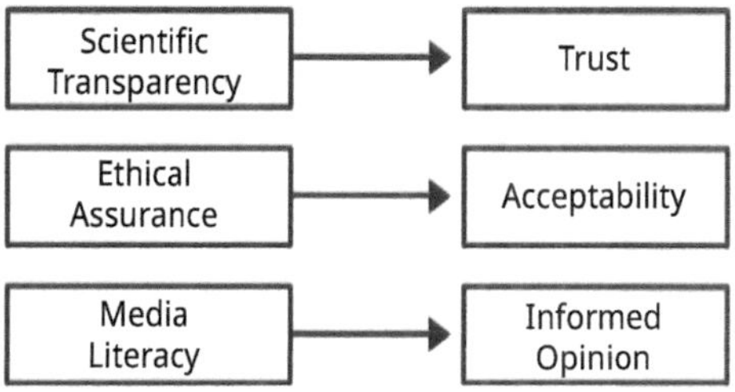

Figure 15.4: Factors influencing public perception of bioprinting.

15.6.2 Media Representation and Hype

Media portrayal plays a critical role in shaping societal understanding and expectations of bioprinting. Popular media has often sensationalized the technology, presenting futuristic and sometimes misleading narratives – such as instant organ printing or fully functional human clones [39]. Examples of bioprinting in media coverage are shown in table 15.5.

15.6.2.1 Positive Aspects

- Increases public interest in biomedical research
- Attracts funding and investment
- Promotes awareness of organ shortage issues

15.6.2.2 Negative Consequences

- Creates unrealistic expectations
- Contributes to ethical panic and regulatory pressures
- Undermines legitimate scientific progress by overhyping timelines

Table 15.5: Examples of bioprinting in media coverage.

Media Outlet	Headline	Type of framing
BBC News	"3D Printing Human Organs: The Future is Here"	Utopian/techno-optimism
The Guardian	"Should We Be Creating Synthetic Life?"	Ethical alarmism
Nature News	"Bioprinting Progress Faces Regulatory Maze"	Balanced/informed

15.6.3 Cultural and Religious Considerations

Different cultures and religions hold varying views on the sanctity of the human body, medical intervention, and the acceptability of synthetic or lab-grown tissues.

15.6.3.1 Religious Viewpoints

- **Christianity:** Generally supports medical innovation when used to preserve life, but conservative factions may oppose interventions perceived as unnatural or hubristic.
- **Islam:** Accepts tissue engineering if it aims to save life and does not violate Islamic jurisprudence regarding bodily integrity and consent [37].
- **Hinduism:** Emphasizes the cyclical nature of life and karma; generally permits biomedical interventions unless they involve animal cruelty or disrespect to the body.
- **Buddhism:** Supports alleviation of suffering but opposes harm to sentient beings, including animals used for bioink sources. Figure 15.5 shows religious acceptance.

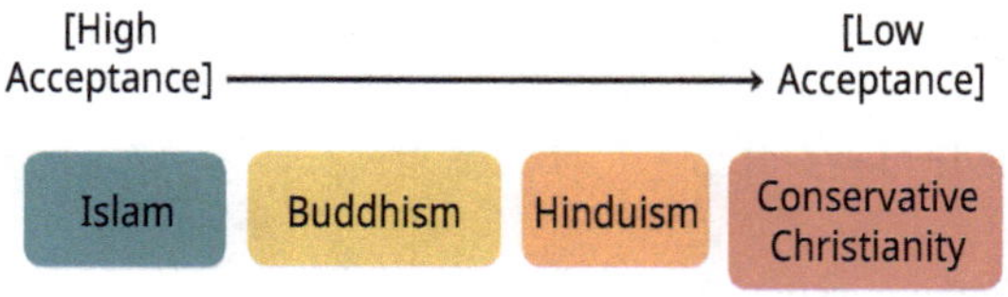

Figure 15.5: Religious acceptance spectrum of bioprinting technologies.

15.6.3.2 Cultural Issues to Consider

- Body Autonomy: In some cultures, the body is considered sacred and should not be altered artificially.
- Death and Rebirth Concepts: Influence how new organs and regenerative technologies are interpreted.

- Collectivist vs. Individualist Values: Affect decision-making in organ donation and bioprinting ethics.

15.6.4 Impact on Organ Donation Systems

Bioprinting has the potential to dramatically alter existing organ donation systems by reducing reliance on human donors. This development brings both opportunity and challenge.

15.6.4.1 Opportunities

- **Reduction in Organ Shortages:** Bioprinted organs could alleviate the global donor organ scarcity.
- **Improved Matching:** Personalized tissues eliminate immune rejection risks.
- **Elimination of Illegal Organ Trade:** Technological alternatives could reduce demand for black-market organs.

15.6.4.2 Challenges

- **Disincentivizing Donation:** If bioprinted organs become widespread, public motivation to register as donors may decline.
- **Ethical Triage:** Questions about who receives bioprinted versus donated organs could introduce new inequalities.
- **Transition Period:** During the adoption phase, both systems shown in table 15.6 (donation and printing) will coexist, necessitating ethical and logistical coordination.

Table 15.6: Comparison of traditional organ donation versus bioprinted organs.

Criteria	Traditional donation	Bioprinted organs
Source	Human donors	Lab-based biofabrication
Immune compatibility	Variable	Customizable
Availability	Scarce	On-demand (future goal)
Ethical concerns	Consent, commodification	Enhancement, ownership
Cost (current estimates)	Moderate (public health systems)	High (experimental phase)

15.7 Case Studies and Real-World Examples

Real-world case studies of bioprinting not only illustrate the technical potential of the technology but also highlight its current limitations, ethical complexities, and diverse applications across medicine and pharmaceutical research. This chapter reviews several landmark examples and pilot implementations that have shaped the field, as well as a visionary look into future possibilities.

15.7.1 Bioprinted Skin for Burn Victims

One of the most advanced and clinically relevant applications of bioprinting to date is the development of bioprinted skin for the treatment of burn injuries. Traditional skin grafting methods require healthy donor sites, which may be unavailable in severe burns. Bioprinting circumvents this issue by using the patient's own cells – keratinocytes and fibroblasts – to fabricate skin layers using a bioink-based extrusion process. In 2019, researchers at the Wake Forest Institute for Regenerative Medicine successfully demonstrated an **in-situ skin bioprinting** system that printed skin cells directly onto the wound site. The printed skin showed rapid integration, reduced scarring, and a significant decrease in recovery time [41]. This approach not only minimizes graft rejection but also addresses concerns of immune compatibility and patient discomfort. However, regulatory hurdles remain, particularly regarding long-term safety and uniform vascularization, which are critical for full-thickness skin regeneration.

15.7.2 3D-Printed Bone and Cartilage Implants

Bioprinting has also seen promising applications in orthopedics, especially in the reconstruction of bone and cartilage. Researchers have successfully developed scaffolds composed of biodegradable polymers, such as polylactic acid (PLA) **or** polycaprolactone (PCL), integrated with osteogenic or chondrogenic cells. In 2021, a team in South Korea successfully implanted a 3D printed cartilage graft into a patient's nasal defect, leading to functional and aesthetic recovery [43]. Similarly, bioprinted mandibular implants have been trialed in veterinary settings, showing high biocompatibility and mechanical stability. What distinguishes these applications is their capacity for patient-specific customization using imaging data, enabling precise anatomical matches. Still, challenges such as limited vascularization, long-term degradation behavior of scaffold materials, and load-bearing capacity under physiological stress must be addressed before widespread clinical use.

15.7.3 Liver and Kidney Tissue Models for Drug Testing

Beyond therapeutic applications, bioprinted organoids and tissue models have transformed preclinical drug testing. The pharmaceutical industry has increasingly adopted liver and kidney tissue models to simulate organ-level responses **in vitro**. For example, **Organovo Holdings Inc.** developed a 3D bioprinted liver tissue platform that mimics native hepatic structure and function, enabling more accurate prediction of hepatotoxicity during drug screening [40]. The models provide physiologically relevant data while reducing reliance on animal testing, aligning with the 3R principle (replacement, reduction, and refinement). Bioprinted kidney proximal tubule tissues are similarly being explored for nephrotoxicity studies. These models offer a scalable, high-throughput platform for evaluating drug metabolism and toxicity in a human-relevant system. Despite these advantages, the lack of systemic interactions, immune responses, and full organ functionality still limits their use to supplementary roles rather than complete alternatives to **in vivo** trials.

15.7.4 Future Case: Bioprinted Hearts

Among the most ambitious goals in the field is the bioprinting of a fully functional, vascularized human heart. In 2019, researchers at **Tel Aviv University** revealed a landmark achievement: a **miniature bioprinted heart**, complete with chambers, vessels, and beating cardiac cells [42]. Though it was only the size of a cherry and lacked full pumping function, the prototype demonstrated the feasibility of using patient-derived cells to print anatomically accurate cardiac tissue. The ultimate goal is to produce transplantable hearts that eliminate the need for donor organs and immunosuppressive drugs. Such advances would revolutionize cardiac transplantation, where donor shortages are dire and waitlist mortality remains high. However, multiple barriers persist: achieving synchronized contractions, establishing a functional conduction system, and ensuring long-term mechanical durability are scientific and engineering feats yet to be fully solved. Moreover, regulatory and ethical questions about organ enhancement and access equity will grow more pressing as this frontier approaches reality.

15.8 Environmental and Sustainability Aspects

As bioprinting technologies become more integrated into biomedical research and clinical practice, it is essential to evaluate their environmental impact. Sustainability considerations, including material sourcing, energy consumption, waste generation, and comparative eco-efficiency, are often overlooked but increasingly critical in shaping future bioprinting infrastructure. This chapter evaluates the environmental and sustainability dimensions of bioprinting across its production and operational lifecycle.

15.8.1 Resource Consumption in Bioprinting

Bioprinting requires a range of physical, biological, and chemical resources. These include bioinks (often derived from animal or human ECM), cell culture media, growth factors, and materials for scaffold fabrication such as gelatin, alginate, collagen, and synthetic polymers like PCL.

While some of these materials are renewable or biodegradable, others involve high environmental costs, as shown in table 15.7. For instance, gelatin and collagen often originate from animal tissues, raising concerns about sourcing ethics and carbon-intensive production. The production of high-grade bioprinting reagents often requires water-intensive purification processes and the use of single-use plastics in sterile lab settings [44].

Table 15.7: Major resource inputs in bioprinting processes.

Resource type	Common examples	Sustainability concern
Biomaterials	Collagen, GelMA, and PCL	Animal sourcing and biodegradability
Cell culture components	FBS, DMEM, and L-glutamine	Animal use and sterilization waste
Scaffolding substrates	PLA, PEGDA, and alginate	Synthetic origin and nonrenewable input
Printing hardware	Nozzles, cartridges, and tubing	Disposable and plastic-based

15.8.2 Waste Generation and Disposal

Bioprinting laboratories generate both biological waste and chemical waste, including leftover bioinks, used culture media, cell waste, and polymer debris. Additionally, sterile operation protocols lead to high use of disposable plastics (e.g., pipette tips, Petri dishes, and cartridges), contributing to lab waste.

The biological components – especially those derived from human or animal cells – require specialized disposal methods to avoid contamination and comply with biosafety regulations. Some bioinks are not fully biodegradable and must be incinerated as biomedical waste [44].

15.8.3 Energy Use and Carbon Footprint

Although often perceived as a clean and digital process, bioprinting can involve substantial energy use, especially in tissue maturation and environmental control sys-

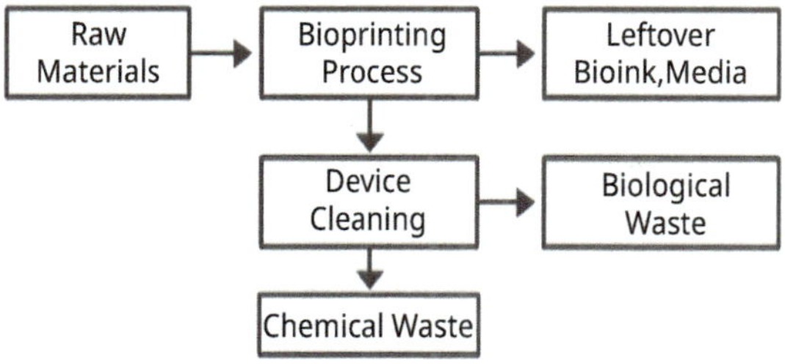

Figure 15.6: Waste stream in a typical bioprinting workflow.

Table 15.8: Types of waste produced in bioprinting.

Waste type	Examples	Disposal method
Biological waste	Spent bioink, cells, and tissues	Autoclaving or incineration
Chemical waste	Fixatives and solvents (e.g., IPA)	Hazardous chemical waste disposal
Plastic waste	Pipette tips, gloves, and tubes	Nonbiodegradable lab waste
Scaffold remnants	Unused PLA/PCL fragments	Controlled landfill or incineration

tems. Bioprinters themselves consume relatively low energy during extrusion or inkjet-based printing. However, bioreactors, incubators, and sterile air-handling units require continuous operation, often 24/7, to maintain cell viability and contamination-free environments. Waste stream in a typical bioprinting workflow is shown in figure 15.6. Types of waste produced in bioprinting is shown in table 15.8.

Studies comparing tissue culture laboratories with standard office spaces have shown that energy consumption can be 5–10 times higher per square foot, driven by HVAC (heating, ventilation, and air conditioning), sterilization systems, and autoclaves) Zhang et al., 2021a.

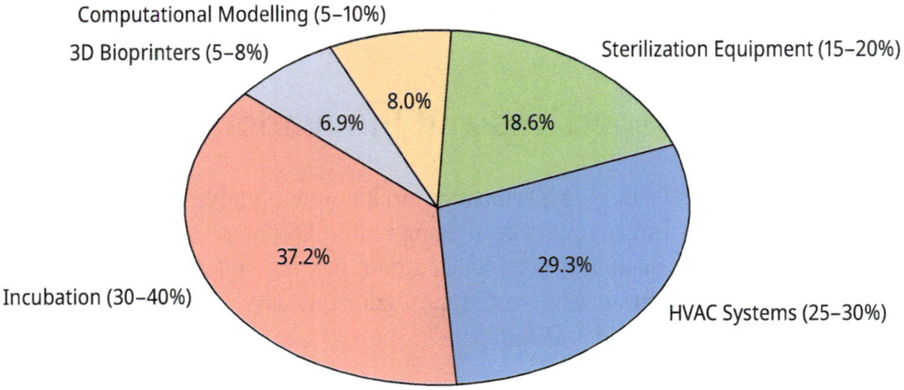

Figure 15.7: Primary contributors to energy use in bioprinting labs.

Given this, carbon offsetting or renewable energy sourcing should be considered in any scale-up of bioprinting operations [45].

Primary contributors to energy use in bioprinting labs is shown in figure 15.7.

15.8.4 Bioprinting Versus Traditional Biomedical Approaches

A crucial sustainability debate centers on whether bioprinting is more or less environmentally intensive than conventional biomedical methods, such as organ donation, synthetic graft manufacturing, or animal testing.

In some areas, bioprinting offers environmental advantages:

- It reduces animal use, aligning with global 3Rs (replace, reduce, refine) principles in scientific research.
- On-demand printing of tissues can reduce waste associated with expired or unsold synthetic implants.
- Customization can minimize inventory and logistics burdens.

Environmental comparison: bioprinting versus conventional approaches are shown in table 15.9. However, in early stages of development, bioprinting may be less efficient due to high rejection rates, small batch sizes, and energy-intensive lab conditions [45].

Table 15.9: Environmental comparison: bioprinting versus conventional approaches.

Aspect	Bioprinting	Traditional biomedical techniques
Animal use	Reduced (in vitro models)	High (especially in drug testing)
Material efficiency	Moderate (custom production)	Low (standardized but wasteful)
Energy use (per unit)	High (controlled environments)	Variable
Waste output	Moderate to high (lab-scale)	High (hospital waste and donor organs)
Transportation footprint	Low (on-site fabrication)	High (organ transport and logistics)

15.9 Future Perspectives and Innovations

As bioprinting evolves from an experimental discipline to a viable clinical and commercial technology, its future hinges on dynamic interplays among stem cell innovation, AI, computational modeling, personalized therapeutics, and democratized innovation. The following sections explore the most transformative trajectories that will shape bioprinting in the decades ahead.

15.9.1 Advancements in Stem Cell Technology

Stem cells serve as the foundational building blocks for tissue engineering in bioprinting. Progress in iPSCs and MSCs has significantly expanded the potential for creating patient-specific tissues with enhanced functional outcomes [49].

15.9.1.1 Emerging Directions

- **Reprogramming Efficiency:** Optimizing the conversion of somatic cells into iPSCs.
- **Lineage-Specific Differentiation:** Engineering protocols to direct stem cells into tissue-specific phenotypes for heart, liver, or neural constructs.
- **Stem Cell Banking:** Facilitating bioprinting through standardized stem cell biobanks. Workflow of bioprinting using patient-derived iPSCs is shown in Figure 15.8.

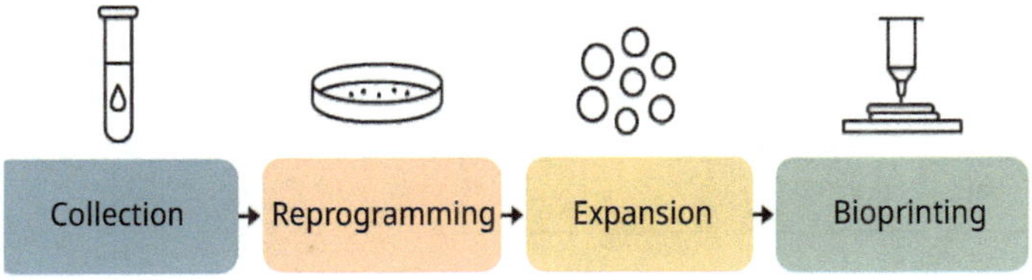

Figure 15.8: Workflow of bioprinting using patient-derived iPSCs.

Table 15.10: Comparative characteristics of stem cell types used in bioprinting.

Stem cell type	Source	Differentiation potential	Immunogenicity	Common applications
iPSCs	Adult tissue	Pluripotent	Low (autologous)	Cardiac and neural
MSCs	Bone marrow and fat	Multipotent	Low	Bone and cartilage
ESCs	Embryos	Pluripotent	High (ethical concerns)	Liver and skin

15.9.2 Role of Artificial Intelligence and Machine Learning

AI and ML are redefining the design, optimization, and prediction processes in bioprinting. AI-driven approaches are enabling smarter, faster, and more precise workflows [46].

15.9.2.1 Applications

- **Print Path Optimization:** AI algorithms can enhance precision and reduce material waste.
- **Cell Viability Prediction:** ML models predict cell fate and survival based on scaffold geometry and bioink properties.
- **Automated Quality Control:** Deep learning facilitates defect detection in real-time during layer deposition.

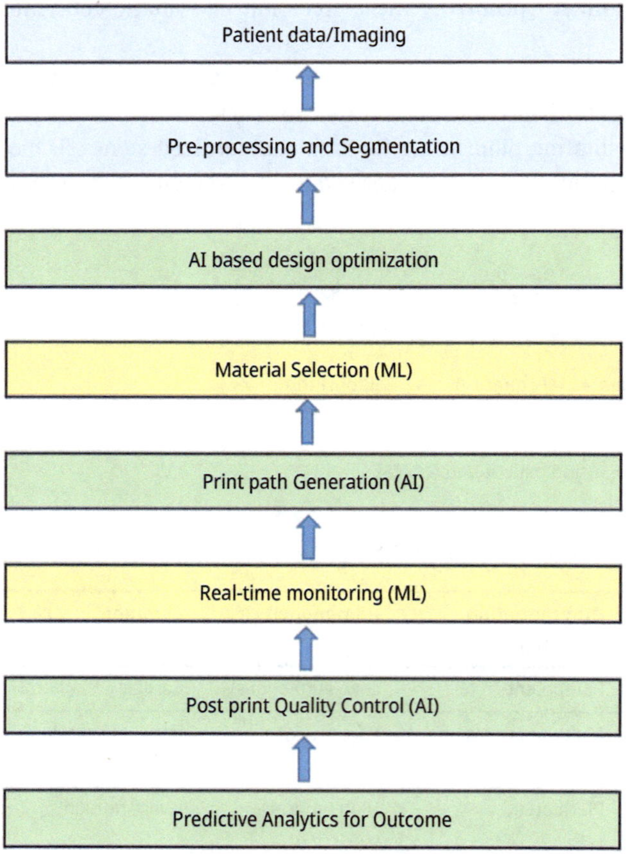

Figure 15.9: Integration of AI and ML in the bioprinting workflow.

Table 15.11: AI Applications in bioprinting.

AI application	Description	Technology used
Print fidelity prediction	Detects print errors and adapts nozzle control	CNN-based models
Scaffold optimization	Suggests optimal design for cell growth	Reinforcement learning
Bioink formulation	Predicts best composition for tissue type	Decision trees/MLP

15.9.3 Organ-on-a-Chip Systems

Organ-on-a-chip (OoC) platforms are miniaturized models of human physiology. When integrated with bioprinting, they offer high-fidelity systems to simulate complex organ functions, enabling more accurate disease modeling and pharmacological testing [51].

15.9.3.1 Advantages of Integration

- **Drug Testing:** Provides real-time responses of printed tissues to pharmacological agents. A schematic diagram of a bioprinted liver-on-a-chip platform is shown in figure 15.10.
- **Disease Modeling:** Helps replicate disease states, such as fibrosis or cancer microenvironments.
- **Microfluidic Enhancement:** Bioprinted tissues can be interfaced with perfusable microchannels for long-term viability.

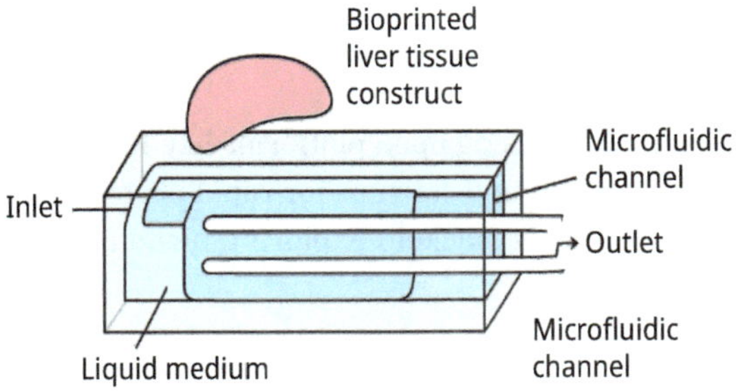

Figure 15.10: A schematic diagram of a bioprinted liver-on-a-chip platform.

15.9.4 Personalized Medicine and Bioprinting

Bioprinting aligns naturally with the goals of personalized medicine by enabling customized tissue constructs derived from a patient's own cells [48].

15.9.4.1 Key Innovations

- **Patient-Specific Implants:** Bioengineered grafts tailored for congenital defects or reconstructive surgery.
- Example of personalized applications in bioprinting is shown in table 15.12.
- **Pharmacogenomic Testing:** Bioprinted tissues used for testing drug compatibility with a patient's genome.
- **Regenerative Therapeutics:** Functional tissues for chronic conditions like diabetes, osteoarthritis, and cardiovascular diseases.

Table 15.12: Examples of personalized applications in bioprinting.

Application	Bioprinted tissue	Personalization aspect
Skin grafts	Dermal equivalents	Cell source and wound topography
Cardiac patches	Myocardial tissue	Autologous iPSCs and geometry
Cancer models	Tumor spheroids	Patient-derived cells

15.9.5 Open-Source and DIY Bioprinting

The democratization of bioprinting is facilitated by open-source hardware/software and grassroots innovation. The movement is rapidly expanding in educational and hobbyist spaces [47].

15.9.5.1 Key Drivers

- **Cost Reduction:** Affordable bioprinters built using open platforms like RepRap.
- **Educational Innovation:** Used in universities and startups for rapid prototyping.
- **Community Science:** Citizen scientists and biohackers exploring niche applications.

15.9.5.2 Risks and Challenges

- Lack of regulatory oversight
- Biohazard and contamination concerns
- Ethical ambiguity in home-based tissue engineering

Figure 9.4: Open-source bioprinting system architecture.

15.9.6 Ethical Frameworks for the Future

With rapid innovation comes an urgent need for adaptive and anticipatory ethical governance. Bioprinting raises novel dilemmas that will require multidisciplinary approaches to resolve [50].

15.9.6.1 Emerging Ethical Considerations

- **Ownership of Bioprinted Tissues:** Who owns the rights to bioprinted organs – patients, scientists, or institutions?
- **Equity in Access:** How can healthcare systems ensure fair access to expensive bioprinting procedures?
- **Human Enhancement and Boundaries:** Risks of using bioprinting for nontherapeutic or enhancement purposes. Emerging ethical questions in bioprinting is shown in 15.13

Table 15.13: Emerging ethical questions in bioprinting.

Ethical issue	Key question	Proposed framework
Tissue ownership	Who retains IP and custody rights?	Bioethics + patent law
Access and affordability	Who will benefit from bioprinting first?	Global health ethics
Enhancement versus therapy	What limits should be set?	Precautionary principle

15.10 Recommendations and Best Practices

As bioprinting technologies advance toward widespread clinical application and commercialization, it is essential to implement foundational principles that promote ethical integrity, collaboration, transparency, inclusivity, and equity. This chapter outlines key recommendations to guide researchers, clinicians, policymakers, and innovators in navigating the complex landscape of bioprinting.

15.10.1 Establishing Ethical Guidelines

The rapid pace of bioprinting innovation necessitates the establishment of proactive and flexible ethical guidelines. Given the emergence of complex dilemmas – such as tissue ownership, human enhancement, and potential commodification of organs – there is a pressing need to develop dynamic ethical standards that adapt to technological advancements [50]. Institutions such as the International Society for Biofabrication (ISBF) and

World Health Organization (WHO) should collaborate to create globally recognized protocols addressing safety, consent, reproducibility, and post-implantation responsibility. Ethical dimension of bioprinting is shown in figure 15.11. The table 15.11 shows components of a comprehensive ethical framework.

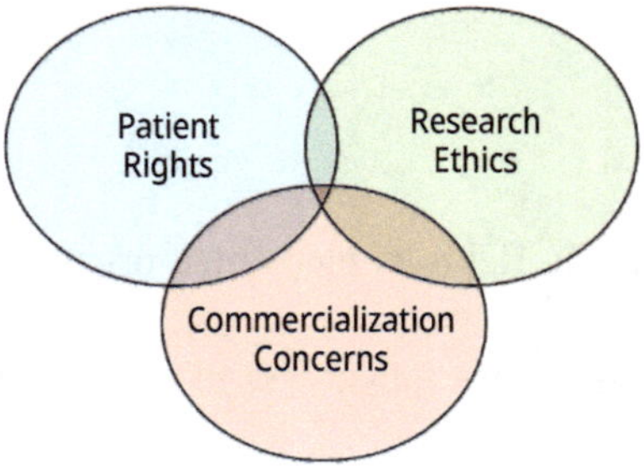

Figure 15.11: Ethical dimensions of bioprinting.

Table 15.11: Components of a comprehensive ethical framework.

Component	Description
Informed consent	Patients must be fully aware of bioprinted implant risks
Ownership rights	Clarifies who holds IP and tissue rights
Use restrictions	Limits nontherapeutic applications (e.g., enhancement)
Monitoring and safety	Post-implantation tracking protocols

15.10.2 Multidisciplinary Collaboration

Bioprinting lies at the confluence of biology, materials science, computer engineering, clinical medicine, and ethics. Hence, multidisciplinary collaboration is not just desirable – it is essential. Scientists, bioengineers, ethicists, regulatory experts, and patient advocates must jointly define project goals and implementation pathways as shown in figure 15.12 [8]. Collaborative research accelerates innovation while ensuring regulatory compliance, ethical integrity, and clinical relevance.

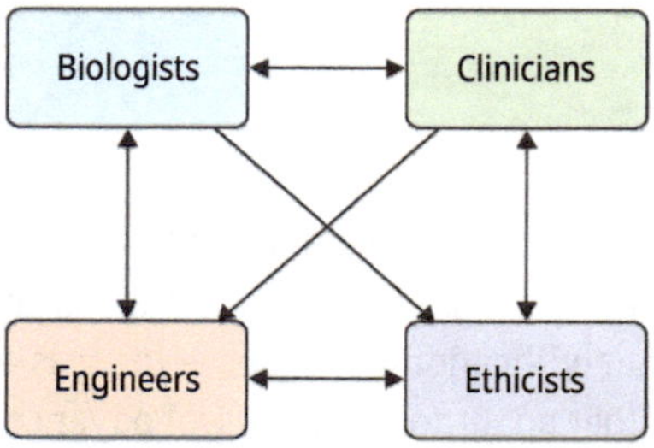

Figure 15.12: Multidisciplinary matrix in bioprinting.
Insert an interlinked flowchart showing input from biologists, clinicians, engineers, ethicists, etc.

15.10.3 Transparency in Research and Development

Transparency across the bioprinting research continuum – from material sourcing to clinical trials – is vital for fostering trust, reproducibility, and public acceptance. Open-access databases and standardized reporting (e.g., bioink composition, cell viability data, and printing resolution) promote reproducibility and peer validation Moroni et al., 2018a. Journals, funding agencies, and research institutions should mandate the publication of detailed protocols and negative results, which are often underreported.

Table 15.15: Key transparency metrics in bioprinting research.

Parameter	Description	Recommended practice
Bioink composition	Full list of materials and sources	Include supplier and formulation
Cell viability rates	Pre- and post-printing survival data	Visual and numerical data sharing
Clinical data sharing	Access to long-term outcomes	Open clinical trial registries

15.10.4 Inclusive Public Engagement

Bioprinting's societal implications extend beyond the lab, demanding inclusive dialogue with the public to align innovations with community values and expectations. Public forums, citizen science initiatives, and patient advisory boards can democratize science, provide feedback loops, and ensure cultural sensitivity [52]. This engagement is particularly crucial in shaping public policy and regulatory frameworks that govern access, funding, and usage.

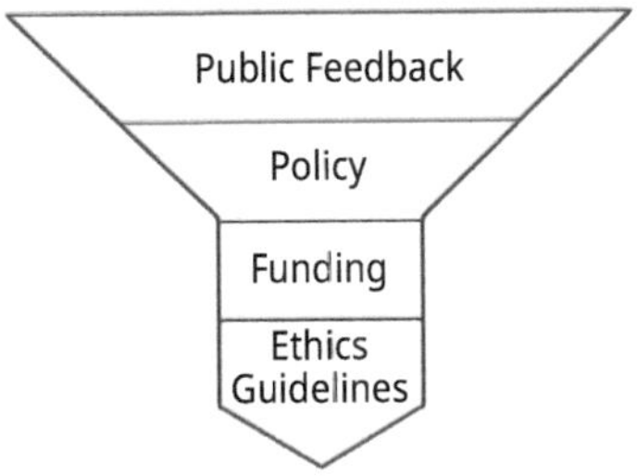

Figure 15.13: Public engagement funnel in bioprinting policy.

15.10.5 Promoting Global Equity

While bioprinting holds immense promise, its benefits may not be equally distributed. High costs, limited infrastructure, and weak regulatory systems in low- and middle-income countries (LMICs) risk deepening existing healthcare disparities [53]. To ensure global equity, international funding mechanisms, technology transfer partnerships, and capacity-building programs must be prioritized. Open-source hardware and decentralized production models offer potential solutions.

Table 15.16: Strategies for promoting global equity in bioprinting.

Strategy	Description	Example implementation
Technology transfer	Sharing blueprints and protocols	WHO-supported bioprinter kits
Open-source initiatives	Accessible tools and software	Open bioeconomy lab
Regional training programs	Build local expertise	UNDP biotech accelerator grants

15.11 Conclusion

Bioprinting sits at the crossroads of innovation and ethics. To harness its full potential, it is essential to anticipate and address the challenges posed by this technology. A balanced approach, combining technological progress with ethical reflection, legal clarity, and societal engagement, will ensure responsible advancement in the field. The future of bioprinting lies at the intersection of biology, engineering, computing, and ethics. To harness its full potential, innovations must be accompanied by robust ethical frameworks and equitable access strategies. The developments outlined in this chapter signal a transformative era for regenerative medicine and biomedical science. To guide the future of bioprinting in a socially responsible, ethically robust, and globally equitable direction, a framework based on ethical principles, interdisciplinary cooperation, public inclusion, and open science is essential. These best practices serve as a blueprint for policymakers, researchers, and practitioners as they collectively shape the next generation of medical biomanufacturing.

References

[1] Gungor-Ozkerim, P. S., Inci, I., Zhang, Y. S., Khademhosseini, A. & Dokmeci, M. R. (2018). Bioinks for 3D bioprinting: An overview. Biomaterials Science, 6(5), 915–946. https://doi.org/10.1039/C7BM00765E

[2] Heinrich, M. A. et al. (2019). 3D-bioprinted mini-brain: A glioblastoma model. Advanced Materials, 31(14), 1806590. https://doi.org/10.1002/adma.201806590.

[3] Jakab, K. et al. (2008). Tissue engineering by cell assembly. Tissue Engineering Part A, 14(3), 413–421. https://doi.org/10.1089/tea.2007.0173.

[4] Kolesky, D. B. et al. (2014). Vascularized tissue constructs. Advanced Materials, 26(19), 3124–3130. https://doi.org/10.1002/adma.201305506.

[5] Ma, X. et al. (2016). Bioprinted liver models. PNAS, 113(8), 2206–2211. https://doi.org/10.1073/pnas.1524510113.
[6] Mao, A. S. & Mooney, D. J. (2015). Regenerative medicine. PNAS, 112(47), 14452–14459. https://doi.org/10.1073/pnas.1508520112
[7] Mirdamadi, E. et al. (2020). FRESH 3D bioprinting. Micromachines, 11(9), 849. https://doi.org/10.3390/mi11090849.
[8] Ozbolat, I. T. (2016). 3D Bioprinting: Fundamentals, Principles and Applications, Academic Press.
[9] Sharma, R. et al. (2020). Bioprinting of stem cells. Materials, 13(17), 4201. https://doi.org/10.3390/ma13174201.
[10] Skardal, A. & Atala, A. (2015). Biomaterials for 3-D bioprinting. Annals of Biomedical Engineering, 43(3), 730–746. https://doi.org/10.1007/s10439-014-1207-1
[11] Huang, Y., He, K., Wang, G. & Li, X. (2021). Applications of organoids in 3D bioprinting. Bio-Design and Manufacturing, 4(2), 370–384.
[12] Kolesky, D. B., Truby, R. L., Gladman, A. S., Busbee, T. A., Homan, K. A. & Lewis, J. A. (2014). 3D bioprinting of vascularized, heterogeneous cell-laden tissue constructs. Advanced Materials, 26(19), 3124–3130.
[13] Mandrycky, C., Wang, Z., Kim, K. & Kim, D. H. (2016). 3D bioprinting for engineering complex tissues. Biotechnology Advances, 34(4), 422–434. https://doi.org/10.1016/j.biotechadv.2015.12.011.
[14] Nguyen, A. K., Narayan, R. J. & Shirwaiker, R. A. (2018). Materials and techniques for in situ tissue regeneration via emerging 3D bioprinting technologies. Progress in Biomedical Engineering, 1(2), 022001.
[15] Norotte, C., Marga, F. S., Niklason, L. E. & Forgacs, G. (2009). Scaffold-free vascular tissue engineering using bioprinting. Biomaterials, 30(30), 5910–5917.
[16] Ouyang, L., Highley, C. B., Rodell, C. B., Sun, W. & Burdick, J. A. (2016). 3D printing of shear-thinning hydrogels with secondary cross-linking for biomedical applications. ACS Biomaterials Science & Engineering, 2(10), 1743–1751.
[17] Ozbolat, I. T. & Hospodiuk, M. (2016). Current advances and future perspectives in extrusion-based bioprinting. Biomaterials, 76, 321–343.
[18] Ozbolat, I. T., Yu, Y. & Moncal, K. K. (2021). Bioprinting toward organ fabrication: Challenges and future trends. IEEE Transactions on Biomedical Engineering, 68(5), 1865–1875.
[19] Skylar-Scott, M. A., Uzel, S. G. M., Nam, L. L., Ahrens, J. H., Truby, R. L., Damaraju, S. & Lewis, J. A. (2019). Biomanufacturing of organ-specific tissues with high cellular density and embedded vascular channels. Science Advances, 5(9), eaaw2459.
[20] Zhang, Y. S., Arneri, A., Bersini, S., Shin, S. R., Zhu, K., Goli-Malekabadi, Z. & Khademhosseini, A. (2020). Bioprinting 3D microfibrous scaffolds for engineering endothelialized myocardium and heart-on-a-chip platforms. Advanced Materials, 28(14), 2764–2770.
[21] Zhao, H., Xu, X., Zhang, Y. S. & Xu, C. (2022). Advanced strategies in engineering vascularized 3D tissue constructs. Biofabrication, 14(2), 022002.
[22] Cattapan, A. (2021). The ethical challenges of 3D bioprinting: Morality, status, and justice. Health Care Analysis, 29(1), 37–53. https://doi.org/10.1007/s10728-021-00433-3
[23] Caulfield, T. & Murdoch, C. J. (2011). Genes, cells, and biobanks: Yes, there's still a consent problem. PLoS Biology, 9(7), e1001081. https://doi.org/10.1371/journal.pbio.1001081
[24] Farahany, N. A., Greely, H. T., Hyman, S., Koch, C., Grady, C., Pascual-Leone, A. . . . Yuste, R. (2018). The ethics of experimenting with human brain tissue. Nature, 556(7701), 429–432. https://doi.org/10.1038/d41586-018-04813-x
[25] Hyun, I. (2010). The bioethics of stem cell research and therapy. The Journal of Clinical Investigation, 120(1), 71–75. https://doi.org/10.1172/JCI40531
[26] Kempeneers, P., Meesen, R. & Dom, G. (2018). 3D bioprinting: A disruptive technology to reshape human identity?. Ethical Perspectives, 25(4), 533–557. https://doi.org/10.2143/EP.25.4.3285735

[27] Lavazza, A. & Massimini, M. (2018). Cerebral organoids: Ethical issues and consciousness assessment. Journal of Medical Ethics, 44(9), 606–610. https://doi.org/10.1136/medethics-2017-104487
[28] Morrison, M. (2019). Anticipatory bioethics: Future-proofing ethical governance in bioprinting. Bioethics, 33(6), 729–738. https://doi.org/10.1111/bioe.12611
[29] Patel, A. R., Da Silva, M. D. & Anand, A. (2020). Bioprinting in low-resource settings: Global health justice implications. Journal of Global Health Reports, 4, e2020071. https://doi.org/10.29392/001c.14208.
[30] Petersen, A. (2017). Stem cell markets and the global bioeconomy: An ethics critique. Regenerative Medicine, 12(7), 783–792. https://doi.org/10.2217/rme-2017-0068
[31] European Medicines Agency. (2022). Advanced therapy medicinal products: Overview. https://www.ema.europa.eu/
[32] Food and Drug Administration. (2017). Technical considerations for additive manufactured medical devices. https://www.fda.gov/
[33] Indian Council of Medical Research. (2023). Draft guidelines on biomedical and health research involving human participants. https://www.icmr.nic.in/
[34] Organovo v. Cellink, U.S. District Court for the District of Delaware (2021).
[35] Pharmaceuticals and Medical Devices Agency. (2020). Guidelines for regenerative medicine products in Japan.
[36] Supreme Court of the United States. (2013). Association for Molecular Pathology V. Myriad Genetics, Inc., 569 U.S. 576.
[37] Al-Aidaros, A. H., Shamsudin, F. M. & Idris, K. M. (2019). Ethical perspectives of Islamic scholars on biotechnology and biomedical sciences. Journal of Islamic Ethics, 3(1), 43–57.
[38] Jones, D. A. (2020). Public attitudes toward bioprinting and regenerative medicine. Bioethics Today, 34(3), 212–220.
[39] Lee, S. & Choi, Y. (2022). Media framing of bioprinting: Between technological optimism and ethical fears. Journal of Science Communication, 21(4), A02.
[40] Kolesky, D. B., Homan, K. A., Skylar-Scott, M. A. & Lewis, J. A. (2016). Three-dimensional bioprinting of thick vascularized tissues. PNAS, 113(12), 3179–3184. https://doi.org/10.1073/pnas.1521342113
[41] Min, D., Lee, W., Bae, I. H., Moon, S. & Chung, M. (2019). In situ skin bioprinting for covering deep burn wounds. Science Translational Medicine, 11(493), eaaw7962. https://doi.org/10.1126/scitranslmed.aaw7962
[42] Noor, N., Shapira, A., Edri, R., Gal, I., Wertheim, L. & Dvir, T. (2019). 3D printing of personalized thick and perfusable cardiac patches and hearts. Advanced Science, 6(11), 1900344. https://doi.org/10.1002/advs.201900344
[43] Zhang, Y., Yu, Y., Chen, X. & Sun, W. (2022). Bioprinted scaffolds for cartilage and bone repair. Bioactive Materials, 12, 189–206. https://doi.org/10.1016/j.bioactmat.2021.11.017.
[44] Sharma, R. & Gupta, M. (2022). Bioprinting and biosafety: A review on waste management and sustainability. Biomedical Engineering Letters, 12(1), 33–48. https://doi.org/10.1007/s13534-021-00210-0
[45] Wang, L., Lee, V. & Kim, B. (2020). Life-cycle environmental impact assessment of bioprinted organs versus traditional donor-based transplantation. Environmental Health Perspectives, 128(10), 107004. https://doi.org/10.1289/EHP7161
[46] Lee, A., Hudson, A. R., Shiwarski, D. J., Tashman, J. W., Hinton, T. J., Yerneni, S. . . . Feinberg, A. W. (2019). 3D bioprinting of collagen to rebuild components of the human heart. Science, 365(6452), 482–487. https://doi.org/10.1126/science.aav9051
[47] Liberski, A. R. & Gorkin, R. (2021). Open-source hardware for 3D bioprinting. Advanced Healthcare Materials, 10(7), 2001341. https://doi.org/10.1002/adhm.202001341

[48] Murphy, S. V. & Atala, A. (2014). 3D bioprinting of tissues and organs. Nature Biotechnology, 32(8), 773–785. https://doi.org/10.1038/nbt.2958

[49] Takahashi, K. & Yamanaka, S. (2016). A decade of transcription factor-mediated reprogramming to pluripotency. Nature Reviews Molecular Cell Biology, 17(3), 183–193. https://doi.org/10.1038/nrm.2016.8

[50] Varkey, M. & Atala, A. (2021). Ethics of 3D bioprinting for human application. Annual Review of Biomedical Engineering, 23, 203–227. https://doi.org/10.1146/annurev-bioeng-092220-065016.

[51] Zhang, B., Korolj, A., Lai, B. F. & Radisic, M. (2018). Advances in organ-on-a-chip engineering. Nature Reviews Materials, 3(8), 257–278. https://doi.org/10.1038/s41578-018-0034-7

[52] Moir, C., Brennan, M. & Harle, R. (2020). Participatory futures: Engaging communities in the development of emerging biotechnologies. Journal of Responsible Innovation, 7(sup1), 163–187. https://doi.org/10.1080/23299460.2020.1788995

[53] World Health Organization. (2022). Global Strategy on Digital Health 2020–2025, Geneva: WHO. https://www.who.int/publications/i/item/9789240020924.

Index

 | https://doi.org/10.1515/9783111719993-016

De Gruyter Series in Advanced Mechanical Engineering

Already published in the series

Volume 20
5D Printing. Sustainable Manufacturing
Rupinder Singh, Ranvijay Kumar, J. Paulo Davim (Eds.), 2026
ISBN 978-3-11-159256-5, e-ISBN (PDF) 978-3-11-159265-7,
e-ISBN (EPUB) 978-3-11-159304-3

Volume 19
Green Manufacturing with Artificial Intelligence Applications
Yashvir Singh, Nishant Kumar Singh, J. Paulo Davim (Eds.), 2026
ISBN 978-3-11-163095-3, e-ISBN (PDF) 978-3-11-163150-9,
e-ISBN (EPUB) 978-3-11-163157-8

Volume 18
Advances in Coating Technologies
Kaushik Kumar, Chikesh Ranjan, 2025
ISBN 978-3-11-069215-0, e-ISBN (PDF) 978-3-11-069219-8,
e-ISBN (EPUB) 978-3-11-069256-3

Volume 17
CAD/CAM. Computer-Aided Design and Manufacturing
Panagiotis Kyratsis, Athanasios Manavis, J. Paulo Davim (Eds.), 2025
ISBN 978-3-11-158467-6, e-ISBN (PDF) 978-3-11-158506-2,
e-ISBN (EPUB) 978-3-11-158555-0

Volume 16
Flow Dynamics and Heat Transfer. Computational Fluid Dynamics, Thermal Analysis, Numerical Simulations
Mukesh Kumar Awasthi, Dhananjay Yadav, J. Paulo Davim (Eds.), 2025
ISBN 978-3-11-166059-2, e-ISBN (PDF) 978-3-11-166167-4,
e-ISBN (EPUB) 978-3-11-166405-7

Volume 15
High-Performance Metallic Biomaterials. Surface Modification and Coating of Implants
Arbind Prasad, Manoj Kumar Sinha, J. Paulo Davim (Eds.),2025
ISBN 978-3-11-157137-9, e-ISBN (PDF) 978-3-11-157142-3,
e-ISBN (EPUB) 978-3-11-157212-3

www.degruyterbrill.com

Volume 14
Machine Learning for Medical Applications.
Ranjith Rajamanickam, Amit Sharma, Dhivya Ranjith, J. Paulo Davim (Eds.):
Volume I: Computational Drug Discovery, Bioimaging, Smart Biomaterials, 2025
ISBN 978-3-11-150318-9, e-ISBN (PDF) 978-3-11-150320-2,
e-ISBN (EPUB) 978-3-11-150374-5
Volume II: Computer Vision, Image Processing, Disease Detection, 2025
ISBN 978-3-11-914782-8, e-ISBN (PDF) 978-3-11-220519-8,
e-ISBN (EPUB) 978-3-11-220529-7

Volume 13
Compressors and Blowers. Maintenance, Practical Guidance, Energy-Efficient Technologies
Raj Kumar Arya, George Verros, J. Paulo Davim (Eds.), 2025
ISBN 978-3-11-136335-6, e-ISBN (PDF) 978-3-11-136395-0,
e-ISBN (EPUB) 978-3-11-136417-9

Volume 12
Machining and Tribology of Advanced Materials. From Coatings, Lubrications, Surface Treatments to Modeling and Simulation
Nishant Kumar Singh, Rajesh Kumar Verma, Virendra Kumar, J. Paulo Davim (Eds.), 2025
ISBN 978-3-11-137642-4, e-ISBN (PDF) 978-3-11-137729-2,
e-ISBN (EPUB) 978-3-11-137772-8

Volume 11
Microfabrication and Nanofabrication. Precision Manufacturing
Kanak Kalita, Ranjan Kumar Ghadai, J. Paulo Davim (Eds.), 2024
ISBN 978-3-11-133543-8, e-ISBN (PDF) 978-3-11-133553-7,
e-ISBN (EPUB) 978-3-11-133559-9

Volume 10
3D Printing. Polymer, Metal and Gel Based Additive Manufacturing
Kanak Singh, Ranvijay Kumar, Vinay Kumar, J. Paulo Davim (Eds.), 2024
ISBN 978-3-11-108061-1, e-ISBN (PDF) 978-3-11-108163-2
e-ISBN (EPUB) 978-3-11-108206-6

Volume 9
Sustainable Hydrogen Energy. Production, Storage & Transportation
Raj Kumar Arya, Anurag Kumar Tiwari, George Verros, Prashant Malik, J. Paulo Davim (Eds.), 2024
ISBN 978-3-11-124641-3, e-ISBN (PDF) 978-3-11-124647-5
e-ISBN (EPUB) 978-3-11-124728-1

Volume 8
Soft Computing in Smart Manufacturing. Solutions toward Industry 5.0
Tatjana Sibalija, J. Paulo Davim (Eds.), 2022
ISBN 978-3-11-069317-1, e-ISBN (PDF) 978-3-11-069322-5
e-ISBN (EPUB) 978-3-11-069325-6

Volume 7
Nonconventional Machining
J. Paulo Davim (Ed.), 2023
ISBN 978-3-11-058410-3, e-ISBN (PDF) 978-3-11-058447-9
e-ISBN (EPUB) 978-3-11-058415-8

Volume 6
Manufacturing in Digital Industries
J. Paulo Davim (Ed.), 2020
ISBN 978-3-11-057507-1, e-ISBN (PDF) 978-3-11-057542-2,
e-ISBN (EPUB) 978-3-11-057526-2

Volume 5
Rapid Prototyping, Rapid Tooling and Reverse Engineering
Kaushik Kumar, Divya Zindani, J. Paulo Davim, 2020
ISBN 978-3-11-066324-2, e-ISBN (PDF) 978-3-11-066490-4,
e-ISBN (EPUB) 978-3-11-066345-7

Volume 4
Additive and Subtractive Manufacturing
J. Paulo Davim (Ed.), 2019
ISBN 978-3-11-054816-7, e-ISBN (PDF) 978-3-11-054977-5,
e-ISBN (EPUB) 978-3-11-054833-4

Volume 3
Drilling Technology
J. Paulo Davim (Ed.), 2017
ISBN 978-3-11-047863-1, e-ISBN 978-3-11-048120-4,
e-ISBN (EPUB) 978-3-11-047871-6

Volume 2
Progress in Green Tribology
J. Paulo Davim (Ed.), 2017
ISBN 978-3-11-037272-4, e-ISBN 978-3-11-036705-8,
e-ISBN (EPUB) 978-3-11-039252-4

Volume 1
Metal Cutting Technology
J. Paulo Davim (Ed.), 2016
ISBN 978-3-11-044942-6, e-ISBN 978-3-11-045174-0,
e-ISBN (EPUB) 978-3-11-044947-1, Set-ISBN 978-3-11-045175-7